T0383362

Handbook of
Avian Medicine

SecondE dition

For Elsevier:

Commissioning Editor: Joyce Rodenhuis
Development Editor: Ewan Halley
Project Manager: Joannah Duncan
Designer: Charlotte Murray
Illustrator: Samantha Elmhurst

Handbook of
Avian Medicine
Second Edition

Edited by

Thomas N. Tully, Jr, BS, DVM,
MS Dipl ABVP (avian), ECAMS
Professor Zoological Medicine, School of Veterinary Medicine,
Louisiana State University, Baton Rouge, Louisiana, USA

Gerry M. Dorrestein Prof Dr, Dr hc, DVM
Director, Dutch Research Institute for Avian and Exotic Animals
(NOIVBD), Veldhoven, The Netherlands

Alan K. Jones BVetMed, MRCVS
AlanK . Jones & Associates, Aviana ndE xotic
Veterinary Practice, Sussex & Kent, UK

Forewordb y
John E. Cooper DTVM, FRCPath, FIBiol, FRCVS,
Diplomate of The European College of Veterinary Pathologists
Professor of Pathology, School of Veterinary Medicine,
The University of the West Indies (UWI),
St Augustine, Trinidad and Tobago, West Indies

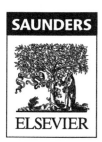
SAUNDERS

ELSEVIER

Edinburgh London New York Oxford Philadelphia St Louis Sydney Toronto 2009

SAUNDERS
ELSEVIER

An imprint of Elsevier Limited

Firstp ublished2 000
Reprinted2 003,2 005
Seconde dition2 009

ISBN 978 0 7020 2874 8

British Library Cataloguing in Publication Data
A catalogue record for this book is available from the British Library

Library of Congress Cataloging in Publication Data
A catalog record for this book is available from the Library of Congress

Notice
Knowledge and best practice in this field are constantly changing. As new research and experience broaden our knowledge, changes in practice, treatment and drug therapy may become necessary or appropriate. Readers are advised to check the most current information provided (i) on procedures featured or (ii) by the manufacturer of each product to be administered, to verify the recommended dose or formula, the method and duration of administration, and contraindications. It is the responsibility of the practitioner, relying on their own experience and knowledge of the patient, to make diagnoses, to determine dosages and the best treatment for each individual patient, and to take all appropriate safety precautions. To the fullest extent of the law, neither the Publisher nor the Authors assume any liability for any injury and/or damage to persons or property arising out or related to any use of the material contained in this book.

The Publisher

Contents

Acknowledgements

It is satisfying as editors to have a work be well received by the veterinary community after the intense effort of compiling the material. Our goal in editing the first edition was to produce a basic avian medical text that brought forth the collective knowledge and expertise of a respected group of international authors. Based on the response through multiple printings and a request to publish a second edition we believe the goal was attained. We as editors also know that veterinary medicine and in particular avian veterinary medicine is a moving target as scientific discoveries and medical advances are frequently achieved. As with the first edition, we have called upon many of the original authors as well as new contributors to exceed the expectations of the veterinary community regarding a basic avian medicine text. We wish to thank existing authors for their continued commitment to this text as well as those participating for the first time. To our colleagues in the Association of Avian Veterinarians, we thank you for contributing to and demanding quality avian medicine. The advances noted in this book can be directly attributed to the enthusiastic members of this worldwide organization.

Again the support staffs for the three editors were invaluable assets: at LSU, Harry M. Cowgill, medical photographer, and Michael L. Broussard, graphic artist, who aided in figure development; at the NOIVBD laboratory, Marianne van der Zee for photographic support. We are also grateful to the collegial support from associates and staff members that is so important on a daily basis, but never more so than when working on a medical textbook: Drs Javier Nevarez, David Guzman, and Shannon Shaw at LSU; Gail and the two Emmas at Dr Alan Jones' Clinic; and Anita Visser at the NOIVBD laboratory and Tonnie van Meegen (NOP) were all instrumental in their support during the formulation and completion of this text.

The editors would also like to thank our publishers Elsevier for their commitment to a second edition. As always, patience and support are cornerstones to publisher/editor/author sanity during the writing process and we were fortunate to work with the best: Joyce Rodenhuis, Commissioning Editor Veterinary Medicine; Rita Demetriou-Swanwick, Development Editor; and especially Ewan Halley, our Development Editor, who guided the book through the majority of the editing process. Thank you for the early mornings, long days, and late nights, not to mention the continual stimulation for results!

Two of the editors would be remiss for not thanking a colleague and friend who has contributed more than his share of editorial duties, Dr Alan Jones. Alan, thank you for joining this group in a project that we feel is a labour of love; your work was professional, first class, and added significantly to the timely production of the book.

Finally, a heartfelt thank you for the unswerving loyalty of our wives Susie Tully and Elaine Jones, partner Marianne van der Zee, plus our families who accept our professional ambitions to advance avian medicine in the face of added stress associated with editing an international avian medical text.

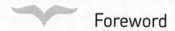

Foreword

...look into the clear bright eyes of the bird whose body equals yours in physical perfection, and whose tiny brain can generate a sympathy, a love for its mate, which in sincerity and unselfishness suffers little when compared with human affection.

William Beebe,
The Bird 1906

Birds have long enthralled the human race and thereby influenced diverse cultures and civilizations. Thousands of years ago the Incas in South America and the then denizens of Mesopotamia (present-day Iraq) kept birds of various types. At about the same time, the Ancient Egyptians were probably the first to *collect* birds; in 1500 BC Queen Hatshepsut organised an expedition to add new species to her private collection. A thousand years or so later Greek and Roman scholars such as Aristotle, Pliny and Varro studied birds, including parrots, and published detailed observations on their biology. Science flourished under Arab scholars during the so-called Dark Ages in Europe and this period spawned seminal writings on numerous aspects of the natural world, including birds and other animals, as well as medicine, geology and astronomy. With the Renaissance came renewed scientific interest in Europe and Leonardo da Vinci, followed by anatomists in England, Germany, Italy and the Netherlands, carried out painstaking dissections of many animal species. These and others produced scholarly descriptions and drawings of birds that are, in many respects, unequalled today. In the 18th century John Hunter, the great surgeon, anatomist and champion of the veterinary profession, explored the links between structure and function in animals. Amongst many other great discoveries, Hunter described the air-sac system of birds and studied avian matters as diverse as the production of crop-milk in pigeons, the seasonal development of the gonads in sparrows and the healing and misalignment of fractures in an eagle.

Neither is medical care for birds a novel concept. In 1486 in England, for example, advice on the diagnosis and treatment of diseases of trained hawks was given in the *Boke of St Albans*. This was written by Dame Juliana Berners; a reminder of the prominent role played by women in avian science, even 500 years ago! The popularity of the sport of falconry in Europe over the succeeding three centuries ensured that publications on raptors continued to appear. There was also a growth of interest in the keeping of pigeons, parrots, finches, crows and other birds as pets. Much affection was often lavished upon these birds, even during periods when the human population was beset by rumours of war and social unrest, as exemplified by the following entry in one of the famous diaries (1665) of Samuel Pepys:

This night when I came home I was much troubled to hear that my poor Canary Bird, that I have kept these three or four years, is dead.

It was not, however, until the 19th and early 20th centuries, with the genesis of the understanding of pathogens, that serious attention started to be paid in Europe and North America to the diagnosis and control of diseases of captive birds. Even so, progress was slow and the input by veterinarians remained limited.

The situation has now changed beyond recognition and over the past three decades our knowledge and understanding of bird diseases has advanced extraordinarily. Much of the credit for this is owed to the 'pioneers' of avian medicine, amongst them the editors and many of the contributors of this book, who have helped to transform avian medicine into a *bona fide*, state-of-the-art, scientific discipline.

I was honoured to be asked to write the foreword to the first edition of this book in 2000 and am delighted to have been invited to do so again for the second, in 2009. As before, my first comment on the book is to applaud its international orientation. The editors hail from three different countries and the twenty contributors from seven. This spread – Australia, Europe and North America – is not global but it is an important reminder of the international significance of avian medicine, in terms not only of treating individual sick birds but also of monitoring and promoting the health of wild (free-living) populations. The latter is a pressing need for a number of reasons, not least because of current concerns about avian influenza and other diseases that are a threat to the health of humans and domestic stock. In addition, of course, there is a desperate need for more information about the part that infectious and non-infectious diseases play in the regulation of numbers of wild birds, particularly those that are under pressure for other reasons. It is now widely accepted that veterinarians and others with specialist knowledge of avian health and host/parasite relations can play a vital part in the conservation of endangered and threatened species. Their contribution in this respect is much enhanced if they have an understanding of aviculture as well as sound professional knowledge of pathology, parasitology, medicine or surgery. In my own work overseas over four decades I have witnessed many such contributions to conservation. For example, the survival and recovery of the Mauritius kestrel (*Falco punctatus*), the pink pigeon (*Columba mayeri*) and other Indian Ocean species, the populations of which were in a parlous state in the 1970s, owe much to close, unselfish, collaboration between veterinarians and biologists, some of them self-funded. There have been similar successes in avian species-conservation elsewhere and I have been fortunate to have seen some of these projects for myself – in New Zealand, for example, where many endemic birds are now relatively safe. It is encouraging that young people, some with a veterinary background, some from other disciplines, want to involve themselves in such conservation projects and thereby contribute to the protection of wildlife and their habitats. This usually means serving in different, sometimes difficult, parts of the world and being willing and able to collaborate with local communities. Examples of such enterprise are to be found documented in various publications, including Notes from the Field in the *Journal of Avian Medicine and Surgery* and project reports in the *Bulletin of the British Veterinary Zoological Society.*

The editors and authors of this book are familiar names to those who keep or treat birds. They are all veterinarians but, without exception, have a personal affinity for birds as animals and an awareness that those from other backgrounds, such as animal behaviourists, ecologists and nutritionists, can also contribute to avian health, welfare and conservation.

Those of us who keep or tend members of the class Aves owe Tom Tully, Gerry Dorrestein and Alan Jones a debt of gratitude for compiling this work and bringing together such a talented team of contributors. In so doing, they have helped to promote a better understanding of birds and the requirements of these unique animals if they are to remain healthy in captivity or in the wild. Their book will do much to encourage others to contribute to the challenging, but exciting, field of avian medicine.

John E. Cooper, DTVM, FRCPath, FIBiol, FRCVS
The University of the West Indies, 2009

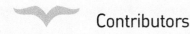

Contributors

Brian H. Coles BVSc, FRCVS, Dipl ECAMS
4 Dorfold Way, Upton, Chester, Cheshire, UK

Lorenzo Crosta DVM, PhD
Clinica Veterinaria Valcurone, Missaglia, Italy

Luis A. Cruz-Martinez DVM
Post-Doctoral Fellow, The Raptor Center, Veterinary Clinical Sciences, University of Minnesota, St Paul, Minnesota, USA

Peter De Herdt DVM, DVSc
Professor of Veterinary Medicine, University of Ghent, Director of Clinic for Poultry and Special Animal Diseases, Merelbeke, Belgium

Gerry Dorrestein Prof Dr, Dr hc, DVM
Director, Dutch Research Institute for Avian and Exotic Animals (NOIVBD), Veldhoven, The Netherlands

Nigel Harcourt-Brown BVSc, FRCVS, Dipl ECAMS
30 Crab Lane, Bilton, Harrogate, North Yorkshire, UK

Don J. Harris DVM
Avian and Exotic Animal Medical Center, Pinecrest, Florida, USA

Alan K. Jones BVetMed, MRCVS
Alan K. Jones & Associates, Avian and Exotic Veterinary Practice, Sussex & Kent, UK

Maria-Elisabeth Krautwald-Junghanns PD Dr Med Vet, Dr Med Vet Habil, Dipl ECAMS FTA
Clinic for Birds and Reptiles, University of Leipzig, Leipzig, Germany

Patricia Macwhirter BVSc (Hons), MA, FACVSc
Principal, Highbury Veterinary Clinic, Burwood, Victoria, Australia

Glenn H. Olsen DVM, MS, PhD
Veterinary Medical Officer, US Department of Interior, US65 Patuxent Wildlife Research Center, Laurel, Maryland, USA

Frank Pasmans DVM, PhD, MSc
University of Ghent, Belgium

Michael Pees DrVetMed, Dipl ECAMS
Clinic for Birds and Reptiles, University of Leipzig, Leipzig, Germany

Patrick T. Redig DVM, PhD
Associate Professor and Director, The Raptor Center, University of Minnesota, St Paul, Minnesota, USA

Ian Robinson BVSc, Cert. SAP, MRCVS
International Fund for Animal Welfare–UK, London, UK

Andrew Routh BVSc, MRCVS
Senior Veterinary Officer, Veterinary Department, London Zoo, Regents Park, London, UK

Stephanie Sanderson MA, VetMB, MRCVS
Veterinary Manager, Chester Zoo, Upton-by-Chester, Cheshire, UK

Linda Timossi DrVetMed
Clinica Veterinaria Valcurone, Missaglia, Italy

Thomas N. Tully, Jr BS, DVM, MS Dipl ABVP (avian), ECAMS
Professor Zoological Medicine, School of Veterinary Medicine, Louisiana State University, Baton Rouge, Louisiana, USA

Amy B. Worell DVM, Dipl ABVP (avian)
Director, All Pets Medical Centre, West Hills, California, USA

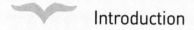

Introduction

The editors and authors are pleased to bring you this 2nd edition of the *Handbook of Avian Medicine*. In the introduction to the 1st edition, we stated that the specific purpose of the text was to provide a resource for the veterinary student, general practitioner and allied staff who have an interest in treating the avian patient. We, as contributors, feel that this goal was accomplished, but much has happened regarding the advancement of avian medicine in the 8 years since the publication of that 1st edition.

What has not changed in that 8 years is the never-ending need for up-to-date basic information for the increasing number of veterinary students, veterinarians and allied staff seeking expertise in the field of avian medicine. Advances in this edition are the inclusion of all colour images and clinician's notes. Colour images are not only pleasing to the eye but often are important in evaluating patients and sample materials collected. Clinician's notes are important highlighted tips (indicated by the flying bird icon in the margin) that will give the reader rapid access to information relevant to the case in question. More tables, highlighted by colour background, are resources to make text referencing quick and easy.

We have tried to fulfil a need with this text by calling on the worldwide expertise of our authors and editors. The multi-authored content utilizes the international expertise of the avian veterinary community. This clinically oriented text again focuses on the basic components of avian medicine at the beginning, progressing to group-specific chapters. If a veterinarian treats birds it is very likely that the specialty is not confined to one order: this text covers canaries to ostriches. As an underlying teaching text it allows for teaching and practice of sound avian medicine.

There is a new chapter in this edition that goes into the development of avian species. The first chapter will give readers an understanding of the formation of these wonderful animals. The next five chapters cover the basic medical information needed to treat avian species in a veterinary hospital. Again this information has been updated to incorporate the latest in technological and scientific advances. As stated in the first edition, the focus of the text is on introductory material and the average companion animal practice. If you are a veterinary student or see between one and five birds a week, this text is for you. The information in this book will allow the veterinarian a comfort zone of knowledge in order to evaluate, treat, and/or refer.

Only through knowledge and confidence in the veterinary skills provided will the general public trust in medical care for their birds. Competent veterinary skills start with the basics, knowing what one can do and what one's limitations are regarding avian practice. We hope this book provides a resource of avian medical information for veterinarians to formulate the educated medical decisions that the bird-owning public has come to demand.

Our wish is for this book to reach veterinarians, allied technical staff, and veterinary students, who need it the most. It has been a pleasure compiling the information contained in the 2nd edition of the *Handbook of Avian Medicine*, and we feel the authors have provided the veterinary community with the most up-to-date basic avian information for the successful hospital.

Thomas N. Tully, Jr
Gerry M. Dorrestein
Alan K. Jones

The development of avian species

Patricia Macwhirter

Fossil evidence since the 1800s has suggested that birds are descended from reptilian ancestors. More recent evidence places avian species as descendants of the theropod dinosaurs, the bipedal group that also gave rise to the iconic predators *Velociraptor* and *Tyrannosaurus*. Based on phylogenic criteria birds should be considered a subgroup of the class Reptilia, albeit a specialized and very successful subgroup, rather than being a class of their own. **A working knowledge of the ongoing debate on how birds evolved is helpful in making sense of the ways in which modern birds are structured, how they function and the diseases they contract.**

If a species is to survive and multiply, evolutionary change needs to confer immediate advantage for the next generation. Key events in the emergence of birds from reptiles have included the development of feathers along with changes in thermoregulation, reproduction, nesting behaviour, respiration, renal function, vision and musculoskeletal structure. Bird bones are fragile and do not preserve well, so it is not surprising that there are gaps in the fossil record, particularly from the Mesozoic era. Currently known and dated bird fossil species do not grade linearly from one to another in stratigraphic context. However, workers have analysed primitive and more modern features of Mesozoic birds (Chatterjee 1997) and in so doing have constructed a cladogram based on a single, most parsimonious tree (Fig. 1.1). By comparing this cladogram with dated fossils it is possible to construct a broad picture of avian evolution with some confidence. Knowledge about the palaeogeographical history of the earth, the species and ecosystems existing when early birds began to emerge, and the biomechanics of flight are all important in understanding bird evolution (Table 1.1; Figs 1.2, 1.3, 1.4, 1.5; Boxes 1.1, 1.2). Key sources for the model described here are listed in the references, but this is an active area of research and details are changing and becoming refined as more material emerges.

The amniote egg

Since multicellular organisms first emerged on earth some four billion years ago, periods of gradual diversification of life-forms have been punctuated with periods of abrupt extinctions (De Duve 1995). In the Carboniferous period (Fig. 1.2), from around 360 mya, crocodile-shaped amphibians called labyrinthodonts dominated a landscape vegetated with primitive psilophytes and horsetails. The continent of Laurasia, which included Europe and parts of North America, had emerged from the sea, moved south and coalesced with the southern continent of Gondwana to become a single land mass, Pangaea. Life-forms between the two land masses intermingled, enabling a vastly increased pool of natural variation and selection pressures that favoured organisms able to reproduce independently of an aquatic environment. In this context the amniotes emerged. These were vertebrates that produced eggs containing specialized membranes that provided the developing embryo with a liquid environment, gave oxygen in exchange for carbon dioxide, stored food as yolk and isolated nitrogenous waste (Box 1.3).

The earliest amniotes were *anapsids* without any lateral openings on the side of the cranium posterior to the orbit. Tortoises and turtles have been traditionally classified as members of the Anapsida. Independently from primitive anapsids the *synapsids* (mammals) evolved with a single lower opening on the skull posterior to the orbit and the *diapsids* (reptiles) evolved with two lateral openings, one above the other. These openings allowed for larger, more powerful jaw muscles for chewing and capturing prey. Birds subsequently evolved an avidiapsid cranium in which the two lateral cranial openings merged into a single opening, allowing for cranial kinesis (i.e. movement of the upper jaw relative to the brain case) (Figs 1.9 and 1.10).

Mesozoic birds

Approximately 250 mya, a wave of global extinctions occurred, wiping out large amphibians over most of Pangaea and marking the end of the Palaeozoic era (Table 1.1). Descendants of the small reptiles survived and evolved to fill a wide range of ecological niches as the warm humid climate of the Mesozoic era progressed. These included the progenitors of turtles, lizards and snakes as well as the archosaurs, a group that gave rise to the crocodile family, the pterosaurs and the dinosaurs (Box 1.4; Fig. 1.13).

Precisely when 'birds' first emerged is an open question. Molecular evidence (Table 1.2), places the emergence of birds at around 183 mya, a date consistent with most fossil finds, except for *Protoavis texensis*, a Texan bird fossil putatively dated *c.* 225 mya. Whatever the outcome of this debate, timing would depend on which features were included in the definition of 'bird'. Phylogenetic analysis and analysis of fossils with possible pro-avian features suggest that birds are embedded in the bipedal dinosaur class Theropoda, probably descendant from the Maniraptora, a group that also gave rise to dromaeosaurs. A dromaeosaur with a bird-like furcula (clavicle) has been found in Montana but theropod dinosaurs occurred across Pangaea, and therefore a Eurasian or American origin for the earliest birds could both be consistent with existing fossil evidence (Chatterjee 1997, Martin 2002) (Fig. 1.14).

Possible evolutionary steps between ectothermic reptiles and the wide diversity of endothermic, flighted and non-flighted avian species of today have generated much speculation. Critical bio-geographical events since the early Mesozoic era when feathered reptiles made their first appearance in the fossil record have included:

- the gradual break-up of Pangaea and Gondwana due to tectonic plate movement
- the expansion of winged insects and emergence of flowering plants, c. 120 mya

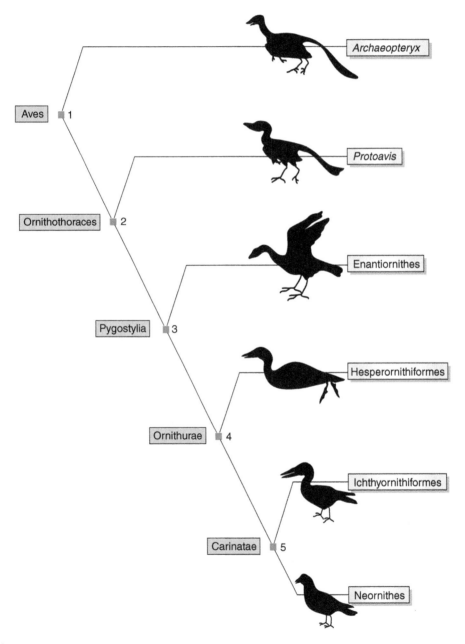

Fig 1.1 Aves cladogram.

- the Cretaceous–Tertiary ('K-T') boundary disaster that marked the end of the Mesozoic era, possibly due to a meteor crash near present-day Mexico, *c.* 65 mya
- *La Grande Coupure* – the separation of South America and then greater Australia from Antarctica with resultant circumpolar currents, global cooling and increased winds, *c.* 33 mya

- the establishment of the Panama land bridge, *c.* 2.5 mya, reconnecting North and South America
- ongoing sea level changes
- fluctuating climates
- the emergence and global expansion of mammalian species, especially pinnipeds, felids, canids and humans.

For any species, evolution is not linear but rather a continuum of a much-branching tree. Genome, lifetime behaviours ('flock culture') and landscape weave together to create a future that, in time, becomes the past. Some signposts along the journey may be marked in the fossil record. Evidence of other changes comes from current geographical distribution, anatomy, physiology and behavioural patterns of present-day species. Stages in the emergence of modern birds that have been reflected in the fossil record are described below.

Table 1.1 Earth's palaeogeological timeline (authorities vary regarding exact dates)

Geological era	Period	Epoch	Commenced – million of years ago
Cenozoic	Quaternary	Holocene	0.01
		Pleistocene	1.6
	Tertiary	Pliocene	5
		Miocene	23
		Oligocene	36
		Eocene	53
		Palaeocene	65
Mesozoic	Cretaceous		145
	Jurassic		205
	Triassic		250
Palaeozoic	Permian		290
	Carboniferous		360
	Devonian		405
	Silurian		436
	Ordovician		510
	Cambrian		560
Proterozoic			

Stage 1 – a bipedal stance, swivel wrist joint and long forelimbs (Maniraptora/Dromaeosaurs)

Members of the Maniraptora family, the prime ancestral dinosaurs for modern birds, were small agile carnivores that probably hunted in packs and were adapted for running and climbing. This was reflected in the bipedal stance they shared with other theropod dinosaurs as well as unique characteristics including swivel wrist joints, lengthened forelimbs and caudally directed pubic bones. Their rigid stiffened tails could be used as a prop when climbing vertical trunks while skin folds on their forearms might assist in clinging to branches when ascending trees or if parachuting down from branches to other

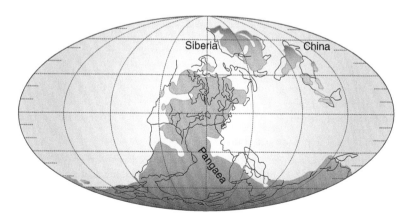

Fig 1.2 Late Carboniferous circa 290 million years ago. The joining of land masses to form the single continent of Pangaea may have favoured the emergence of reptiles from amphibians around this time. Reptiles, including their descendants the birds, utilize insoluble uric acid as their key waste product in the protein breakdown and lay amniote eggs containing specialized membranes to keep toxic waste products away from the sensitive developing embryo. These developments, which are fundamental to both reptile and bird physiology, allowed reptiles to hatch eggs away from water and to take advantage of new land-based ecological niches.

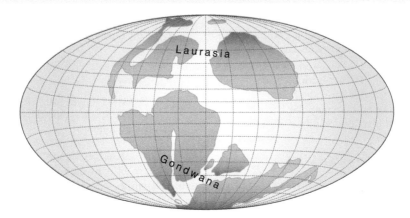

Fig 1.3 Late Jurassic circa 150 million years ago. Most molecular and fossil evidence points to the emergence of feathered birds in the Jurassic period, probably less than 185 mya. Primitive fossil finds have come from marine and freshwater wetlands in Europe (*Archaeopteryx*) and Asia (*Confuciusornis*). The single exception is a controversial fossil, *Protoavis* from Texas, a bird with remarkably advanced features but putatively dated to over 220 million years ago, in the Triassic. See text.

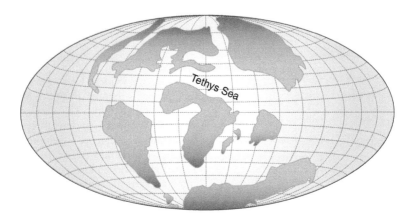

Fig 1.4 Late Cretaceous circa 65 million years ago. Birds were present globally before the K-T boundary extinction event of around 65 mya. Enantiornithines, Hesperornithiformes and Ichthyornithiformes were wiped out, along with all other dinosaurs, except for the Neornithes, the group to which all modern bird families belong. Fossil and molecular evidence suggests that the southern hemisphere was probably the place of origin of the Neornithes and that, for most bird orders, global repopulation and expansion in the Tertiary originated from this region. Land connections from Antarctica to South America, to Australia and, via island chains, to Africa were critical in this repopulation.

branches or to the ground (Fig. 1.15). Dromaeosaurs are currently known only from Cretaceous fossils but are considered to be of greater antiquity. They had skeletons with these additional basic features:

- skull – numerous teeth, a rigid upper jaw, diaspid openings on their skull
- vertebral column – tall neural spines on their cervical vertebrae, a flexible thorax and a long tail
- pelvis – separate ilium, ischium and pubis and a broad, footed pubis
- pectoral girdle – broad scapula, fused scapulocoracoid, short coracoid, flat sternum
- forelimb – separate carpal and metacarpal bones with 3 digits and a phalangeal formula of 2-3-4
- hindlimb – separate tibia, tarsal and metatarsal bones.

Compared with other theropod dinosaurs, dromaeosaurs were small and the pubic foot of the pelvis was caudally, rather than cranially, directed. Compared with their larger, more land-bound relations, these features may have been adaptations that helped them to climb and manoeuvre up trees and shrubs which would have better enabled them to escape predators and take advantage of a rich, emerging aerial food source, the

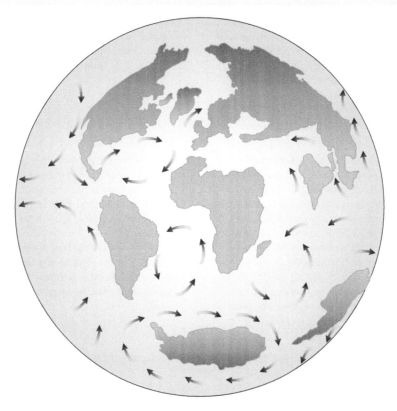

Fig 1.5 Oligocene circa 30 million years ago. *La Grande Coupure*, the great cut of around 35–33 mya saw South America and then Australia unzipped from Antarctica and circumpolar currents beginning to flow. This was associated with global cooling and increased winds. While almost all orders of modern birds had emerged before this time, these climatic conditions would have favoured endothermic metabolism and flight and facilitated global expansion of modern birds.

fl ying insects. The fl at-toed, digitigrade structure of both dromaeosaurs and early fossil birds suggests they leaped, waded, walked or ran on two legs rather than perched on small branches as practised by their more curved-toed avian descendants. In common with other theropods, most birds have the phalangeal formula of 2-3-4-5 with absence of the fifth digit.

Stage 2 – add feathers for insulation and gliding (Troodontids/Aves/Archaeopteryx)

In general, ectotherms are at an advantage in hot climates where food sources are scarce. Endotherms perform better when the climate is cooler and food is abundant. Winged insects pre-date the emergence of birds. Such insects, along with aquatic creatures, could have provided an abundant food source for birds in the warm wetlands of the Triassic and Jurassic periods (Fig. 1.3). In the swampy areas where early bird fossils have been found, they perhaps leaped or hang-glided, using long necks and faces, with their mouths still containing reptilian teeth, to catch fl ying prey. Their forelimbs

remained free to balance and perform other functions. Aerial agility and acute vision would both have been advantageous to feathered proto-avian species such as the troodontids (Long & Schouten 2008) (Fig. 1.16).

Feathers do not appear to be modified scales but rather emerged among the theropod dinosaurs as independent tubular structures that became progressively more complex. Feathers, hair, nails and scales all grow by proliferation and differentiation of keratinocytes which die and leave behind deposited masses of keratin, filaments of protein that polmerize to form solid structures. Feathers are made of beta-keratins, which are unique to reptiles and birds. Skin and the outer sheath of growing feathers are made of alpha-keratins, which are found in all vertebrates (Figs 1.17, 1.18).

Insulation, balance and perhaps buoyancy, rather than flight, may have been key initial benefits that feathers provided. This is demonstrated in the wide diversity of species of feathered theropod dinosaurs that have recently emerged from the fossil record in China (Prum & Brush 2004) (Fig. 1.19).

Archaeopteryx, a bird that lived on the islands that comprised Europe around 150 mya, is one of the earliest avian fossils identified; its features were transitional between the Maniraptora and birds and it is thought to be a relic species. Critically, it had typical flight feathers, each with a long, tapering central shaft (rachis) and

broad, flexible, asymmetric vanes. The vane on the leading edge of the feather was thicker but narrower than the vane on the trailing edge, giving a typical aerofoil shape. The tail was long and bony but feathered bilaterally.

Box 1.1 Biomechanics of flight

For birds or planes there are four forces involved in flight: *lift, weight, thrust* and *drag*. An aerofoil, such as a wing, has a cambered or convex upper surface with a concave, less cambered or flat lower surface. It is thicker at the front or leading edge and narrows towards the rear or trailing edge. As the aerofoil moves through air, relative airflow is created across the top and bottom surfaces. Because the top surface is convex the air travelling over the top surface must travel a greater distance relative to that of air travelling under the wing. The pressure on the top surface of the aerofoil is therefore reduced, producing the upward force *lift* to oppose the downward force of *weight* produced by gravity acting on the airframe or bird's body.

Thrust is the force that moves the airframe forward. In planes it is produced by the propeller; in birds it is produced by the downstroke of the wing, with the outer primary feathers being twisted and tilted downward and outward in relation to the direction of the airflow and 'swimming' through the air. Thrust is opposed by *drag*, the force produced by resistance of the airframe, or bird's body, to the airflow. **In volant (flying) birds an evolutionary trend has been toward design features that facilitate flight by improving lift and thrust while reducing weight and drag (Fig. 1.6 – aerofoil wing).**

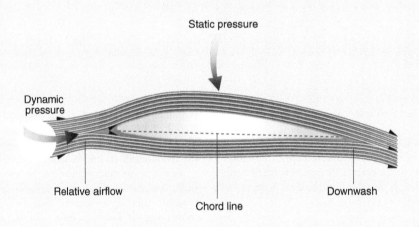

As dynamic pressure increases, static pressure decreases

Static pressure

Dynamic pressure

Relative airflow

Chord line

Downwash

Bemoulli's Theorem:
Dynamic pressure + static pressure = total pressure

Fig 1.6 Aerofoil cross-section (see Box 1.1).

Box 1.2 Emergence of sexual reproduction

Giardia is a flagellate parasite associated with 'cow plop' diarrhoeal syndromes in birds and mammals. The two 'eye-like' nuclei that can be seen when examining the protozoan microscopically are haploid, each containing a single complement of chromosomes (Fig. 1.7). This contrasts with the double

complement of chromosomes typically seen in a single nucleus when meiosis, sexual reproduction, has been fully completed.

Meiosis, sexual reproduction, was an important evolutionary step that emerged over 600 million years ago (mya) and facilitated mixing of genetic material between organisms and vastly increased variation from one generation to the next. **In birds, females are heterogametic (XY or 'ZW'), while males are homogametic (XX or 'ZZ').** Avian sperm, such as the budgerigar sperm illustrated in Figure 1.8, often have elongated heads and may be seen in droppings. They should not be mistaken for flagellates.

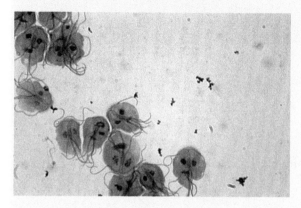

Fig 1.7 *Giardia* (see Box 1.2).

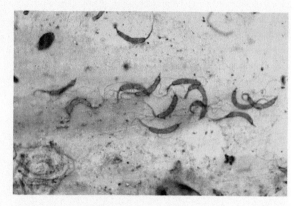

Fig 1.8 Budgerigar sperm (see Box 1.2).

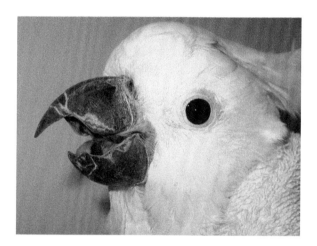

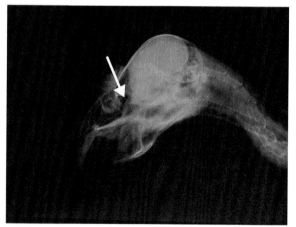

Figs 1.9 and 1.10 Jugal bar fixation in a sulphur-crested cockatoo. Streptostyly is a sliding action of the quadrate bone pushing the jugal bar cranially which in turn pushes the upper jaw so that it pivots around a craniofacial hinge joint and opens the upper jaw independently of the lower. In this bird the jugal bar dislocated, preventing the bird from closing its upper jaw. The problem was resolved by extending and manipulating the beak around a soft rod.

Box 1.3 Which came first, the chicken or the egg?

The first amniote eggs were laid some 300 million years before the first chickens hatched out. The novel use in the amniote egg of a partially pervious, calcium-impregnated shell along with insoluble uric acid as the key metabolic pathway to isolate nitrogenous waste has had far-reaching effects on the anatomy, physiology and disease processes in birds and reptiles compared with other vertebrates. Although modern bird eggs have harder shells, the internal structure of the egg has remained much the same as that of early eggs studied from the fossil record.

In pectoral girdle structure, relative to the non-flying dromaeosaurs, *Archaeopteryx*'s scapula was strap-like and formed a flexible joint set at an acute angle with a larger, caudally reflexed coracoid. The glenoid cavity was located laterally and the biceps tubercle was large and cranial. There was no sternum, rather a series of gastralia behind the coracoids, but there was a rudimentary furcula ('wish bone') (Fig. 1.20).

Dromaeosaurs, troodontids and *Archaeopteryx* all had swivel wrist joints and two long and one shorter finger on their hands. All had teeth and long bones with thin cortices (see Fig. 1.27). In *Archaeopteryx* the brain

Box 1.4 Tarsal joint structure in the Crurotarsi and Ornithodira

Tarsal joint structure is an important distinguishing feature between the Crurotarsi group from which crocodiles descend and the Ornithodira from which pterosaurs, theropod dinosaurs and birds descend (Fig. 1.11). The former have a rotary crurotarsal joint between the astragalus (tibiotarsal) and calcaneum (fibular tarsal) bones with a heel on the calcaneum and a plantigrade stance. In the Ornithodira, the astragalus and calcaneum are fused and form the proximal end of a mesotarsal hinge joint opposing the distal tarsal bones. Stance is digitigrade (standing on the toes, without a heel) (Fig. 1.12).

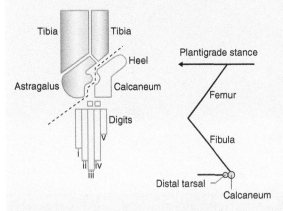

A Crurotarsal (rotary) joint (Crocodyliformes)

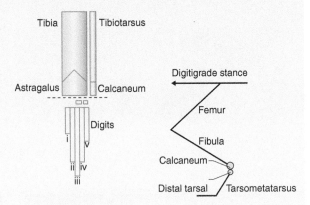

B Mesotarsal (hinge) joint (theropod dinosaurs and Aves)

Fig 1.11 Comparative tarsal joint structure (see Box 1.4).

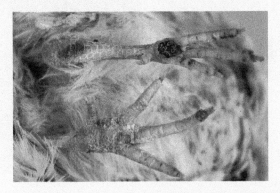

Fig 1.12 Pododermatitis. Because birds stand on their toes and do not have a 'heel', they can be prone to pressure sores, calluses and secondary infections on their feet and legs. These most commonly occur on the interdigital pad or (if the bird 'squats') the plantar surface of the intertarsal joint (see Box 1.4). Walking or perching on rough or hard substrates, obesity, restricted exercise and diets low in vitamin A are predisposing factors that should be avoided.

was enlarged and the ascending process of the jugal bar reduced so that there was partial confluence of diapsid openings on the lateral skull allowing for large eyes surrounded by a ring of scleral ossicles and partial stereoscopic vision. Probably to help cushion landings, the femur was 80% of the size of the tibia, and the tibia, fibula and proximal tarsal bones were partially fused, as were the distal tarsal and metatarsal bones. The hallux (first digit) was reversed. Pectoral girdle structure did not allow for a triosseal canal through which the supracoracoideus muscle could pass to elevate the wing. Consequently *Archaeopteryx* could run and glide freely but manoeuvrability would have been poor, powered flight rudimentary and taking off from the ground would have been difficult.

Confuciusornis, a pigeon-sized bird fossil found in rock formations in north-east China dating to the Jurassic–Cretaceous boundary (*c.* 145 mya), showed contour feathers, suggesting that the bird was endothermic. In common with *Archaeopteryx*, *Confuciusornis* had a retroverted pubis and a reversed hallux. It also had a large premaxilla with a nasofrontal hinge and an edentulous (toothless)

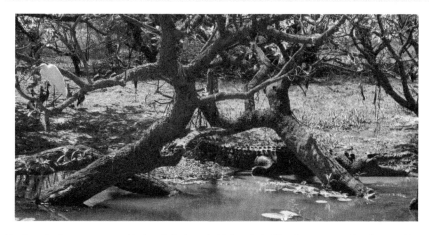

Fig 1.13 An extended family gathering: a great egret (*Ardea alba*), plumed whistling ducks (*Dendrocygna eytoni*) and a crocodile, on the banks of the Yellow River, Kakadu, Northern Territory, Australia. Archosaurs gave rise to crocodilians, pterosaurs and dinosaurs. Birds descend from dinosaurs. As pterosaurs and non–avian dinosaurs became extinct around 65 million years ago, crocodiles are now birds' closest living relative.

Table 1.2 Dating estimates for early avian divergences based on molecular data calibrated with penguin/stork fossils at 62 mya (after Harrison et al 2004)

Groups	mya
Palaeognaths/neognaths	101
Ratite/tinamou	84
Ostrich/other ratites	75
Gallianseres/Neoaves	90
Magpie goose/duck + goose	66
Owl/other neoavians	80
Passerines/other neoavians	80
Oscines/suboscines	70
Falconiformes/parrot	72
Shorebirds/penguin, stork	74
Penguin/stork	**62 (fixed)**
Birds/crocodilian	183
Archosaurs/turtles	199

beak. Its hands showed unfused carpal elements, long fingers and long curved claws, suggesting it was a good climber. Its tail was short with long tail feathers allowing increased manoeurability in flight.

Stage 3 – add stereoscopic vision, brain development and a supracoracoideus pulley for rudimentary powered flight (Ornithothoraces/ Protoavis)

While fossilized bird remains are sparse, possible tracks dating to the late Triassic and early Jurassic have been found in Africa, Europe and North America, suggesting

that birds may have been global species before *Archaeopteryx*. *Protoavis*, a species that lived in North America, controversially dated *c.* 225 mya, was ahead of its time when compared with *Archaeopteryx* and other Mesozoic bird fossils, so much so that some scientists doubt its validity. It had a spring-like furcula joined ventrally by a hypocleidium, dorsally directed glenoids, strut-like coracoids and a sternum. Rudimentary triosseal canals formed at each shoulder at the confluence of the furcula, coracoid and scapula, through which could pass the pulley-like supracoracoideus muscles which were used to elevate the wings. These features all suggest that this bird was capable of limited powered flight (Fig. 1.21). Fossil feathers for *Protoavis* have not been found but knobs identified on the ulna suggest they existed in life. There were three carpal and four separate metacarpal bones.

Protoavis had large eyes, stereoscopic vision, a partially toothed beak and an avidiaspid cranium that allowed a nasofacial hinge joint to open by the action of the quadrate bone pushing the jugal bar, much as it does in modern birds. Olfactory lobes were reduced but the cerebrum, optic lobes and cerebellum were increased and a visual Wulst bulge (thought to be involved with prehensile abilities and eye–foot coordination) could be identified on the dorsal cerebrum. Also like modern birds, the number of cervical vertebrae was increased, bones were pneumatic and the bodies were saddle-shaped (heterocoelous), enabling the head to be moved in all directions and the beak to be used as a universal tool. At rest the neck was S-shaped so that the head could be retracted back close to the centre of gravity (Figs 1.22 and 1.23). The tail was long, enabling control of pitch and roll on a level course of flight but making turning, climbing or diving difficult.

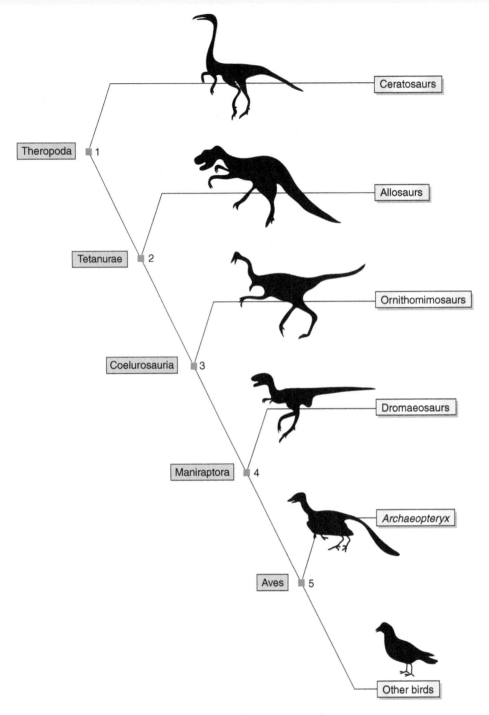

Fig 1.14 Cladistic relationships of the major groups of theropod dinosaurs (after Gauthier 1986).

Protoavis showed fusion of the ilium and ischium caudally, features that would have strengthened the pelvis and helped to withstand the impact of landing from a height. There were renal fossas indicating that the kidneys were streamlined into the pelvis. The ischium and pubis were open ventrally without a symphysis, which would allow the passage of large, hard-shelled eggs. On the tibia there was a cranial cnemial crest as in modern birds, but the tibia was not fused with fibula and proximal tarsal bones to form what we call the tibiotarsus. The distal tarsal bones were not fused with the metatarsal bones. The foot was ansiodactyl with a large, opposable,

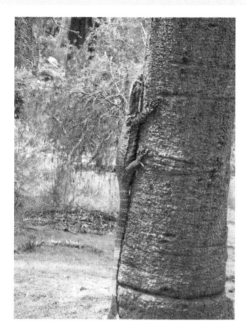

Fig 1.15 A goanna (*Varanus varius*) climbing vertically up a tree trunk. Pro-avian dinosaurs had long tails and long fingers on their hands. As demonstrated by this goanna in a picnic ground in South Eastern Australia, these anatomical features could have enabled them to climb up tree trunks with ease. A patagial fold between the wrist and the shoulder in pro-avians may have served as an elastic band to keep the animal close to the trunk when climbing upwards as well as slowing speed and softening their landing if parachuting down from a height.

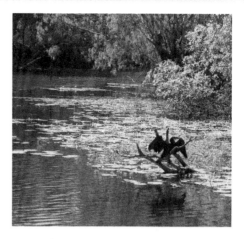

Fig 1.16 A darter (*Anhinga melanogaster*) with wings outstretched, Kakadu, Northern Territory, Australia. Early birds could have also used this behaviour for camouflage, protecting their nests or drying feathers before advances in barbule configuration in the feathers improved waterproofing. Warm wetland areas, such as this, are the habitat in which early birds are believed to have evolved.

fully reversed hallux indicating *Protoavis* had a grasping foot with a capacity for both walking and climbing.

Stage 4 – add a locked coracoid-scapula, a carpometacarpus, an alula and a pygostyle for manoeuvrability (Pygostylia/Enantiornithines)

This group of birds first appeared in the fossil record in Cretaceous times around 120 mya (Fig. 1.4). The proximal coracoid formed a peg to fit into the socket of the scapula, locking in a solid airframe configuration against which wings could flap. The tail was reduced to a short pygostyle from which tail feathers emerged. The carpal and metacarpal bones fused to form major and minor carpometacarpi and the alula (Fig. 1.24). Pelvic formation utilized the ilium and ischium fused posteriorly to enclose a large ilioischiadic fenestra. This constellation of features improved manoeuvrability and capacity for powered flight and controlled landings.

By the time Enantiornithines became widespread, Pangaea had fractured and the continents were moving apart. However, these birds were not confined to single land masses as they would have been able to use their ability to fly, wade and/or swim across water to reach other land masses. Some genuses included: *Enantiornis leali*, the type species from Argentina, *Avisaurus* from

North America, *Iberomesornis* from Europe, *Nanantius* from Australia and *Gobipteryx* from Mongolia. Nests of *Gobipteryx* have been found, showing that some of these birds hatched precocial chicks from eggs incubated in the ground.

Flightless land birds allied with the Enantiornithines, such as *Patgopteryx* from Patagonia, also emerged in the fossil record from the late Cretaceous period. The wings were highly atrophied; the ilia formed a pelvic shield with the synsacrum while posteriorly the ilia and ischium separated without enclosing an ilioischiadic fenestra. A large antitrochanter was present on the rim of the acetabulum, the femur was robust and the distal tarsal and metatarsal bones fused to form the tarsometatarsus. These features resemble present-day ratites.

Stage 5 – add ossified uncinate processes to the ribs to strengthen the 'fuselage' and more pelvic fusion (Ornithurae/Hesperornithiformes)

The Hesperornithiformes were flightless, foot-propelled diving birds whose stronghold was an inland sea that bisected North America in late Cretaceous times. The Hesperornithiformes and several other species of toothed birds were first described in 1880 by O.C. Marsh in an excellently illustrated text that attracted Charles Darwin's praise (Fig. 1.25). *Hesperornis*, the best-known genus, parallels modern loons and grebes in many skeletal features and the possession of salt glands. It was a much larger bird than its modern counterparts, about 2 metres long, covered with soft, hair-like plumaceous feathers. Like many subsequent species that evolved in geographically isolated areas in the absence of predators, it did not fly. The uncinate processes on the ribs were ossified. The

As in hair, nails and scales, feathers grow by proliferation and differentiation of keratinocytes. These keratin-producing cells in the epidermis, or outer skin layer, achieve their purpose in life when they die, leaving behind a mass of deposited keratin. Keratins are filaments of proteins that polymerize to form solid structures. Feathers are made of beta-keratins, which are unique to reptiles and birds. The outer covering of the growing feather, called the sheath, is made of the softer alpha-keratin, which is found in all vertebrates and makes up our own skin and hair.

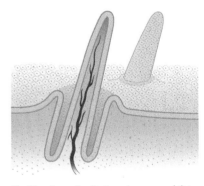

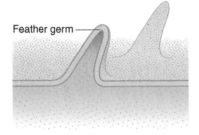

Feather germ

The placode then forms a unique elongated tube, the feather germ.

Proliferation of cells in a ring around the feather germ creates the follicle (detail below), the organ that generates the feather. At the base of the follicle, in the follicle collar, the continuing production of keratinocytes forces older cells up and out, eventually forming the entire, tubular feather.

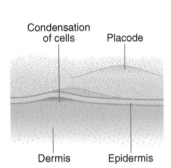

Condensation of cells

Placode

Dermis

Epidermis

Feather growth begins with the placode, a thickening of the epidermis over a condensation of cells in the dermis.

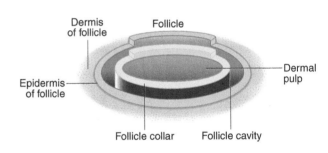

Dermis of follicle

Follicle

Epidermis of follicle

Dermal pulp

Follicle collar

Follicle cavity

Fig 1.17 Feather formation (after Prum & Brush 2004, with permission from Patricia J. Wynne).

synsacrum was enlarged with the incorporation of more than eight vertebrae and the pelvic elements were fused, with the ilium, ischium and pubis more or less parallel. These features would help 'strengthen the fuselage' for travel through either air or water. As in present-day paddling waterfowl, the cnemial crest on the tibia was large (in this case derived from the patella), the femur was short and held horizontal and the paddling leg movement was predominantly a function of the stifle joint.

Stage 6 – add a deeper keel bone, a complete triosseal canal and fused tibiotarsus and tarsometatarsus for controlled, powered flight and safer landing (Carinatae/Ichthyornithiformes)

Ichthyornis and *Apatornis* were toothed birds of the late Cretaceous period in North America that were also first described by O.C. Marsh in 1880. They resembled present-day gulls and terns and had expanded brains and salt glands. The sternum had a large carina and there was a triosseal canal, the humerus had an enormous deltoid crest and a brachial depression at the

distal end. Both the tibiotarsus and the tarsometatarus were fused (Fig. 1.26).

Stage 7 – add skull bone fusion (Neornithes/ Gobipipus and modern birds)

By the close of the Mesozoic era Enantiornithines were found on all continents, Hesperornithiformes were swimming in northern hemisphere seas and Ichthyornithiformes were found along the shore lines. While the location of their ancestral population is unclear, modern birds (Neornithes) in which the individual bones in the skull were fused were beginning to appear globally in the fossil record. In North America transitional shorebirds were emerging in coastal areas, and in Eurasia there was *Gobipipus*, a land bird known from late Cretaceous Mongolia. Its fossilized nests included an egg containing a precocious chick on the point of hatching. In the southern hemisphere, swimming off an island near western Antarctica in a shallow marine environment alongside plesiosaurs was *Polarornis*, the oldest loon (Gaviiformes).

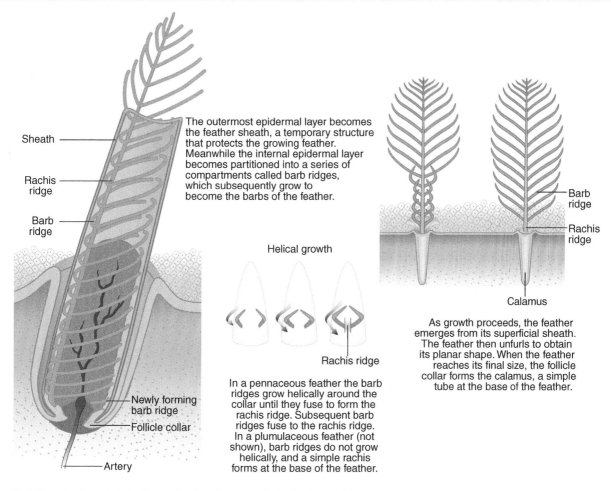

Sheath

Rachis ridge

Barb ridge

The outermost epidermal layer becomes the feather sheath, a temporary structure that protects the growing feather. Meanwhile the internal epidermal layer becomes partitioned into a series of compartments called barb ridges, which subsequently grow to become the barbs of the feather.

Newly forming barb ridge

Follicle collar

Artery

Helical growth

Rachis ridge

In a pennaceous feather the barb ridges grow helically around the collar until they fuse to form the rachis ridge. Subsequent barb ridges fuse to the rachis ridge. In a plumulaceous feather (not shown), barb ridges do not grow helically, and a simple rachis forms at the base of the feather.

Barb ridge

Rachis ridge

Calamus

As growth proceeds, the feather emerges from its superficial sheath. The feather then unfurls to obtain its planar shape. When the feather reaches its final size, the follicle collar forms the calamus, a simple tube at the base of the feather.

Fig 1.18 Feather formation (after Prum & Brush 2004, with permission from Patricia J. Wynne).

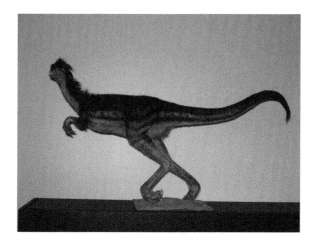

Fig 1.19 *Mononykus*. There have been a number of finds in recent years of feathered, bird-like theropod dinosaurs. *Mononykus*, a feathered, non-flighted theropod dinosaur from the late Cretaceous period in China, had avian skull characteristics. Model from the 'Dinosaurs of China' exhibition, Melbourne Museum, 2005.

Alongside fossil evidence, evidence from nuclear and mitochondrial DNA hybridization is now placing the origin of modern birds in the late Cretaceous period, with more than 13 extant modern orders emerging prior to the K-T boundary disaster.

Tertiary birds

The Cretaceous–Tertiary (K-T) boundary, 65 mya, was marked by a global extinction event, thought to have been triggered by a meteorite whose main crash site was in present-day Gulf of Mexico. As with other animals, it is likely that birds living near the impact would have had little chance of surviving the initial explosion, fires and the ensuing long dark winter. Birds living at higher latitudes might have been better adapted to the cool, dark conditions and could provide bird populations from which other areas could be repopulated. The ability to fly, swim, wade or walk would have

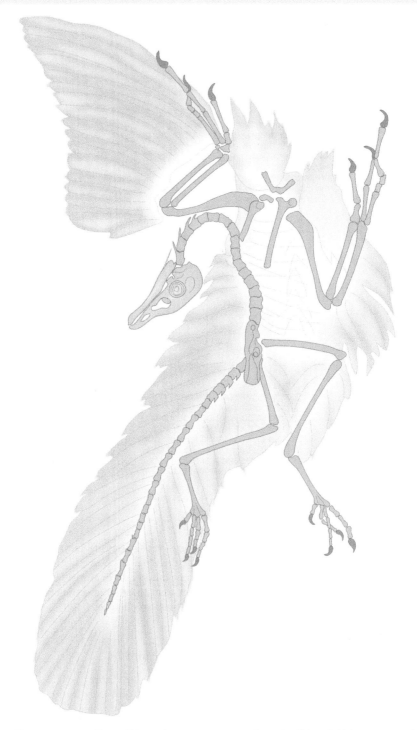

Fig 1.20 *Archaeopteryx*. Even when it lived in Europe 150 mya, *Archaeopteryx* was a relic species. This early bird was not strongly built, it had teeth, separate bony fingers on its hands, no sternum, a long tail and multiple metatarsal bones. However, it also had typical flight feathers, a strap-like scapula set at an acute angle with a large reflexed coracoid and a rudimentary furcula. It was capable of gliding but taking off from the ground would have been difficult. (Engraving by Zittel 1887.)

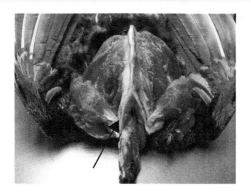

Fig 1.21 Pectoral girdle structure in volant birds. Because extended wings have an aerofoil configuration (see Box 1.1), birds can rely on the force of lift to maintain altitude while in flight and they do not need strong muscles to raise their wings on the upstroke. However, they do need strong muscles for the downstroke and to generate thrust. The tendon of the supracoracoideus (deep pectoral) muscle acts like a pulley, travelling from muscle attached to the sternum, through the triosseal canal (see arrow) to insert on the head of the humerus and raise and extend the wing. The overlying superficial pectoral muscle provides power for the downstroke and forward thrust. The strap-like scapula and strut-like coracoid are firmly attached and form part of the triosseal canal. In conjunction with the supracoracoideus, they help to maintain the aerofoil configuration of the wing. The spring-like furcula, the third bone of the triosseal canal, makes the downstroke easier and also provides support for the shoulder.

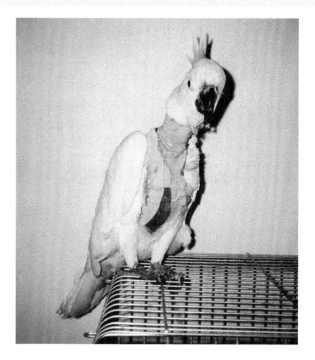

Fig 1.23 The cervical subluxation of the sulphur-crested cockatoo was reduced by manipulation and the neck placed in a brace attached to a body harness (as shown) for several weeks. He made a full recovery.

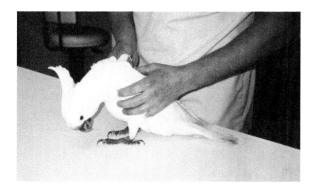

Fig 1.22 Cervical subluxation in a sulphur-crested cockatoo. To compensate for not having hands, birds have long necks with many heterocoeleus (saddle-shaped) vertebrae which enable the head and beak to be moved in all directions and used as a universal tool. This leaves them vulnerable to neck injury, for example as occurred here when this bird caught his head in cage wire then tried to pull it out.

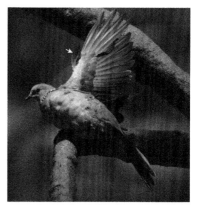

Fig 1.24 Alula. When extended, the alula ('thumb') (see arrow) acts as a 'slot', maintaining laminar air flow over the dorsal surface of the wing as the bird slows and hence enables a smoother, more accurate landing at slow speeds.

aided dispersal. Enantiornithines, Hesperornithiformes and Ichthyornithiformes did not survive the extinction event, nor did the pterosaurs, but Neornithes birds survived and went on to fill ecological niches on land, sea and air across the globe (Figs 1.28, 1.29).

Perhaps there were soft tissue differences, for instance in brain development, navigational ability or instinctive behaviour, nesting or migration patterns, that gave the Neornithes an edge over the archaic birds. Both DNA and fossil evidence indicate that all modern birds fall into this monophyletic clade but the bony differences between the Ichthyornithiformes and the Neornithes do not seem to be dramatic enough to account for the

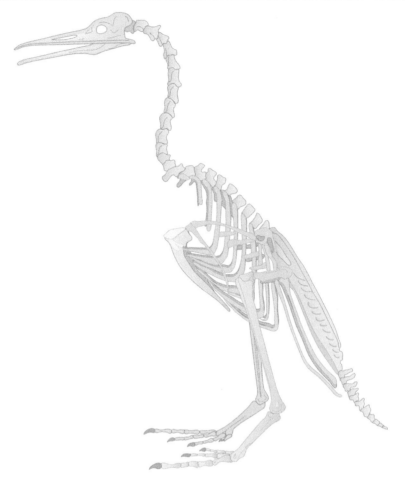

Fig 1.25 *Hesperornis*. The Hersperornithiformes were specialized, toothed, flightless, foot-propelled diving birds that lived in northern hemisphere waters in Cretaceous times. Like modern diving birds their bodies were streamlined and strengthened by ossified uncinate processes on the ribs and fusion of vertebrae to form the synsacrum. They had large cnemial crests derived from the patella and paddling leg motion was predominately a function of the stifle joint. The group did not survive the K-T boundary extinction event 65 mya. (From Marsh 1872.)

Neornithes' global dominance. Neornithes subsequently split into Palaeognathae (the ratites and tinamous) and Neognathae (all other modern birds). Palaeognathae palate structure shows features similar to primitive archosaurs while in the Neognathae there is a development of a flexible joint between the pterygoid and palatine. There are also differences in sternal structure, with the neognaths generally showing deeper carinae enabling stronger flight.

Relationships amongst the living orders of neognaths have been problematic to unravel and are still much debated. Present-day southern hemisphere continents now have the largest diversity of endemic bird families (South America: 31, Australia: 15 and Africa: 6) (see Fig. 1.32). Early modern bird fossils from at least five groups, including the stone curlew, penguin, transitional

wader and magpie goose/duck, have now been found dating to around 66 mya from Vega Island, off Antarctica. Molecular and palaeogeological evidence dates New Zealand's endemic parrot and passerine lineages to before the islands' split from Gondwana, over 80 mya. These findings lend support for a southern hemisphere origin for modern birds perhaps around 100 mya. Table 1.2 gives estimates for early avian divergences based on molecular data for these groups calibrated against penguin fossils from North Canterbury, New Zealand dating to 62 mya and supported by the more recent bird fossil finds from Vega Island mentioned above.

Land connections between South America, Antarctica and Australia continued from the K-T boundary until *c.* 35–33 mya, while intermittent, much more tenuous,

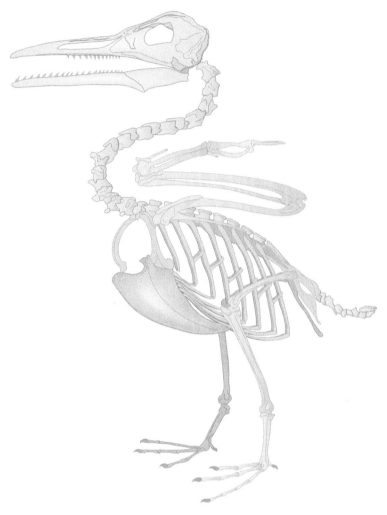

Fig 1.26 *Ichthyornis.* The Ichthyorniformes were toothed, gull-like shorebirds of late Cretaceous times in North America. They had many features in common with modern volant birds including a large sternum, a pectoral girdle structure with a triosseal canal, fused major metacarpus and fused tibiotarsus and tarsometatarsus. The group did not survive the K-T boundary extinction event 65 mya. (From Marsh 1872.)

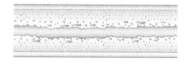

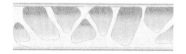

Fig 1.27 Left: mammalian long bone. Right: avian long bone. Unlike non-avian reptile bones, bird bones have evolved for lightness and strength: they are pneumatic with thin cortices and wide medullas that are crossed by strategically placed trabeculae for reinforcement. This produces challenges for avian orthopaedic surgeons as such bones splinter easily and do not lend themselves to fixation with plates and screws. On the other hand, bird wings fold snugly against the body. Braille or figure-of-eight bandages and tie-in techniques for fracture repair are some of the procedures that have been developed because of these unique features of avian patients.

island chain connections existed between Antarctica and the east coast of Africa via the Keuguelen plateau over the same period. While still speculative, these connections could have provided a corridor for modern birds to populate Africa and Eurasia from the south after the 65 mya K-T disaster. Alternatively, some orders, such as Strigiformes (owls), may have re-emerged from remnant high latitude northern populations.

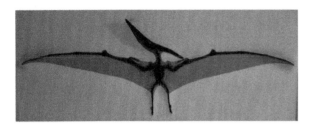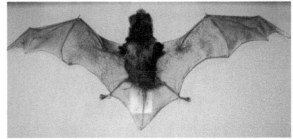

Figs 1.28 and 1.29 Apart from birds, winged flight has evolved independently in two other vertebrate groups: pterosaurs and bats: In pterosaurs the fifth digit became elongated and supported a membranous skin fold. Pterosaurs did not survive the KT boundary extinction event. In bats, flying mammals that emerged in the Tertiary Period, skin folds form between elongated digits. Photos taken at the British Museum and Melbourne Museum, 2005.

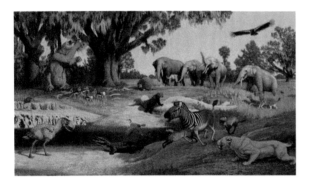

Fig 1.30 Florida 2 million years ago. Large flightless land birds related to Gruiformes (cranes and bustards) and Anseriformes (waterfowl) emerged as dominant herbivores and predators following the demise of the non-avian dinosaurs at the time of the K-T boundary disaster around 65 mya. They became extinct as sharp-toothed placental mammal predators emerged. South America was a later-day stronghold of the giant land birds as it was largely isolated from these placental mammals until the development of the Panama land bridge 2.5 mya. *Titanis*, illustrated here, moved from South to North America at this time but the species was subsequently wiped out in both places. Illustration by Carl Buell, Florida Museum of Natural History.

In the warm, subtropical, Palaeocene times (65–53 mya), the era that followed the demise of non-avian dinosaurs, an 'evolutionary relay' seemed to develop as birds and mammals competed for dominance. There are fossil records from France of *Gastronis*, an early ratite. Strigiformes emerged in North America and bony-toothed Pelicaniformes were found globally. Most spectacularly, giant flightless birds of the Gruiformes (crane, rail and bustard) family rose to become dominant herbivores (e.g. *Diatryma* of North America and Europe) and predators (e.g. the phorusrhacids of South America). As time moved on, these large flightless birds were vulnerable to emerging apex predators

amongst the placental mammals, who could move rapidly on land, raid nests for eggs and attack the adults with their sharp teeth and claws (Fig. 1.30). Flightless birds disappeared from the fossil record in Eurasia and North America as the placental mammals took over but, as evidenced by the present-day distribution of ratites, flightless birds were able to hold their own on land masses where placental mammal predators had not reached. Stratigraphic evidence suggests that recent-day palaeognaths:

- the Tinamidae of South America
- the kiwis and extinct moas of New Zealand
- the extinct elephant birds of Madagascar
- the emu and cassowaries of Australia
- the ostrich of Africa and
- the rhea of South America

derived from smaller ancestors that could, with difficulty, fly/swim or wade across the bodies of water that separated the southern hemisphere land masses (Fig. 1.31). The distances involved were much shorter than exist today. Of these birds, only ostriches initially co-evolved with large placental mammal predators.

Sphenisciformes (penguins), probably derived from a loon-like ancestor, are known only from the southern hemisphere with Antarctica their stronghold. Fossils of giant penguin-like birds have been found in South Australia dating to the Eocene epoch (Vickers-Rich 1996). While loons are known to have been present in Antarctic regions in the late Cretaceous and early Tertiary periods they are now only found in the northern hemisphere. Perhaps proto loon species were outcompeted by the emerging penguins or pinnipeds (seals) or adversely affected by local climate change.

Of the present-day orders of Neognathae birds there is general consensus that the 'Galloanserae' were an

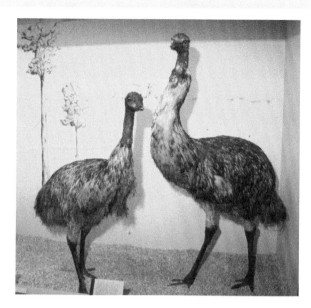

Fig 1.31 Mainland and dwarf emus. Fossil evidence suggests that ratites were once found globally, probably descendant from small, flighted ancestors resembling present-day tinamous. In historical times their stronghold has been the southern hemisphere. There have been many examples of island extinctions of ratites coinciding with the arrival of humans, e.g. the moas of New Zealand, the elephant birds of Madagascar and, as illustrated here, the dwarf emus of the Bass Strait Islands of Australia. These emus were isolated when global sea levels rose 14 000 years ago and they developed into dwarf forms on several islands. They were easily caught and became extinct shortly after the arrival of Europeans. This specimen was brought to France as a live bird in 1804 and was stuffed when it died. There are no specimens of dwarf emus left in Australia. (Photo by Elliot Forsyth.)

early offshoot and derived from common ancestry. This group includes:

- the Anseriformes: screamers of South America, ducks, geese and other waterfowl and
- the Galliformes: chickens, quail and pheasants.

The remaining Neognathae, the Neoaves, fall into three main groups:

1. The Gruiformes (cranes).
2. The Chardriormorphae, a shorebird-derived complex that, in addition to present-day shorebirds, gave rise to the 'Ciconiimorphae':
   - Phoenicopteriformes (flamingoes)
   - Ciconiiformes (storks)
   - Pelicaniformes (cormorants, shags, pelicans)
   - Gaviformes (loons)
   - Sphenisciformes (penguins)
   and the 'Columbimorphae':
   - Turniciformes (button quail)
   - Pteroclidiformes (sand grouse)
   - Columbiformes (doves and pigeons)
   - Psittaciformes (parrots and cockatoos).
3. 'The land bird assemblage', which gave rise to:
   - Opisthocimiformes (hoatzins)
   - Falconiformes
   - Cuculiformes (cuckoos)
   - Musphagiformes (touracos)
   - Strigiformes (owls)
   - Caprimulgiformes (goatsuckers, frogmouths)
   - Apodiformes (swifts and hummingbirds)
   - Bucerotiformes (hornbills)
   - Piciformes (woodpeckers)
   - Passeriformes, which now comprise over half of present-day bird species.

The Piciformes were amongst the last modern bird orders to emerge in the fossil record, with first recordings currently dating to the Oligocene epoch, 53–36 mya.

La Grande Coupure c. 33 mya

Following the K-T crisis, another critical biogeographical event for evolving avifauna was *La Grande Coupure* – the great cut, so coined by the Swiss palaeontologist Hans Stehlin. Beginning about 60 mya, Australia began to unzip itself from Antarctica as tectonic plate movement slowly drew the continent northwards. By 40 mya, India had crashed into southern Asia and the Himalayan mountains began rising, as they continue to do today. The Drake Passage between South America and Antarctica opened *c.* 35 mya and finally, *c.* 33 mya, a long submarine rise that stretched from Australia to Antarctica severed, allowing bottom water of the Antarctic circumpolar current to flood between the two continents for the first time. This caused global cooling and strengthened coastal and trade winds. The effect was magnified as polar ice caps expanded, winds strengthened, temperatures dropped and global cold water currents carried rich marine food sources northwards (Flannery 2000). While present-day orders of birds emerged prior to *La Grande Coupure*, it was after this time that a dramatic expansion of volant bird families occurred.

North and South America were rejoined by the Panama land bridge *c.* 2.5 mya and with this there was interchange of bird and animal species from the two continents. Large flightless birds made their way briefly to North America from the south but, in the end they were wiped out (Fig. 1.30). Apex placental mammal predators, the large cats, bears and canids, were probably the cause of their extinction. These, however, were exceptions; globally birds thrived under diverse circumstances, including Ice Age conditions during the Pleistocene epoch.

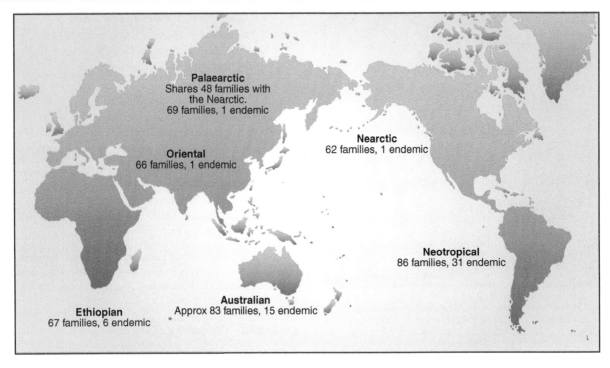

Palaearctic
Shares 48 families with
the Nearctic.
69 families, 1 endemic

Nearctic
62 families, 1 endemic

Oriental
66 families, 1 endemic

Neotropical
86 families, 31 endemic

Australian
Approx 83 families, 15 endemic

Ethiopian
67 families, 6 endemic

Fig 1.32 Present-day global distribution of bird families. South America and Australia currently have the largest number of endemic bird families but fossil evidence suggests birds such as the megapodes and psittacines were formerly present elsewhere. Present-day distribution lends support to a Gondwana/southern hemisphere origin for modern birds.

The end of the Ice Age brought the global expansion of humans, who have had a devastating effect on bird diversity. Around the world, local extinction of bird species has followed the arrival of humans and our domestic dogs, cats, rats, livestock and machines. The scale of these extinctions has been enormous, especially for island populations. It is estimated that over 2000 species of birds have disappeared from the islands of the Pacific since the arrival of the Polynesians and the Europeans. Large flightless birds have been particularly vulnerable. The moas of New Zealand, the elephant bird of Madagascar, and the dodo of Mauritius are just a few examples. Continental birds, like the passenger pigeon, Carolina parakeet and great auk, have also suffered extinctions. From a peak of over 12 000 species before the start of this human-induced crisis there are currently around 9650 living species. The number of avian species worldwide continues to diminish (Fig. 1.33).

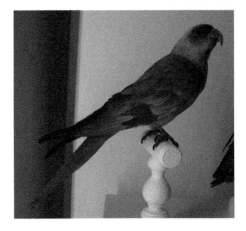

Fig 1.33 Carolina parakeet (*Conuropsis carolinensis*), the only indigenous parrot species in eastern United States, became extinct in the early 1900s from habitat loss, hunting by farmers who considered them a pest species and possibly from disease. Currently numerous other parrot species throughout the world are also threatened or endangered. Avian veterinarians have a role to play in reversing this trend. Stuffed specimen, Audubon Exhibition, Museum of Natural History, Nantes, France, 2005.

Behavioural and soft tissue adaptations

Fossils can tell only part of the story of avian evolution. Behavioural, urogenital and other soft tissue adaptations were critical in the emergence of structure and function of modern birds. These features leave little trace in the stratographic record, so estimation of the time of emergence of these features can be difficult. However, they are reflected in anatomy, physiology, behaviour, diversity and distribution of present-day bird species.

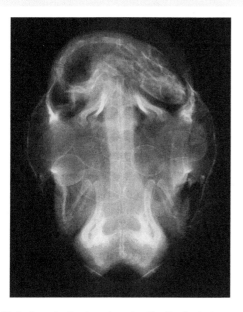

Fig 1.34 Radiograph of turtle on the point of lay. Reptiles lay large clutches of soft eggs concurrently and the eggs are incubated in soil. Avian ancestors evolved to lay eggs one at a time as birds would not be able to fly and carry such a large number of eggs internally. (Photo by Anne Fowler.)

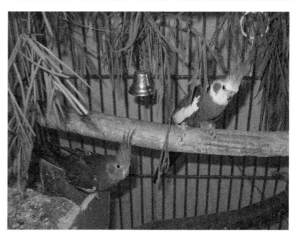

Fig 1.35 Cockatiels with an egg. Endothermy and feathers enhanced the capacity for birds to incubate eggs against their bodies compared with their dinosaur ancestors. Dinosaur nest-protecting behaviour could have gradually become modified into egg-incubating behaviour. Smaller clutch sizes would allow eggs to be incubated against the body and the incubation period, and hence the risk of nest predation, to be reduced. Brood patches, vascular areas that develop on the ventrum of egg-incubating birds, also assist in maintaining warmth and shortening the incubation period.

Reproductive adaptations

Birds' reptilian ancestors had two ovaries and laid large clutches of eggs (Fig. 1.34). These eggs were incubated in nests on the ground in warm, moist conditions and gave rise to precocial young. Crocodilians still nest in this manner. For early birds, using body heat to shorten the incubation time (and later developing specialized brood patches) would have been an advantage in reducing risk of predation and enhancing survival of their young, particularly in cool climates. It would have also favoured birds having small clutches to incubate against the parents' bodies. Ducks or swans that nest in reeds or build floating nests might be a model for this type of incubation. Alternatively, feathered, partially endothermic avian ancestors may have nested in burrows as, for example, some penguins (another ancient avian family) do today (Kavanau 1987).

The ability of early birds to use their own body heat to speed up the incubation process may have been advantageous in the short term in enabling birds to make use of nest sites in tree hollows, branches or bushes. The evolution of avian incubation also required a change in egg structure to enable the embryos to survive in conditions with lower humidity (Fig. 1.35). Laying small clutches of eggs individually rather than as a simultaneous clutch, as in reptiles, eliminated a need for two ovaries and birds' bodies could be aerodynamically streamlined to contain a single ovary and oviduct. The emergence of medullary bone lay-down of calcium in egg-laying females would have assisted this process. Flight and the avian reproductive 'package' developed hand in hand (Figs 1.36, 1.37, 1.38).

Eggshell structure

For both birds and reptiles an excretory system based on the production of insoluble urates (rather than soluble urea) enabled waste material to be compartmentalized within the egg but away from the developing embryo in a non-toxic form. The development of insoluble urates gave birds the capacity to lay eggs that could survive out of water. Both the non-avian theropod dinosaurs and the Enantiornithines produced eggshells with an internal mammillary layer composed of numerous, tightly packed conical knobs. External to this was the thicker, squamate or spongy zone composed of calcite crystals arranged on a protein matrix. Neoaves also have these layers, but in addition there is also an external zone composed of smooth, shiny, protein cuticle and the spongy zone has vertical palisades separated by minute pore canals. With these innovations, modern bird eggs were less prone to desiccation and parent birds were better able to exploit nesting sites above the ground (Fig. 1.39).

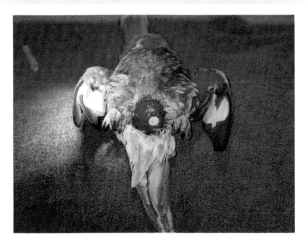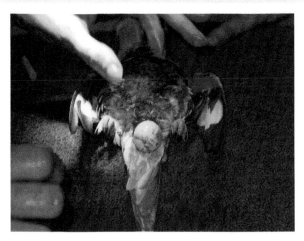

Figs 1.36 and 1.37 Egg binding in a lorikeet. Compared with their dinosaur ancestors, laying eggs one at a time and having smaller clutch sizes would have facilitated parent birds being able to fly to seek food while caring for their offspring. However, large, heavily calcified eggs that can be incubated above ground without desiccation can also be difficult to pass, as shown with this egg-bound lorikeet. Warmth, calcium and fluid therapy are medical treatments that can be helpful to relieve egg binding from a large egg. If not resolved, egg implosion or salpingotomy may be needed to treat the reproductive problem.

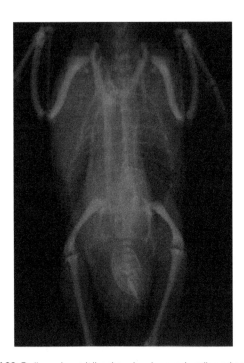

Fig 1.38 Radiograph, medullary bone lay-down and a collapsed egg. As a means to store calcium to satisfy their high metabolic calcium requirements during egg laying, birds have evolved a mechanism for oestrogen-dependent medullary bone lay-down ('polyosteotic hyperosteosis'). Increased long bone density is seen in both normal, reproductively active females as well as those showing pathology, such as illustrated here. In males it may be an indication of an oestrogen-producing Sertoli cell tumour of the testicle.

While primitive birds hatched large, downy feathered, precocial young (as evidenced by *Gobipipus*, ratites, Anseriformes and Galliformes), it is possible for altricial (small, featherless, helpless) chicks to be produced from smaller eggs relative to the size of the adult bird. For some species, benefits of this appear to offset the greater parental care required to rear altricial young (e.g. Columbiformes, Psittaciformes and Passeriformes).

Respiratory adaptations

Crocodilians have multi-chambered lungs with complex, branching bronchi leading into high-density parenchyma. There is neither diaphragm nor alveoli. Birds also lack a diaphragm and have air capillaries rather than alveoli and there is extensive development of the air sacs which provide a reservoir of air for release into the air capillaries and into pneumatic bones. These features generally make for lighter bodyweight and efficient respiration, both of which are cornerstones for leaping, running, swimming or flight. Penguins and emus have paleopulmonic parabronchi in which airflow is caudocranial, unidirectional and linked with air sacs. Other birds also have neopulmonic parabronchial networks, in which airflow is bi-directional, in addition to paleopulmonic parabronchi. Birds' abdominal muscles and intercostal muscles act as a diaphragm for the whole coelomic cavity with both inspiration and expiration. The cone-shaped skeletal torso of modern birds appears to function as a bellows-like apparatus in

External zone

Squamate zone

Mammillary layer

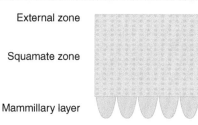
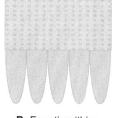
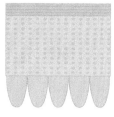
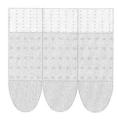

A. Nonavian theropod eggshell

B. Enantiornithine eggshell

C. Ratite eggshell

D. Neognath eggshell

Fig 1.39 Eggshell structure in early and modern birds. Both birds and theropod dinosaurs produced eggs with an internal mammillary layer and an external, thicker spongy layer of calcite crystals arranged on a protein matrix. In addition to this, modern bird eggs have an external layer of a protein cuticle and vertical palisades separated by minute pore canals. This innovation aided in respiration and minimized the risk of eggs desiccating when kept in nests above the ground.

breathing while at the same time streamlining and lightening birds' bodies for swimming, gliding or flight.

Digestive adaptations

Avian digestive systems reflect diet diversity, weight constraints of powered flight and evolutionary origin. For example, while all present-day birds lack teeth, large caeca are present in the Galliformes and Anseriformes (closely related, generally herbivorous, families) but are reduced or absent in Columbiformes, Psittaciformes and Passeriformes. In the absence of teeth, a muscular ventriculus with grit is used as an alternative for grinding food.

'The flight package' of modern birds

In volant birds the centre of gravity needs to be below the extended wings rather than above them. With rotation of the coracoid to the front of the chest and the scapula to the flat of the back, the glenoid socket of the scapulo-humeral joint moved to a dorsolateral position. This positioning of the scapula facilitates the attachment of the wing and it is also seen in mammalian climbers, including primates. However, in the avian model the scapula is strap-like, narrow and fixed, compared with the broad triangular scapula of climbing animals. Once in flight, birds do not require strong muscles to raise their wings as lift performs this function, but they require strong muscles for the down beat – a function performed by the superficial pectoral muscles. The tendon of the deep pectoral muscle (supracoracoid) passes through the triosseous canal and inserts on the humerus, thereby assisting in lift by adjusting curvature of the dorsal aerofoil surface of the wing through an indirect effect on the patagial membranes and by altering the angle of attack of the wing.

In addition to the change in the centre of gravity, reduction and fixation of the scapula and emergence of the supracoracoid/triosseous canal pulley system, skeletal refinements useful for flapping flight in birds include:

- swivel carpal joints for wing folding
- the enlargement of the coracoid
- development of flight feathers with asymmetrical, closed pennaceous vanes
- enlargement of the ulna to which secondary wing feathers attach
- fused clavicles forming the furcula
- pneumatic bones
- fusion and strengthening of bones of the limbs, spine and synsacrum
- development of the alula
- shortening of the tail to become the pygostyle
- development of uncinate processes on the ribs
- development of the keeled sternum
- replacement of teeth with lighter beaks.

These changes could be seen to gradually emerge through dromaeosaurs, troodontids *Archaeopteryx*, *Protoavis*, Enantiornithines, Hesperornithiformes, Ichthyornithi-formes and Neornithes, but the upsurge and expansion of birds capable of controlled, manoeuvrable, flapping flight occurred when the 'whole package' of musculoskeletal, soft tissue, reproductive and behavioural features was refined and became widespread. The 'package' was versatile, however, and did not just depend on flapping flight. This is evidenced by the diversity of present-day bird species that range in size from the hovering 6.3 cm bee hummingbird of Cuba (3 g) to the flightless 2.5 m tall ostrich (135 kg) of Africa.

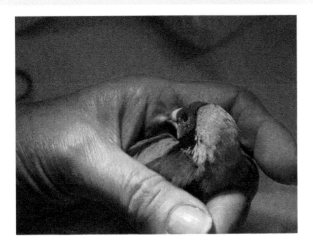

Fig 1.40 Being bitten by a flying dinosaur. Passeriformes, such as this Gouldian finch (*Erythrura gouldiae*), now comprise over half of the species of birds in the world. Like many other species, Gouldian finches in the wild are threatened by disease, habitat clearance and human activity in their range. We are currently witnessing the greatest number of global extinctions since the K-T boundary disaster of 65 mya and our species is the cause. The future of birds is in human hands.

Our generation of humans is the first generation of living, thinking, beings who, working collectively, have been able to unlock the story of over 200 million years of bird evolution. In a practical sense, understanding the developmental stages in the 'flying dinosaur' model helps us to understand diverse avian anatomy and physiology and so aids in day-to-day veterinary practice. In a wider sense the story is humbling. Our own species has been given the keys to this amazing story, yet at the same time we have thoughtlessly orchestrated the greatest mass extinctions since the K-T boundary disaster of 65 million years ago. We need to appreciate the diversity of life-forms with which we share the planet, temper the massive destructive powers we hold and act as responsible custodians to halt this unsustainable trend (Fig. 1.40).

References

Chatterjee S 1997 The rise of birds, 225 million years of evolution. Johns Hopkins University Press, Baltimore, MD, p 1–224

De Duve C 1995 Vital dust, the origin and evolution of life on Earth. Basic Books, New York, p 1–8

Flannery T 2000 The eternal frontier. Text Publishing Company, Melbourne

Gauthier J 1986 Saurischian monophyly and the origin of birds. In: Padian K (ed) The origin of birds and evolution of flight. California Academy of Sciences Memoir, San Francisco, p 1–55

Harrison G L, McLenachan P A, Phillips M J et al 2004 Four new avian mitochondrial genomes help get to basic evolutionary questions in the Late Cretaceous. Molecular Biology and Evolution 21(6):974–983

Kavanau J L 1987 Lovebirds, cockatiels and budgerigars, behaviour and evolution. Science Software Systems, Los Angeles, p 373–640

Long J, Schouten P 2008 Feathered dinosaurs: the origin of birds. CSIRO Publishing, Melbourne, p 151–165

Marsh O C 1872 Notice of a new and remarkable fossil bird. American Journal of Science 4:344

Martin L 2002 An early archosaurian origin for birds. IOC Proceedings, Beijing, p 9

Prum R, Brush A 2004 Which came first, the feather or the bird? Scientific American, Special edition, p 72–82

Vickers-Rich P 1996 The Mesozoic and Tertiary history of birds on the Australian Plate. In: Vickers-Rich P, Monoghan J M, Baird R F, Rich T H (eds) Vertebrate palaeontology of Australasia. Monash University Publications, Melbourne, p 721–808

Suggested reading

Baird R 1996 Avian fossils from the Quaternary of Australia. In: Vickers-Rich P, Monoghan J M, Baird R F, Rich T H (eds) Vertebrate palaeontology of Australasia. Monash University Publications, Melbourne, p 809–870

Sereno P 2002 Birds as dinosaurs. IOC Proceedings, Beijing, p 10

Simkiss K 1963 Bird flight. Hutchinson Educational, London, p 13–46

Vickers-Rich P, Hewitt-Rich T 1993 Wildlife of Gondwana. Reed, Sydney

Warheit K 2001 The seabird fossil record and the role of paleontology in understanding seabird community structure. In: Schreiber E A, Burger J (eds) Biology of marine birds. CRC Press, Boca Raton, p 17–56

Wilson B 1979 Birds, Readings from Scientific American. W H Freeman, San Francisco, p 1–148

Basic anatomy, physiology and nutrition

Patricia Macwhirter

2

Introduction

In companion animal practice, veterinarians traditionally treat dogs and cats – species that are significant because of the bonds they form with their human owners. Avian practice shares that focus on the human–animal bond, but in addition avian practitioners treat cage and aviary birds, zoo birds, wild birds, racing and fancy pigeons, ducks, raptors, ratites and poultry. A fundamental challenge for the avian practitioner is to offer quality patient care across this wide range of species as well as understanding the needs and expectations of their owners.

Because of the diversity of species encountered, avian medicine is best mastered by learning about one family of birds in some detail and then drawing comparisons. In this chapter, avian anatomy, physiology and nutrition are reviewed using psittacine species as a basic model; however, where appropriate, there are comparisons with other avian species likely to be encountered in veterinary practice. When studying or treating birds, it is important to consider how each species has evolved and take every opportunity to observe birds in their natural habitat. By thinking beyond the examination room, veterinarians will gain insight into medical and behavioural problems of individual patients as well as playing a role in trying to preserve avian biodiversity for future generations to experience and enjoy.

Feathers

From an evolutionary perspective birds are warm-blooded reptiles with feathers as one of their key, unique distinguishing features. Feathers contain a different type of keratin and appear to have evolved separately from reptilian scales (Prum & Brush 2004). On the body feathers are arranged in tracts called pterylae with unfeathered areas between the pterylae called apteria (Fig. 2.1).

New feathers develop from the epidermal collar at the base of the feather follicle, and grow upward. This development process is sensitive, and nutritional deficiencies, stress or exogenous cortisone can cause horizontal fault lines to occur on the emerging feather.

The central stalk or shaft of the feather (the quill) is termed the calamus from the follicle to the point where the barbs emerge and then it is termed the rachis. In developing feathers there is a nutrient artery that traverses the centre of the shaft and is surrounded in the calamus by feather pulp ('blood feather'). The feather pulp and artery regress as the feather matures, but keratinized pulp caps remain as horizontal bars across the lumen of the shaft (Figs 1.17, 1.18, 2.2). **A 'blood feather' is an early stage in the moulting process of every normal emerging feather. If cut or damaged, blood feathers may bleed profusely from the nutrient artery.**

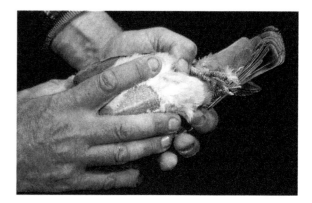

Fig 2.1 The unfeathered apteria may provide skin exposure without removing feathers to provide a site for subcutaneous fluid administration.

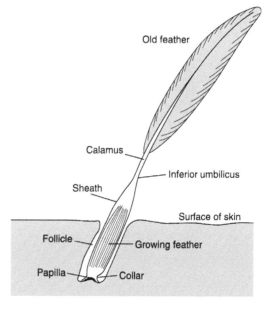

Fig 2.2 Line drawing of a developing feather.

As the feather emerges its external keratin sheath disintegrates, producing a dandruff-like material. Unfurling helically at 45° to the rachis are the barbs, and emerging from the barbs at 45° are barbules. These interlock with each other by a system of hooks (or barbicels), which enables waterproofing. Preening is needed to restore interlocking if the barbules become dislodged. The vane is the portion of the feather extending either side of the rachis, and may be plumulaceous (soft and fluffy) or pennaceous (closely interlocked), depending on the individual type of feather (Fig. 2.3).

Contour feathers cover the bird's body. They have well-developed shafts with plumulaceous and pennaceous components to the vane. Covert feathers are small contour feathers present on the wings and tail.

Flight feathers, or remiges, are pennaceous and, in volant birds, asymmetric to allow for an aerofoil shape to facilitate lift. The leading edge of the flight feather is thicker while the trailing edge is broad and flat. Primary remiges are those that emerge from the periosteum of the metacarpus, secondary remiges are those that emerge from the ulna, and tertiaries emerge from the humerus. Primary remiges are numbered from the carpus distally, while secondary remiges are numbered from the carpus proximally. The tail feathers (retrices) are structurally similar to remiges, but are symmetrical. They are numbered from the centre laterally (Fig. 2.4).

Birds have other feathers adapted for special purposes. Plume (or down) feathers have a rachis shorter than the longest barb, and non-interlocking barbules. These provide an undercoat for insulation. Specialized powder down feathers are located anterior to the hips,

and produce a keratin material that performs a dry lubrication function. Powder down feathers grow continuously and are often the first to develop abnormalities if a bird is infected with circovirus. They are prominent in cockatoos, cockatiels and African grey parrots, so people prone to feather allergies should avoid close contact with these species. Overgrowth of powder down feathers will occur if a bird cannot preen (i.e. if the animal is collared or suffering from beak damage). Semiplume feathers have fluffy vanes, but the rachis is longer than the longest barb. These usually lie near feather tracts to aid in insulation. Filoplumes are hair-like, with a long rachis and short barbs at the end. Bristles have a stiff rachis with few or no barbs at the end, and function like whiskers. After feathers (hypopnea) are small remnant feather structures attached to the shaft at the superior umbilicus, the position where the calamus emerges from the skin.

Integument

Bird skin is thinner and more delicate than that of mammals and sweat glands are absent. In most cases the subcutaneous layer is insufficient to surgically suture (Fig. 2.5). The only epithelial glands are the uropygial glands and holocrine glands of the external ear canal, but the keratinocytes produce lipid, essentially making the entire skin an oil-producing holocrine gland. Since birds lack sweat glands, they dissipate heat by increasing their rate of respiration and holding the wings away from the body. Cold birds 'fluff' their feathers and crouch to retain heat. Normal body temperature for birds is higher than for mammals (depending on species, generally 39–42°C).

The bilobed uropygial gland is found dorsally at the base of the tail on some Columbiformes and most

Fig 2.3 A typical avian feather showing (**A**) pennaceous and (**B**) plumulaceous vane structure.

1 cm

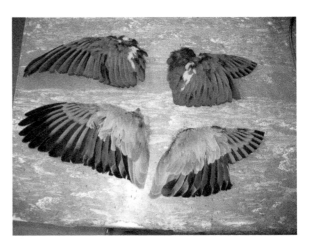

Fig 2.4 Wings showing one commonly used style of wing clipping. By clipping remiges distal to the covert feathers the risk of cutting too close and damaging the skin is minimized. Retrices (tail feathers) should NOT be clipped.

psittacine species, except for Amazon parrots (Fig. 2.6). Each lobe is drained by a single duct, which empties into a lone papilla. The gland, which is not essential, secretes a lipoid sebaceous material that is spread over feathers during preening to help with waterproofing. Impaction or neoplasia are two of the more common disease presentations associated with this structure. If impacted the uropygial gland can be manually expressed or removed surgically. **A brood patch forms on birds incubating eggs. The dermis on the chest becomes thickened and vascular, and feathers are lost. This structure should not be mistaken for a pathological condition.**

Legs, claws and feet

In psittacine species, digits II and III point anteriorly while digits I and IV are oriented posteriorly. In passerines, digit I points posteriorly while digits II–IV point anteriorly.

A bird's feet and legs are covered with scales – raised areas of highly keratinized epidermis separated by a fold

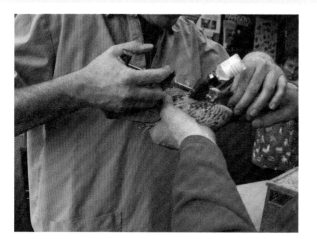

Fig 2.5 Birds rely on the force of lift to raise their wings so dorsal musculature is not well developed. Between the shoulders is a useful place to give subcutaneous injections, for example with Newcastle disease vaccination in a pigeon.

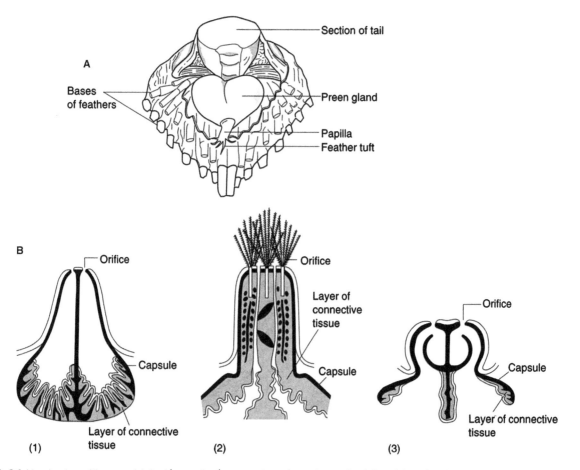

Fig 2.6 Line drawings of the uropygial gland (preen gland) representing various avian species. **A** Dorsal view of the gland on a white leghorn chicken. **B** Details of papilla: (1) delicate type; (2) compact type; (3) unique passerine type.

of less keratinized skin. Claws have a strongly keratinized dorsal plate and a softer ventral plate that grows more slowly, thus producing the curved claws for perching. Vitamin A deficiency, as seen in birds fed all-seed diets, or paradoxically vitamin A excess, can both result in hyperkeratosis. Scaly mite (*Cnemidocoptes* sp.) may also induce hyperkeratosis, typically with a dysplastic 'honeycomb' appearance.

Senses

Sight

Birds possess great visual acuity. 'An eye attached to a wing' is an often quoted but apt description of flighted avian species. Most birds' eyes have a very large, asymmetrical globe, and 10–18 ossicles (eyebones) that overlap to form a ring encircling the sclera. **The sphincter and dilator muscles of the pupil are striated; therefore, unlike mammals, voluntary control may be possible and atropine has no effect.**

A soft lens, which has an annular pad, allows for rapid accommodation by the avian patient. The ciliary body is in direct contact with the lens. The retina is thick and has no direct blood vessels but many cones, allowing for excellent colour vision. Vision is tetrachromic and includes sensitivity in the ultraviolet range. The fovea is well developed and, in raptors, there are multiple foveae enabling two planes of vision without head movement. The pecten projects into the vitreous body from the optic nerve and consists of capillaries and extravascular pigmented stromal cells. It provides nutrients to the avascular retina (Fig. 2.7). In some birds, small regular torsional movements of the eye sweep the pecten through the vitreous. **Birds can discern more rapid light flicker than humans. Fluorescent light that appears constant to human eyes can appear flickering to birds and may cause stress. Natural or non-flicker globes are preferable light sources within an avian environment.**

Birds' dorsal and ventral eyelids do not blink, and there are semiplumes rather than eyelashes. There are no meibomian glands, and the third eyelid blinks in a nasal to temporal direction. Eye movements are limited, but this is compensated for by greater head and neck mobility. The septum between the eyes is very thin and light may penetrate, making it difficult to accurately test consensual pupillary light reflexes.

Hearing

Birds have no pinna. Instead, specialized contour feathers (ear coverts) cover the meatus. There is a short horizontal ear canal and the tympanic membrane projects outwards rather than inwards, resulting in otitis externa being an uncommon avian disease presentation. The columella is the only bony ossicle (compared with three ossicles in mammals). The cochlear duct is short when compared to that of mammals. Because of these differences, birds have good discrimination of pitch (frequency) but are less sensitive to higher and lower tones

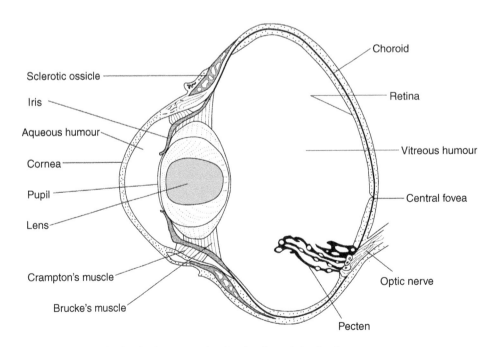

Fig 2.7 Cross-section of the avian globe showing the pecten as it projects into the posterior chamber.

than humans. Temporal resolution is about 10 times faster than in humans (Fig. 2.8).

Taste

Taste buds, which are usually associated with salivary gland openings, are present on the roof and floor of the oropharynx, but not on the tongue. Taste appears to differ between individual birds and between species but is generally less developed than in mammals. Parrots, budgerigars, hummingbirds and nectar feeders actively select sugar solutions, while other insectivorous and granivorous species may not be particular in selecting food for taste. **Birds are relatively tolerant to acidic and alkaline solutions but will move their tongue and beak and shake their head in response to bitter medication and will avoid drinking unpalatable medicated water or mash.**

Smell

Birds have a fully developed olfactory bulb but lack a vomeronasal organ. The size of the olfactory bulb relative to the cerebrum broadly reflects olfactory acuity. The sense of smell in psittacines, passerines and pigeons is, in general, poorly developed, while in albatrosses, vultures, kiwis and waterfowl olfactory acuity is more sensitive. Olfactory discrimination by starlings shows a strong correlation with nest building, suggesting a hormonal influence. (Mason & Clark 2000.)

The digestive system

Beak

The beak (rhamphotheca) consists of the maxilla (upper) and mandible (lower) jaw bones and their horny, keratinized sheaths (Fig. 2.9). Both jaws are connected to the skull by kinetic joints and can move independently. The sheath covering the maxilla is called the rhinotheca and that on the mandible is the gnathotheca. These are composed of modified epidermis, with cells of the stratum corneum containing free calcium phosphate and hydroxylapatite crystals as well as abundant keratin. Beak tissue extends outwards towards the surface, over much of the beak, extending to the edges and tip. In cases of chronic nasal discharge or injury to the germinal layer of the beak below the nares, permanent vertical defects in the rhinotheca leading from the nares to the tomia (the cutting edge of the beak) may develop.

Oropharynx

Birds have no soft palate. The opening to the nasal passageway, the choana, is a slit between the palatine folds of the roof of the mouth that closes during swallowing (Fig. 2.10). Caudally directed papillae are abundant in

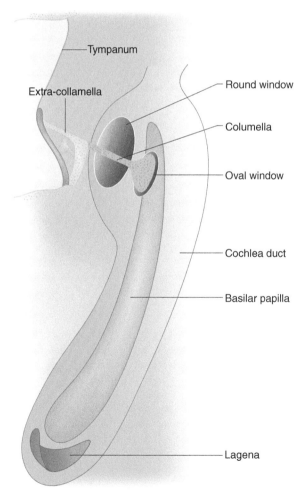

Fig 2.8 Diagram of the avian ear. Birds have a single bony ossicle, the columella, and the cochlear duct is short.

- Tympanum
- Extra-collamella
- Round window
- Columella
- Oval window
- Cochlea duct
- Basilar papilla
- Lagena

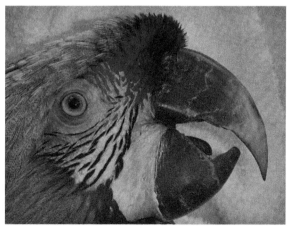

Fig 2.9 The large beak of a green-winged macaw (*Ara chloroptera*).

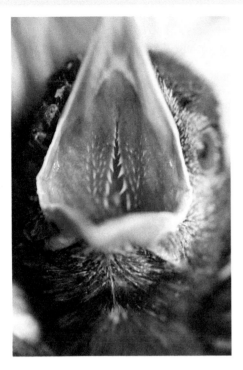

Fig 2.10 The choanal slit is the oral nasal interface located in the dorsal aspect of the oral cavity.

and thickening of the cervical oesophageal and ingluvial tissue. During the breeding season parent birds will regurgitate food stored in the crop to feed their chicks. In Columbiformes, under the influence of prolactin, the stratified squamous epithelial lining of the crop thickens and sloughs to form 'crop milk', a nutrient rich in protein and essential fatty acids that parents of both sexes regurgitate to feed their chicks.

Food is evacuated from the crop as a result of complex contractions of the crop wall. These are increased by acetylcholine or vagal (parasympathetic) stimulation and unaffected by sympathetic nerve stimulation. Crop dilatation occasionally occurs in older birds, but is more commonly observed in hand-fed juveniles. Chilling, ingestion of substrate bedding, inappropriate hand-feeding formula, overfilling or microbial infections have been identified as problems that lead to crop dilatation. The role of neurohumeral mechanisms in the development of the condition is unclear. **A full crop can be viewed under the skin at the base of the neck in nestlings without feathers, or in adults that have lost feathers. Alarmed owners will sometimes present birds, not realizing that this structure is normal.**

Aspiration of crop contents is recommended for avian patients that present with a full crop prior to anaesthesia but withholding food for too long in small birds can lower blood glucose and also increases the surgical risk. Always palpate the crop prior to inducing anaesthesia.

Stomachs

Most birds have two well-defined stomachs. The cranial proventriculus (glandular stomach) is thin-walled and lined with mucus-secreting columnar epithelial cells and oxynticipeptic cells, which secrete hydrochloric acid and pepsinogen. The caudal ventriculus (gizzard) lies in a ventral position on the left side of the mid-coelomic cavity, with the pylorus joining the duodenum right of the midline. The myenteric plexus is generally located immediately under the serosal surface rather than between muscle layers. The outer longitudinal muscle layer of the stomach wall is poorly developed in most birds while the innermost circular muscle layer is well developed. **The proventricular–ventricular junction, the isthmus, is a common site for inflammation, neoplasia, and infection associated with avian gastric yeast (AGY)** (*Macrorhabdus ornithogaster*, also known as 'megabacteria'). The isthmus appears to contain a pacemaker for the gastrointestinal cycle as destruction of the myenteric plexus in this area (e.g. with proventricular dilatation syndrome) will eliminate proventricular contractions and reduce ventricular and duodenal contractions by 50%.

The evolutionary development of a bird species' stomach depends on diet. In granivorous birds, glands in the thick, biconvex, muscular ventricular wall secrete

this region. The infundibular cleft, which opens to the auditory tube, is situated immediately caudal to the choana. Parrots have intrinsic muscles in the tongue, while other birds have only extrinsic muscles. Salivary glands produce mucus rather than a more serous secretion, and are abundant on the walls of the oropharynx. **When breathing, air moves from the nares through the choana, pharynx, laryngeal mound and trachea. If flushing nasal passages, be sure to keep the bird's head lower than the body and the mouth wide open to prevent flushing solution entering the trachea.**

Oesophagus and crop

The oesophagus goes down the right side of the neck – opposite to its anatomic position in mammals. The crop (ingluvies) is a dilatation of the oesophagus in which food is stored and softened with mucus prior to its passage into the proventriculus. In most bird species, very little if any digestion takes place in the crop. Food enters the crop on the right and exits caudally on the midline, where the oesophagus extends to the proventriculus. Enlarged thyroid glands or lesions caused by *Trichomonas* spp. can cause obstructions in this region. Pressure on the oesophagus in the cervical area can induce respiratory distress, vomiting, or crop dilatation. Trichomoniasis can also cause abscessation a hard, proteinaceous, cuticular lining, the koilin. This cuticular layer helps protect the sensitive underlying tissue as food is ground in preparation for digestion and absorption in the intestinal tract. The koilin is usually yellow or green due to bile pigment reflux and catalysed into the tough protective lining by hydrochloric acid influx from the proventriculus. In bird species with a well-developed ventriculus, this organ usually contains grit. In finches, gizzard worms (*Acuaria* spp.) are sometimes found beneath the koilin lining.

Birds that consume predominately soft food or nectar, such as the lorikeets, have poorly developed ventricular muscles. Conversely birds consuming large prey items compared to their body size (e.g. penguins) may have enormous stomachs relative to their body size. As a normal digestive process, owls and several other avian species egest (regurgitate) castings composed of undigested remains of bones and fur of their prey from the ventriculus (Fig. 2.11).

Intestines, liver and exocrine pancreas

The duodenum, jejunum and ileum are located on the right side of the coelomic cavity. Peristaltic as well as retroperistaltic waves occur, allowing chyme to move back and forth to the ventriculus. The pancreas lies in the U-shaped duodenal loop, near the body's midline, in a position than can be easily accessed for biopsy. In some species, there is an additional, 'splenic head' to the pancreas. The jejunum begins after the ascending loop turns back on itself and finishes at the vitelline (formerly Merkel's) diverticulum, the remnant of the yolk duct, located opposite the cranial mesenteric artery. The ileum ends at the rectal caecal junction. There is no difference histologically between the different sections of

the small intestine. Intestinal folds and villi do not contain lacteals, but have a well-developed capillary system instead. Amylase, maltase, sucrase, enterokinase, peptidases and lipase are produced by the intestinal mucosa. The exocrine pancreas produces amylase, trypsin, chymotrypsin and lipase.

The liver consists of two lobes that are joined at the cranial aspect of the organ. The gall bladder is usually absent in psittacines and ostriches, but is present in many other avian species. The gall bladder receives bile from the hepatocystic duct from the right lobe only. The cyticoenteric (birds with gall bladders) or hepatoenteric (birds without gall bladders) duct enters the distal rather than the proximal duodenum as is the case in mammals.

Many species, including poultry, ducks and quail, have large paired caeca, but these anatomic structures are absent or vestigial in psittacines, passerines and Columbiformes. Caeca are the site of blackhead (histomoniasis) infection in gallinaceous birds (e.g. turkeys, quail or peacocks). The rectum is usually short and straight and exhibits marked retroperistalsis carrying urine from the urodeum back to the level of the caeca, providing a key mechanism for water resorption. The rectum terminates in the coprodeum of the cloaca. **Canary breeders sometimes describe a disease they call 'blackspot', because chicks with this presentation show a large black spot under the skin on their cranial abdomens. This 'spot' is an enlarged liver, which may be observed as a clinical sign related to several diseases (e.g. atoxoplasmosis, circovirus, bacterial infections).**

Cloaca and vent

The cloaca is the common terminal chamber of the genital, urinary and gastrointestinal systems. It consists of:

- the cranial coprodeum, which receives faeces from the rectum
- the middle urodeum, into which the ureters enter dorsolaterally on both sides; in males the ductus deferens enter near the ureters, while in females a single oviduct enters the urodeum dorsolaterally on the left side
- the caudal proctodeum, on the dorsal surface of which, in juveniles, is located the bursa of Fabricius and on the floor of which is located the phallus if present (not in psittacines) (Fig. 2.12).

Urine is not concentrated in the kidneys. A colloidal suspension of urate in dilute urine is deposited in the urodeum. From there the urine moves retrograde into the coprodeum, rectum and caeca where it is mixed with chyme, and resorption of water, sodium and chloride takes place. Birds on low sodium diets show increased height and density of microvilli on the coprodeal epithelial cells, allowing for an enhanced absorptive surface area.

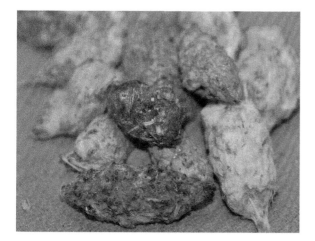

Fig 2.11 Regurgitated casts of undigested bones and fur are 'egested' from the ventriculus of owls and some other species as a normal part of the digestive process.

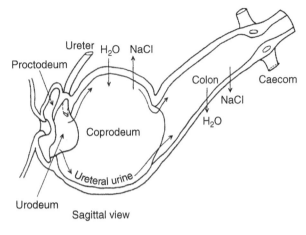

Fig 2.12 Cross-section of the cloaca.

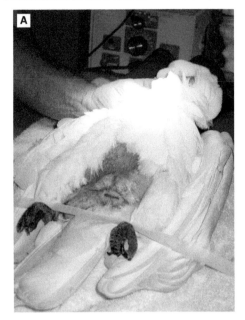

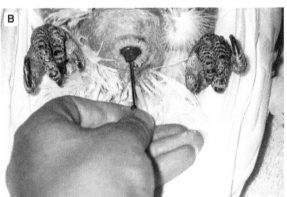

Normal bird droppings have three distinct components: liquid urine, semi-solid white or cream urate, and faeces. The vent is the external opening of the cloaca. When droppings are passed the urine/urate component of the dropping from the urodeum is evacuated first and then the opening of the coprodeum aligns closely with the vent so that the faecal component can be evacuated without contaminating the urodeum. A suddenly stressed bird (i.e. an avian patient being examined) may have an increased urine component to its droppings because the droppings pass before lower intestinal water resorption occurs. In most avian species the vent is horizontally flattened (i.e. shaped like 'lips' rather than being circumferential like a mammalian anus) (Figs 2.13A and 2.13B). In cases of avian cloacal or oviductal prolapse, one or two transverse sutures, adjusted to maintain reduction while still allowing the bird to pass droppings, are generally preferred to a pursestring suture because of the slit-like shape of the vent. A cloaca that has prolapsed past an atonic vent may look like a growth. To further identify the disease condition one may carefully attempt to pass a probe.

Fig 2.13A, B In most avian species the vent is horizontally flattened, i.e. shaped like 'lips' rather than being round like a mammalian anus. Because of this, in cases of rectal or oviductal prolapse, one or two transverse sutures, adjusted to maintain reduction while still allowing the bird to pass droppings, are generally preferred to a pursestring suture. A rectum prolapsing past an atonic vent can look like a growth; always attempt to pass a probe if there is any doubt.

Respiratory system

The nares are fixed and located above the beak and may be surrounded by feathers. In budgerigars the cere is generally blue or pink, smooth in males and brown and lumpy in females. The variation in budgerigar beak presentation depends on the bird's age, colour, health and reproductive status (Fig. 2.14). Paired nasal cavities communicate in psittacines, but not in passerines. A cornified flap of tissue, the operculum, is located immediately behind the nares in the nasal cavity. Care must be taken not to mistake this normal anatomical structure for a nasal foreign body (Fig. 2.15). There are three conchae in the upper respiratory system of avian species: the rostral, middle and caudal. The caudal nasal concha does not connect directly with the nasal cavity, but instead opens dorsally into the infraorbital sinus.

The infraorbital sinus is an irregular cavity that runs extraosseous and rostroventral to the eye. This single sinus has two communication outlets, both dorsal; one to the nasal cavity and the other to the caudal nasal concha. The anatomical structure of the sinus adversely affects the drainage of exudates, particularly in birds with partial blockage of these passages. In some birds with blocked sinuses lancing and surgical drainage may be needed, along with other treatments.

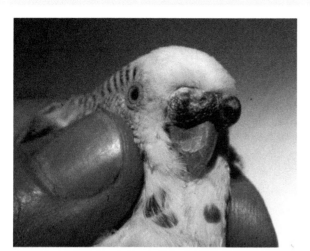

Fig 2.14 Brown cere hypertrophy in a budgerigar. This is a normal feature of some mature females under the influence of oestrogens. It should not be mistaken as pathological. The excess keratin may be gently peeled off if first softened with paraffin (mineral) oil, but it rarely causes problems and this is generally not necessary.

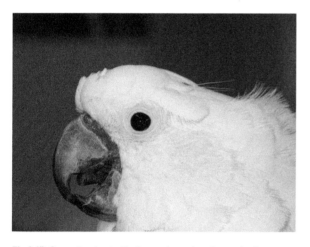

Fig 2.15 Operculum located in the nasal opening of an umbrella cockatoo (*Cacatua alba*).

In birds, the epiglottis is absent and the larynx lacks vocal cords and plays no part in vocalization. The cricothyroid cartilage is combined. The trachea is located on the left side of the cervical area, is mobile throughout its length and contains complete cartilaginous rings (360°). The syrinx is located at the caudal bifurcation of the trachea, and produces voice by vibrations of bilateral tympaniform membranes during the expiratory phase of respiration. Successful surgery to devocalize parrots has not yet been devised as in these birds the tympaniform membranes are obscured by intricate muscles and are difficult to access. Devocalization by cauterizing the tympaniform membrane is possible in gallinaceous birds but the surgery has risks and is not always successful and therefore not recommended. Male ducks have a cartilaginous out-pocketing of the trachea at the level of the syrinx called the syringeal bulla. This should not be mistaken for an abnormal structure on radiographs or when grossly observed during a post-mortem examination.

Cuffed endotracheal tubes should be avoided or used with caution. With complete cartilaginous rings, avian patients have suffered tracheal necrosis due to vascular compromise associated with the pressure exerted against the tracheal lining by the inflated cuff. Tracheal strictures have occurred in birds intubated with endotracheal tubes previously soaked in chlorhexidine. This disinfectant should be avoided due to the possible correlation of tracheal pathology with using chlorhexidine disinfectants.

The lungs are small and recessed between the ribs. There are no lobes or alveoli; consequently expansion of the thorax during inspiration is minimal and occurs by extension of the intracostal joints. Instead of inspired air being drawn by negative pressure directly into the lungs, the bulk of inspired air is drawn via the primary bronchi with a bellows-like action into the caudal air sacs. From the caudal air sac the volume of air is pushed back into the lungs so that airflow within the lung tissue is predominantly unidirectional, caudal to cranial (Fig. 2.16).

Psittacines have paired caudal air sacs (caudal thoracic and abdominal) and paired cranial air sacs (cervical and cranial thoracic), as well as one unpaired medial sac with several diverticula (clavicular). Gas exchange does not occur in the air sacs, which are hollow spaces with thin walls consisting of simple squamous epithelium supported by a small amount of connective tissue. Delivery of therapeutic levels of drugs to air sacs can be problematic since they have poor vascularity. Nebulization or surgical drainage are other therapeutic options to treat diseases involving the air sac system (Fig. 2.17).

Primary bronchi form at the tracheal bifurcation, while four groups of secondary bronchi connect with the air sacs. Parabronchi (tertiary bronchi) anastomose with other parabronchi and connect with the air sacs. Rather than alveoli, each parabronchus has anastomosing 'air capillaries' that exit centrifugally (outwards) and are surrounded by blood capillaries in which blood flows centripetally (inwards). There are two types of parabronchi: (1) unidirectional flow of air through the air capillaries (paleopulmonic); (2) bidirectional flow (neopulmonic). Gaseous exchange occurs between the air capillaries and blood capillaries. The counter-current flow of blood and air through these adjacent capillaries allows for very efficient oxygen exchange in birds compared with mammals.

In the absence of a diaphragm, the triangular shape of the coelomic (combined thoracic and abdominal)

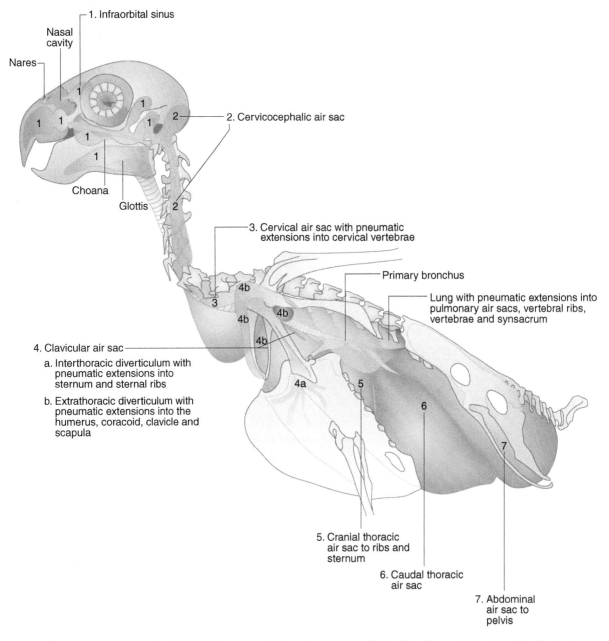

- 1. Infraorbital sinus
- Nasal cavity
- Nares
- 2. Cervicocephalic air sac
- Choana
- Glottis
- 3. Cervical air sac with pneumatic extensions into cervical vertebrae
- Primary bronchus
- Lung with pneumatic extensions into pulmonary air sacs, vertebral ribs, vertebrae and synsacrum
- 4. Clavicular air sac
  - a. Interthoracic diverticulum with pneumatic extensions into sternum and sternal ribs
  - b. Extrathoracic diverticulum with pneumatic extensions into the humerus, coracoid, clavicle and scapula
- 5. Cranial thoracic air sac to ribs and sternum
- 6. Caudal thoracic air sac
- 7. Abdominal air sac to pelvis

Fig 2.16 The avian respiratory tract. As with other body systems, birds' respiratory tracts are lightweight, efficient and adapted to flight. They do not have a diaphragm; rather there are paired air sacs throughout the coelomic cavity that are connected with the lungs and with diverticula leading into pneumatic bones. Lungs are small and recessed into the ribs. The abdomen is large relative to the size of the thorax and acts like a bellows drawing air into the abdominal air sacs on inspiration and pushing air out through the lungs on expiration. See text.

cavity allows for a bellows-like effect during breathing. Both inspiration and expiration require active muscle contraction. Birds with space-occupying coelomic masses (e.g. tumour, egg) may present with laboured respiration because of air volume reduction. Particular care should be taken to avoid restricting an avian patient's respiration by applying pressure on the chest during restraint or when bandaging.

Breathing

Air takes two complete breathing cycles to pass through the avian respiratory system.

1. First breathing cycle
   - Inspiration 1: the air goes into the trachea, through the primary and intrapulmonic bronchi

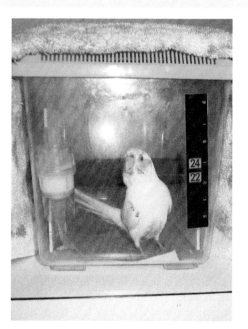

Fig 2.17 Nebulization therapy can be useful in delivering drugs to the syrinx and respiratory tract.

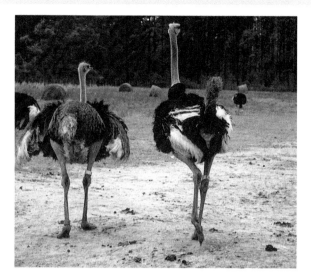

Fig 2.18 Protruding phallus of a male ostrich.

and into the caudal air sacs; a minor amount of air volume stays in the lungs, moving directly into the secondary bronchi and parabronchi to undergo gas exchange.

- Expiration 1: most of the air volume goes from caudal air sacs to the lungs, parabronchi and then to the air capillaries, where gas exchange occurs. A minor amount of air escapes from the primary bronchus up the trachea.

2. Second breathing cycle
   - Inspiration 2: air goes from the lungs to the cranial air sacs.
   - Expiration 2: air is expelled via the primary bronchus and trachea.

It is possible to respirate birds via a breathing tube placed in the abdominal air sacs or the clavicular air sac. These options are useful in anaesthetizing birds with upper airway disease, when allowing upper airway injuries to heal, when performing tracheal endoscopic procedures and/or when performing surgery on the head.

Male reproductive system

Birds have paired internal testes that may be white, cream, yellow or melanistic (e.g. cockatoos, rosellas). They are located craniomedial to the cranial pole of the kidneys and caudal to the adrenal glands. In some species, the testicles may enlarge over 50-fold during breeding. Daylight hours and other environmental triggers

are important in initiating gonadotrophin release, testicular development and testosterone production. For example, lengthening daylight hours stimulate testosterone production and singing in male canaries.

The epididymis lies dorsal to the testes, and is a system of ductules to collect sperm. Sperm storage and maturation occurs in the convoluted ductus deferens, which leads from the epididymis to the urodeum. There are no accessory sex glands.

A phallus, comprised of erectile lymphatic tissue, is present in some species (e.g. ducks, geese and ratites) but not in psittacine species (Fig. 2.18). The phallus is solely reproductive in function and is not associated with urination. The semen travels via the seminal groove on the external surface of the phallus. Lacerations, abscesses and paralysis of the phallus are occasionally encountered, particularly in ducks, when several males attempt to mate with the same female and the organ gets injured in the fray. **The phallus can be amputated without any adverse effect on the passage of urine.**

Semen

Birds produce sperm of high density and viscosity (see Fig. 1.8). Capacitation is not necessary for fertilization. Once ejaculated into the oviduct, sperm is stored in the spermatic fossulae at the uterovaginal junction and the glandular grooves and tubular glands of the infundibulum. Semen may remain fertile for many days to weeks, depending on the species and the individual bird.

Female reproductive system

In most avian species, apart from raptors and kiwis, only the left ovary and left oviduct develop. The immature ovary is small and triangular, and resembles pancreatic tissue. It is primarily cream or white but may be melanistic, particularly in macaws, rosellas and cockatoos. The mature ovary looks like a cluster of grapes as primary oocytes develop into follicles and mature (Fig. 2.19).

After ovulation, the large oocyte (egg yolk) is engulfed by the fimbria of the oviduct and formation of an egg begins. There is no corpus luteum, and progesterone levels drop rapidly after ovulation. This stimulates additional luteinizing hormone secretion, which promotes ovulation of the next mature follicle. The postovulatory follicle is believed to secrete non-steroidal hormones that are involved in oviposition and nesting behaviour (King & McLelland 1984). Fertilization is not required for egg formation. **The oviduct is composed of five sequential regions; it enlarges tremendously during egg laying, and occupies much of the left abdomen.** The five segments of the oviduct are:

- the infundibulum – the funnel-shaped anterior opening where fertilization and formation of the yolk membrane and the outer and chalaziferous layer of albumen occur
- the glandular magnum, which secretes thick albumen, along with sodium, magnesium and calcium
- the isthmus, which produces the shell membranes; its glandular tissue is less well developed than that of the magnum
- the uterus, which has leaf-like longitudinal folds and is the site of shell formation; it typically takes around 5 hours for an egg to pass from the infundibulum to the uterus, where it remains for 20–26 hours before being expelled through the vagina and vent

- the vagina, which can be everted through the vent so that the egg is laid with minimal contamination by cloacal contents (Fig. 2.20).

In birds the female is heterogametic ('**ZW**' sex chromosomes) and thus determines sex, while the male is homogametic ('**ZZ**' sex chromosomes). Aviculturalists will sometimes talk about a cock bird being 'split' for a particular recessive sex-linked gene (i.e. a normal green Indian ringneck 'split for lutino'). It is not possible for a hen to be 'split' for a sex-linked gene, as whatever gene is present on the 'z' chromosome will phenotypically manifest in the bird.

Urinary system

Birds have paired kidneys recessed into renal fossae, bony depressions in the fused vertebrae of the synsacrum. There are three lobes, anterior, middle and posterior, in which there is no renal pelvis but renal lobules comprising a medullary cone and the region of the cortex that it drains. Desert species often have smaller kidneys with less cortex and more medulla than those species found in non-desert areas. Avian kidneys have both reptilian and mammal-like features, with renal lobules containing two main types of nephrons as well as transitional forms:

1. The predominant cortical, 'reptilian' type (RT) nephrons which have no loop of Henle and are uricotelic (i.e. produce uric acid as the end product of nitrogen excretion).

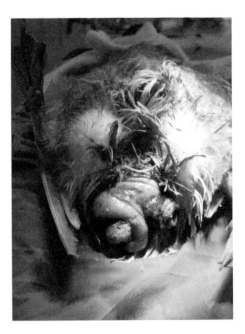

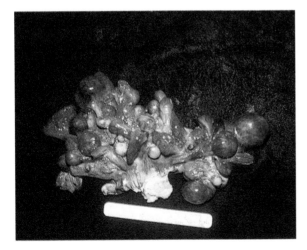

Fig 2.19 Mature ovary from ostrich hen.

Fig 2.20 Prolapse in a duck showing the rectum with faeces on the right side and the oviduct on the left.

2. The less common, long-looped, medullary type (MT), which comprise about 10–30% of nephrons. These have a loop descending into the medullary region of the lobule, they produce urine and have almost double the glomerular filtration rate of RT nephrons.

The blood supply to avian kidneys is complex, receiving about 10–15% of cardiac output. Arterial blood from the aorta is the only source of blood for the renal corpuscle and the renal medulla. Birds have a juxtaglomerular apparatus and a renin-angiotensin system (RAS) responsive to sodium depletion and haemodynamics. The role of the RAS in aldosterone secretion is less precise than is the case in mammals. **Avian kidneys receive over half of their blood supply from the renal portal system, which comes as venous blood from the large intestines and pelvic limbs via the internal and external iliac veins, the ischiadic vein and the caudomesenteric vein.** The renal portal valve, a smooth muscle sphincter under combined adrenergic (causing valve closure) and cholinergic (allowing valve opening) control, is located between the renal portal vein and the common iliac artery. If the valve is open blood flows directly into the vena cava. If the valve is shut blood is forced into the renal portal vein and from there to the peritubular capillary network within the cortical region of the lobule, In this cortical region of the lobule it mixes with arterial blood from the renal corpuscle then passes via efferent veins to the common iliac vein and caudal vena cava. Alternatively venous blood may be rerouted out of the kidney without traversing a capillary plexus via the caudal mesenteric vein to the liver or via the cranial renal portal vein, the cerebral to venous sinuses, the jugular vein and then back to the heart (Maina 1996) (Fig. 2.21).

Infections of the feet, legs or lower intestines may drain to kidneys and induce renal disease. Renal neoplasia or infection may cause venous stasis of the pelvic limbs or leg paralysis due to pressure on the sciatic nerves, which pass through the kidneys.

Uric acid is produced by the liver, transported in the blood, and excreted by means of glomerular filtration and tubular secretion. In the collecting tubules it forms a colloidal solution with mucopolysaccharides and glycoprotein, which allows transport through the kidney without precipitation. Urine is drained by ureters, which empty into the urodeum; it is then moved by retroperistalsis into the rectum, where resorption of water and salt takes place. Birds have no urinary bladder.

Osmoregulation involves not only the kidneys but the interaction of the kidneys with the intestinal tract, salt glands (when present), the surface epithelium and respiratory tracts as routes of evaporative water loss. Water-deprived desert birds, such as budgerigars, will generally cease to concentrate urine beyond a specific gravity of around 1.007 and instead pass dry droppings with solid urate, having resorbed the fluid component in the lower intestine. While not recommended husbandry, healthy budgerigars have survived on a seed diet without water for over 6 weeks, yet, paradoxically, I have seen budgerigars with uncontrolled diabetes insipidus that would regularly drink more than their own body weight in water over a 24 hour period.

Endocrine system

The pituitary gland

As in mammals the pituitary gland is intimately connected with the hypothalamus at the base of the brain and lies near the optic chiasma. Tumours are occasionally encountered, particularly in budgerigars, and affected birds may present with blindness and neurological signs because of pressure on nearby anatomical structures as well as signs referable to over-production of specific pituitary hormones.

The neurohypophysis forms the pars nervosa (equivalent to the posterior pituitary gland), the infundibular stalk and the median eminence. The median eminence contains neurosecretory terminals for pituitary hormone releasing and inhibiting neuropeptides, arginine vasotocin (AVT) and mesotocin (MT), all of which are synthesized in hypothalamic cell bodies. AVT is analogous to mammalian antidiuretic hormone and MT is analogous to oxytocin. AVT and oxytocin will induce uterine contractions in birds but not as effectively as MT. There is no separate pars intermedia in the avian pituitary gland.

The pars distalis produces the range of pituitary hormones found in mammals under the control of releasing and inhibiting neuropeptides carried via hypophyseal portal vessels from the median eminence. There is complex interplay between various endocrine axes. Adrenal corticotrophic hormone (ACTH) and melanin-stimulating hormone (MSH) are secreted by the corticomelanotrophic cells of the adenohypophysis. Growth hormone, gonadotrophins (luteinizing and follicle-stimulating hormones), thyroid-stimulating hormone and prolactin are also produced by the avian pituitary gland. **In adult male and female birds prolactin stimulates proliferation and sloughing of crop wall mucosal cells, resulting in the production of 'crop milk'.** This prolactin stimulation of the ingluvial lining occurs in parents of both sexes just before the eggs hatch. Prolactin also contributes to broodiness and incubation behaviour of the parent birds.

The thyroid

Paired thyroid glands, histologically comparable to those of other vertebrates, are located within the thoracic inlet

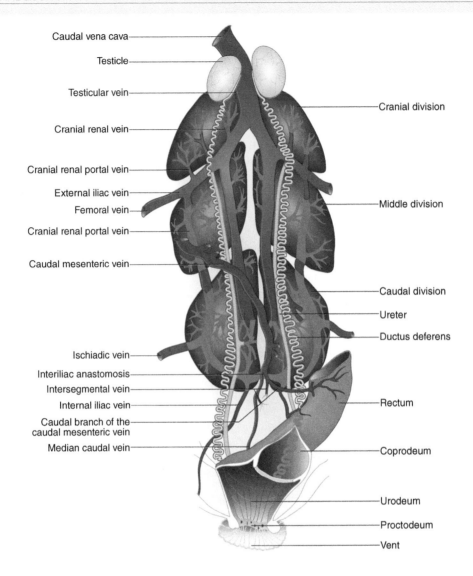

Caudal vena cava

Testicle

Testicular vein

Cranial renal vein

Cranial renal portal vein

External iliac vein

Femoral vein

Cranial renal portal vein

Caudal mesenteric vein

Ischiadic vein

Interiliac anastomosis

Intersegmental vein

Internal iliac vein

Caudal branch of the
caudal mesenteric vein

Median caudal vein

Cranial division

Middle division

Caudal division

Ureter

Ductus deferens

Rectum

Coprodeum

Urodeum

Proctodeum

Vent

Fig 2.21 The avian urogenital tract (male). Birds have testicles within the abdominal cavity and kidneys recessed into the pelvis. There is no urinary bladder; ureters carry a slurry of insoluble urates and urine from the kidneys to the urodeum from where it is retrograded into the coprodeum/rectum and water resorption takes place. Normal bird droppings comprise three distinct components: clear liquid urine, solid cream-coloured urates and solid or semisolid faeces.

and are not palpable. **Enlargement of thyroid glands due to goitre or neoplasia may cause wheezing respiration and crop dilatation in budgerigars due to mechanical pressure on the trachea and/or the oesophagus.**

Thyroid hormones play a key role in controlling oxygen consumption and metabolic heat production. Avian thyroid receptors are sensitive to T3 but T4 is readily converted to T3 and shows similar potency. In general, exposure to cold will increase thyroid hormone production via the hypothalamic-pituitary-thyroid axis while decreased food consumption will lower thyroid production. There is a complex interplay between reproductive hormones, growth hormone and thyroid hormone in regulating

hatching, moult and reproductive cycles. T3 and T4 levels rise dramatically around the time of hatching in precocial chicks such as domestic poultry but this is not seen in altricial chicks. Thyroid hormones are necessary for reproductive function but high concentrations can have antigonadal effects. Oestrogen decreases are important in initiating moult while an increase in thyroid hormone/oestrogen ratio is important for new feather formation.

The adrenal glands

The adrenal glands are not clearly divided into a cortex and medulla; rather, the cortical and chromaffin tissues are intermingled. Corticosterone is the most important corticoid hormone in birds. Potassium and angiotensin II stimulate the synthesis of aldosterone from corticosterone. About half of the circulating noradrenaline (norepinephrine) and all of the circulating adrenaline (epinephrine) is derived from chromaffin cells of the adrenal glands. **Birds possessing nasal salt glands (e.g. marine birds) are able to tolerate hyperosmotic drinking water, as the cardiovascular effects of salt and water depletion stimulate atrial natriuretic peptide thereby activating salt secretion. Corticosterone is not directly involved with the salt-secreting process. Birds without a nasal salt gland are unable to tolerate hyperosmotic drinking water; thus mineral regulation occurs via aldosterone, as in mammals.**

The pancreas

The pancreas generally lies within the duodenal loop, just inside the ventral abdomen. It can be readily accessed for biopsy via endoscopy or exploratory laparotomy. The exocrine pancreas consists of compound tubuloacinar cells which secrete amylase, lipase, proteolytic enzymes and sodium bicarbonate. Duct(s) drain from the pancreas into the distal ascending duodenum.

Regulation of carbohydrate metabolism differs significantly in birds and mammals. Birds normally have blood glucose levels 150–300% above those of mammals. If the pancreatic tissue is removed from a mammal the animal will die of hyperglycaemia resulting from insulin depletion. Birds also die if pancreatic tissue is removed, but these patients develop a hypoglycaemic state, most likely due to a lack of glucagon and its glucose-elevating effect. It is possible that there is a source of insulin or insulin-like hormone apart from the pancreas but this has not yet been identified. As in mammals, the islet cells of the pancreas are important in glucoregulation and consist of four main cell types that synthesize endocrine hormones: A-cells, glucagon; B-cells, insulin; D-cells, somatostatin; PP-cells, pancreatic polypeptide. Glucagon occurs at levels 10 times higher than in mammals and serves to keep blood glucose levels elevated. Free fatty acids and cholecystokinin trigger glucagon release while glucose has an inhibitory effect. Somatostatin is also present at higher levels than those found in mammals. Insulin occurs at only one-sixth of mammalian levels but avian insulin is two to four times more potent than equivalent amounts of mammalian insulin. Glucose is not a major trigger of insulin release; rather B-cells are more sensitive to cholecystokinase, glucagon and a mixture of absorbed amino acids. Diabetes mellitus or 'deranged carbohydrate metabolism resulting in hyperglycaemia' is encountered in avian patients but the pathogenesis of the condition has not been clearly defined. In our clinic some birds have reverted to normal glucose levels after treatment with amoxicillin, conversion to a pelleted diet or with

the passage of time. Others can be controlled with oral hypoglycaemic drugs (e.g. glipizide) or insulin injections.

Nervous system and circadian pacemaker

The avian cerebrum has minimal convolutions (lissencephalic) and the cerebral cortex is thin. Olfactory lobes are small and there are few olfactory nerves. The corpus callosum is absent while the corpus striatum is large, which is the opposite to that found in mammalian species. Important areas of the avian brain include a slight dorsal bulge, the Wulst, which receives both visual and somatosensory input and is thought to be involved with prehensile abilities (e.g. gripping with the feet). The dorsal ventricular ridge contains the 'high vocalization centre', linked with a complex of neurological pathways, including connections with the ear and the syrinx to control learning and maintenance of song. Ventromedially, the paleostrial complex is thought to integrate input from visual and other sensory systems to coordinate body position with object location in space. The cerebellum has a role in motor neuron control, especially of learned movements. In common with dinosaurs, the spinal cord lacks a cauda equina but has both a lumbosacral and a smaller cervical glycogen body, which in birds consists of glial cells that contain a high content of glycogen. The function of these glycogen bodies is uncertain.

The autonomic nervous system has sympathetic components which are catecholamine based and prepare the body for 'flight or fight' and parasympathetic components which are acetylcholine based. Both are linked with functional neural pathways in the brain, particularly the visceral forebrain system, the limbic system and strategically placed circumventricular neuroendocrine organs. This arrangement allows for background homeostatic mechanisms to control cardiovascular, respiratory, gastrointestinal and reproductive functions as well as the capacity to entrain or override these homeostatic mechanisms in response to environmental stimuli.

The pineal gland is located on the dorsal surface of the brain in the triangle between the hemispheres of telencephalon and the cerebellum. Avian pinealocytes, which produce the hormone melatonin, are controlled by an endogenous circadian oscillator as well as being photosensitive. Acting in concert with changing binding sites (the effect of which varies between species), melatonin decreases body temperature and metabolic rate and facilitates sleep at night. Melatonin receptors occur throughout the brain and also in peripheral organs, with high concentrations found in parts of the limbic system associated with arousal and vocalization, the retina and the gastrointestinal tract. The retina and gastrointestinal tract also produce melatonin and, together with the pineal gland, are key components of the circadian pacemaker system. The most important synchronizer ('zeitgeber stimuli') of circadian rhythms in birds is periodic alteration of light intensity, but food availability, temperature and social interaction may also affect the pacemaker system. Removal of the pineal gland of sparrows held in constant darkness abolished daily circadian locomotor and body temperature rhythm. Circannual cycles of gonad development, moult and migration behave similarly to circadian cycles but neither the eyes nor the pineal gland are essential for seasonal effects of photostimulation. These appear to be controlled by deep encephalic photoreceptors linked with circumventricular neuroendocrine organs, most probably the infundibular nuclear complex and the lateral septal organ (Kuenzel 2000).

Circulatory system

The typical avian heart is four chambered and is larger and beats faster than that of a mammal of the same size. Arterial pressure is high in spite of lower peripheral resistance. The heart is surrounded by the liver caudally and the lungs dorsally. Unlike the mammalian configuration, there is an atrioventricular ring of Purkinje fibres that forms a figure of eight around the heart and aorta. **The atrioventricular ring of Purkinje fibres results in the mean electrical axis of the QRS wave lying close to minus 90 degrees (i.e. cranially along the long axis of the body rather than caudally as is typically the case in mammals).** The aorta is derived from the right rather than the left fourth arterial arch and the internal carotid, rather than the common carotid, is the major artery in the cervical region. Birds lack a cerebral arterial circle of Willis but there is extensive intercarotid anastomosis to provide collateral circulation, as well as cranial anastomosis between the jugular veins. Both hepatic and renal portal systems are present with the capacity to reroute renal portal blood to the liver, brain or directly to the heart. In the tarsal and axillary regions there are arteriovenous networks of vessels that serve as heat exchange mechanisms, potentially reducing heat loss to the environment. **The right jugular vein is much larger than the left, and is a useful site for blood collection in many bird species. It is found beneath an apteria on the neck and can be accessed with minimal feather plucking by wetting or parting feathers. Other useful sites for blood collection include the brachial vein on the ventral aspect of the elbow and the medial metatarsal vein (Fig. 2.22).**

Blood

Birds have large, oval, nucleated erythrocytes that live around 30 days (compared with 120 days in most mammals). There are also nucleated thrombocytes rather than platelets, and heterophils rather than neutrophils. Erythropoiesis takes place in the yolk sac initially and, after the bird hatches, in the bone marrow. The extrinsic

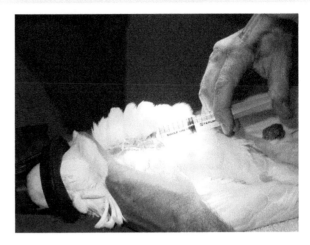

Fig 2.22 Jugular vein catheterization in a sulphur-crested cockatoo.

pathway is of greater importance than the intrinsic pathway in blood clotting. Blood glucose is typically more than double that of mammals while plasma protein is lower.

Lymphatic and immune systems

The cloacal bursa (of Fabricius) is a diverticulum on the dorsal surface of the proctodeum, unique to juvenile birds, that actively collects antigenic material from the environment. Following exposure to antigens in the bursa, blood-borne stem cells, possibly derived from embryonic aorta or coelomic epithelium, differentiate into immunologically competent B-lymphocytes, which colonize secondary lymphoid tissue, including the spleen, the caecal tonsil and Peyer's patches in the intestines, Merkel's diverticulum, the pineal gland and Harderian glands. The bursa regresses in adult birds. Some viruses, particularly circovirus, selectively attack the bursa and can impair the immune competence of young birds.

Avian B-cells produce immunoglobulins, IgA, IgM and IgG. IgE has not been identified in birds but avian IgG has characteristics intermediate between mammalian IgG and IgE and is sometimes termed IgY. Birds show reactions on intradermal skin testing but reactions are not as pronounced as in mammals and response to histamine positive control is not consistent. (Macwhirter & Mueller 1998.)

The thymus is located alongside the jugular vein in juvenile birds and, like the bursa, is colonized with blood-borne progenitor cells but these cells differentiate into immunologically competent T-cells that regulate cellular immunity. T-cells go on to colonize secondary lymphoid tissue.

The spleen does not serve as a reservoir for blood. It is small, spherical and located dorsal to the liver in psittacines and pigeons. It can show marked enlargement in response to antigenic stimulation, particularly when the bird is infected with *Chlamydophila psittaci*. In canaries and finches, the spleen is comma-shaped.

Lymphatic vessels follow blood vessels and empty into large veins and are less numerous in birds than in mammals. Avian species have two thoracic ducts. Variable amounts of lymphoid tissue occur in virtually all avian tissues and organs, but lymph nodes occur in only a few species (not psittacines).

Musculoskeletal system

The avian skeletal system has intricately evolved as an efficient, strong, lightweight and aerodynamic apparatus. It has specific adaptations, which, along with the bird's feathers, muscles and specialized circulatory and respiratory systems, enable flight.

There are two main types of bones:

1. Pneumatic bones, linked with air sacs and filled with air, found in the skull, vertebrae, pelvis, sternum, ribs, humerus and sometimes the femur.
2. Medullary bones, long bones with large medullary cavities and thin cortices. Interconnecting spicules grow from the endosteal surface of the cortex and extend across the medullary cavity. This arrangement improves strength while adding minimal weight and provides a place to store calcium. **With their strong lightweight nature avian bones have a higher calcium content and tensile strength than their mammalian counterparts. When fractured, avian bones are brittle and easily shatter.** The large medullary cavity can make achieving rotational stability with fractures a challenge. Reproductively active females lay down medullary calcium in response to oestrogens. These bone densities (polyosteotic hyperosteosis) should not be considered pathological on radiographs of egg-laying birds but could reflect a pathological rise in oestrogenic activity in other birds (e.g. with Sertoli cell tumours in males) (see Figs 1.27, 1.38).

Many avian bones are fused to decrease weight, increase strength and improve aerodynamics. The spine is divided into cervical, thoracic, synsacral (fused lumbar, sacral and caudal vertebrae), free caudal and fused caudal (pygostyle) sections. The number of vertebrae varies with the species (Fig. 2.23).

Their extremely mobile necks enable birds to use their heads as a 'universal tool'. There is a single, mobile occipital condyle and more cervical vertebrae than in mammals. The individual cervical vertebrae have heterocoelous (saddle-shaped) centra and weakly developed neural spines.

Caudal cervical and thoracic vertebrae have attached ribs. The cervical ribs are short and fused to the vertebrae, while the thoracic ribs articulate dorsally with vertebrae and (in most cases) ventrally with a large central carina or sternum (the keel bone). Uncinate processes anchor the caudal edges of some of the ribs to the cranial edge of the subsequent rib and lend strength to the thoracic cage and improve its function as a fuselage, but make surgical access to the thoracic cavity difficult. Blood supply courses along the cranial edge of the ribs.

There is generally only one mobile joint in the lower back (between the sixth and seventh thoracic vertebrae in budgerigars), and it is at this point that fractures and soft tissue injuries most commonly occur, particularly in birds with metabolic bone disease. Damage to this mobile site in the lower back should be considered in birds that present with bilateral leg paresis. The seventh and eighth thoracic vertebrae are fused to the lumbar vertebrae as well as to the overlapping ilia.

There are two main types of avian skeletal muscle:

- White, or twitch, fibres with fibrillar appearance similar to mammalian muscle. These are focally innervated by one or only a few nerve fibres.
- Red, or tonic, fibres with a granular and indefinite appearance that have multiple innervated slow contracting fibres. These fibres have large numbers of mitochondria and more profuse capillarization, and their red colour is due to large amounts of myoglobin.

Individual muscle groups generally contain a combination of these two muscle types (including several subtypes) and proportions may change seasonally or with exercise. Normal contractile activity is essential for post-hatching growth and development, while in adult birds muscle atrophy is reversible. For example, if a fledgling's wings are clipped before it learns to fly it may never be able to fly even when feathers regrow on subsequent moults. If clipping of wing feathers is delayed until after the fledgling learns to fly, the lack of muscle control does not seem to be a problem.

The thoracic limb

The thoracic girdle is comprised of strap-like scapulae, strong coracoid bones which act as struts for the wings, and clavicles which fuse medially at the hypocleidium to form the spring-like furuncula ('wishbone'). In most species, as an adaptation to flight, the triosseal foramen is formed by the articulation of these three bones. The tendon to the supracoracoideus (deep pectoral muscle) passes through this foramen to attach onto the head of the humerus (see Fig. 1.21). The glenoid cavity is dorsally rotated. Contraction of the supracoracoideus raises the wing and, working in concert with the propatagialis muscle complex and the extensor metacarpi radialis,

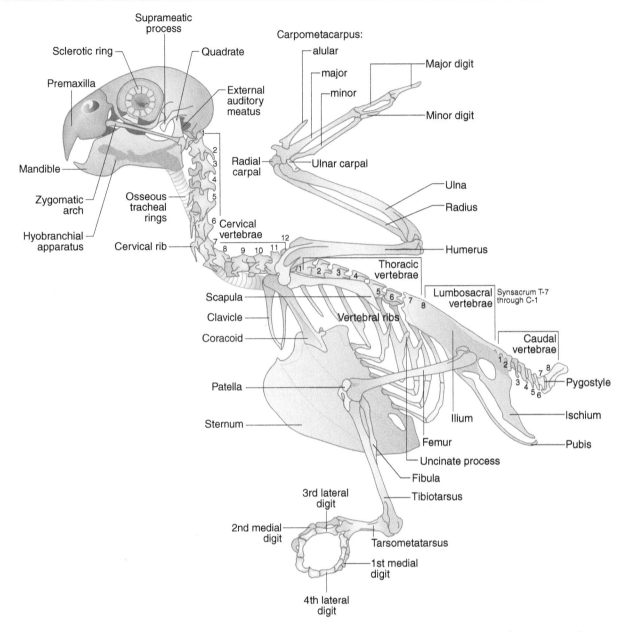

Fig 2.23 Skeleton of a typical parrot. Almost every aspect of a bird's skeleton shows adaptations for flight, e.g. bones are often fused and generally reduced in number for strength and lightness, some are pneumatic. Caudal vertebrae are reduced to a pygostyle from which retrices (tail feathers) emerge but there are 12 mobile cervical vertebrae that allow birds to extend their necks for grasping as well as retracting their head when at rest to a position closer to their centre of gravity. Stance is digitigrade.

it enables the wing to configure to an aerofoil shape with an appropriate angle for flight. Once laminar airflow across the wing is established, greater air pressure under the wing is achieved relative to that above the wing. This air pressure gradient generates upward lift, an essential element for flight (see Box 1.1). Clavicular or coracoid fractures may impair flight with minimal wing drooping observable upon presentation.

Complex, interrelated soft tissue structures are also critical to flight. The propatagium ('wing web') is the skinfold between the shoulder and the wrist and contains tendons of the propatagialis muscle complex, which inserts onto the tendon of the extensor carpi radialis and extends the metacarpus while flexing the elbow. The metapatagium is the skinfold at the trailing edge of the wing between the elbow and the body wall. Caution should be observed when bandaging wings to prevent damage to the propatagium or flight may be impaired even though there is adequate musculoskeletal healing.

The large superficial pectoral muscle which overlies the supracoracoideus generates wing downstroke and forward thrust. Working in conjunction with the biceps brachii (flexing the elbow) and flexor carpi ulnaris (flexing the wrist), contraction causes the wing to lower and, depending on species, the distal primary flight feathers to act as propellers and 'swim' through the air. The well-developed superficial pectoral muscles provide a convenient muscle mass to be used as an injection site even in small birds. However, injecting irritant solutions can impair fast flight and should be avoided in racing pigeons or other performance birds.

The humerus is short, stout and pneumatic, containing an extension of the clavicular air sac in its proximal end. The ulna, situated at the leading edge of the wing, is larger than the radius. The secondary remiges (flight feathers) emerge from the periosteum at the caudal border of the ulna. The distal ulna is a useful site for intraosseous fluid administration. Fractures of either the radius or ulna may respond to external co-aptation if the opposing bone is undamaged and able to act as a splint to maintain length. However synostosis is a risk with fractures of the antebrachial region, especially if immobilization is prolonged.

The wrist joint swivels craniocaudally to allow the wings to be folded against the body when at rest. When the wings are extended the joint is rigid in the dorsoventral plane. Two proximal carpal bones, distal carpal bones and three metacarpal bones fuse to form the carpometacarpus. There are three digits: the alula or 'bastard wing', the major digit (with two large phalanges), and the minor digit. The alulas are extended as flight speed slows, acting as 'slots' to reduce air turbulence over the dorsal surface of the wing, and are used for controlled landings (see Fig. 1.24).

The pelvic limb

A bird's stance is bipedal and digitigrade, walking on two hind legs and standing on the toes. The need for strength and balance while running, perching, landing and, in some species, swimming has influenced the positioning and structure of the bones that make up the pelvic limb. Most avian species can retract their legs and feet to streamline their bodies during flight. The ilium, ischium and pubis comprise the pelvis. These three bones are partially fused to each other and to the synsacrum as a strengthening mechanism. The pubic bones are not fused ventrally, thus allowing for the passage of eggs.

The femur is held subhorizontally and movement is almost exclusively cranial and caudal; lateral rotation is limited. The tibiotarsus, a useful site for intraosseous fluid administration, is formed by the fusion of the tibia and proximal tarsal bones, while the tarsometatarsus is formed by the fusion of the distal tarsal bones to the three main metatarsal bones. The intertarsal (hock) joint is formed between the tibiotarsus and the tarsometatarsus. Limb tendons may be ossified in birds (see Fig. 1.11).

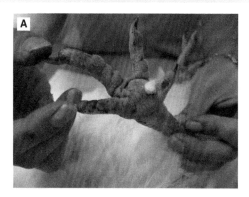

Fig 2.24A The interdigital pad is a common site for pododermatitis ('bumblefoot'). Pressure sores from unsuitable perches or substrate, hypovitaminosis A and infection can be contributing factors.

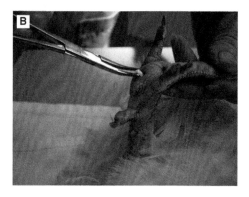

Fig 2.24B Treatment of pododermatitis with slow-release antibiotic-impregnated methyl methacrylate beads.

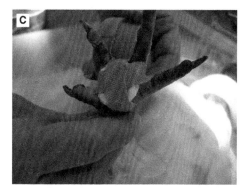

Fig 2.24C Bandaging the foot with a 'corn pad' style doughnut bandage to take pressure off the lesion.

Birds' toes radiate from the distal end of the single tarsometatarsal bone. The interdigital pad, which protects and cushions the plantar surface of the tarsometatarsal-phalangeal joints, bears the bulk of the bird's weight when standing or perching. The interdigital pad and plantar foot surface are common sites of pododermatitis ('bumblefoot') lesions. **In psittacine species, two, three, four and five phalanges are usually found in digits I, II, III and IV respectively (Figs 2.24A, B, C).**

Nutrition

With over 9000 species of birds worldwide, it is not surprising that birds have a diversity of specific dietary requirements. Nutritional deficiencies or imbalances resulting in primary or secondary disease are commonly diagnosed. When treating birds, veterinarians need to consider individual species' requirements, as well as individual variation due to age, reproduction, exercise and disease conditions. While some nutritional imbalances will cause specific clinical abnormalities, they are often only one aspect of a multifactorial problem. Poor nutrition may suppress a bird's ability to resist disease, prolong recovery from illness or decrease reproductive performance.

Increased information has been presented in recent years regarding the nutritional requirements of individual species, and formulated foods have improved substantially as problem areas have been identified and addressed. However, comprehensive data are still lacking, and manufacturers' claims may not reflect this paucity of information. It is vital to understand that there is considerable interspecies variation regarding nutrient requirements. Extrapolating nutrient requirements (particularly minerals) from poultry data to other species may cause health problems. For example, finches may consume up to 30% of their body weight daily, whereas poultry consume only 6%. Where essential nutritional information is lacking, rather than relying on first principles to resolve a suspected nutritional imbalance, a practical approach is empirically to change the bird to a formulated diet or supplementation regimen considered to be successful for that particular species. If health problems continue to occur, adjustments can be made based on the species of bird, history of the problems, and presenting clinical abnormalities.

Specific nutrients

Water

Avian species that have evolved in arid regions, such as budgerigars and zebra finches, can survive several months without drinking, apparently relying on water derived from metabolic sources. Avian species that significantly utilize metabolic sources of water are an exception, and most companion birds consume water daily and become distressed or possibly die within 48 hours if it is withheld. Clean water should be available at all times. Thirst will increase if there are young in the nest or when exposed to warm environmental temperatures. The addition of any compound to the drinking water that renders it unpalatable may reduce water consumption and result in dehydration and death, particularly in diseased birds. Drinking water medication may be an inaccurate, and potentially dangerous way of delivering drugs. It is preferable to avoid this method, or at least carefully monitor the patient when administering medications or vitamin supplementation via drinking water. Bacterial contamination of water or of foods with a high moisture content ('soft foods') is also a health risk. Water containers should be regularly cleaned and disinfected.

Protein and amino acids

As a guide only, recommended nutritional allowances for granivorous companion birds are listed in Table 2.1. A generally recommended minimum protein allowance for maintenance in granivorous companion birds is about 12%, depending on bioavailability and essential amino acid content. Substantial species variation occurs, with insectivorous birds having higher protein requirements. While there is some tolerance for protein level variation, both excess and deficiency of proteins and amino acids can be problematic.

Clinical signs such as lateral deviation of the metacarpi ('aeroplane wings' or 'angel wings') in growing water fowl or leg deformities in other species may be associated with protein excess if birds are fed rations too high in protein and weight gain occurs too quickly (e.g. when turkey starter pellets containing 30% protein are fed to ducks or geese). Disease conditions associated with elevated protein levels in the feed are especially problematic when the diet is also low in calcium and high in energy. Renal disease, behavioural changes such as biting, feather picking, nervousness, rejection of food, and regurgitation have been noted with the intake of excess dietary protein. The end products of nitrogen excretion in birds include urate, ammonia, urea and creatinine. Urates are by far the most prevalent end product of nitrogen excretion in birds. Renal function will impact on the bird's capacity to break down nitrogenous waste and tolerate protein excess; so too will protein composition. Cockatiels, for example, can have 70% of their diet as plant-derived protein without ill effects while animal protein sources can be problematic (Roudybush 1986).

Essential amino acid composition of the protein supplement is important because of functions performed by the essential amino acids and their effect on food intake. In the breeding season, provided essential amino acid levels are optimal, birds may increase their total protein by increasing their total food consumption without necessarily requiring higher dietary protein levels. In non-breeding birds, where energy requirements are lower, obesity can result if there is an attempt to overeat, thereby compensating for amino acid deficiencies (Underwood et al 1991).

Protein and amino acid deficiencies may be associated with poor weight gain, poor feathering, stress lines on feathers, plumage colour changes and poor reproductive performance.

Table 2.1 Recommended nutritional allowances for granivorous companion bird diets (Brue 1994, Debra MacDonald, personal communication 2006)

Nutrient	Recommended allowance for maintenance	Good source
Protein (%)	12[a]	Fish and meat by-products, eggs, milk, oil seeds
Fat (%)	4[a]	Animal and vegetable oils, oil seed, eggs, animal fat
Energy (kcal/kg)	3000	Same as above
Vitamins		
Vitamin A (IU/kg)	2000–4000[a] (less than 1000 IU/kg for some lorikeets)	Greens, carrot, fish liver oil, liver, eggs, dried milk
Vitamin D (IU/kg)	400[a]	Fish liver oil, eggs, dried milk
Vitamin E (mg/kg)	200[a]	Vegetable oils, sunflower, safflower, wheatgerm
Vitamin K (IU/kg)	1 Fig parrots – 300 µg/bird daily	Green vegetables, eggs
Thiamine (ppm)	5	Yeast products, sunflower, wheatgerm, carrots
Riboflavin (ppm)	10	Yeast products, dried milk, eggs
Niacin (ppm)	75	Yeast products, sunflower, meat and fish by-products
Pyridoxine (ppm)	10	Yeast products, sunflower, eggs, wheat germ
Pantothenic acid (ppm)	15	Yeast products, sunflower, eggs, wheat germ
Biotin (ppm)	0.2	Eggs, safflower, dried milk
Folic acid (ppm)	2	Yeast products, wheat germ
Vitamin B_{12} (ppm)	10	Yeast products, eggs, fish and meat by-products
Choline (ppm)	1000[a]	Yeast products, fish and meat by-products
Minerals		
Calcium (%)	0.5[a]	Bone meal, calcium carbonate (cuttle fish, egg shell)
Phosphorus (total) (%)	0.4[a]	Bone meal, fish and meat products, yeast products
Sodium (%)	0.15	Salt, dried milk, fish meal
Chlorine (%)	0.15	Salt, dried milk, fish meal
Potassium (%)	0.4	Dried fruit, yeast products, wheat germ
Magnesium (ppm)	600	Yeast products, wheat germ, sunflower
Iron (ppm)	80	Bone meal, fish and meat products, yeast products
Zinc (ppm)	50	Bone meal, fish and meat products, wheat germ
Copper (ppm)	8	Yeast products, nuts, oil seeds
Iodine (ppm)	0.3	Dried whey, yeast products, eggs
Selenium (ppm)	0.1	Fish meal, yeast products, oil seeds
Amino acids		
Lysine (%)	0.6	Yeast products, wheat germ, fish and meat meals. Protein meal should include 1.5% lysine
Methionine (%)	0.25	Yeast products, wheat germ, fish and meat meals
Tryptophan (%)	0.12	Yeast products, wheat germ, fish and meat meals
Arginine (%)	0.6	Yeast products, wheat germ, fish and meat meals
Threonine (%)	0.4	Yeast products, wheat germ, fish and meat meals

Other amino acids are sufficient in common diets. These allowances are general approximations only, appropriate for granivorous passerines and psittacines. Variation in requirements will occur between species and depending on life cycle, life stage and general health.

[a] *These nutrients should be increased in growing and breeding birds.*

Insectivorous birds are prone to deficiencies as these species have higher than average protein requirements, particularly during the breeding season. If signs of possible deficiency are observed, protein sources and intake should be scrutinized closely and compared with what is known about preferences and requirements for that particular avian species.

Fats and essential fatty acids

Fats are needed as an energy source. Essential fatty acids (linoleic and arachidonic) are required for the formation of membranes and cell organelles, as hormone precursors, and as the basis of psittacofulvins (i.e. feather pigments found in psittacine species). A commonly recommended minimum fat allowance for granivorous companion bird diets is about 4% (Table 2.1). In mammals lipogenesis occurs mainly in adipose tissue, while in birds it takes place predominantly in the liver. This is the pathophysiology involved with the liver that results in the development of duck and chicken liver paté. Illness may be associated with hepatic lipidosis in pet birds fed high energy diets, especially if exercise is restricted.

Depending on other dietary components, birds can tolerate a wide range of fats. For example, young cockatiels grew normally if given fat levels from 1 to 60% of the diet, but half of the birds fed 60% died (Roudybush 1986). Excess fats have been associated with obesity, hepatic lipidosis, diarrhoea, oily feather texture, interference with the absorption of other nutrients such as calcium, and atherosclerosis (with diets high in saturated fats and cholesterol).

Fat deficiency has been associated with weight loss, poor growth and reduced disease resistance, especially if other adequate sources of energy are not provided. Linolenic acid deficiency has been associated with decreased metabolic efficiency, decreased growth, hepatomegaly, decreased reproduction and poor hatchability.

If fats become rancid (e.g. fish liver oil), essential fatty acids may be destroyed. Lipid peroxidation will also destroy vitamin E, a potent antioxidant. Dietary fats that develop a fetid odour may reduce amino acid availability and block the activities of fat- and water-soluble vitamins, leading to neurological abnormalities.

Carbohydrates

Carbohydrates provide an energy source that is readily converted into fats in the liver and vice versa. Glucagon, rather than insulin, is the principal director of carbohydrate metabolism in birds. Diets high in simple sugar have been associated with clostridial infections in insectivorous birds and lorikeets. Gas fermentation in the intestines, which can be detected as abnormal radiolucent areas on radiographs, may be a consequence of clostridial infections. Intra-intestinal gas is not typically observed on radiographic images of normal psittacine patients, while it may be noted in other avian species (e.g. poultry).

Carbohydrates are the only source of energy utilizable by the nervous system; therefore neurological abnormalities may indicate deficiency in a diet that is otherwise adequate in kilojoule content. Raptors and small birds are prone to collapse from hypoglycaemia if deprived of food. Vitamin B deficiencies may exacerbate the problem, as these vitamins are involved in carbohydrate metabolism. All-meat diets are low in carbohydrates, vitamin A, B vitamins (particularly thiamine), and calcium. **Birds presenting with neurological signs that have been fed an all-meat diet should be given glucose, B vitamins, vitamin A and calcium supplementation to address these multiple deficiencies.**

Vitamins and minerals

General principles regarding vitamin requirements for birds are comparable to those for mammals, except that the active form of vitamin D birds require is vitamin D_3 (cholecalciferol) rather than vitamin D_2 (ergocholeciferol). Vitamin C is only essential in some fruit-eating species (e.g. bulbuls), but it may be useful in debilitated birds where the ability to synthesize the vitamin is reduced and the requirements are higher.

Antibiotics may induce vitamin deficiencies by interfering with normal intestinal microflora. Intestinal infections (e.g. giardiasis) may block vitamin absorption from the intestine (e.g. vitamin E, vitamin A). Hypervitaminosis has become an increasing problem, as clients may over-supplement formulated food or multivitamin preparations, thereby causing renal failure due to hypervitaminosis D. Hypervitaminosis A can also result in disease problems, especially in nectarivorous birds.

Fat-soluble vitamins
Vitamin A

Vitamin A is needed in mucopolysaccharide biosynthesis, for the formation of normal mucous membranes and epithelial surfaces, for growth, vision, vascular development, adrenal hormone production and immune response. Vitamin A precursors, carotenoids, are needed for the formation of red and yellow feather pigments in passerines. In psittacines these feather pigments are derived from psittacofulvins, which do not require dietary carotenoids.

Vitamin A deficiency may cause squamous cell metaplasia of mucous membranes and deranged keratosis of epithelial surfaces. Parenteral administration is the recommended administration protocol for the initial treatment for hypovitaminosis A since intestinal absorption may be poor. Excess vitamin A may cause weight loss, dermatitis, hepatopathy, inflammation of the nares and mouth, haemorrhaging and decreased bone strength. Unfortunately signs of hypervitaminosis A are sometimes similar to signs of vitamin A deficiency. It is essential to obtain a correct diagnosis of the nutritional problem in order to determine the appropriate dietary balance. A study in cockatiels showed that they need about 2000–4000 IU/kg but as little as 10 000 IU/kg can be toxic. Careful analysis of the diet in consideration of the individual species' requirements is needed to determine the nature of the disease problem and devise an appropriate correction. In lorikeets, disease has been associated with nectar mix formulations that contain excessive levels of dietary vitamin A. Iron storage disease in frugivorous and nectarivorous birds has also been correlated with excessive vitamin A intake. To circumvent the risk of vitamin A toxicosis, it may be safer to supplement the bird's diet with natural foods that contain provitamin A carotenoids if requirements of the individual species are unclear. Cockatiels need 2.4 mg/kg carotene for to meet their vitamin A requirements, and these levels can be obtained from feeding 0.15% spirulina.

Clinical signs of vitamin A deficiency are listed in Box 2.1.

VitaminD

Ingested vitamin D precursors (e.g. ergocalciferol) are converted to the active form (vitamin D_3-1,25 dihydrocholecalciferol) through the action of ultraviolet light on non-feathered parts of the skin or oil from the preen gland. Vitamin D_3 works in concert with parathyroid hormone (PTH) to stimulate the absorption of calcium from the intestinal tract, increase calcium reabsorption in the renal tubules, and increase mobilization of calcium from medullary bone.

Clinical signs of vitamin D_3 deficiency (which may be triggered by lack of intake or lack of conversion of precursors because of lack of UVB light) and of excess vitamin D_3 are listed in Box 2.2.

VitaminE

Vitamin E is an antioxidant, and acts in concert with sulphur-containing amino acids and selenium to prevent peroxidase damage to cell membranes. Increased demand for vitamin E may occur with malabsorption syndromes – for example, in intestinal protozoan infections (Harrison & Harrison 1986). Rancid fats in the diet may also increase the demand for vitamin E, as these induce higher antioxidant requirements. This has been seen in lorikeets fed with liquid formulas, inducing spastic leg paralysis (Wilson 1994), and in *Neophema* parrots fed on diets containing rancid dog food and showing neurological signs (Campbell 1987). Excessive levels of vitamin A in the diet may also induce clinical

Box 2.1 Clinical signs of vitamin A deficiency

- White pustules along the mouth, oesophagus, crop and nasal passages.
- Caseous nodules blocking salivary glands or accumulating under the eyelids.
- White caseous material, which may block the infraorbital sinuses (especially in gallinaceous birds).
- A caseous plug, which may block the syrinx.
- Polyuria/polydipsia and gout (associated with damage to ureters).
- Reduced egg and sperm production (associated with squamous cell metaplasia along the reproductive tract).
- Loss of footprint and hyperkeratosis of the plantar surface of the feet, which predisposes to pododermatitis.
- Feather coloration may become muted yellow and red if these are dependent on carotenoid precursors (although not necessarily provitamin A carotenoids).
- Immune response may be affected, leading to increased susceptibility to disease – particularly aspergillosis.
- Xero-ophthalmia due to damage at lacrimal glands.

Box 2.2 Clinical signs associated with vitamin D deficiency or excess

Deficiency, which is exacerbated by concurrent calcium deficiency, causes:

- decreased calcium absorption, hypocalcaemia, increased PTH
- demineralized soft bones, bent bones, pathological fractures
- thin-shelled and soft-shelled eggs.

Treatment should be by parenteral supplementation initially. Calcium requirements need to be addressed concurrently.

Excess vitamin D_3 (4–10 times the requirement) causes:

- increased calcium absorption, increased bone resorption
- hypercalcaemia, decreased PTH
- mineralization of soft tissue
- nephrocalcinosis, polyuria.

Macaw and black cockatoo chicks can be particularly susceptible to hypervitaminosis D_3. It is important not to over-supplement vitamin D.

signs of vitamin E deficiency. Lack of vitamin E in laying hens may result in decreased hatchability in their chicks as vitamin E is required for healthy pipping muscle formation and contraction. Affected chicks may present as dead in shell at term or die shortly after hatching.

Clinical signs of vitamin E deficiency vary depending on the species, age and concurrent health/nutritional problems (Box 2.3). Recommended treatment for vitamin E deficiency is parenteral supplementation and correcting the diet or eliminating the inciting cause. Hypervitaminosis E is unlikely to be a problem with companion avian species, as toxic levels exceed normal requirements by 100-fold.

Vitamin K

Vitamin K is needed for synthesis of prothrombin and clotting factors. Intestinal bacteria are a natural source of vitamin K_2 but the small size of the large intestines in many avian species may not support a large bacterial population. Plant-derived vitamin K_1 obtained from leafy green plant tissue is an alternative source. Naturally occurring deficiencies of vitamin K_1 are rare in birds but have been reported in certain fig parrots, possibly because of their dependence on bacterial K_2, which relies on a different absorption mechanism than either K_1 or synthetic K_3. Deficiencies in poultry have been associated with sulphonamide treatment interfering with normal intestinal flora (Calnek et al 1991). Care must be taken in using warfarin derivatives to control rodents in the vicinity of aviaries as these compounds, which block the action of vitamin K, are also toxic to birds.

Box 2.3 Clinical signs associated with vitamin E deficiency

- Poor muscle function (this may induce elevated creatinine kinase levels):
  - muscular dystrophy/spastic leg paralysis (e.g. in lorikeets)
  - undigested seed in droppings due to poor gizzard muscle function
  - degeneration of pipping muscle in neonates, causing poor hatchability
  - spraddle legs
  - exertional rhabdomyolysis
  - muscle twitching, localized wing paralysis (e.g. in cockatiels with concurrent giardiasis)
- Neurological abnormalities:
  - encephalomalacia
  - incoordination, abnormal body movements and torticollis
- Reproductive abnormalities:
  - testicular degeneration in males
  - infertility in hens
  - early embryonic mortality and poor hatchability
- Steatitis (in birds fed fish with a high fat content)
- Exudative diathesis (in poultry).

Water-soluble vitamins

Unlike fat-soluble vitamins, water-soluble vitamins can be excreted in the urine; therefore toxicity is much less likely to occur and, except in the case of niacin, suspected deficiencies can be addressed by supplementation with little risk of adverse side-effects. Often it is not possible to identify the precise water-soluble vitamin deficiency, in which case multiple B vitamins are indicated.

Thiamine (B_1)

Thiamine is needed for nerve transmission, and deficiencies are associated with loss of appetite, opisthotonus, seizures and death. This vitamin is found in a number of plant food sources, but only at low levels. All-meat diets may be marginal in thiamine content. Compounds with antithiamine activity include: drugs such as amprolium, which act as competitive inhibitors; some bacteria and food preservatives; thiamine agonists such as tannic acid and enzyme-splitting thiaminases contained in raw fish (Brue 1994). **Fish thiaminases can deplete an entire store of thiamine within 90 minutes of death so even feeding 'fresh fish' will contribute to a B_1 deficiency.** Birds fed marginal dietary levels of thiamine may show acute deficiency signs if their diets also contain antithiamine components.

Clinically, thiamine deficiency is most commonly observed in juvenile animals consuming all-meat diets (e.g. in hand-reared baby Australian magpies, raptor species) or with piscivorous birds fed raw fish containing high thiaminase levels. Marginal thiamine levels, in conjunction with a possible thiamine agonist present in natural foods, have been associated with deaths in honey-eaters.

Treatment for thiamine deficiency is urgent, and the response often dramatic. Suspected cases should be given thiamine by intramuscular injection, and the diet supplemented with vitamin B_1. Thiamine supplementation is recommended for all avian cases that present with non-specific neurological signs. Toxicity from overdose has not been reported and any delay while trying to definitively diagnose the cause of the neurological signs may result in death of the patient.

Riboflavin (B_2)

In cockatiels, riboflavin (B_2) deficiency has been associated with failure to incorporate pigment into feathers (Roudybush 1986). Riboflavin deficiency has been associated with poor growth, weakness and diarrhoea, rough dry skin and curled toe paralysis in poultry and other species (Lowensteine 1986). Hens may show fatty infiltration of the liver and decreased egg hatchability. In chronic cases of B_2 deficiency permanent nerve damage will occur, but other clinical signs are responsive to riboflavin supplementation.

Niacin, pyridoxine

Deficiencies of niacin and pyridoxine have been reported in poultry and other avian species but not in Psittaciformes. When poor growth, nervousness and neurological signs are observed in a psittacine patient, niacin and pyridoxine deficiency should be considered as a possible contributing factor to the disease process.

Pantothenic acid, biotin

Deficiencies of pantothenic acid and biotin, which are needed in the formation of critical enzymes in carbon dioxide metabolism, cause similar clinical signs. These include dermatitis around the face and feet, perosis (slipping of the gastrocnemius tendon from the hock), poor growth, poor feathering and ataxia. Egg white contains avidin, a biotin antagonist; therefore egg whites should be cooked before feeding to inactivate the avidin, or additional biotin should be provided. Egg yolk and dried milk are good sources of pantothenic acid and biotin (see Table 2.1).

Folic acid, vitamin B_{12} and choline

Folic acid is needed for carbon transfer in the biosynthesis of amino acids and nucleotides. Folic acid deficiency has been associated with poor feathering, embryonic mortality, poor growth, anaemia and perosis. Folates are widespread in grains and other common foods.

Vitamin B_{12}, or cyanocobalamin, is involved in single carbon unit transfer, and is a critical component in a variety of metabolic pathways, including nucleic acid, protein, fat and carbohydrate synthesis. Its utilization is interrelated with folate and choline; as a result signs of vitamin B_{12} deficiency parallel those of folic acid deficiency. Unlike folate, however, vitamin B_{12} is produced by bacterial biosynthesis and must be obtained by consuming a bacterial source, animal tissues or the few plants that accumulate this compound. Sources of cyanocobalamin include liver, muscle, peas, beans and spirulina.

Choline is required for acetylcholine, phospholipid and cartilage production, and prevents hepatic lipidosis by promoting fatty acid transport and utilization. While essential, choline is commonly found in a variety of foodstuffs and deficiencies are rarely diagnosed. Deficiencies may be associated with poor growth and perosis in juveniles, or fatty liver infiltration in adults. Over-supplementation has been associated with mortalities and should be avoided.

Minerals

Calcium, phosphorus and magnesium

Calcium is essential for bone and eggshell formation, for blood coagulation and nerve and muscle function. Its absorption from the intestinal tract and deposition in bone is regulated by vitamin D_3 and parathyroid hormone. Calcitonin controls hypercalcaemia by decreasing calcium resorption from bone. Diets high in fats, phytate (in grain), oxalates (in spinach as well as other leafy green vegetables) and phosphates will decrease calcium absorption by forming insoluble soaps or complexes.

Secondary nutritional hyperparathyroidism (SNH) due to calcium deficiency and/or calcium/phosphorus imbalance is commonly encountered in birds. High phosphate levels will interfere with calcium absorption from the intestinal tract. The calcium to phosphorus ratio should be around 2:1, but seeds, fruit, vegetables, meat and day-old chicks or mice are extremely calcium deficient and unbalanced (e.g. corn has a 1:37 ratio, sunflower 1:7, muscle meat 1:20). Juveniles on low calcium diets are likely to develop SNH, particularly if exacerbated by vitamin D_3 deficiency.

Phosphorus deficiency is unlikely to occur in avian species because it is widespread in plant food and meat diets. If phosphorus deficiency is diagnosed, investigation of that patient's diet is recommended because much of plant phosphorus may be bound as phytate and not available through intestinal uptake. Calcium deficiency may result in poor mineralization of bone, pathological fractures, bent bones, 'aeroplane wings' (rotation of the distal metacarpi), soft-shelled eggs, leg deformities in ratites, egg binding and neurological signs.

Osteoporosis is a common problem in egg-laying chickens whose exercise is restricted, and it is occasionally seen in egg-laying psittacines. Affected birds may suffer paralysis due to spinal compression of the caudal thoracic vertebrae. Egg-laying birds on low calcium diets may also show muscle tetany or seizures that are responsive to injectable calcium supplementation.

Birds suspected of calcium deficiency should be given immediate parenteral calcium support, and the overall suitability of the diet and lighting regimens assessed and modified based on the husbandry evaluation. Hypocalcaemia in African grey parrots is a clinical syndrome associated with an inability to mobilize calcium from bone in response to stress or immediate physiological demands. Affected birds will often present with seizure activity or show signs of ataxia. Adequate, life-long UVB light and calcium supplementation is critically needed for these birds.

Magnesium serves as an activator for many enzymes involved with phosphate transfer. High levels of either calcium or phosphorus will increase magnesium requirements. Magnesium deficiency may cause poor growth, lethargy, convulsions and death, while excess may cause diarrhoea, irritability, decreased egg production and thin-shelled eggs. Hypomagnesaemia will cause concurrent decrease in serum calcium levels. Low serum magnesium levels may be correlated to the African grey hypocalcaemic disease syndrome.

Iron

Iron is needed for the production of haemoglobin, which is needed for cellular respiration. While there is negligible excretion, body reserves are efficiently recycled and intestinal absorption is controlled to prevent excess accumulation. Iron deficiencies may cause hypochromic microcytic anaemia and poor feather pigmentation.

Iron storage disorders (ISDs) are diagnosed in avian patients fed diets with high iron levels, but have also been noted in other cases where the dietary iron levels are low. Clinically affected birds present with liver failure, and liver biopsy shows haemochromatosis and haemosiderosis. Serum iron levels or total iron-binding capacity do not correlate very well with the occurrence of the disease. Toucans and mynahs may have a genetic predisposition to the problem, and are commonly affected by this disease process. ISDs have been correlated with diets high in vitamin A.

Recommended treatment options for iron storage disease that may lower the serum iron level are: iron-binding agents such as tannins; administration of vitamin C; restriction of vitamin A; giving provitamin A carotenoids; and if necessary, regular phlebotomy therapy. Response to treatment may be poor, and ISD is often associated with sudden death.

Copper

Copper is needed for haemoglobin synthesis and in the formation of several enzymes, including those involved in the formation of elastin and melanin synthesis. Deficiency has been associated with aortic rupture, bone fragility, poor feather pigmentation, decreased egg production and shell abnormalities.

Zinc

Zinc is needed for the formation of insulin and many enzymes. Deficiency may cause hyperkeratosis and bone deformities, but this is clinically rare. Zinc toxicosis is a common presentation to veterinary hospitals, as aviary birds are exposed to this metal by chewing the zinc-impregnated galvanized coating off the cage wire. Clinical signs may include vomiting, diarrhoea, neurological abnormalities and death.

Selenium

Selenium is part of an enzyme that acts as an antioxidant. It has a vitamin E sparing effect but cannot be used as a substitute for vitamin E. Selenium is linked with pancreatic exocrine function and the production of thyroid hormones. While selenium deficiency may cause poor growth and feathering, impaired fat digestion, and pancreatic atrophy; excess may reduce hatching success, and contribute to teratogenic development of the embryo.

Manganese

Manganese is needed for chondroitin sulphate production, normal eggshell and bone formation, growth and reproduction. Deficiency of manganese in the diet may cause perosis, limb deformities, delayed growth, and ataxia in poultry and waterfowl. Excess dietary calcium may interfere with manganese absorption.

Iodine

Iodine is needed for the formation of thyroxine and related compounds in the thyroid gland. Iodine deficiency may result in goitre (particularly in budgerigars) and/or hypothyroidism (reported in pigeons). Iodine toxicity may induce goitre, antagonize chloride, depress growth rates, and cause CNS signs and death.

Clinical signs of goitre in budgerigars are associated with the space-occupying effect of the enlarged thyroid gland, which lies just within the thoracic inlet (e.g. wheezing respiration, crop dilatation and vomiting, sudden death due to respiratory obstruction or aspiration of vomitus). Budgerigars suffering with goitre are considered emergency cases, and should not be stressed during examination and treatment. Initial treatment of a suspected goitre patient should include dilute iodine supplementation. For long-term treatment, iodine may be administered into the drinking water or the patient placed on an iodine-supplemented diet.

Sodium and chloride

Salt deficiency may cause weight loss, poor egg production and cannibalism, and may be associated with self-mutilation syndromes. Excessive amounts of salt may be acutely toxic, with affected birds showing intense thirst, muscle weakness and convulsions.

Sea birds have a nasal salt gland controlled by an ATPase pump. Oil contamination may suppress the pump and cause clinical signs of salt toxicity.

Practical nutrition

Avian nutrition has been an active area of research; while debate regarding optimal diets for birds is ongoing, the connection between some feeding practices and illness are now well established.

Health problems due to deficiencies and imbalances associated with all-seed diets are common and such diets should be avoided. In particular, oil seeds such as sunflower and safflower contain excessive levels of fat but may be deficient in vitamin A as well as provitamin A carotenoids, vitamin D_3, E, B_{12} and K, riboflavin, pantothenic acid, niacin, biotin, choline, iodine,

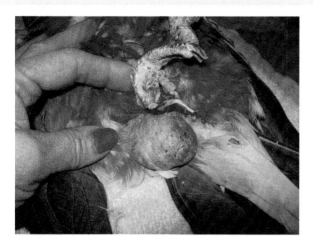

Fig 2.25 Lipoma, overgrown, twisted claws, excessive scale and loss of plantar footprint in a galah kept for many years in a small cage on a sunflower seed diet. Such a diet contains excessive fat but is deficient in vitamin A and a range of other vitamins, trace minerals and essential amino acids.

iron, copper, manganese, selenium, sodium, calcium, zinc and some amino acids (e.g. lysine, and methionine) (Fig. 2.25).

Appropriate diets will vary between species but, if feeding seed, supplementation should be offered to address these imbalances. Leafy green and yellow vegetables such as spinach, silver beet and carrot are good sources of most of the deficient vitamins and minerals, but a variety of fruits and vegetables are useful to add a psychological stimulus to the diet. Sprouted seed and cooked and sprouted pulses will also increase digestibility and availability of nutrients. Avoid avocado, as some varieties have been reported to be toxic. Chocolate, caffeine and alcohol may also be toxic and should be avoided (Bauck & LaBonde 1997).

A calcium source such as cuttlefish bones or calcium blocks should be available, particularly for growing or breeding birds. Grit is not essential for captive psittacine species but studies in poultry and pigeons suggest that it may increase the digestibility of feed by as much as 10%. Occasionally birds may ingest too much grit and become impacted. The problem of grit impaction has been noted more frequently in North America than appears to be the case in Australia. The reason for the regional variation is uncertain but some veterinarians advocate withholding grit because of this risk (Clipsham 1996, Macwhirter 1994). There do not appear to be any adverse consequences from withholding grit from captive psittacine species.

Commercial formulated diets designed for individual avian species have been available for many years and the best of them are backed by scientific research, extensive feeding trials and field experience. They are convenient for owners and many birds will thrive on them. Low iron pellets have been found especially useful for avian species such as mynahs and toucans that are prone to iron storage disease. Commercial nectar food, fed either wet or dry, is convenient for lorikeets and other nectarivorous birds However, these commercially formulated diets are not without potential problems and deaths have been seen in birds fed exclusively on formulated foods inappropriate for the species, particularly those high in vitamin A or in situations where the bird finds the food unpalatable and will not eat, or ingests inadequate amounts, of the formulated food. Availability can also be an issue and a single formulation will not suit all birds at different life, moult and reproductive stages. A diet based on a combination of some seed, dark leafy green and yellow vegetables, fruit and formulated food allows for flexibility and is generally recommended.

If feeding live food, the diet and life stage of the food item species needs to be considered. For example, if crickets and other insects to be used as a food source for birds are fed on vegetable matter or bran alone, their protein and calcium content may be low. Also pinhead (juveniles) crickets have lower protein compared with adult crickets (55% versus 64%) but higher calcium (1.29% versus 0.14%) and much of the protein in adults may be unavailable chitin. Rearing insects on high protein diets and gut loading with calcium supplements can help to improve their nutritional value as an avian food source. Day-old chicks, mice or rats are usually calcium deficient compared with appropriately fed juveniles. Alternative calcium sources need to be provided if very young animals are being used as food items.

Tips on getting birds to eat a balanced diet

Birds often develop strong preferences for unbalanced diets, and even if they are offered appropriate nutrients they may choose inappropriate items (e.g. they may select sunflower seeds exclusively over other more nutritious offerings). Ideally birds should be provided with a wide variety of foodstuffs from the time of weaning. Birds can be encouraged to accept a new food by:

- offering the new food first thing in the morning when the appetite is greatest
- mixing the new food with the bird's normal diet
- allowing birds to watch other birds and people eating the new food
- hand-feeding, if the bird is attached to a human
- making a game of fossicking food items
- only offering the new food.

Care must be taken when attempting to change a bird's diet, and weight should be regularly monitored. If the bird becomes ill, return to what the bird is willing to eat and attempt dietary change at a later date. Ketosis has been seen in cockatoos that starve themselves, breaking down body fat too rapidly, because they will not accept the dietary change.

Nutritional disorders

Nutritional imbalances may cause digestive and respiratory disorders, skin changes, skeletal and muscular disorders, neurological signs, reproductive disorders, and general ill health or sudden death. These disorders and possible causes are listed below.

Digestive disorders

Digestive disorders are treated initially by giving appropriate parenteral medication, then by addressing the underlying nutritional imbalance and/or disease condition. They include:

1. White plaques in the mouth or lumps around the choana or salivary ducts – associated with squamous metaplasia due to vitamin A deficiency.
2. Partial paralysis of the muscles of mastication or other body muscles – vitamin E deficiency, associated with malabsorption due to giardiasis in cockatiels.
3. Crop impaction:
   - high fibre diets
   - foreign material ingestion
   - excess grit consumption
   - in hand-fed babies, it can be associated with cold food, a cold environment, infrequent feeding, food of an inappropriate consistency (usually too thick), or microwaved food that has been inappropriately mixed.
4. Regurgitation:
   - high protein diets in cockatiels
   - iodine-deficient diets (in budgerigars, where an enlarged thyroid obstructs the outlet to the crop).
5. Crop liths (concretions) – in birds on marginal diets, high protein supplementation or birds who eat droppings and form urate liths.
6. Diarrhoea:
   - in birds fed high fat, low fibre diets of human processed food
   - bacterial contamination of food may occur if feed dishes are positioned so that faecal contamination can occur.

7. Polyuria/polydipsia:
   - hypo- or hypervitaminosis A
   - hypocalcaemia
   - excess dietary protein
   - hypervitaminosis D_3
   - excessive salt intake
   - dry seed diets
   - formulated diets or a high percentage of dietary fibre.
8. Passing undigested food in the faeces – may be associated with vitamin E/selenium deficiency, lack of grit, excess oil in the diet or dehydration.

Polyuria alone may occur in birds fed semi-moist foods, fruit or vegetables. B vitamins, berries and some foodstuffs can alter urine colour without causing concurrent health problems.

Respiratory disorders

Respiratory disorders associated with nutritional imbalances include:

1. Wheezing/squeaking respiration (partial airway obstruction)
   - iodine deficiency where enlarged thyroid glands present as space-occupying masses (goitre)
   - vitamin A deficiency, inducing squamous cell metaplasia of the tracheal mucosa; in these cases obstruction most commonly occurs at the level of the syrinx.
2. Airway obstruction – aspiration of feeding formula or incorrect tube feeding. Millet or wheat seeds may also be aspirated and typically lodge in the trachea or at the syrinx.

Skin changes

Skin changes associated with nutritional imbalances include:

1. Plantar corns, loss of papillae and/or pododermatitis – biotin and hypo- or hypervitaminosis A.
2. Oedema of subcutaneous tissues – vitamin E and selenium deficiencies.
3. Exfoliative dermatitis on the face and legs – biotin, pantothenic acid, riboflavin or zinc deficiencies.

Skeletal and muscular disorders

Skeletal and muscular disorders associated with nutritional imbalances include:

1. Demineralized, curvature of the long bones with concurrent pathological fractures – hypovitaminosis D or deficiencies of calcium, phosphorus or manganese.
2. 'Aeroplane/angel wing' (rotation of the distal metacarpi). High protein and/or low calcium in rapidly growing waterfowl with emerging heavy primary flight feathers causes torsion of the distal wing.
3. Slipped tendon of the hock (perosis) – manganese, biotin, pantothenic acid or folic acid deficiencies.
4. Enlargement of the hock (without tendon slipping) – zinc or niacin deficiency.
5. Spastic leg paralysis – vitamin E, calcium, chloride or riboflavin deficiencies.

Neurological signs

Neurological signs associated with nutritional imbalances include:

1. Sudden collapse, fainting or seizures:
   - hypoglycaemia in malnourished raptors and other species
   - hypocalcaemia, particularly in African grey parrots or egg-laying birds.
2. Opisthotonus and seizures – characteristic of thiamine deficiency.
3. Aggressiveness and nervousness – high protein diets.

Change to formulated diets is sometimes associated with decreased biting and screaming and increased activity and playfulness.

Reproductive disorders

Many nutritional disorders may result in poor reproductive performance. Calcium, vitamin E and selenium deficiencies may be associated with egg binding. Vitamin E deficiency has also been linked with peri-hatching deaths because of poor development of the pipping muscle.

General ill health or sudden death

Sudden death in avian patients may be caused by:

1. Fatty infiltration of the liver
   - high energy diets in exercise-deprived birds
   - high fat diets
   - vitamin B deficiencies.
2. Ascites – an iron storage disease which may be associated with high dietary levels of iron in susceptible birds.
3. Gout:
   - high dietary protein or calcium, hypervitaminosis D_3

- dehydration and vitamin A deficiency causing squamous metaplasia of the ureters.
4. Atherosclerosis – high fat and cholesterol.
5. Aortic rupture – copper deficiency.

Specific nutritional disorders

Obesity/lipomas

Birds gain weight if the energy content of the diet is excessive for the energy demands of normal metabolic functions and the amount of exercise. This can occur if the energy content of the food is too high or if birds overeat either to satisfy deficiencies of other essential nutrients (e.g. a protein deficiency in a seed diet) or simply for behavioural reasons. Restricted exercise will exacerbate the problem. Many (but not all) lipomas are the result of obesity and can be addressed simply by dietary and lifestyle change without the need for surgery.

Strategies to address obesity will vary with the individual patient and owner, but the following are general principles:

1. The diet should be balanced and the kilojoule intake decreased by using food of lower kilojoule content (i.e. white millet seed and fresh fruit and vegetables) or by restricting feeding to meal times rather than ad lib. Using appropriate formulated diets can make a dramatic difference in some cases.
2. Exercise should be increased – move the bird to a larger cage or aviary and encourage flight or just walking if not able to fly.

Low body weight/poor growth

Poor growth may be caused by inadequate or inappropriate food intake, infrequent feeding, progressing to an adult diet too early, loss of appetite, maldigestion or malassimilation. The underlying problem should be corrected and the bird placed on a balanced, high energy diet. Digestive enzymes, sprouted seeds and fibre hemicellulose (Metamucil®) may be useful in increasing digestibility.

Polyphagia

Young birds suddenly introduced to new food items may overeat fibrous food or grit, causing proventricular or gizzard impactions. Vitamin E and selenium deficiencies, hepatopathies, renal dysfunction and exocrine pancreatic deficiency have also been suggested as causes of polyphagia. Feigned polyphagia, where a bird hulls seed and appears to be eating but the crop remains empty, may occur with birds that are weak or offered inappropriate food items. Faecal output and weight gain, rather than apparent eating, should be used to determine food consumption. The underlying cause of feigned polyphagia should be corrected and the bird placed on an appropriate balanced diet. Laxatives or surgery may be necessary in the case of impactions. Treatment with multivitamins or pancreatic enzymes should be considered if needed.

Immune response

Low vitamin A levels may result in a suboptimal immune response, and have been associated with the occurrence of aspergillosis in psittacines. Adequate levels of B vitamins (particularly pantothenic acid and riboflavin) and vitamin E have been shown to improve the body's response to pathogens.

Plumage abnormalities associated with nutritional imbalances

Fault (stress) marks, which are horizontal linear defects across the vane, are associated with cortisone release at the time of feather formation, and can be caused by disrupted feeding schedules and nutritional deficiencies – particularly protein or methionine.

Muted feather colours in passerines may be caused by deficiencies of carotenes and xanthophylls, which originate from plant material. These pigments are found in fat globules in the feathers, and give rise to yellow, red and orange colours.

Dark coloured feathers may become lighter in birds on tyrosine- or copper-deficient diets, as these nutrients are required for melanin formation.

Blue/green/grey feather colour changes

Blue is a structural colour, and depends on the scattering of light by the spongy layer of the feather rami rather than the occurrence of pigments. Amino acid deficiencies that alter the structure of keratin may alter blue feather coloration, but the exact nature of the deficiency has not been clarified. Green coloration is generally due to a combination of structural blue and yellow combined. A green to yellow colour change is a common occurrence in birds, and can be due to loss of structural blue coloration. Most often this is associated with liver disease, but it may also be associated with nutritional deficiencies. A blue or grey to black colour change is sometimes seen with liver disease or malnutrition, and is thought to be due to altered keratin structure in the spongy layer preventing normal light scattering; hence melanin granules (if present) absorb all wavelengths of light to give the visual effect of black.

Feather picking may be initiated by dry, flaky pruritic skin, which may be associated with deficiencies of sulphur-containing amino acids, arginine, niacin, pantothenic acid, biotin, folic acid and salt; and/or deficiencies and excesses of vitamin A. Fatty acid imbalance or excessive dietary fat have also been incriminated as causes of self-mutilation, along with many other medical and psychological causes.

References

Bauck L, Labonde J 1997 Toxic diseases. In: Altman R B, Clubb S L, Dorrestein G M, Quesenberry K E (eds) Avian medicine and surgery. W B Saunders, Philadelphia, PA, p 604–613

Brue R N 1994 Nutrition. In: Ritchie B, Harrison G, Harrison L (eds) Avian medicine: principles and application. Wingers, Lake Worth, FL, p 70–85

Calnek W B, Barnes H J, Beard C W et al 1991 Diseases of poultry, 9th edn. Iowa State University Press, Ames, IA

Campbell T W 1987 Hypovitaminosis E: its effects on birds. In: Proceedings of the 1st International Conference on Zoo and Avian Medicine, Hawaii, p 75–78. Issued by the Association of Avian Veterinarians

Clipsham R 1996 Psittacine pediatrics, gastrointestinal tract. In: Rosskopf W R, Woerpel R (eds) Diseases of cage and aviary birds, 3rd edn. Williams & Wilkins, Baltimore, MD, p 334–338

Harrison G L, Harrison L R 1986 Nutritional diseases. In: Harrison G L, Harrison L R (eds) Clinical avian medicine and surgery. W B Saunders, Philadelphia, PA, p 397–407

King A S, McLelland J 1984 Birds – their structure and function, 2nd edn. Baillière Tindall, London

Kuenzel W J 2000 The autonomic nervous system of avian species. Sturkie's Avian physiology, 5th edn. Academic Press, New York, p 101–122

Lowensteine L J 1986 Nutritional disorders of birds. In: Fowler M (ed) Zoo and wild animal medicine. W B Saunders, Philadelphia, PA, p 202–212

Macwhirter P J 1994 Malnutrition. In: Ritchie B, Harrison G, Harrison L (eds) Avian medicine: principles and application. Wingers, Lake Worth, FL, p 842–861

Macwhirter P J, Mueller R 1998 Comparison of immediate skin test reactions in clinically normal and self-mutilating Psittaciformes. Proceedings of the Association of Avian Veterinarians – Australian Committee Conference, Canberra, October 1998, p 1–8

Maina J N 1996 Perspectives on the structure and function in birds. In: Rosskopf W, Woerpel R (eds) Diseases of cage and aviary birds, 3rd edn. Williams & Wilkins, Baltimore, MD, p 163–217

Mason J R, Clark L 2000 The chemical senses in birds. In: Sturkie's Avian physiology, 5th edn. Academic Press, New York, p 39–53

Prum R, Brush A 2004 Which came first, the feather or the bird? Scientific American, Special edition, p 72–82

Roudybush T. 1986 Growth, signs of deficiency and weaning in cockatiels fed deficient diets. Proceedings of the Association of Avian Veterinarians, p 333–340

Underwood M S, Polin D, O'Handley P, Wiggers P 1991 Short term energy and protein utilization in budgerigars (Melopsittacus undulatus) fed isocaloric diets of varying protein concentration. Proceedings of the Association of Avian Veterinarians, p 227–236

Wilson P 1994 Nutritional myopathy in free-living lorikeets. Proceedings of the Association of Avian Veterinarians, p 229–234

Suggested reading

Calnek W B, Barnes H J, Beard C W et al 1991 Diseases of poultry, 9th edn. Iowa State University Press, Ames, IA

Evans H E 1996 Anatomy of the budgerigar and other birds. In: Rosskopf W R, Woerpel R (eds) Diseases of cage and aviary birds, 3rd edn. Williams & Wilkins, Baltimore, MD, p 79–162

King A S, McLelland J 1984 Birds – their structure and function, 2nd edn. Baillière Tindall, London

Krautwald M, Tellhelm B, Hummel G et al 1992 Atlas of radiographic anatomy and diagnosis of cage birds. Paul Parey Scientific Publishers, Berlin

McLelland J 1991 A color atlas of avian anatomy. W B Saunders, Philadelphia, PA

Orosz S, Ensley P, Haynes C 1992 Avian surgical anatomy, thoracic and pelvic limbs. W B Saunders, Philadelphia, PA

Rubels G A, Isenbugal E, Wolvekamp P 1992 Atlas of diagnostic radiology of exotic pets. W B Saunders, Philadelphia, PA

Schubot R M, Clubb K, Clubb S et al 1992 Analysis of psittacine diets fed at ABRC. In: Schubot R M et al (eds) Psittacine aviculture, perspectives, techniques and research. ABRC, Loxahatchee, FL, p 52–59

Smith S A, Smith B J 1992 Atlas of avian radiographic anatomy. W B Saunders, Philadelphia, PA

Whittow G C 2000 Sturkie's Avian physiology, 5th edn. Academic Press, New York

The physical examination

Alan K. Jones

3

Introduction

In common with all animals dealt with in veterinary practice, competent handling of the avian patient in the clinic will inspire confidence in the client that the veterinarian is able to deal with birds. The converse – incompetent handling – may prove a danger to the bird, the owner, the veterinarian, the clinic staff, and even the environment, as well as ensuring that the client will not return.

A thorough, systematic clinical examination is essential to a proper diagnosis, but this should be preceded by a number of stages to be described further before the bird is handled. The approach will be governed by the urgency of the case – is the bird acutely ill or injured; is it chronically sick or perhaps clinically normal but sub-clinically infected; or is this a routine health check in a normal bird?

Proper steps taken at this stage will give important clues to a diagnosis, and will indicate further tests that may be required, and a probable treatment regimen. A confident, efficient and skilful approach at this stage will also convince the client of your expertise!

There is an innate fear among veterinarians about handling birds, engendered by lack of experience and tuition at veterinary schools, and apocryphal tales of beloved pet canaries dying in the hand. Plus, of course, those beaks and claws! This chapter should address those fears and enable a confident approach to avian examination. Much of what follows appeared in this chapter written by Martin Lawton in the first edition of this book, and where necessary the text has been updated and revised.

Equipping the practice for avian patients

In order to deal appropriately with avian cases, there are several basic items required that may not routinely be used in small animal practice (Lawton 2000). Some of these may be available if the practice currently deals with other exotic species, and there is obvious crossover with equipment already used for dogs and cats (such as radiography and an in-house laboratory or access to an outside lab that can provide fast but accurate results and interpretations). Although it is advantageous in an avian practice to have endoscopes, radiographic restraining devices, radiotherapy, operating micro-scopes, ophthalmic surgical instruments and nebulizers, to name but a few, these are not included here because they are not considered 'basic'.

The following items are required to practise avian medicine at an acceptable basic standard:

1. *Towels.* There should be a ready supply of towels of various sizes and thicknesses for the examination and handling of many birds, primarily psittacines. A new, clean towel should be used for each bird to prevent the possibility of disease spread. It is acceptable to keep a towel (provided it remains clean) for an individual bird if it is to be hospitalized (Fig. 3.1).

2. *Gloves or gauntlets.* **These will be required for birds of prey, but should *not* be used on psittacine patients. They are too inflexible and insensitive to allow comfortable handling of such birds, and may cause a tame pet bird to become hand-shy.**

3. *Digital scales.* Essential equipment to record accurate weights of all avian patients, not only to allow precise dosing of drugs, but also to enable weight loss or gain to be monitored. All hospitalized patients should be weighed at least once a day to establish if they are eating and to indicate any requirement for supplementary feeding or fluid therapy (Fig. 3.2). Scales should be of various ranges and sensitivity. The standard platform scales used for dogs and cats are not accurate enough for smaller patients. Scales should have an accuracy of 1 g for weight ranges up to 100 g, and 2–5 g for weight ranges up

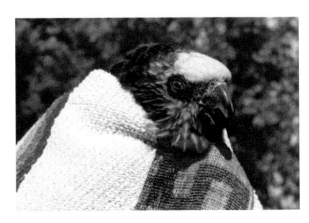

Fig 3.1 Hawk-headed parrot restrained in towel. Body under control, head exposed but safely restrained.

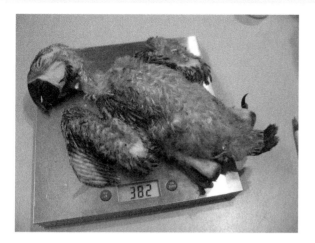

Fig 3.2 Digital scales for accurate weighing of avian patients.

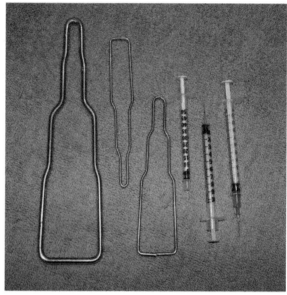

Fig 3.3 Stainless steel mouth gags and syringes with needles suitable for avian patients.

to 500 g. Over 500 g body weight an accuracy of 5–10 g may be acceptable. It is necessary to have some means to support the bird whilst it is being weighed. Hand-reared tame birds may be placed directly onto the platform of the scales. For others a small cage, bag or perch is required. Ideally, scales should have the ability to be zeroed on placement of the receptacle, and to maintain this 'memory' when removed. Alternatively, the weight of the container should be written on it to ease calculation of the weight of the bird. Body weight should never be guessed, as inaccuracy could lead to under- or overdosing – often with dire consequences.

4. *Insulin or other low-dose syringes.* These allow small but accurate doses of drugs to be administered, based on calculations made using the correct weight of the birds. The needle used should also be the smallest available that will deliver the medication, to reduce the trauma involved in the injection process (Fig. 3.3).

5. *Paediatric blood tubes and swabs.* It is inappropriate to place small blood samples in standard mammalian tubes, as the amount of anticoagulant supplied is calculated for a set volume. Tubes designed to take 0.5 mL or less are readily available, and should be available in the practice. For other sample collections, the use of paediatric or nasopharyngeal swabs is advised, as the head of the swab is smaller than that of a standard bacteriological swab and allows more accurate sampling.

6. *Cages.* These are essential for the confinement of birds admitted for hospitalization and treatment. Although many patients will be brought in their own cages, some will come in a box or cage

unsuitable for longer-term housing. Some permanent caging should therefore be available, and this should be easily cleaned and disinfected, and sited away from dogs and cats. Although not a basic requirement, it is advantageous to have a cage that can be used for nebulization of any bird with respiratory disease.

7. *Nets.* Any veterinary practice intending to see avian patients should have a selection of nets of several sizes suitable for the species likely to be encountered. There will be occasions when avian patients escape from the cage, and there is nothing more embarrassing and time-consuming than chasing a bird around a consulting room, with the owner losing faith in proportion to the length of time that it takes to catch the bird. The appropriate net and expertise in its use will help in recapturing the escaped patient, and also substantially reduce the chances of injury in the process. There are specialized avian nets available, with padded rims to prevent damage and cloth bags. Open-meshed fishing nets are *not* suitable, as small birds may break through the mesh, or toes and legs may get caught.

8. *Heat.* An appropriate supply of additional heat is beneficial for the sick bird. All birds have a higher metabolism than mammals of the same body weight, and this increased metabolism means that there is a greater risk of chilling, especially in the sick bird. The effort of maintaining body temperature diverts energy from recovery. Suitable heating sources range from dedicated hospital

cages with built-in heating and thermostats to an infrared heat lamp pointed at a cage. Where an external heat source without a thermostat is used it is important to prevent overheating, which can also be very stressful or even damaging to the patient.

9. *Crop tubes.* These may be purpose purchased or practice prepared. For most avian species it is preferable to use a metal crop tube with a ball end to reduce trauma to the mouth and oesophagus, and to avoid the risk of the bird biting through plastic tubing and swallowing it. The latter will require retrieval of part of the tube from the oesophagus or crop – or worse still, surgical intervention. The technique of crop tubing is easy with practice, and is invaluable both for administering medications or liquid food, and for obtaining samples from the crop ('crop wash').

10. *Spinal needles.* The suggestion that spinal needles should be considered a 'basic' requirement may at first seem strange; however, these are essential for the provision of intraosseous fluid therapy. No veterinary practice should consider it is ready for avian patients unless it is also prepared to deal with the dehydrated or moribund case. Although it is possible to use standard hypodermic needles, they will frequently be blocked with osseous material associated with the placement and therefore require repeated 'stabs' or will completely prevent establishment of a patent intraosseous route (Lawton 2000).

11. *Microscope.* Access to a microscope is essential to allow the investigation and diagnosis of many avian conditions. It is not acceptable solely to use an outside laboratory, as the assessment of protozoal infections (including trichomonads), for example, requires evaluation of a fresh wet preparation. A faecal sample may be evaluated by performing a direct smear (looking for evidence of parasites) and a Gram's stain. This is a quick, simple technique, readily performed by the veterinarian or nurse/technician, and will give rapid, valuable information.

12. *A library and access to further information.* All practices should have a basic in-house library. Some textbooks considered 'small animal' may contain useful chapters or information on avian conditions, but there are now many textbooks dedicated to avian medicine and surgery. It is not essential for every practice to have all the avian textbooks or publications, but it is vital to know how to obtain further information. All veterinary practices should have the ability to perform a basic literature search (this may include access

to the internet or a subscription service via a veterinary library). It is also of utmost importance that staff should be aware of where to refer cases that are beyond their expertise or unresponsive to treatment. Very few veterinarians lose clients by referring early or at an appropriate time – unlike those that do not refer or leave it too late.

13. *Isoflurane (or sevoflurane).* This is an essential basic requirement for safe avian anaesthesia (see later).

14. *Trained staff.* Although it is accepted that almost all veterinary practices have trained nurses/ technicians, these staff may not be experienced in the handling, care and treatment of birds. Any practice that intends to hospitalize and treat avian patients should ensure that staff are trained in the basics of handling, administering medication (including fluid therapy) and the nutritional requirements of the common species.

Preparation

Further education and experience in the field of avian medicine is essential. This can be acquired by joining local bird clubs and societies, and attending their meetings to become acquainted with bird keepers and the species kept. The Association of Avian Veterinarians (www.aav.org) is an invaluable source of knowledge and information on avian medicine, and includes an international network of approachable experts in this field.

Avian veterinarians deal with a vast number of disparate species and subspecies, with many of those bred in captivity occurring in an infinite number of varieties. Some of the more common types are described in more detail in other chapters of this book, but the ability to recognize at least the genus of a bird to be examined is important. Again, client confidence in the veterinarian's abilities will fade quickly if basic questions like 'what is it?' and 'what does it eat?' are asked at the beginning of the consultation.

The receptionist should receive training in asking the right questions when scheduling the appointment. A note of the species and a brief description of the problem(s) should be made so that the veterinarian is forewarned and may, if necessary, do some basic reading on the species and the condition beforehand. It is often the case, though, that many owners do not know the species of their pets – the 'Amazon green', or even an 'African green' are commonly encountered! The receptionist should be able to assess the urgency of the case – a sick bird should always be considered as serious and urgent, as opposed to a budgerigar needing a nail clip, or a chronic feather picker. The client should be advised about transporting the bird(s), and bringing samples of food and droppings where appropriate (Lawton 2000).

Timing of consultation (Lawton 2000)

Avian cases should *not* be examined during a normal busy small animal clinic. Most birds will view cats and dogs as potential predators, thus increasing the stress of the visit. A totally separate waiting area is the optimum. Appointments should be scheduled outside dog and cat hours, and extra time allowed. The avian consultation generally requires more time than the average small animal case. Attempting to deal with any case when rushed will probably not do the veterinarian or the bird justice. In view of the extra time required, a realistic practice policy should be sought on charging for such visits. Although most pet bird owners are prepared to pay for a thorough examination and comprehensive therapy, there is a tendency for the keepers of small cage-birds to believe that they are doing the veterinarian a favour by bringing the bird in, and to resent any form of charge at all! The quoting of realistic fees in advance (especially for possible diagnostic tests) is strongly recommended, as this can avoid many misunderstandings.

Examination room

The room used for avian consultations should have lockable doors and windows, and window blinds. Extractor fans should be covered, and any ceiling fans should be turned off. Staff should be trained not to enter the room whilst patients are being examined, unless specifically requested to do so. Lights should be controlled by a dimmer switch, or be capable of being switched off from inside the room. All equipment for restraint, handling, sampling and treatment should be prepared and available prior to catching the bird (Lawton 2000).

Expertise at handling different species is acquired by working with experienced avian veterinarians, or other professional bird handlers such as falconers, pigeon fanciers, bird breeders, or zoo keepers. Owners vary in their ability to handle their birds, with falconers on the whole being competent, whilst most pet parrot keepers are incapable of controlling their charges. Beware the client that comes in with their pet on their shoulder or arm!

Pet bird owners are often reluctant to be involved in the direct medication or treatment of their birds (Lawton 2000). Psittacine species have excellent memories, and undoubtedly bear a long-term grudge against any persons who they feel have invaded their privacy, handled them roughly, or inflicted pain upon them. If the owner is present at the time the bird is restrained and treated, that bird may well consider the owner as responsible as the veterinarian. For this reason, owners should be offered the opportunity to leave the room prior to the handling, but the reasons should be explained, otherwise the owner may assume the veterinarian is trying to conceal incompetence or cruelty!

Transportation

Depending on species, the bird should be brought to the clinic in its normal cage. If this is not possible, then the owner should be encouraged to bring photographs to allow visual assessment of its normal environment (Lawton 2000). Most owners and breeders will have photographs of their pets and will be delighted to bring these. Modern digital cameras and mobile (cell) phone cameras make this easy, and short video clips of behavioural patterns can also be taken.

The cage should not have been cleaned out prior to the visit, so that diagnostic clues may be provided (see below). It should be wrapped with a cloth in order to darken the environment, reduce stress and prevent draughts. A transport container other than the bird's home cage must be suitable for the task. For all species it should be escape-proof and unlikely to cause damage during transportation (Figs 3.4, 3.5). Cardboard boxes are seldom suitable, as larger birds may bite their way out in minutes; and trying to capture a small lively bird from a cardboard box is likely to lead to its escape. Small mammal carriers with top or front opening access are strong, but again it is often difficult to extract the patient without it escaping.

There is a lot of advantage in examining a bird in its own environment, especially when a collection is involved. Many more clues as to husbandry, management, feeding regimen, environmental hazards and the like can be gleaned by a site visit rather than checking a single stressed bird in a pet carrier at the clinic.

Prior to handling

The veterinarian should not rush into handling the bird. There is a great tendency for parrot owners particularly

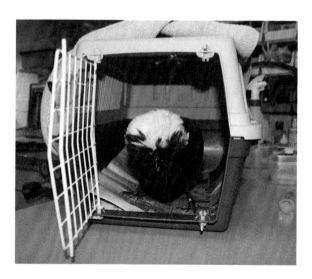

Fig 3.4 Pet carrier with bantam hen. Secure, safe temporary transport.

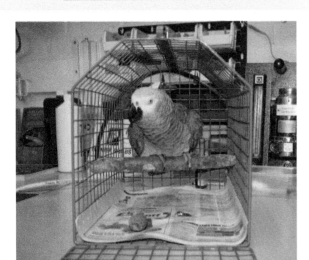

Fig 3.5 Pet carrier with grey parrot. Secure transport, provided with perch.

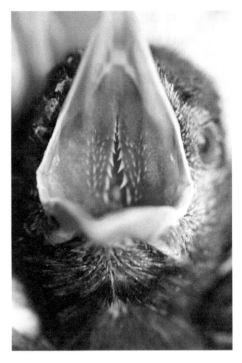

Fig 3.6 Fledgling magpie chick begging for food. Shows choanal slit with edging papillae.

to place the carrier on the table and immediately remove the bird and thrust it at the veterinarian, or worse still, allow it to climb on their shoulder. Birds have a survival instinct to look fit and normal, so can give misleading signals. Allowing the bird to relax and settle may reveal useful diagnostic signs.

Clinical history

While allowing the bird to settle, the veterinarian should be questioning the owner to establish the answers to the following points:

1. Are we dealing with a collection of birds, or an individual? Group species such as waterfowl, pigeons and doves, aviary parakeets or breeding parrots may have intrinsic monetary value (top racing pigeons, some macaws and cockatoos), or rarity value (mutation parakeets, rare poultry breeds). Many of these may be considered domesticated, modified genetically from their wild ancestors (ornamental poultry and doves, canaries and parakeets). Avian medicine in these species is often administered on a flock basis, with preventative treatments (vaccinations in pigeons and poultry; anthelmintics in many species) and the sacrificing of an individual bird for post-mortem examination being commonplace.

   Individual pet birds may have a high monetary value, but usually also a very high emotional attachment. These are family members (and often child replacements) with names and individual characters. At the same time, since most such birds are psittacine species, they are not genetically far removed from their free-living ancestors, and as

such may be subject to considerable behavioural and mental problems resulting from their confined lifestyle coupled with owners' ignorance of their needs and behaviour patterns. Other pet birds would include canaries and mynahs.

   Veterinarians will also be called upon to examine and treat wild native birds, generally 'abandoned' fledglings, or accident cases (Fig. 3.6). A broad knowledge of the species found in the area is useful, together with handling techniques, dietary requirements, and liaison with the local wildlife rehabilitation centre.

2. The species and numbers of birds involved. As stated before, we are dealing with a very large number of different species, and there are disease conditions that may affect one type and not another – for example species-specific viruses like duck viral enteritis. If many birds are affected, we may be dealing with a contagious disease or an environmental toxin, whereas a single isolated pet is more likely to be suffering from a dietary-, age- or husbandry-related condition.

3. Are the birds housed outside or indoors? Outdoor aviary or enclosure birds will be exposed to intestinal parasites and infectious diseases carried by wild birds, to predator attack as well as to environmental factors such as bonfire or barbecue smoke. Indoor birds may be exposed to cooking

fumes, cigarette smoke or an excessively dry atmosphere, the possibility of toxic houseplants, plus the effect of other household members such as children and mammalian pets.

4. How long have the birds been owned, and were they imported or bred in captivity? If newly purchased, they may be suffering from stress-induced exacerbation of subclinical infections such as chlamydophilosis ('psittacosis'), or carrying other infectious diseases such as salmonellosis or polyomavirus. Newly imported birds especially could be infected with *Salmonella*, *Chlamydophila*, or viruses such as Pacheco's disease in parrots. Long-established birds are *more* likely to be suffering illness resulting from management, environment, or diet, although the veterinarian must check the possibility of recent contact with other birds (such as pet-shop visits, or boarding during holidays). One should also be aware that many infectious conditions such as chlamydophilosis, psittacine beak and feather disease (PBFD), or proventricular dilatation disease (PDS) have a long incubation period or can remain dormant for many months.

5. What is the age of the bird? All animals will have disease syndromes that will affect only infant, juvenile, adolescent, adult or geriatric individuals, and birds are no exception. Young birds of many species may be determined by eye colour (grey irises in young African grey parrots or large macaws, becoming yellow with adulthood) (Figs 3.7, 3.8, 3.9, 3.10); plumage (bald eagles (Figs 3.11, 3.12), many thrushes); cere colour (budgerigars) (see Fig. 3.15); beak shape, colour, and proportions (macaws (Figs 3.9, 3.10), eclectus parrots). Many birds are fitted with a closed leg

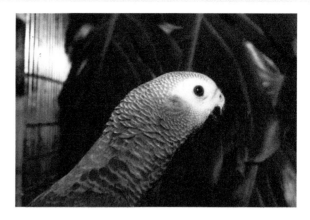

Fig 3.8 Juvenile grey parrot, showing grey iris. Both this bird and the one in Fig. 3.7 show white facial skin.

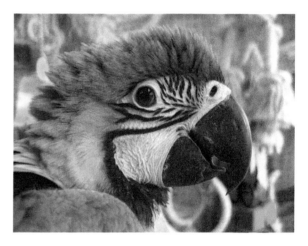

Fig 3.9 Juvenile blue and gold macaw, showing grey iris, round head, small maxillary beak, white facial skin and facial feather lines.

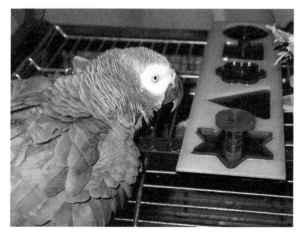

Fig 3.7 Adult grey parrot, showing yellow iris. Also defensive posture, with neck feathers raised.

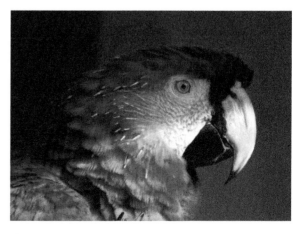

Fig 3.10 Very old scarlet macaw showing yellow iris with pigment spots, unsheathed head feathers, proportionally larger maxillary beak, with groove resulting from chronic nasal discharge.

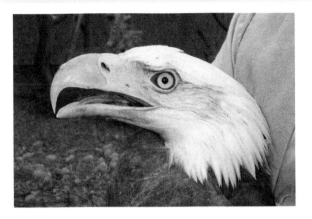

Fig 3.11 Adult bald eagle, with all head feathers white, yellow iris, yellow beak.

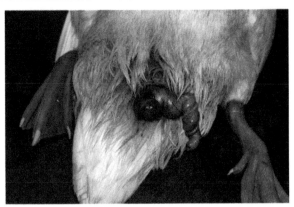

Fig 3.13 Prolapsed phallus in male duck.

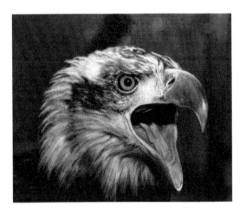

Fig 3.12 Juvenile bald eagle, brown feathers in head, darker iris and beak. Also shows epiglottis at base of tongue and feathers raised in threat.

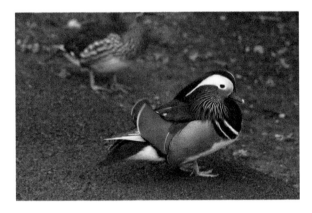

Fig 3.14 Obvious plumage dimorphism in mandarin ducks, the male being flamboyantly coloured.

ring (band) a few days after hatching, which will carry the year of hatch as a suffix (see Fig. 3.28). Once reaching sexual maturity, most birds change little in the adult years (although many birds have different plumage in and out of the breeding season), until signs of old age become evident. These may include senile cataracts, arthritis (evidenced by difficulty in manoeuvring and hence reduction in preening), pigment spots in the iris (Fig. 3.10), and general coarsening of the scales on feet and legs. Further details with reference to psittacine species are given in Chapter 7.

6. What is the sex of the bird? Obviously conditions relating to egg production can only occur in females, while sex-related aggression, masturbation and prolapse of the phallus (Fig. 3.13) in those species that have this organ (ducks and geese) will be found in males. Birds are broadly divisible into sexually *dimorphic*,

where male and female are visibly different; or *monomorphic*, where the sexes appear identical. (At least to the human eye: birds' ability to perceive colours at the ultraviolet end of the spectrum probably means that there are subtle differences in appearance of plumage or skin not visible to us.) Monomorphic species (this would include most commonly kept parrots) will require scientific techniques to determine their sex: either endoscopy ('surgical sexing'), or DNA analysis of a blood or feather sample.

Dimorphic species may be so by virtue of plumage differences (obvious in most ducks (Fig. 3.14), game birds and eclectus parrots, more subtle in others such as ring-necked parakeets and cockatiels); cere colour (budgerigars) (Fig. 3.15) or size (swans); or body weight (many birds of prey); eye colour (white cockatoos) (Fig. 3.16). Some of these differences are obvious at an early

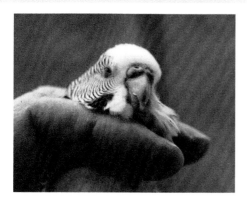

Fig 3.15 Blue cere in male budgerigar. Also showing hand position for restraint, and blood streak in beak, usually indicative of liver disease.

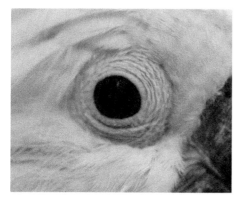

Fig 3.16 Red iris colour in adult female sulphur-crested cockatoo. External opening to ear canal just visible through feathers on side of face.

age (plumage colour in eclectus parrots being primarily red in the hen and green in the cock is evident as soon as the chick fledges), while most show only at sexual maturity.

An indication of the bird's sex may also be given by behavioural characters such as singing and displaying, defending territory, nest building and decoration, although some species knowledge is required to recognize these more subtle signs.

7. What is the bird's diet? It is important to establish not only what the owner *gives* to the bird, but also how much of this the bird *actually eats* (see also below). Ask the owner to bring along samples of the food and any supplements given. Have there been any recent changes to the diet or the source of supply? Are the supplements appropriate for birds, or are they intended for dogs, cats or humans? Is the food being properly stored, with regard to possible contamination by

vermin, becoming overheated, or kept past its 'best by' date? So many disease conditions we see in birds are the result of inadequate, unbalanced, deficient or downright dangerous dietary items, that this provides a good opportunity to discuss with the client their feeding regimen. The veterinarian or practice nurse should point out the dangers of inappropriate food items such as junk food and avocado, alcohol and chocolate, especially in pet parrots (Lawton 2000).

Examination of the transport container

If the normal 'living accommodation' of the bird is produced, an opportunity is provided to assess its suitability or otherwise, and to check the size and types of perches and food and water containers (Lawton 2000). This allows an assessment of the level of hygiene, the knowledge of the owner, diet provision and water availability. The food present helps to confirm the owner's description of the diet offered. Many owners believe the bird is eating exactly what they give the bird, but many birds are selective feeders and will search through the container and discard what is not liked on to the bottom of the cage. As discussed above and elsewhere in this volume, imbalance or deficiency in the diet is a cause of many disease problems in birds, especially parrots (Lawton 2000). **Budgerigars with megabacteriosis or trichomoniasis may spend hours over their food bowls apparently eating seed, but in fact have difficulty in prehending and dehusking the seed, so end up eating very little, losing weight, and dropping whole seeds back in the bowl or on the floor.**

Unsuitable toys may cause trauma, gastrointestinal obstruction or even toxicosis. If the cage is custom-made bear in mind the possibility of 'new cage' disease, which is associated with zinc toxicity and is more likely to occur when galvanized wire has been used. Most countries will also have their own legislation about cage sizes, usually with regard to wing span (Lawton 2000).

This time may be used to advantage to assess the owner's knowledge and abilities in aviculture, and where necessary provide advice and further education. The preparation of practice handouts on various aspects of bird care is valuable.

Examination of the bird's droppings

Many important aspects of a bird's health may be assessed from a thorough inspection of its droppings (Lawton 2000). Birds defecate frequently, and can almost be guaranteed to oblige when stressed or excited, so will undoubtedly produce a sample whilst discussing the history and management. Owners may be advised to place a sheet of white paper or plastic film in the floor of the carrier to collect a sample uncontaminated with other cage coverings such as shavings.

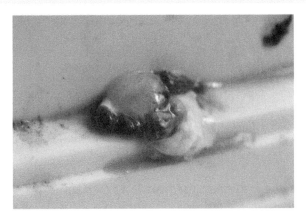

Fig 3.17 Fledgling bird (magpie) dropping, showing white urate, brown faecal component and mucous sac.

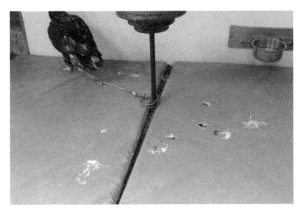

Fig 3.19 Raptor dropping, showing higher proportion of urate and liquid, the urate in this case stained green.

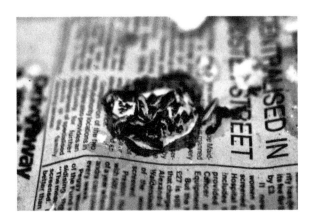

Fig 3.18 Normal parrot dropping, showing white urate, dark faecal material and some liquid urine.

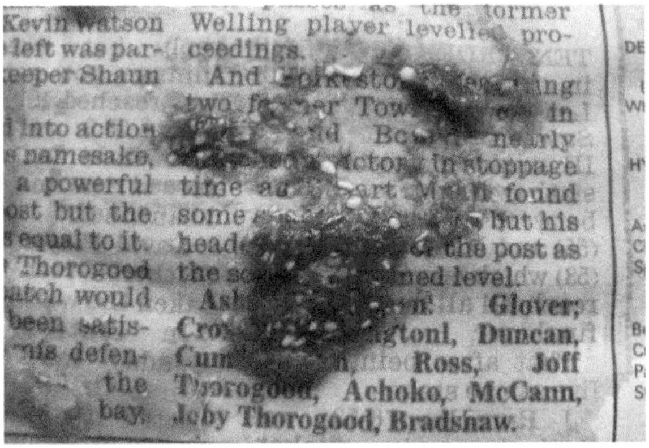

Fig 3.20 Droppings containing pepper seeds and coloured red with pepper content.

In common with reptiles, birds produce a 'dropping' formed of combined waste from the bowel (faeces) together with waste from the kidneys (urates and urine) (Figs 3.17, 3.18, 3.19). The relative proportion, colour, consistency and quantities of these components will vary considerably between species, diet consumed, time of day or state of breeding cycle, and various disease processes. A sound knowledge of the *normal* appearance and the reasons for normal variation is therefore important before suggestions may be made as to the cause of abnormalities. There is often a mucous sac encasing the whole dropping, especially evident in nestlings, which enables the parent bird easily to remove the whole dropping from the nest site (Fig. 3.17).

Faeces should be formed and uniform in character, with no obvious blood or undigested food (Lawton 2000). The colour, volume and consistency will vary with the species and with dietary content and composition. They will be dry and almost black in small seed-eating species from arid areas, such as budgerigars, through dark green in seed-eating parrots, to brown with a protein-rich diet (raptors), and very pale and liquid in fruit and nectar feeders. Pigments from food items will colour both faeces and urates – e.g. black- or blueberries, beetroot, pepper seeds (Fig. 3.20). The presence of blood is always important (Lawton 2000), and can signify gastrointestinal disease (enteritis, neoplasia etc.), renal disease, testicular or ovarian tumours, coagulopathies, cloacal papillomata, calculus, cloacitis or other cloacal pathology, oviduct abnormalities (pre- or post-egg laying), liver disease, heavy metal toxicity or malnutrition. Acute haemorrhagic syndrome should be considered in Amazon species. Dark, digested blood (melaena) (Fig. 3.21) suggests haemorrhage higher in the digestive tract, while fresh red blood will appear from the distal bowel or cloaca.

If the faeces are clay-coloured, this may indicate maldigestion or malabsorption. Kaolin medication or a barium meal, however, may also cause this appearance.

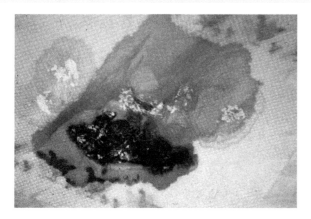

Fig 3.21 Droppings showing melaena – partially digested blood in the faecal component.

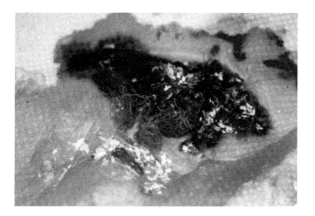

Fig 3.22 Droppings from a roseate cockatoo containing many nematode worms.

Large intestinal parasites such as roundworms or tapeworm segments may be voided and will be obvious (Fig. 3.22).

Faecal volume is a useful indicator of the state of health:

1. Reduced faecal volume usually indicates a decreased food intake, a decreased gastrointestinal transit time or food deprivation. This should be distinguished from small dry faeces, which are usually associated with water deprivation or liver disease.

2. **Voluminous faeces can be normal and occur in situations where there is a high vegetable or fluid content in the diet. However, any cause of malabsorption (e.g. gastrointestinal disease, pancreatitis, parasitism, peritonitis, diabetes, renal disease or neoplasia, or liver disease) can also cause an increase in bulk. The presence of any undigested food (to be differentiated from regurgitation) is** *always* **abnormal and**

is an indication for further investigation and confirmation of malabsorption, maldigestion, hypermotility (due to inflammation, infection or parasitism), pancreatitis, proventriculitis or ventriculitis, or proventricular dilatation syndrome/disease (PDS/PDD). (Lawton 2000).

The quantity is increased in the first void of the day, following overnight accumulation, and also in mature egg-laying hen birds, since the cloaca is expanded and will hold more. The hen will retain droppings while sitting on the nest, and void an enlarged quantity when she moves. The faecal component may be loose or even absent at times of stress such as travelling, or following handling and medication.

It is a simple matter to examine a fresh faecal sample under the practice microscope:

- A wet preparation should be checked for motile protozoa.
- A flotation technique may be used for the identification of parasite ova or coccidia.
- A Gram's-stained sample should be examined for bacteria, fungi, yeasts and anti-inflammatory cells (Lawton 2000). Faecal samples are seldom worth culturing, but a Gram's stain will yield an assessment of the number of bacteria present and whether there are predominantly Gram-positive or Gram-negative organisms (Harrison & Ritchie 1994, p. 151).

Faecal samples can also be tested for evidence of chlamydial shedding, and this should be undertaken for all sick birds (Lawton 2000).

Urates are normally white or cream in colour, but may absorb blue or purple pigments from dietary items. There is a higher urate content in birds eating a high protein diet, such as birds of prey (Fig. 3.19). Any green or yellow coloration indicates the presence of bile pigments such as biliverdin, and will be associated with haemolysis, hepatitis or renal disease. Such disease may result from malnutrition, toxic damage, neoplasia, or chlamydial, bacterial or viral infections. **The presence of green urate is always an indicator for further diagnostic tests.** A total *absence* of urates may also indicate liver or kidney disease (Lawton 2000).

Liquid urine is present in all bird droppings, but may be in infinitesimal quantities in seed-eating birds from arid areas. Conversely, there will be a normal large volume in nectar feeders and waterbirds. Increased volume over what is normal for the species may be produced in a number of situations, and is usually linked to increased drinking – polyuria and polydipsia (PUPD). Polyuria may be *physiological* or *pathological* (Box 3.1).

The urine fraction is easily examined on an impervious surface as soon as possible after being passed, using

Box 3.1 Causes of PUPD

Physiological causes of PUPD

- Stress – handling and examination
- Travelling
- High environmental temperature

Pathological causes of PUPD

- *Primary* – renal failure

  Infection

  Neoplasia

  Toxins

- *Secondary* – diabetes mellitus or insipidus

  Pituitary disease

  Adrenal disease

  Iatrogenic

     Corticosteroids

     Progestogens

     Aminoglycosides

  Calcium imbalance

  Hypovitaminosis A

  Hypervitaminosis D

  Excess dietary salt

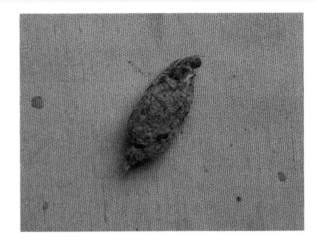

Fig 3.23 Pellet regurgitated by tawny owl, containing fur, feather, small bone fragments and beetle exoskeletons.

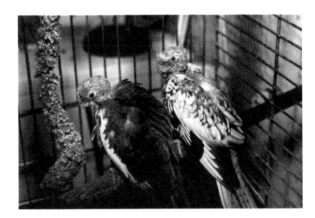

Fig 3.24 Nestling cockatiels with heads and necks plucked by frustrated parents wanting to start another breeding cycle.

standard dip sticks. Microscopic examination may follow, looking for crystals or abnormal cells.

Pellets are regurgitated by birds of prey, comprising indigestible portions of hair, feather, or bone from their prey. These may also be examined for the presence of abnormal contents, excessive blood or mucus, or parasites (Fig. 3.23).

While taking the history, talking with the owner, and examining the cage, the veterinarian should be observing the bird. As it begins to relax in the consulting (examination) room after the journey, it may show signs that were masked in its earlier stressed state. These may include lifting of a leg or drooping of a wing, closing of an eye, open-beaked breathing, sneezing, coughing or retching, dyschezia; excessive preening or scratching, etc., all of which may give pointers to the underlying problem.

Once again, knowledge of what is *normal* for the bird is essential before one can investigate something *abnormal*. Many birds pant or hold their wings away from the body when hot; young birds or inferior birds in a group may have head and neck feathers plucked out by parents or dominant companions (Fig. 3.24). Birds that are aggressive or fearful will constrict and dilate their pupils (this is striated muscle under voluntary control), fan their tail feathers, or raise their wings and head/neck feathers in order to appear larger than they really are (Figs 3.7, 3.12, 3.25).

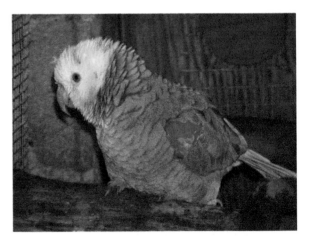

Fig 3.25 Yellow-headed Amazon showing threat display, with ruffled neck feathers, constricted pupils, and fanned tail. (Photo: Jan Hooimeier.)

The importance of taking a full history cannot be over-emphasized. The information obtained and the observations of the bird and its surroundings as discussed above may result in 50% or more of the diagnostic detail. The veterinarian may have sufficient information to make a presumptive diagnosis at this point, and should certainly have an idea about the course of the examination, any required diagnostic tests, and a possible treatment regimen.

The physical examination

Having established all the above background information and mentally planned a possible diagnostic and treatment protocol, the patient at last needs to be examined. As with any veterinary examination, this should proceed in a systematic fashion, so that nothing is missed or neglected. All doors and windows should be closed, and staff warned not to enter the room, and extractor fans should be turned off, *before* removing the patient from its container. Dimmed or subdued lighting may make the catching of a small, nervous diurnal bird easier. All necessary equipment and possible medications should be prepared and to hand, together with appropriate handling materials. Stout gloves are essential when handling larger raptors, to protect the handler against their talons, but these are *not* suitable for passerine or psittacine species. They do not allow sensitivity of touch, so the handler will be unaware of the pressure applied, and will not be able to palpate parts of the patient. They will also make such birds subsequently hand-shy.

The examination should be as brief as possible, while still being thorough. This is especially important in dyspnoeic birds, where handling time should be minimal, allowing the bird to rest and recover if necessary before proceeding with the next stage. The previous history-taking and observation of the patient will prepare the veterinarian for the important features of examination, diagnostic sampling and initial therapy. Although it is possible for a small bird to die in the hand, this should really only occur with an extremely sick or dyspnoeic bird. The most common reason for a bird to die during handling by an inexperienced veterinarian is the method of restraint, which results in the inability of the bird to move its keel and thus prevents adequate respiration.

Do not refer to books in front of the client at this stage – it will not inspire confidence! Research may be done before the scheduled appointment, or the bird may be admitted 'for further investigation' to allow necessary consultation with literature or more experienced colleagues.

There is no secret to the successful examination, recognition and diagnosis of diseases or injury in birds (Lawton 2000). Once the bird is restrained, the clinical examination should be carried out in exactly the same way as with a cat or dog. A methodical approach must

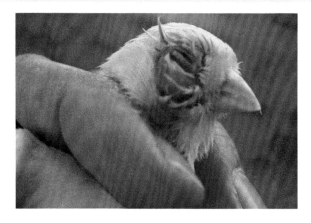

Fig 3.26 Canary showing suborbital swelling resulting from sinus infection. Also shows handling technique.

be employed, starting with the head and working down the body. Once the clinician is experienced at examining birds, it should take no more than 3–4 minutes. All parts of the body should, where relevant, be symmetrical; one side should always be compared with the other.

The head

The eyes, sinuses and rhinarium are all anatomically interrelated, hence infection of any one may lead to or be indicative of infection in all three. The eyes should be clear, round, centrally placed, moist and shining, with no epiphora or ocular discharge or caking around the eyelids. There should be evidence of normal tear production. An abnormal tear film could indicate xerophthalmia associated with hypovitaminosis A. There should be no evidence of periocular or periorbital swellings (Fig. 3.26). Swelling medial to the eye may be associated with a primary sinusitis; swellings above or below the eye are usually associated with hypovitaminosis A, and sterile inspissated material with squamous cell metaplasia of the lacrimal glandular epithelial tissues. Any swelling should be investigated further by taking swabs, a needle biopsy or flushings to submit for cytology, bacteriology or histopathology. A routine examination with an ophthalmoscope should disclose abnormalities of the lens or the cornea; however, assessment of fundic lesions requires more experience.

The nares should be clear and open, with a centrally placed shiny operculum. The shape does vary with the species being examined, and in some it may not be possible to visualize the operculum. Discharge, occlusion or rhinoliths may be present (chlamydophilosis is always a differential diagnosis). Any rhinoliths should be removed for a further examination of the nares and the taking of samples, if considered necessary. Any abnormal discharge from the nostrils warrants further sampling for cytology and culture and sensitivity as required. The cere, where present, should show no sign of trauma or excessive scaling as

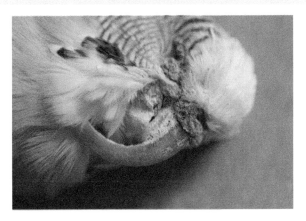

Fig 3.27 Budgerigar showing severe hyperkeratosis and tunnel formation following chronic infestation with the mite *Cnemidocoptes pilae*. The beak is overgrown and the cere is discoloured (compare Fig. 3.15).

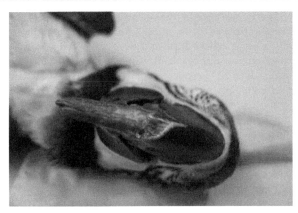

Fig 3.29 Blue and gold macaw beak showing flaking, overgrowth and interlaminar infection, often resulting from chronic nutritional deficiency.

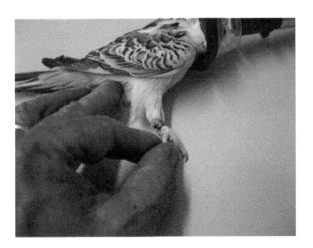

Fig 3.28 Budgerigar leg with aluminium leg ring (band) showing year of hatch, but also hyperkeratosis on leg resulting from cnemidocoptic infection. This will have the effect of constricting blood supply under the ring.

occurs with *Cnemidocoptes* spp. infestation in budgerigars (Figs 3.27, 3.28).

The beak assumes a variety of shapes and colours depending on the type of bird and its diet. In most species it would appear smooth and shiny, but in cockatoos there should be evidence of a white powder down (Fig. 3.16), as excessively shiny beaks may be an indication of lack of down feathers and possibly an early suggestion of psittacine beak and feather disease (Lawton 2000). The maxillary and mandibular portions of the beak should meet evenly. The beak should then be examined for signs of excessive growth or abnormal wear. Cracks in the keratin may be indicative of nutritional deficiencies. Abnormal positioning (malocclusion) of the beak is commonly associated with incorrect diet early in growth, and may require surgical intervention

or lifelong trimming. Aspergillosis and candidiasis of the beak are not uncommon, frequently secondary to vitamin A deficiency (Fig. 3.29).

The beak should then be opened and the mouth examined. The oral cavity is best examined with the assistance of an auriscope operculum, a stainless steel gag (Fig. 3.3), or in small birds a paper clip gag. All areas of the mouth, especially the tongue, sublingual tissues, choana, oral membrane and glottis, should be viewed. In cases of hypovitaminosis A, there may be abscesses on the tongue or between the mandibles; this is particularly common in psittacines. The choana should be clear with no sign of inflammation or discharge (Fig. 3.6). If there is a discharge, samples should be taken for further cytological and microbiological investigation. In pigeons and raptors, any caseous material should be examined as a wet preparation under a microscope to rule out trichomoniasis.

Birds' ears have no pinnae but consist of an auricular opening and aural canal situated ventrocaudal to the lateral canthus (Fig. 3.16). The auricular openings should be assessed for signs of inflammation or discharge. Clinical problems are usually polyps, neoplasia or infections (Lawton 2000).

At this time, the feathers on the rest of the head should also be examined and assessed. Abnormalities of the head feathers in a bird with body feather abnormalities indicate it is not a behavioural problem, and suggest that further investigation should be undertaken. In many species, the presence of large amounts of unsheathed pinfeathers could indicate a very sick bird that is not grooming itself, or problems such as arthritis that make grooming difficult (Fig. 3.10).

Birds with no facial feathering such as macaws and grey parrots may show bruising easily if handled roughly or for long periods, and the owner should be warned of this possibility (Figs 3.7, 3.8, 3.9).

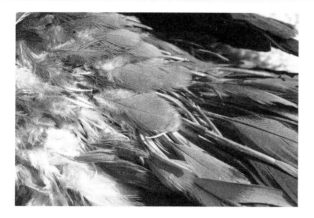

Fig 3.30 Poor feather quality and persistent quill sheaths in an Amazon parrot, the result of severe and long-term nutritional imbalance (cf. retained sheaths because of inability to preen in old macaw, Fig. 3.10).

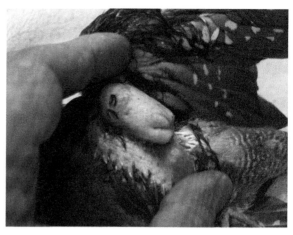

Fig 3.31 Xanthoma under wing of cockatiel.

The neck

The neck should be examined systematically and always palpated (especially on the right side) for any abnormal swellings, including distension of the crop (in birds where this is present). The oesophagus should be palpated and the mucosal thickness assessed. To aid examination, the overlying skin can be wetted with surgical spirit and, if necessary, transilluminated; alternatively, endoscopy can be performed. If on palpation regurgitation occurs, the material should be examined microscopically as a wet preparation for the presence of protozoa. Trichomonads are particularly common in budgerigars. If no protozoa are revealed, a Gram's-stained slide should be examined for evidence of megabacteriosis.

The limbs

The wings should be stretched out to assess mobility, and should be of even length. There should be no drooping at rest. If there is any drooping then radiographs should be taken to assess the shoulder joint, clavicular, coracoid and scapular bones. The feathers should be examined for signs of damage or loss. The carpal areas should be free of trauma or swelling. Any white or yellowish swelling of the wing joints should be treated as suspected gout, and appropriate blood samples obtained to assess the uric acid, calcium and phosphorus levels. Other conditions causing swelling of the wings include xanthomatosis (yellow fatty swelling) (Fig. 3.31) and wing tip oedema in birds of prey.

The keel musculature should then be assessed, as this is an indication of body condition. Different species will normally have varying degrees of pectoral covering over their sternum (keel). The clinician should be familiar with expected degrees of pectoral mass for the species being examined. Ratites (rheas, emus and ostriches) have very little musculature here; racing pigeons are

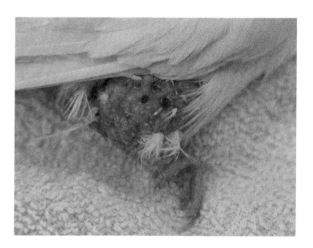

Fig 3.32 Xanthoma on leg of budgerigar.

well muscled. Domestic backyard poultry have much less pectoral muscle than the familiar chicken reared for the table. Loss of condition will give some indication of the severity and chronicity of the process. All patients should be routinely weighed and recorded at each consultation, as this provides baseline data for that individual. In obese birds the keel bone will not easily be felt and the skin may assume a yellowish tinge, which is associated with subcutaneous fat deposition or, in extreme cases, xanthomata (Figs 3.31, 3.32). In birds with a very prominent keel, this could be an indication of poor condition or underlying disease. Due to the presence of the feathers, it is often possible for a bird to lose substantial weight without this change becoming obvious to the owner. All birds should be scanned at this time to assess if a microchip is present.

The legs should then be examined, and particular attention paid to the joints of the digits so that lesions suspicious of articular gout may be identified (Fig. 3.33).

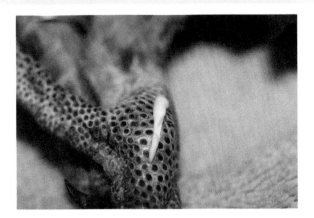

Fig 3.33 Articular gout in a grey parrot. There is obvious swelling over the joint, and the skin has been excised to expose the urate deposits.

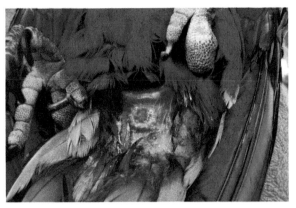

Fig 3.34 Cloacal papilloma in a green-winged macaw. Stainless steel leg band also visible.

There should be no sign of self-mutilation or pain on extension or flexion of these limbs. Any abnormalities or swellings require radiographic evaluation and further investigation. The plantar aspect of the foot should be examined for signs of bumblefoot, calluses or excessive wear. Raptors, waterfowl and cockatiels appear to be particularly prone to bumblefoot associated with incorrect environment or perches. Any rings present should be noted and checked to ensure that they are freely movable on the leg and there is no build-up of keratin under the ring that could eventually lead to constriction of the blood supply (Fig. 3.28).

The body

The abdomen should then be palpated for signs of abnormalities or swellings (especially in females). If there is a swelling of the abdomen, it should be established if this is fluid or a solid mass. If there is fluid, then aspiration and examination of the fluid is indicated. Any other abnormalities should be investigated using radiography or endoscopy.

Examination of the cloaca can often reveal signs not evident on examination of the faeces. Chronic soiling of the vent plumage may be caused by cloacitis, cloacal uroliths, cloacal papillomata, diarrhoea, polydipsia, etc. Following gentle eversion, the cloacal mucosa can be examined for signs of papillomata (Fig. 3.34). Digital examination through the cloaca may also be useful, especially in larger birds, for palpation of the kidneys. Endoscopy may be useful for the further investigation, or samples may be collected using a cloacal swab. Owners should be warned that after such sampling, the bird is likely to pass blood-streaked droppings for up to 24 hours.

Prior to turning the bird over, the pectoral and abdominal areas should be auscultated with a stethoscope. Auscultation is relatively unrewarding in avian patients. Very few sounds are heard over the abdominal area, unless there is an air sacculitis. The heart can also be assessed, although the rapid heart rate usually makes it difficult to distinguish murmurs unless they are severe. The heart is better assessed by an electrocardiogram (ECG) (100 mm/second paper speed is required) or heart monitor, should the clinical history or physical examination indicate a possible cardiovascular problem.

On turning the bird over, the lungs should be further evaluated by placing the stethoscope diaphragm between the wings; this is usually the best area for listening to the lungs. The lung field of birds is small and fixed compared to that of mammals. It is often possible to hear a faint short inspiratory noise in the normal bird. If other noises are heard they are likely to be associated with diseases of the nares or sinuses, restricted airflow in the trachea (e.g. syringeal aspergilloma) or severe air sac disease (always suspect chlamydophilosis or aspergillosis). Upper respiratory disease should be clinically differentiable from air sac disease. If the latter is suspected, radiography and endoscopy are indicated. If air sacculitis is present and endoscopy is performed, an air sac swab or biopsy should be taken for bacteriology, histopathology, cytology or ELISA. Any bird showing respiratory signs should always be screened for chlamydophilosis.

The back and tail base should then be examined. The uropygial (preen) gland is present and well developed in most species, but is absent in some others (e.g. Amazons). It is situated on the dorsal body wall, immediately anterior to the insertion of the central tail feathers. The gland is responsible for producing the oil used during preening to assist with feather condition and waterproofing. When present, the gland should be symmetrical and smooth, and it should be possible to express a small volume of oily secretion. Birds can suffer from dysfunction, abscessation or neoplasia of the gland (Fig. 3.35).

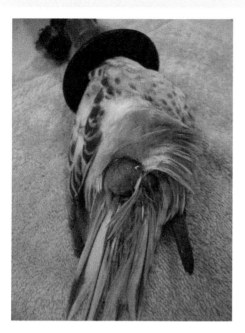

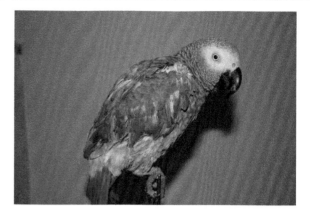

Fig 3.36 Grey parrot showing abnormal pink, stunted feathers associated with infection with psittacine beak and feather disease (PBFD) virus.

Fig 3.35 Budgerigar showing enlarged uropygial (preen) gland on dorsal tail base. Possibly infected, may be obstructed, cyst or tumour. Also shows anaesthetic face mask and towel for warmth.

Plumage and skin

Throughout the whole of the physical examination, the condition of the feathers and skin should be assessed for any signs of abnormality or loss. The condition of the plumage and skin may give clues as to the overall health of the bird (Fig. 3.30) or if there is evidence of underlying disease such as PBFD (Fig. 3.36), hepatopathy or nutritional deficiencies (essential amino acids or vitamin A). Feathers vary at different sites of the body. Over the head, trunk and limbs they are known as general feathers, while those found over the wings and tail are flight feathers. A basic understanding of a normal feather is required in order to assess any abnormal feathers (Jones 1998). All feathers emerge from the skin as a calamus or quill. The shaft (or rachis) is the main body of the feather; fine branches (barbs) arise from the shaft at 45° on either side and from these barbs smaller branches (barbules) arise at an angle of 45°. Flight feather barbules are locked together by small hooks, resulting in a flat, firm feather. If the barbules are not locked together, then the feather appears as a 'fluffy' feather. Powder is produced by disintegration of the tips of the powder down feathers. This powder helps to make the rest of the feathers waterproof, and also helps to lubricate them. At the time of examination, check for the presence of new growing (pin) feathers (Fig. 3.10). If they are present, then it is unlikely that a hormonal disturbance is the cause of any feather loss. New growing feathers show that the normal feather growth cycle is active following feather loss or moults.

Feather loss is one of the most common reasons for bringing pet birds (especially psittacines) to the veterinary surgeon. At the time of examination it should be established whether the feather loss is throughout the body or confined to certain areas. The areas that are showing signs of feather loss must be carefully examined for signs of damage or deformity to the remaining feathers. Signs of trauma to the feathers or the skin are often associated with neurosis and self-inflicted mutilation. Deformation of feathers, however, can be associated with viral infection or nutritional problems. Where there is damage to the skin, this should be assessed to determine whether it is self-inflicted or due to parasitic or infectious causes (see later). In behavioural feather plucking, the head is likely to show normal feathering while the rest of the body shows varying degrees of feather loss or damage.

If there is generalized feather loss with deformed feathers in psittacine birds (especially cockatoos), which also involves the head, the papovavirus associated with psittacine feather and beak disease (PFBD) should be suspected (Fig. 3.36). Diagnosis is by a PCR test on a blood sample, examination of a biopsy specimen or electron microscopy of a plucked feather (some epithelial tissue should still be attached to the feather follicle to allow examination of macrophages for the viral intranuclear inclusion bodies).

Owners often consider parasites to be the cause of any feather loss. In single pet birds, which have not had recent contact with other birds, this is an unlikely possibility. They are, however, common in poultry, pigeons, raptors and canaries. Where parasites are suspected, it is a good idea to use some form of magnification to examine the bird's skin and feathers. Only on finding a parasite (or the type of pathology associated with a particular parasite) can a diagnosis of parasitism be made (Fig. 3.37). The parasite *Cnemidocoptes pilae* produces

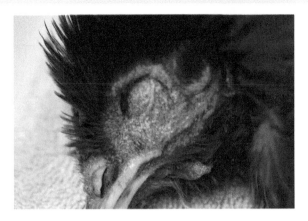

Fig 3.37 Hyperkeratosis on the face of a chicken produced in response to louse infestation. Needs to be differentiated from dermatomycosis.

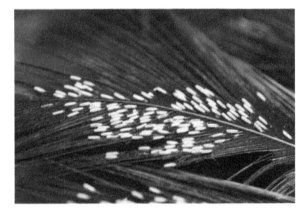

Fig 3.38 Eggs of lice on vulture feathers.

classic hyperkeratosis of the skin and excessive scaliness, usually around the beak and eyes or legs and feet (Figs 3.27, 3.28), and results in a substantial feather loss. While *C. pilae* is the most common species of this mite found, passerines may be infested with *Cnemidocoptes mutans* or *Cnemidocoptes jamaicensis*, and *C. laevis* is the depluming mite of parrots (especially macaws). Other parasites that may be found include the quill mites (*Syringophilus bipectinatus* and *Dermoglyphys elongatus*), which destroy feathers early in development. These may also cause dermal cysts. The mites are easily seen, as they are quite large and deposit their eggs along the feather shaft (Fig. 3.38).

The red mite (*Dermanyssus gallinae*) is not usually found on the bird during the physical examination, as it feeds only at night. During the day the mite lives within the cage in recesses or even under droppings. Diagnosis during the day requires very careful examination of the cage. Nocturnal examination of the bird may demonstrate the mite, but is not normally appreciated by the veterinarian! Even if the mite is not visible, there are often signs of pruritus and restlessness in the bird.

Lice are commonly found on raptors, poultry, pigeons and waterfowl. Ticks may be found on aviary-dwelling birds, and may cause sudden death, especially in parakeets.

Whenever there are any noted abnormalities of the skin, biopsy samples may be helpful. They should always be full thickness and include one or two feather follicles. Although routine H&E staining, and light-microscopic examination are helpful, electron microscopy is necessary for diagnosing viral causes. Bacterial skin infection or folliculitis is less common; however, it can be diagnosed on examination of biopsy specimens or a Gram's stain of the feather pulp.

Dermatophytes (mainly *Miscrosporum gallinae*) may also be encountered in fowl (Galliformes) (Fig. 3.37), ducks (Anseriformes), pigeons (Columbiformes), but are very rare. Lesions are limited to fleshy or thin-skinned areas of the head, and are seen as scabs, crust or alopecia. *Candida albicans* can cause similar lesions. Microscopic examination of skin scrapings gives a definitive diagnosis.

Grooming

It is at this stage of the examination in pet birds that grooming techniques of wing clipping and nail or beak trimming, where appropriate or requested by the client, may be carried out. **These apparently simple procedures are in fact fraught with pitfalls, and successful, skilful, stress-free grooming of pet birds can make the reputation of an avian veterinarian, while conversely faulty technique will ensure that the client never returns! Clipping of the wrong wing feathers so that the bird can still fly after the event; the bird being returned to the owner with bleeding claws or beak; or owner, veterinarian and staff being bitten are all commonplace, but undesirable scenarios in inexperienced practices.** Greater detail of techniques is given in AAV articles on wing clipping (Jones 1996).

On beaks and claws, appropriate clippers may be used, and finer finish is provided by a Dremel tool. With the aid of an experienced avian veterinary technician, this procedure may be accomplished in most birds in a few minutes with the patient manually restrained (Fig. 3.39). However, if the bird is excitable and nervous, or if the work required is more extensive owing to deformity or neglect, it is perfectly acceptable to anaesthetize the bird for a short period (see following section) in order to accomplish the procedure more efficiently.

The correction of more significant beak deformities is dealt with elsewhere in this volume.

Sampling techniques

Diagnostic samples may be taken in the form of swabs from eyes, nares, choana, throat or cloaca. Blood samples may be taken easily from the ulnar vein (Fig. 3.40); the jugular vein (Fig. 3.41) – especially accessible in

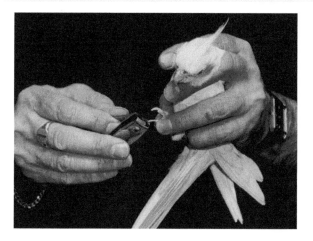

Fig 3.39 Clipping the claws of a cockatiel.

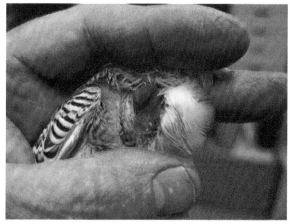

Fig 3.41 Demonstrating the prominent right jugular vein in the neck of a budgerigar.

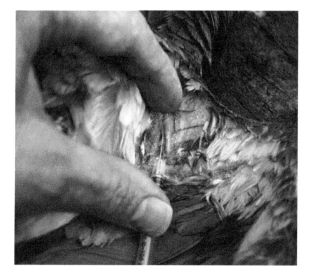

Fig 3.40 Taking a blood sample from the ulnar vein.

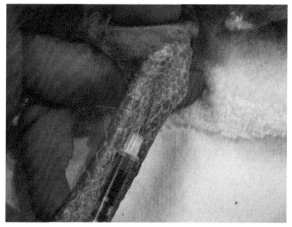

Fig 3.42 Taking a blood sample from the median metatarsal vein.

small birds, **and more prominent on the right side than on the left;** or the median metatarsal vein in waterfowl (Fig. 3.42).

Basic anaesthesia

Modern anaesthetic agents have made the anaesthesia of birds a safe and uneventful procedure. This has allowed longer and more adventurous surgical procedures to be developed, and it is also a legitimate tool to make diagnostic sampling, radiography, or grooming simpler, quicker, and less damaging to all parties.

The progression from halothane to isoflurane and recently sevofl unne has greatly increased the safety margin, and any practice that still uses halothane only should not consider itself equipped to deal with birds.

Halothane, although available in most veterinary practices, has a lower safety margin (3.0) than isoflurane (5.7) and is contraindicated in birds with underlying hepatopathies (a common finding), as well as being more depressive on respiration and of lower analgesic potential than isoflurane (Lawton 2000). The main advantages of isoflurane are two-fold:

- The low blood gas partition coefficient (1.4 at 37°C) means that there is a low solubility of isoflurane in blood and tissues, which leads to a rapid induction and recovery due to less retention following tissue distribution.
- The low metabolism (0.3%) speeds up the elimination of isoflurane from the body solely by expiration and without the production of potentially toxic metabolite products that can cause a hangover effect (Lawton 2000).

The unique avian anatomy and physiology should be understood (see Chapter 2), as these affect anaesthesia and (should the need arise) the emergency procedures necessary for resuscitation. The aims of anaesthesia should be to provide a smooth, reliable induction with adequate restraint, muscle relaxation and analgesia, followed by a fast, full, uneventful recovery (Lawton 1996a, 1996b).

Induction and maintenance (Lawton 2000)

The use of a dedicated vaporizer is recommended for all volatile anaesthetics to allow an exact concentration to be given, immaterial of temperature or air pressure, within certain ranges. It is not possible to use the same vaporizer for both halothane and isoflurane due to the differences in these volatile fluids, unless the vaporizer is cleaned and recalibrated prior to each change.

Isoflurane allows a relatively easy method of induction by face mask (Fig. 3.35) (other than for diving birds, whose breath-holding abilities make such induction tedious), reducing many of the complications of handling and injecting and the stresses that are involved with these procedures. Face masks can be purchased or self-made from disposable items such as syringe cases (for small birds) or soft drink bottles (for macaws or long-beaked birds). The advantage of using disposable face masks is the elimination of the risk of spread of infection between birds; they also often provide a more suitable mask for an avian patient than those currently on the market. If the face mask is not a disposable item, then it is important that it is cleaned well before reusing. A face mask does have disadvantages, especially if examining or operating around the head.

Once induced, it is possible to maintain anaesthesia just with a face mask, although endotracheal intubation should be considered for anything other than the shortest procedure. Intubation of birds is easy, due to the forward placement of the glottis behind the base of the tongue (Fig. 3.12). With the mouth held open and the tongue pulled gently forward, a suitably sized tube can be introduced through the glottis. Various sized endotracheal tubes can be made in the clinic using cut-down urinary or intravenous cannulae or catheters, although small diameter tubes may become blocked with respiratory secretions. Once intubated, a bird should be maintained on a Bethune or Ayre's T-piece system.

An endotracheal tube is likely to restrict access when operating around the beak, head or face. When there is an obstruction, such as that seen with a syringeal foreign body or aspergillic granulomata, intubation may not be adequate for ventilation and maintenance of anaesthesia. In both these situations, the unique air sac system (see Chapter 2) may be utilized to maintain oxygenation and anaesthesia. The site for placement of an air sac tube is one of personal preference, but is usually similar to the site chosen for endoscopic examination. Traditionally this is the left side just behind the ribs, although Sinn (1994) has suggested the insertion of short endotracheal tubes or rubber tubes into the clavicular or caudal thoracic air sacs. The placement of the air sac tube is usually performed after induction by face mask or injection of a suitable anaesthetic agent, although in cases of severe airway obstruction it is possible to place the tube in a physically restrained conscious bird. The placement of the tube in a conscious bird is quick and appears to cause little discomfort or distress; the bird may be restrained with its head in a mask into which 100% oxygen is being delivered (Lawton 1996b). As large a tube as possible (French gauge 14) should be placed and attached to the anaesthetic circuit (see also Chapter 6 and Lawton 2000).

Intermittent positive pressure ventilation (IPPV) via the placed air sac tube or endotracheal tube has a lot of advantages. Birds with air sac intubation will usually stop breathing spontaneously due to the expulsion of all carbon dioxide from the respiratory system (Korbel et al 1993). IPPV for any anaesthetized bird allows not only control of the rate and depth of respiration, but also control of oxygenation and the prevention of hypercapnia. Although a gaseous flow rate of three times the normal minute volume, i.e. approximately 3 mL/g body weight (a 400 g Amazon parrot therefore needs 1.2 L/min) is suggested (Lawton 2000), in practice a standard flow rate of 2–3 L/min irrespective of size is generally adopted. Ventilated birds will not breathe again spontaneously until after perfusion via the air sac is terminated and the blood carbon dioxide levels rise. The tube can be removed postoperatively, or left in situ in cases of dyspnoea (e.g. after surgery to the neck or in cases of aspergillosis plugs of the syrinx).

Alternative injectable anaesthetic agents

Despite the ease and safety of isoflurane anaesthesia, there are occasions when an injectable agent is needed. Such occasions include induction of diving birds, lack of gaseous anaesthetic equipment (such as in the field), and excitability or aggression on handling for face mask induction. In all cases where an injectable agent is to be used, the bird should be accurately weighed. Without a precise weight it is not possible to calculate an accurate dose, and the possibility of an overdose and even a fatality could occur. Suitable injectable agents are listed in Table 3.1.

Anaesthesia monitoring

Despite the safety of isoflurane, there is no excuse for complacency over monitoring during anaesthesia (Lawton 1993). The depth of anaesthesia may only

Table 3.1 Injectable anaesthetic agents

Agent	Dose and route	Comments on use
Alphaxalone/alphadalone	5–10 mg/kg i.v.; 36 mg/kg i.m. or i.p.	A wide safety margin but only a short length of action. Following i.v. administration there is often a transient apnoea
Ketamine	18–50 mg/kg s.c., i.m. or i.v.	Ketamine, historically, was the drug of choice; it is now used less often in avian practice, although it is useful for reducing stress when handling larger species such as swans or other waterfowl. A good sedative but a poor anaesthetic with poor muscle relaxation and little analgesia, although there is little respiratory or cardiovascular depression. There is often wing flapping during recovery, even when used in combination with tranquillizers
Ketamine/diazepam or midazolam	Ketamine 10–30 mg/kg i.v. and diazepam 1–1.5 mg/kg i.m. or 0.2 mg/kg midazolam s.c., i.m.	This combination allows a smooth induction and recovery when compared to ketamine by itself
Ketamine/medetomidine	1.5–2 mg/kg ketamine + 60–85 µg/kg medetomidine i.m. (reversed by atipamezole 250–380 µ/kg i.m.)	Sedative and analgesic properties, with good muscle relaxation but no arrhythmias or respiratory depression. This combination is particularly good in waterfowl
Ketamine/xylazine	4.4 mg/kg ketamine + 2.2 mg/kg xylazine i.v. (reversed by yohimbine 0.1 mg). (Atipamezole 250–380 µg/kg i.m. can be used to reverse the effects of xylazine)	Synergistic action of the combination produces a smooth induction and improved muscle relaxation, without difficulties in recovery due to residual ketamine effect. Unreversed, there is a prolonged recovery and postoperative depression
Propofol	1.33–14 mg/kg i.v.	Very high safety margin and easily metabolized. A smooth rapid induction; good muscle relaxation with a short duration of 2–7 minutes
Tiletamine/zolazepam	5–10 mg/kg i.m.	Tiletamine is more potent than ketamine. Good immobilization
Xylazine	1–20 mg/kg i.m. or i.v. (reversed with yohimbine hydrochloride, 0.1–0.2 mg/kg i.v. or atipamezole 250–380 µg/kg i.m.)	By itself, is unreliable, causes bradycardia and A/V block, and is extremely depressant of the respiratory system

be correctly controlled if the bird is carefully and continuously monitored. Monitoring of birds should be approached in exactly the same way as monitoring of any other species, although it is considered to be more challenging (Flammer 1989).

In any anaesthetized bird, the following should be monitored:

1. *Reflexes* that may be monitored are the palpebral, corneal, cere, toe pinch and wing twitch reflexes, but in the current author's experience a simple pull on a body feather gives the best guidance. As the bird becomes more deeply anaesthetized, the standard reflexes usually slow and decrease in strength or eventually disappear.

2. *Circulatory volume.* Birds are thought to be better able to tolerate blood loss than mammals (Heard 1997), although haemorrhage is still a problem. The amount of blood lost during surgery should be monitored – if necessary by measuring swabs – and fluid therapy or even a blood transfusion should be considered. In an emergency situation pigeon blood can be used

for most species, although there are always risks involved in this procedure – not least from viral infections.

3. *Heart rate.* The use of a cardiac monitor is recommended, although an oesophageal stethoscope can be of use (Lawton 1993). The standard lead placements are over the distal lateral tarsometatarsus and the carpal joints of each wing, using atraumatic clamps or silver needles. As an aid to the assessment of pain, the heart rate is dramatically effective. It is not uncommon for a cockatiel, on feeling pain, to increase its heart rate from 300 bpm to over 700 bpm (Lawton 1996a). The heart rate should never fall below 120 bpm (Doolen & Jackson 1991).

4. *Respiration.* Electronic monitoring of respiration is considered the best indicator of the depth and stability of anaesthesia in the absence of response to pain. However, the majority of respiratory monitors work on thermal changes between inspired and expired gases, and this can lead to difficulty in measurement in small

birds – especially when the flow rates of the cold carrier gases are high. The pattern of respiration is also important; it should be stable and continually monitored during anaesthesia (Lawton 1993). A sudden change in pattern, especially in the depth of respiration (from shallow to deep), may indicate that the bird's plane of anaesthesia is lightening or the bird is feeling pain. Depending on the bird's body size, the respiratory rate should not fall below 25–50 breaths per minute (Doolen & Jackson 1991); below this there is a risk of hypercapnia. Pulse oximeters with a cloacal probe are useful for assessing the oxygenation of the blood and also the rate of respiration.

5. *Temperature.* Warmth should be provided before induction, during anaesthesia, and in the recovery period. Sick or anaesthetized birds may not be able to maintain their core body temperature adequately, and sick birds attempting to maintain their high core temperature may become hypoglycaemic due to hypothermia. Hypothermia can cause peripheral vasoconstriction, bradycardia, hypotension and, when severe, ventricular fibrillation (Heard 1997). The core body temperature of birds is usually between 40 and 44°C (Carter-Storm 1988), with that of smaller birds being 41°C (Cooper 1989). Anaesthetized birds should be placed on a towel (Fig. 3.35) or an insulated 'Vet-bed'; the use of heating pads or lights can also help to reduce heat loss, but care must be taken to prevent overheating or burns. Bubble wrap or space blankets can also be used for wrapping most of the bird to prevent unnecessary heat loss. Cold anaesthetic gases will also have a chilling effect on the bird, but there is little that can be done to prevent this other than keeping the overall length of anaesthesia to the shortest possible.

Summary

Attention to the foregoing should equip the interested veterinary clinician with the confidence to handle, examine and pursue a reasonable diagnostic work-up in avian patients. Further reading and research, linked with the detail provided by ensuing chapters in this book, plus perseverance, will quickly develop expertise in this interesting and rewarding field of avian medicine and surgery.

References

Carter-Storm A 1988 Special considerations for general anesthesia of birds. Clinical Insight 2(3):61–62

Cooper J E 1989 Anaesthesia of exotic species. In: Hilbery A D R, Waterman A E, Brouwer G J (eds) Manual of anaesthesia for small animal practice, 3rd edn. BSAVA, p 182–191

Doolen M D, Jackson L 1991 Anesthesia in caged birds. Iowa State University Veterinarian 53(2):76

Flammer K 1989 Update on avian anesthesia. In: Kirk R W, Bonagura J D (eds) Current veterinary therapy. X. W B Saunders, Philadelphia, PA, p 776–779

Harrison G J, Ritchie B W 1994 Making distinctions in the physical examination. In: Harrison G L, Harrison L R (eds) Clinical avian medicine and surgery. W B Saunders, Philadelphia, PA, p 151

Heard D J 1977 Anesthesia and analgesia. In: Altman R B, Clubb S L, Dorrestein G M, Quesenberry K (eds) Avian medicine and surgery. W B Saunders, Philadelphia, PA, p 807–828

Jones A K 1996 Wing clipping in pet birds: a study and comparison of techniques. In: Proceedings of the Annual Conference of the Association of Avian Veterinarians 1996, p 337–342

Jones A K 1998 The normal moulting process in birds. In: Proceedings of the Annual Conference of the Association of Avian Veterinarians 1998, p 65–70

Korbel R, Milovanovic A, Erhardt W et al 1993 Aerosaccular perfusion with isoflurane – an anaesthetic procedure for head surgery in birds. In: Proceedings of the European Conference of the Association of Avian Veterinarians. AAV, p 9–42

Lawton M P C 1993 Monitoring the anaesthetized bird. In: Proceedings of the European Conference of the Association of Avian Veterinarians. AAV, p 1–8

Lawton M P C 1996a Anesthesia. In: Beynon P H, Forbes N A, Lawton M P C (eds) Manual of psittacine birds. BSAVA, Cheltenham, p 49–59

Lawton M P C 1996b Anesthesia. In: Beynon P H, Forbes N A, Harcourt-Brown N (eds) Manual of raptors, pigeons and waterfowl. BSAVA, Cheltenham, p 79–88

Lawton M P C 2000 The physical examination. In: Tully T N, Lawton M P C, Dorrestein G M (eds) Avian medicine. Butterworth-Heinemann, Edinburgh, p 26–42

Sinn L C 1994 Anesthesiology. In: Ritchie B, Harrison G, Harrison L (eds) Avian medicine: principles and application. Wingers Publishing, Lake Worth, FL, p 1066–1080

Clinical tests

Don J. Harris

4

Introduction

Clinical pathology holds the key to unravelling much of the mystery surrounding the sick avian patient. Although many avian diseases present with identical clinical signs, laboratory data can often distinguish between disease aetiologies and/or tissues affected (e.g. infectious versus metabolic, bacterial versus fungal, renal versus hepatic). As this is a handbook, the focus of the clinical tests chapter is to guide the practitioner in the practical organization of diagnostic protocols. In a clinical situation, an appropriately broad selection of laboratory tests offers the best odds of quickly determining the nature of the patient's problem. Minimal attention will be paid to the materials, methods, biochemistry and physiology behind the tests themselves, except where it serves to clarify the test's usefulness.

Overview

For the sake of organization, laboratory tests can be divided into several basic groups:

1. Indicators of immune system activity – the complete blood count (CBC) and electrophoresis (EPH)
2. Serum biochemistries – indicate the condition or function of various organ systems
3. Serology – tests for antibodies to various diseases
4. Antigen detection tests – tests for the antigens specific to infectious agents
5. Microbiology – methods of propagating and identifying infectious agents
6. Miscellaneous – randomly utilized tests such as urinalysis, heavy metals, cytology, etc.

It is advisable for individuals attempting to formulate a diagnostic protocol always to begin the laboratory profile with general indicators of immune or organ system functions, then to progress toward specific tests to verify or rule out suspect aetiologies.

Complete blood count

The complete blood count (CBC) is arguably the most important component of an avian diagnostic panel, especially in younger patients. Perhaps no other single test provides as much important information regarding the overall health of an avian patient as the CBC. For analytical purposes the CBC may be divided into

classifications describing: the volume and character of the red blood cells; the numbers, percentages and characteristics of the white blood cells; the concentration of solids in the plasma; the relative number of thrombocytes; and the presence or absence of blood-borne parasites. While many other tests provide information not demonstrated by the CBC, no other single test provides such a broad range of information. Differences exist between avian and mammalian blood but, once these differences are recognized, the similarity in functions of the various components becomes evident.

The primary differences between mammalian and avian blood are that:

- normal mature avian red blood cells are nucleated
- regenerative anaemia is demonstrated by polychromasia among the red cells in a stained smear
- white blood cell types parallel mammalian cells except that birds possess heterophils instead of neutrophils
- platelets are replaced in avian blood by thrombocytes.

Unlike dogs and cats, total cell counts of birds may vary widely among members of a given species. To determine normal total cell count values for an individual, baseline data must be collected during periods of apparent good health. Reference values for various species have been published, but these tables should only be used as rough guidelines. Published ranges will typically be wide, therefore subtle patient variations may not be apparent.

Beyond the above mentioned differences, the functions of the various cellular components in avian blood are roughly comparable to those of mammals. One must remember that an increase in the total white count in the presence of an elevated heterophil population is an indication of inflammation. Inflammation may or may not be associated with infection. Infections, non-infectious inflammation, necrosis, neoplasia are examples of disease processes that may cause a leucocytosis. A moderate heterophilia often indicates the presence of an infectious disease or cellular necrosis, and an extremely high heterophil count often accompanies avian chlamydiosis, aspergillosis or tuberculosis. Increases in the heterophil count are usually characterized by varying degrees of toxic changes in the white cells. Subtle-to-moderate heterophilias, without toxic changes in the white cells, may reflect stress leucograms. Sometimes, the degree of toxicity among the white cells is more important than the actual white cell count itself.

An overwhelming bacterial infection or a severe viral infection may result in a leucopenia with a heteropenia or occasionally a lymphopenia. The leucopenic episode may be due to decreased production or increased consumption of the cell line. Increased consumption is evidenced by the presence of immature and toxic cells, findings not present with decreased production.

In some avian species the relative lymphocyte count may be higher than in others. An absolute lymphocytosis suggests a viral infection or certain stages of chlamydiosis. Certain leukaemias may produce an elevation of a particular line of lymphocytes.

A lymphopenia may occur in severe viral infections, such as avian circovirus in young African grey parrots.

A monocytosis implies the presence of chronic granulomatous disease or extensive necrosis in which a large amount of phagocytosis is occurring. Classic examples conditions that contribute to a monocytosis include chronic inflammatory diseases such as aspergillosis, tuberculosis, and avian chlamydiosis.

Eosinophil functions have not been clearly defined. Although speculated, intestinal parasitism in avian species does not appear to produce a consistent eosinophilia. There has been no scientific evidence at this time that allergic conditions result in a peripheral eosinophilia.

Basophils are uncommon findings in normal avian haemograms. Conditions that increase circulating basophils include respiratory infections, resolution of tissue damage, parasitism and some avian chlamydiosis infections.

Electrophoresis (EPH, SPE)

The fractionation of plasma proteins via protein electrophoresis is analogous to the separation and identification of white blood cells in the differential cell count. Just as different families of white cells are separately quantitated, so are the relative percentages of the plasma proteins measured. **It should be realized that the technique of performing an electrophoresis does not produce absolute values of each protein fraction; rather, it reveals the percentage of each as part of the premeasured total protein.** The absolute values must be calculated after the total protein has been determined through another method. The electrophoresis then yields information regarding a variety of physiological and immunological states of the patient. The primary categorization of avian plasma proteins includes pre-albumin, albumin and globulin components. Globulins are then divided and sometimes subdivided into alpha, beta and gamma fractions.

One aspect of protein determinations that should always be observed is the albumin : globulin (A : G) ratio. More important than the patient's total plasma protein are the relative quantities of pre-albumin, albumin

and globulin. The ratio is calculated using the formula (pre-albumin + albumin)/globulins, and the normal A : G ratio ranges from 1.6 to 4.5. The importance of this ratio is illustrated by the following example:

Snowflake and Peaches each have total plasma proteins of 4.0. At first glance, according to published data, each patient's proteins appear to be normal. Snowflake's albumin is 3.0 and his globulin is 1.0, resulting in an A : G ratio of 3.0, normal. Peaches, however, has an albumin of 1.0 with a globulin of 3.0. Peaches' A : G ratio is 0.33, grossly abnormal. Peaches' albumin is very low and her globulins are very high – an indication of a potentially serious condition. Peaches is losing or failing to manufacture albumin, while at the same time some portion of the globulins is being produced at an accelerated rate.

Pre-albumin and albumin fractions

The significance of the pre-albumin fraction of the serum protein in birds is unknown. It may function as a transport protein, similar to albumin. There does not appear to be a comparable component in mammalian blood. In avian samples it may comprise as much as 40% of the total serum protein. In some species, it appears that low pre-albumin values may have the same significance as low albumin values in other species.

The albumin fraction typically comprises 45–70% of avian serum protein in species that have high pre-albumin values, and tends to be lower in species with low pre-albumin values. **Albumin functions primarily as an osmotic pressure regulator and a transport protein in birds, as it does in mammalian species.**

Globulin fraction

The globulin fraction has alpha (α), beta (β) and gamma (γ) components, and high-resolution electrophoresis will divide the globulins into the protein components listed under the α, β and γ subgroups discussed below. Each of the three primary globulin fractions contains proteins active in different physiological and pathophysiological conditions.

Alpha globulins

Alpha globulins consist of two principal fractions, α1 and α2. Contained within this group of globulins are acute phase inflammatory proteins such as α-lipoprotein, α1-antitrypsin, α2-macroglobin and haptoglobin. The α2-macroglobin sometimes migrates into the β range. One condition associated with elevated alpha globulin levels in birds is parasitism. Other consistent correlations have yet to be identified. Elevations in alpha globulins are somewhat uncommon.

Beta globulins

Beta globulins constitute other acute phase inflammatory proteins, including β2-macro-globulin, fibronectin, transferrin and β-lipoprotein. In some species, namely the African grey parrot, the β component of the EPH consists of two primary components, β1 and β2. Elevated beta-globulin levels may be indicative of chronic liver or kidney disease, or chronic inflammatory diseases such as aspergillosis or avian chlamydiosis. The most common reason for elevated beta globulins in birds, which is attributable to the transferrin component, is egg production. A significantly elevated beta-globulin level, combined with a 1.5–2-fold increase in the blood calcium level, in birds of unknown sex, is highly suggestive that the bird is an ovulating female.

Gamma globulins

In mammals, gamma globulins appear as two primary fractions, γ1 and γ2. In avian species, only one fraction is demonstrated. The primary components of the gamma globulins are antibodies, complement and complement degradation products. Elevated gamma globulins are a common finding in birds suffering from acute *Chlamydophila psittaci* infection.

Serum biochemistries (Fig. 4.1)
Alanine aminotransferase (ALT, SGPT)

Alanine aminotransferase is an enzyme found in the cells of many avian tissues. In other animals elevations have been shown to be associated with hepatocellular disruption, but no such association has been consistently demonstrated in birds. Little clinical significance can therefore be applied to ALT values in avian patients.

Albumin

The function of albumin is discussed above. It should be noted here that an accurate albumin determination is best calculated through electrophoresis. Currently

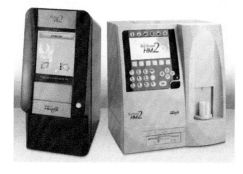

Fig 4.1 Technical advancements have led to the development of plasma chemical analysis machines that can run samples on the very small volumes of blood that can be collected from even the smallest avian patient. (Photo courtesy of Abaxis North America, Union City, CA, USA.)

utilized dry chemistry assays do not provide accurate avian albumin measurements.

Alkaline phosphatase (AP, SAP)

Alkaline phosphatase is found in bone, kidneys, intestine and liver. The hepatic fraction composes only a very small proportion of the total reported in routine testing. Because changes in the hepatic fraction have little and inconsistent influence on the overall value, no correlation can be made between liver disease and AP levels. The inconsistent elevations from variable sources cause AP to be of almost no value in avian diagnostics. Disruption of bone probably causes elevations of AP more than other sources.

Amylase

In birds, the pancreas, liver and small intestine produce amylase. Elevations have been associated principally with acute pancreatitis and, to a lesser extent, enteritis. Because more than one source of amylase exists, an elevation is not in itself diagnostic. Some investigators question the usefulness of amylase in avian diagnostics because of its lack of specificity.

Aspartate aminotransferase (AST, SGOT)

The intracellular enzyme most useful for diagnosing hepatocellular disruption in avian species is aspartate aminotransferase. Although present in liver, skeletal muscle, kidney, heart and brain, elevations are frequently associated with liver disease or muscle damage. When an elevation in AST is detected, a creatine kinase (CK) level should be obtained. An elevated AST without a concurrent elevation in CK is highly suggestive of hepatocellular disruption. It should be emphasized that this does not confirm liver disease; nor does a normal AST positively rule out liver disease. **As with all diagnostics, the AST provides evidence towards a diagnosis but does not in itself determine the diagnosis.** Also, the AST in no way indicates the functional capacity of the liver. The bile acids test, discussed shortly, is more appropriately used to evaluate hepatic function.

Bicarbonate

Measurement of bicarbonate levels provides an indication of the patient's acid–base status. Increases in bicarbonate imply alkalosis, while decreases imply acidosis.

Bile acids

Bile acids are produced by the liver to aid in the digestion of fats. After excretion into the intestinal tract, bile acids are reabsorbed and returned to the liver via the portal circulation. The liver then extracts the bile acids from the blood for recycling. The amount not extracted is therefore inversely proportional to liver function. Elevation of bile acids in the general circulation is associated with decreased ability of the liver to extract the bile acids from the portal circulation, and therefore impaired liver function.

Confusion arises when it is noted that the liver is the organ of bile acid synthesis. It would seem logical that hepatic insufficiency would result in decreased production of bile acids, and therefore in decreased circulating levels. However, **hepatic extraction of bile acids from the portal circulation is apparently more dependent on efficient liver function than is the synthesis of bile acids.** It is reasonable to presume (and it does appear to happen) that at some point the production of bile acids does diminish and values fall. As with aspartate aminotransferase, a normal bile acid level does not absolutely rule out hepatic disease.

It is important to distinguish between the information provided by the AST and bile acids. Aspartate aminotransferase is a leakage enzyme, and therefore an indicator of hepatocellular integrity, while bile acids are indicators of liver function. One is not necessarily dependent on the other. For example, a patient may exhibit a normal AST but elevated bile acids, implying impaired liver function, even though the cells were intact (e.g. hepatic lipidosis, chronic fibrosis). Conversely, many diseases such as salmonellosis or acute avian chlamydiosis may cause hepatocellular damage without impairing overall liver function. Marked elevations in the AST may be observed without concurrent elevations in bile acids. Again, normal values of either or both do not rule out hepatic disease. A totally fibrotic end-stage liver lacks sufficient functional hepatocytes to produce measurable AST or bile acids.

Bilirubin

Since biliverdin is the major avian bile pigment, bilirubin is uncommonly observed in avian serum samples. In occasional cases of severe liver disease, significant bilirubin levels are present; therefore, hepatic pathology may be suspected in patients demonstrating elevated bilirubin levels.

Blood urea nitrogen (BUN)

The usefulness of BUN is limited because of the low measurable levels of urea in avian blood. Also, the avian kidney appears able to excrete most urea as long as the patient's hydration is adequate. Therefore, blood urea may be a better indicator of hydration than renal function, and an elevated urea would imply dehydration.

Calcium

Calcium levels are profoundly influenced by a number of normal as well as pathological conditions, and great care should be exercised in the interpretation of abnormal findings. Almost all pathological changes are secondary to conditions not associated with dietary levels. Because of the effectiveness of the parathyroid gland, dietary deficiencies of calcium will rarely cause subnormal blood levels. Blood calcium levels are also directly linked to albumin levels. Hypoalbuminaemia will result in artefactual depression of measured calcium levels. Other causes of lowered blood calcium levels include hypocalcaemic syndrome in African grey parrots, glucocorticoid administration, hypomagnesaemia and insufficient exposure to full spectrum lighting.

Dehydration will sometimes elevate albumin, and therefore blood calcium. Two-fold or greater elevations typically occur with ovulation. Elevated levels of calcium have been associated with vitamin D_3 toxicity, osteolytic bone tumours, renal adenocarcinoma and dehydration.

Chloride

Changes in chloride levels are rarely observed in avian samples.

Cholesterol

Cholesterol levels in birds may accompany various physiological or pathological conditions, but there is inconsistency and a lack of specificity associated with abnormal findings. Generally, elevations are associated with liver disease, hypothyroidism, high fat diets and starvation, especially in obese birds. Subnormal levels may be observed with endotoxaemia, aflatoxicosis, spirochaetosis and low dietary fat. Unfortunately, there are no clear indicators to determine whether or not an abnormal cholesterol level is associated with a particular condition. For example, if an obese bird were to display elevated cholesterol, it would be unclear whether the elevation was a result of hypothyroidism, excessive dietary fat, hepatic lipidosis, or mobilization of body stores during anorexia. Other tests and observations usually provide evidence of these conditions, with or without the support of the cholesterol level. Again, normal values do not rule out the aforementioned conditions.

Creatine kinase (CK, CPK)

The primary sources of CK include skeletal muscle, cardiac muscle and nervous tissue, and elevations are associated with significant disruptions of these tissues. The primary usefulness of this enzyme is in distinguishing between hepatic and non-hepatic causes of an elevated

AST. Any elevation in AST should be compared with the patient's CK level. If the CK is normal, it is relatively safe to conclude that the liver is the source of the elevated AST. If the CK is elevated, muscle should be considered a possible source of the elevated AST. Other possibilities for the dual elevations would of course be concurrent liver and muscle or liver and neurological disease.

Creatinine

Creatinine levels in avian serum samples typically fall below a measurable range, and are rarely useful in avian clinical pathology. Also, certain technical factors contribute to a high incidence of artefactual changes. Elevations have been associated with kidney disease, but creatinine is not considered to be a reliable indicator of renal function.

Gamma glutamyl transferase (GGT)

Gamma glutamyl transferase activity in birds is low. Various observations have been made by different investigators, giving inconsistent findings. It does not appear to be useful as a diagnostic aid in birds.

Glucose

Elevations in blood glucose levels are the principal pathological change noted in avian species. Hypoglycaemia is extremely rare in birds and, when present, is almost never associated with starvation. The primary cause of hypoglycaemia in pet birds is septicaemia.

Hyperglycaemia occurs commonly due to stress or after meals and, occasionally, diabetes mellitus. Because of the frequency with which hyperglycaemia is caused by stress, a diagnosis of diabetes mellitus should be considered carefully and only if supported by other clinical evidence. A visibly normal hyperglycaemic patient displaying no polydipsia, no polyuria and no weight loss should not automatically be considered diabetic. Repeat testing, other diagnostic investigative tests and observation are necessary to confirm a diagnosis.

Glutamate dehydrogenase (GLDH)

Sources of GLDH in birds include the kidney, liver and brain. Although not widely available, the GLDH level can provide significant information in the investigation of hepatic disease. Elevations are observed when significant cellular destruction occurs.

Lactate dehydrogenase (LDH)

LDH is found in skeletal and cardiac muscle, liver, kidney, bone and erythrocytes. Elevations can be observed with disruption of any of these tissues or in haemolysis, and are therefore extremely non-specific. One benefit of measuring LDH levels may be in following the progress of liver disease, in which LDH levels apparently change more quickly than SGOT levels; lowering LDH values may imply improvement even though SGOT levels remain elevated.

Lipase

Serum lipase levels may be elevated in cases of acute pancreatitis. **Currently, the only reliable ante-mortem confirmation of pancreatitis is by pancreatic biopsy.**

Phosphorus

Less common than in other species, elevated serum phosphorus is occasionally observed in avian renal failure. An elevated phosphorus level resulting from renal disease suggests chronicity and offers a guarded prognosis. Elevations of phosphorus are also observed in hypoparathyroidism and nutritional secondary hyperparathyroidism. Haemolysis may also artefactually elevate serum samples. Malabsorption and vitamin D deficiencies may cause lowered blood phosphorus levels.

Potassium

As with sodium, pathological changes in potassium levels indicate a serious and usually life-threatening clinical situation. Hyperkalaemia develops with advanced kidney disease, adrenal disease, and during episodes of acidosis. Hypokalaemia may result from potassium loss through diarrhoea, and during states of alkalosis.

Sodium

Changes in sodium values usually reflect serious conditions. Elevated levels occur with salt poisoning, water deprivation and dehydration. Decreased levels occur due to sodium loss through renal disease or diarrhoea.

Total protein (TP)

A total serum protein level must be evaluated in light of its components, albumin and globulin. The total value is influenced by various factors but, as discussed previously, a normal value does not rule out abnormalities of the individual protein components. Overall, dehydration and immune stimulation may cause a hyperproteinaemia. Hypoproteinaemia may be caused by overhydration, protein loss associated with renal disease, starvation, hepatic disease or intestinal disease.

As stated earlier, the protein should never be considered normal until the A : G ratio is known to be normal.

Uric acid

The blood uric acid level is the primary indicator of renal function in birds. An elevated uric acid level is a reliable indicator that renal function is impaired. With many tests, substantial elevations are necessary before there is reason for concern; however, even a subtle elevation in the uric acid warrants suspicion of renal disease. Conversely, serial determinations should be made after adequately hydrating the patient before concluding a diagnosis of renal disease. It must be noted that uric acid levels may be artefactually elevated if blood is collected via a toenail trim, due to faecal contamination on the claw which contains uric acid.

Serology

Avian chlamydiosis

Several serological tests for antibodies against avian chlamydiosis have been developed. Various technologies are currently used, including complement fixation, latex agglutination and immunofluorescent antibody. Although each utilizes a different method for detecting antibodies, the presence of antibodies must be interpreted with the same degree of care for each. Specifically, the presence of antibodies does not necessarily relate to the status of infection; a positive antibody titre may indicate present or past exposure in a given patient. Paired serum samples may provide more information, with a rising or falling titre more significant than an unchanging one.

Aspergillus

The detection of antibodies to *Aspergillus* spp. provides inconsistent evidence towards a diagnosis. A positive titre may imply infection, but false positives and negatives are common.

Antigen detection

Avian chlamydiosis

There are two primary technologies (excluding culture) currently used for the detection of chlamydial antigen. Various manufacturers have marketed an in-house ELISA test, which with reasonable consistency demonstrates chlamydial antigen in specimens such as mucosal swabs, faecal samples or tissue preparations. However, the absence of antigen in no way rules out the presence of *Chlamydophila* spp. in the host. Since chlamydial organisms may be shed only for brief periods, a negative test means only that antigen is not present when the sample was tested. False positives do exist but, in conjunction with other data, the ELISA test can be useful.

The second technology currently being utilized involves a DNA probe that theoretically detects a portion of the *Chlamydophila* spp. genome. Because this technology focuses on the agent's unique DNA, it dramatically reduces the incidence of false positives; its sensitivity reduces the incidence of false negatives. The DNA probe may indicate the presence of the organism but does not determine that the disease state exists. **As mentioned before, specific diagnostic testing confirms a diagnosis, it does not by itself create a diagnosis.**

Aspergillus

An IFA test for *Aspergillus* spp. antigen is currently available. Theoretically, this test offers the advantage of detecting circulating antigen instead of antibodies. The presence of antigen in addition to antibodies would provide strong evidence of an active infection, while the presence of antigen in the absence of antibodies could represent either background levels of antigen or an immunosuppressed patient with an active infection. Clinical experience will help to determine which of these scenarios holds true.

Polyoma

The suspected presence of polyomavirus in a patient is best detected through a DNA probe. The technology behind this test is probably one of the most reliable with regard to specificity. In essence, viral DNA patterns are as unique as fingerprints. The probe technology amplifies and labels only the viral DNA for which the test is designed, and the persistence of the label in the suspect sample confirms the presence of the viral DNA.

The test is performed either on cloacal swabs or whole blood, each having different clinical implications. A bird that tests positive via a cloacal swab is infected, shedding the virulent virus, in danger of dying, and represents a threat to susceptible birds. A patient that demonstrates circulating polyoma DNA may either be in the very early phase of infection with active circulating virus, or in a post-infection phase where only inactivated viral particles remain. These post-infection patients usually recover fully and cease to act as a source of infection for other birds.

Psittacine beak and feather disease (PBFD)

The technology behind PBFD testing is identical to that for polyoma, the primary difference being that cloacal swabs are not useful in the diagnosis of PBFD. The PBFD probe may be performed on either whole blood or follicle biopsies, and a positive feather biopsy is prognostically more grave than a positive blood test. **In the absence of clinical signs, a patient testing positive via a blood sample should be treated as a suspect only and retested 30+ days later.** Many of these patients revert to negative and do not pose a threat to themselves or other birds. Feather follicle biopsies that test positive indicate infected patients, which carry very poor prognoses and are highly infective to other birds.

Microbiology

Bacterial culture and sensitivity testing

The harvesting of bacteria from a particular site and their subsequent identification and testing for antibiotic susceptibility is an easy process; more difficult is determining the significance of the findings. In reality, bacterial culture/sensitivity testing has been grossly misused as an indicator of avian health. In the early days of avian medicine it was believed that all Gram-positive organisms were beneficial and all Gram-negative were harmful, but experience has demonstrated that the separation of beneficial from harmful organisms is far less clear. A few species of Gram-negative bacteria such as *Salmonella* spp. are recognized as obligate pathogens, but most have varying degrees of pathogenicity. There are also instances where Gram-positive bacteria such as *Staphylococcus aureus* can be markedly pathogenic.

The best way to interpret bacterial findings is closely to examine the patient, even before attempting to identify a possible pathogen. The first question to be addressed is whether or not there are any visible clinical signs of infection. **A bacterial culture from a perfectly normal oropharynx may be irrelevant, regardless of the bacteria that might be isolated.** If, however, overt clinical signs are present, a culture may identify causative agents. **Rarely should a patient be treated with antibiotics merely because of the presence of suspect bacteria.** Allegedly undesirable bacteria may actually be harmless, or they may be present secondary to another condition (e.g. malnutrition, contamination of the water source). **Only when a specific disease condition can be directly linked to a possible pathogen should a culture be considered significant.**

Fungal culture

The primary fungi of concern to the avian practitioner are *Candida albicans* and *Aspergillus fumigatus*. Other species can be significant but more often exist as contaminants, and standard culture techniques should allow for the appearance of these organisms. When isolated, their significance must be interpreted in light of clinical signs, haematological data etc. Their mere presence does not confirm disease.

Avian chlamydiosis

The only absolute established confirmation of the presence of *Chlamydophila psittaci* in an avian sample is its growth and identification in culture. All other tests carry risks of false positive or negative results. However, culture for the *Chlamydophila psittaci* organism can produce false negative results.

Mycoplasma

Investigations into infectious causes of avian respiratory disease should always include the consideration of *Mycoplasma* as a possible contributing agent. **Although not difficult to propagate, it is necessary to specifically request for a *Mycoplasma* culture.** Most laboratories will overlook the possibility of its presence.

Virology

The true cause of an avian illness is often a virus, and it seems as though there is always an emerging viral disease. Virus isolation will always have a role in the investigation of avian illness.

Miscellaneous

Urinalysis

Because avian urine and faeces are mixed in the cloaca, pure avian urine samples are difficult to obtain. The most useful aspect of avian urinalysis is the analysis of the urine sediment. Often the only clinicopathological evidence of renal disease is the presence of granular or hyaline casts. Polyuria that cannot be determined through other means should be investigated by carefully examining the urine sediment for these casts. **Evidence of ketones in avian urine is a true reading and will be evident in cases of diabetes mellitus.**

Heavy metal assays

Lead and zinc are common causes of heavy metal intoxication in birds. Assays are available for each of these, as well as for copper. Unfortunately other metals also cause toxicity and illness; therefore the absence of lead, zinc and copper in a suspect sample does not completely rule out heavy metal toxicity in a patient.

Cytology

Cytological preparations of avian samples, both ante-mortem and post-mortem examinations, can be extremely useful. By carefully examining the cellular and microbiological content of a given specimen, a tentative diagnosis is often possible.

Faecal examinations for parasites

Gastrointestinal parasites, while rare in pet birds, are occasionally the primary cause of avian illness and death. Suspect cases should be examined through the use of direct saline smears, flotation techniques and specialized assays.

Giardia spp. is one parasite for which there are a variety of diagnostic techniques available. **Direct saline smears are occasionally revealing, although the organisms may be more clearly visible when stained with warmed Lugol's iodine.** Trichrome staining will, on occasion, increase the prominence of the organisms. An ELISA test is now available that shows great promise in identifying *Giardia* spp. cases that are difficult to diagnose.

Gram's staining

At one time, the Gram's stain was the most commonly utilized test in avian medicine. Much controversy now surrounds its significance in assessing avian health.

The Gram's stain itself will always be a useful test; the problem lies not in the test but in its interpretation. Many birds are erroneously diagnosed with Gram-negative bacterial infections due to artefact from poor staining techniques. The findings of a correctly performed test are often misinterpreted as abnormal when in fact they may be acceptable. A common misinterpretation is the assumption of a yeast infection following the identification of yeasts in a Gram's stain. Brewer's yeast from bread products are often the source of such findings. **An understanding of avian bacteriology is a prerequisite for accurate interpretation of avian Gram's stains.** The Gram's stain may then be used as a crude indicator of the major flora in a given faecal sample. Usually, abnormal findings should be validated through bacterial/fungal cultures.

Summary

Laboratory testing is an essential component of avian medicine. When examining avian patients, both routinely and in the face of illness, it is necessary to utilize an appropriate assortment of tests in order to obtain a reasonably complete profile of the patient. Knowing how to interpret the results of diagnostic testing is as important as knowing which tests to utilize. By employing the appropriate tests in relation to the patient's presentation, history and clinical signs, and correctly interpreting the results of these tests, avian patients can be diagnosed and treated with a maximum of accuracy and effectiveness.

Imaging techniques

5

Maria-Elisabeth Krautwald-Junghanns and Michael Pees

Introduction

Imaging techniques are of special importance for diagnosis of diseases in birds. They provide much information about the size, shape, structure and function of the inner organs and support interpretation of clinical and laboratory findings. Due to the unique anatomical features in birds, there are some differences in comparison to mammals when using radiology, ultrasound or endoscopy. However, basic principles of realization and interpretation are similar. The radiological examination is the imaging technique most often used in avian species. Ultrasonography is of special interest in space-occupying processes and suspected cardiac alteration. Whereas 2-D-ultrasonography (B-mode) is well documented, the use of M-mode for avian echocardiography is not possible due to the position of the coupling area. Endoscopic access is easy in comparison to mammals since the air sac system can be used and insufflation of air is normally not necessary.

Radiography

High-quality radiographs are a basic requirement in the use of radiographic imaging as a diagnostic procedure in avian medicine and surgery. The small size of avian patients and their delicate anatomical structures necessitate a high degree of detail in order to recognize and correctly interpret the diagnostic images. To correctly produce and interpret avian radiographs, specific technical factors (such as the type of radiography machine, film–screen combination and film processing) and an experienced clinician are necessary.

Movement is a problem with avian patients, causing poor radiographic detail. Anaesthesia reduces patient motion but does not reduce the high respiratory rates; therefore a short exposure time (0.015–0.05 s) should be used. This is achieved by using a powerful radiography machine of at least 200–300 mA (a two- or multiphase generator). Low kilovolt values are recommended in order to obtain radiographs with high contrast and as many shades of grey as possible. Increasing the kV output in order to reduce the exposure time is not advisable, since this leads to a reduction in contrast. Lowering the dosage by decreasing the focal–film distance is also of limited value (a minimum of 60–70 cm should be used with a high definition film–screen combination), since this leads to a significant loss of definition due to the large size of the focal spot in low performance machines. With the ongoing technical development, the use of digital radiography devices will become more important also in avian medicine. With these devices, short exposure times are possible. However, detail recognition is still reduced in comparison to conventional radiography.

High-definition screen–film combinations have proved most efficient for avian radiographic studies. Significantly higher dosages are required when using non-screen films or dental films, and this means more radiation exposure to the operator as well as a longer exposure time. These films are therefore inappropriate for radiographing the bird's body, despite their advantage of recording greater detail.

Modern mammography films can combine high detail resolution and acceptable exposure times. Nevertheless, the use of screens with a greater intensifying capacity is strongly recommended in order to minimize the exposure time. However, a higher intensifying capacity of the screen is associated with a decrease in sharpness of the image. The development of rare-earth screens has proven to be a major advance when compared to normal calcium tungstate screens. Rare-earth screens have a similar intensifying capacity but significantly improved definition (high sensitivity), and are routinely combined with films giving high resolution and the best possible contrast. The best combination for use in avian radiology seems to be a rare-earth screen at the back of the cassette, providing high definition, and a film emulsified on one side, such as those used to record monitor images in computed tomography. More intensifying rare-earth screens (sensitivity of 200) may be advisable when working with very low performance machines, as the resulting decrease in picture quality will not be as distracting as the motion artefacts incurred with long exposure times. Calcium tungstate screens, which are even more intensifying, are inadequate because of the loss of image detail.

Restraint

There are several possible methods of restraining birds for radiography. It is always best to restrain the patient in a way that does not expose veterinary medical personnel to radiation, and this is possible with the help of a Plexiglas® plate. If the Plexiglas® plate is no thicker than 0.8 cm, it does not adversely affect the definition of the

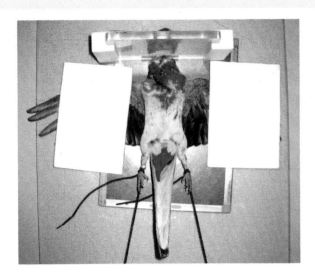

Fig 5.1 Fixation of an Eastern rosella (*Platycercus eximius*) for a radiographic examination, using a fixation plate. With this method, an optimal position of the bid allows examination of the whole body, with optimal radiation protection for the veterinarian.

radiograph (Fig. 5.1). Another method for restraining small birds is with adhesive tape, and crepe tape is used for feathered parts of the body to avoid damage to the skin and feathers when the tape is removed. However, this method may lead to feather destruction, which is critical especially in wild birds, and anaesthesia is normally necessary to reduce the stress during fixation.

It may not always be possible to avoid restraint using the hands, and in these situations it is important adequately to protect the hands of the person holding the bird. It may be impossible to wear lead gloves for manual restraint procedures, particularly when working with very small patients; in these cases the diaphragm must be adjusted so that the hands are out of the primary beam. Lead gloves can then be laid over the operator's hands to help protect them.

The question of whether or not sedation is indicated for radiography in birds must be decided on a case-by-case basis. In routine practice it is often not necessary to sedate an avian patient for radiography. If an inhalation anaesthetic unit is available, isoflurane is the drug of choice. If no inhalation apparatus is available, the radiographic procedures may be finished more quickly in routine practice without spending time on parenteral anaesthesia (weighing the bird, post-anaesthetic supervision, possible over-sensitivities, etc.).

If a contrast medium is administered orally for a radiograph of the gastrointestinal tract, inhalation anaesthesia should be avoided because it can lead to a reduction in the peristalsis of the alimentary tract (xylazine and most barbiturates can have the same effect). On the other hand, blurring due to movement can be avoided with sedation. Sedation may be necessary in

birds unaccustomed to human contact, and especially in raptors, to avoid powerful defence reactions. In cases where birds are restrained by adhesive tape, and in most head/skull evaluations, sedation is advantageous.

Standard views

At least two projections, taken at 90° angles to one another, are recommended for all studies.

The following standard views are suggested:

- body (plus neck and proximal limbs) – laterolateral, ventrodorsal
- head/neck – laterolateral, ventrodorsal, dorsoventral, rostrocaudal
- wing – mediolateral, caudocranial
- leg – mediolateral, dorsoventral.

For the ventrodorsal projection (Fig. 5.2) of the body, the bird is laid in dorsal recumbency on the table; the wings are drawn outwards from the body and the legs extended caudally to avoid superimposition. The sternum and the vertebral column should be directly aligned if the patient is correctly and symmetrically positioned.

For the laterolateral projection (Fig. 5.3) of the body, the bird is usually restrained in right lateral recumbency with the legs extended caudally and the wings pulled dorsally over the body. If the correct symmetrical position has been achieved, the two hip joints should be superimposed in the radiograph.

Sedation is usually necessary to radiograph the head. Restraining the patient with a Plexiglas® plate has a disadvantage in that the shadows of the radio-opaque head clamps obscure the first cervical vertebra and the occipital part of the skull. For the dorsoventral and the ventrodorsal projection of the head, the bird is laid in either ventral or dorsal recumbency on the table with the neck stretched and the head placed straight and in a symmetrical position. In the correct symmetrical position, the two rami of the mandible are parallel to the surface of the table. For the laterolateral projection of the head, the bird is placed in right or left lateral recumbency on the table with the neck stretched. If the patient is correctly and symmetrically positioned, the rami of the mandible should overlap.

Radiographs of the bird in both dorsal and lateral recumbency show the wings in the same plane (mediolateral). For the caudocranial projection of the wing, the bird is turned downward at right angles to the table. The wing must be extended laterally as far as possible, so that the cranial border of the wing lies parallel to the edge of the table (Fig. 5.4).

Positioning for radiography of the legs is easy. Adhesive tape is used to hold the legs. The shadow produced by the tape can be ignored.

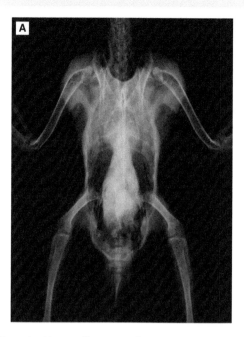
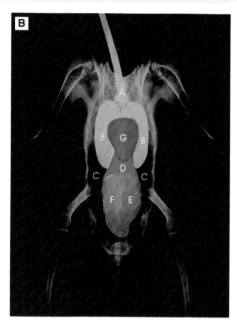

Fig 5.2A, B Blue and gold macaw (*Ara ararauna*), ventrodorsal projection: A = trachea/syrinx, B = lungs, C = air sacs (thoracic and abdominal), D = liver, E = gizzard, F = intestines.

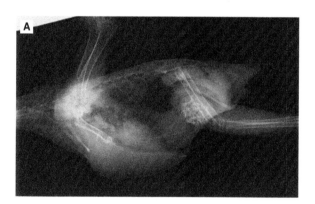
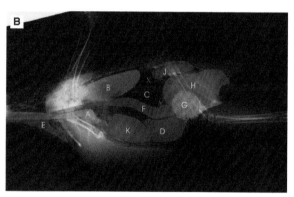

Fig 5.3A, B Citron-crested cockatoo (*Cacatua sulphurea citrinocristata*), laterolateral projection: A = trachea/syrinx, B = lungs, C = air sacs (thoracic and abdominal), D = liver, E = crop, F = proventriculus, G = gizzard, H = intestines, J = kidneys, X = position of the gonads, Y = position of the spleen.

Radiographic contrast studies

Gastrointestinal contrast

In addition to the plain radiograph, gastrointestinal contrast investigations with barium sulphate and, in individual cases, double-contrast of the digestive tract with barium sulphate and air are important diagnostic procedures.

A suspension of barium sulphate, using a dosage of 20 mL/kg body weight and a concentration of 25–45%, is administered as a contrast agent directly into the crop or oesophagus. The concentration of the suspension used depends on the indication; a higher concentration is more effective for demonstrating lesions in the wall of the gastrointestinal tract, while a liquid contrast agent with a more rapid transit time is sufficient for outlining the intestines against neighbouring organs (Fig. 5.5).

Indications for contrast studies are:

- examination of the intestinal size, shape, content and position
- determination of the intestinal function (e.g. transit time)
- assessment of the size of neighbouring organs
- examination of the thickness and the condition of hollow structures.

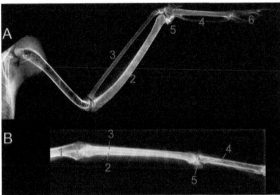

Fig 5.4 African grey parrot (*Psittacus e. erithacus*), wing projections (A: mediolateral projection, B: caudocranial projection); 1 = humerus, 2 = ulna, 3 = radius, 4 = carpometacarpus, 5 = os carpi ulnare, 6 = phalanx).

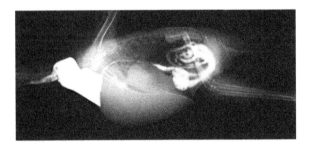

Fig 5.5 Eastern rosella (*Platycercus eximius*), Laterolateral projection. Contrast study with barium sulphate (20 mL/kg, 2 h after administration).

A survey radiograph must always be taken before beginning a contrast study. This is of particular importance for the demonstration of radiodense heavy metal particles, since these could by disguised by the contrast agent. If birds are not severely ill, they should be fasted for about 2 hours prior to the administration of the contrast medium. In dehydrated birds adequate fluid replacement must be achieved prior to the administration of the contrast medium, otherwise inspissation of the contrast medium due to dehydration may occur, leading to delayed passage or even obstruction of the intestines. There is considerable species and individual variation in the emptying time of the gastrointestinal tract in barium studies. The transit time depends on the species' diet, size and length of the digestive tract. It is also influenced by numerous other factors, such as age, nutritional status and stress. Regurgitation of the contrast medium may occur in severely stressed birds, predisposing the patient to aspiration pneumonia. A rapid or accelerated transit is seen in birds living on a soft food diet, in small songbirds, and in cachectic and stressed birds. A slow or prolonged transit of contrast medium occurs in large seed-eating birds, young birds, obese birds and when the stomach is congested with food, as well as in sedated or anaesthetized birds. Prolonged fasting prior to administration of the contrast medium leads to a reduced transit time to the ventriculus and an increased transit time through the rest of the gastrointestinal tract, prolonging the elimination of the contrast medium.

A double-contrast study of the gastrointestinal tract is rarely used in avian practice, but it can be helpful in diagnosing non-perforating wall lesions as well as other changes in the thickness and condition of the gastrointestinal wall. The contrast agents can be administered orally or as an enema; 10 mL/kg positive contrast medium (25% barium sulphate suspension) are given per os or via the cloaca. Air is used as a negative contrast medium, and is introduced immediately after administration of the positive contrast medium. The volume of air used is double that of the positive contrast agent, i.e. 20 mL/kg body weight (oral or cloacal). For better dispersion, the bird is carefully rotated around its own longitudinal axis several times immediately after administration of the contrast medium. For double-contrast radiographs in large birds, the kV is lowered one step. If excessive amounts of contrast agents are used complications may occur, including rupture of the gastrointestinal tract.

Urography

The application of urography in birds is limited; there are significant differences between the urogenital tracts of birds and mammals in that birds do not have a bladder, urethra or renal pelvis, and there is no distinct difference between renal medulla and renal cortex. Therefore there are very few indications for urography in birds, and the demonstration of the kidneys by this method is not as clear as in mammals. Because of the bird's renal portal system, the contrast medium is eliminated very quickly.

Iodine compounds are the best contrast media for urography, and should be warmed to body temperature and administered slowly into the basilic vein. The dosage is 2 mL/kg body weight of a 300–400 mg iodine/mL solution.

The patient should be fasted for about 2 hours prior to administration of the contrast medium. Sedation or anaesthesia is necessary, and in avian patients with renal insufficiency there may be problems since some anaesthetic agents (e.g. ketamine hydrochloride) impose an additional stress on the kidneys. The quality of contrast obtained depends on the renal concentrating ability of the preparation applied and on the iodine concentration of the contrast agent.

Radiography of the skeletal system

Avian bones are characterized by a thin cortex and a very delicate pattern of trabeculae. The long bones of

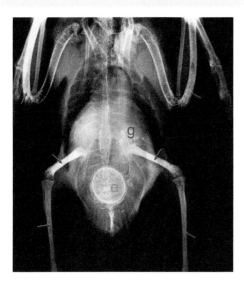

Fig 5.6 Cockatiel (*Nymphicus hollandicus*), ventrodorsal projection. Old egg (e) with roughened calcified shell in the caudal abdominal region; displacement of the ventriculus (g) to the left cranial side; soft tissue shadow in the mid-abdominal region. The soft tissue shadow was due to three laminated eggs in the oviduct. Note: 'medullary bone' (increased radiodensity) of the ulna, the femur and the tibiotarsus on both sides (red arrows).

most birds are pneumatized – as are, to a lesser extent, other parts of the skeleton (e.g. skull, pelvis, vertebrae, coracoid). In young birds the skeleton is poorly demonstrated by radiography, because persistent cartilaginous parts are typical in growing birds (e.g. the distal sternum, the scapula and the diaphyses). Ossification of the skeletal system occurs earlier in smaller avian species. Avian bones have no ossification centres in the epiphyses such as in mammalian bones.

Homogeneous hypercalcification ('medullary bone', Fig. 5.6, in combination with a pathological finding) is a physiological characteristic seen in female birds prior to egg production. This is a physiological calcium storage site, whereas irregular hyperostosis is a result of excessive hypercalcification, often caused by an abnormally high oestrogen level and associated with pathological findings such as laminated eggs, gonadal tumours or cysts.

Periosteal reactions and osteolysis indicate an inflammatory process. Periostitis may occur with fracture healing, or in conjunction with other inflammatory processes – for example, rhinitis and sinusitis with oversecretion may be seen as increased radiodensity of the infra-orbital sinus. Surrounding bones may show osteolytic changes. Septic pododermatitis is visible on radiographs as various degrees of arthritic and osteolytic lesions of the toes, joints and tarsometatarsi.

The diagnosis of fractures or pathological changes of the bones of the shoulder girdle is more difficult than in long bones because of the muscle mass found in this area of a bird's body. In the lateral view it is impossible to distinguish the coracoid from the scapula, but asymmetrical positioning may help radiographic interpretation. Fractures of the vertebral column usually involve the last two thoracic vertebrae and the synsacrum.

Fracture healing in birds should be assessed by the extent of the endosteal callus formation (Bush et al 1976). A large formation of callus is not necessarily a sign of progressing stability, but may be an indication of movement at the fracture site. Increased radiodensity as a result of calcium deposition at the fracture site followed by the formation of new bone, in the absence of signs of inflammation, indicates primary healing.

Multiple deformities of the skeleton are often a consequence of calcium, phosphorus and vitamin D_3 imbalance at the nestling age. The typical appearance in the bird is that of a convex vertebral column (kyphosis) and malformed long bones with pathological fractures. Older birds can succumb to osteomalacia or secondary hyperparathyroidism; the latter can be recognized by increased radiodensity in various parts of the skeleton, mainly in the shoulder girdle and the skull.

Radiography of the respiratory tract

The cartilaginous rings of the trachea are easily demonstrated in radiographs, and the lungs have a typical honeycomb structure. Radiographically, the air sacs have almost the same radiodensity as the surrounding air. Absolute absence of movement blur is necessary to be able to interpret changes of the respiratory tract in a radiograph.

A homogeneous increased density of the lung field and the air sacs can be caused by fat deposits or pneumonia, requiring comparison with a radiograph of a normal bird of the same species for a definitive diagnosis. Mycotic infections manifest as irregularly distributed areas of increased pulmonary density.

Mycobacterial or mycotic granulomata can be seen as irregular focal dense areas.

Overdistension of the axillary air sacs is sometimes seen in birds due to a stenosis of the lower respiratory tract, whereas overdistension of the abdominal air sacs is typical of a stenosis of the upper respiratory tract. The membranes of normal air sacs cannot be demonstrated in radiographs, but in later stages of chronic inflammatory disease, including air sacculitis, they may be well defined. Air sac walls may be thickened by bacterial, chlamydial or fungal infections.

Radiography of the liver

The liver is visible in a ventrodorsal view of the body, along with the heart, as an hourglass-shaped shadow. Hepatic enlargement is easily demonstrated in radiographs (Fig. 5.7). Hepatomegaly is a common finding in birds. In order to differentiate a tumour from an enlarged

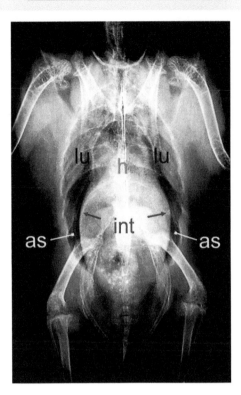

Fig 5.7 Yellow-cheeked Amazon (*Amazona autumnalis*), ventrodorsal projection. This female bird presented with a body weight of 830 g (adiposity). The intestinal/liver shadow (int) is enlarged; lungs (lu) and air sacs (as) show an increased radiodensity (h = heart). A massive enlargement of the liver is suspected, and should be confirmed with a contrast study.

liver of a different aetiology, ultrasonography is necessary. Infections that lead to an enlarged liver include psittacosis, tuberculosis and Pacheco's disease, as well as other bacterial or viral infections. The proventriculus is often displaced dorsally in patients exhibiting hepatomegaly.

Diseases such as haemochromatosis are commonly considered clinically because of the extensive massive ascites. Radiographically, the entire abdomen (except for the air-filled lungs) is uniformly radiodense, and no differentiation of various organs is possible.

Radiography of the spleen

The spleen can sometimes be seen in the indentation between the proventriculus and the ventriculus on a lateral view. An enlargement of the spleen can be suggestive of psittacosis, especially if the liver is also enlarged. Splenic enlargement can also be a sign of mycobacterial or viral disease (e.g. Pacheco's disease). Neoplasia of the spleen is occasionally seen in budgerigars, but rarely in larger psittacines.

Radiography of the gastrointestinal tract

The gastrointestinal tract of birds can best be identified on the lateral view – especially in seed-eaters, where the grit-filled (radio-opaque stones) ventriculus is easily identified. Its physiological location is between the two acetabuli, paramedian on the left-hand side of the body. The proventriculus can be found dorsocranially of the ventriculus. In birds that prefer soft food, it is not always possible to distinguish the proventriculus from the ventriculus. Use of a contrast medium allows differentiation of the gut from other internal organs, tumours and products of the reproductive tract.

Metallic foreign bodies in the alimentary tract are easy to identify, and must be distinguished from normal grit. They are typically found in the ventriculus. In most cases foreign bodies are more radiodense than grit, and identification is straightforward. Excessive grit in the ventriculus may pass into the intestines, and this may be a result of nutritional deficiency or malabsorption caused by enteric infections.

Extensive gas in the intestines may be indicative of parasitic ileus, but it can also be caused by bacterial gastroenteritis or an obstruction of a different aetiology.

Displacement of the ventriculus (Fig. 5.6) always indicates enlargement, swelling or neoplasia of a neighbouring organ. Dorsocranial or caudal displacement suggests hepatic enlargement, ventrocranial or caudal displacement suggests renal or gonadal enlargement. Ventrocranial displacement can also be caused by a laminated egg in the oviduct, ovarian cysts or enlarged intestinal loops.

Dilatation of the digestive tract is easily identified in contrast radiographs. It can be caused by neurogenic infections, neurotoxic poisons, food stasis, worm infestation or ileus of the distal segments. A massive dilatation of the proventriculus can be a symptom of proventricular dilatation disease (PDD). Other characteristics of PDD include a retarded passage time, thinning of the proventricular wall, atrophy and deformation of the ventriculus. Candidiasis should be considered as a less serious differential diagnosis (but might also be a secondary infection), as the radiographic image produced by this disease is similar to that of PDD.

Radiography of the heart and vascular system

In radiographs the heart is partially overlaid by the liver, and these two organs form the shape of an hourglass in the ventrodorsal view. The cardiac apex is directed ventrocaudally and lies between the fifth and sixth ribs. The aorta and other large vessels are projected in an oblique direction, and may be seen as round radiodense structures in the ventrodorsal view. In the lateral view, the brachiocephalic trunk, the pulmonary artery and the caudal vena cava are visible.

An enlargement and/or increased radiodensity of the heart shadow can be caused by different cardiac diseases, and the use of radiography for the diagnosis of pathological processes in the heart is limited. Ultrasonography and electrocardiography are often more precise methods for diagnosing heart and circulatory disturbances.

Radiography of the urogenital tract

The kidneys are only visible in the lateral view. They lie caudodorsally along the vertebral column.

Enlargement of the kidney shadow is frequently seen in combination with an enlargement of other organs as a sign of generalized infection, e.g. psittacosis, or in connection with renal neoplasia (especially budgerigar). Kidney cysts may cause changes in the shape of the kidneys; however, cysts can be better diagnosed by ultrasonography. A contrast medium using organic iodine compounds is indicated if functional disturbances of the urinary organs are suspected, or simply to highlight expected defects.

The gonads are particularly easy to visualize in their active state. On a lateral view, they are seen cranial to the anterior pole of the kidneys. Homogeneous hypercalcification of the bone (medullary bone) is common in females before they begin laying eggs. Eggs can be clearly differentiated by the radiodensity of the calcified shell (Fig. 5.6). When impacted with radiodense crystalline deposits, the kidneys are easily visualized. This is a sign of renal insufficiency, and may be the result of temporary dehydration or chronic infection.

Laminated non-shelled eggs cannot be clearly demonstrated in radiographs. Like other pathological alterations of these organs (e.g. salpingitis, ovarian cysts or tumours), they present as an indistinct soft tissue mass in the abdomen, often accompanied by the presence of medullary bone (Fig. 5.6). An additional ultrasonographic examination may help to differentiate between salpingitis, laminated eggs, tumours and cysts.

Ultrasonography

Ultrasonography is a useful non-invasive diagnostic tool in birds, especially in diagnosing soft tissue alterations. Diseases of the liver, heart and urogenital tract in particular are important indications for the use of ultrasonography in avian medicine.

Modern ultrasound devices used for small mammals are also suitable for use in birds. Due to the limited coupling surfaces in smaller birds, microconvex or phased array probes are preferable (Fig. 5.8). In birds up to 1000 g body mass, frequencies of at least 7.5 MHz are required. Larger probes are of limited use because the area of contact with the bird is normally small. However, in birds with abdominal distension, these

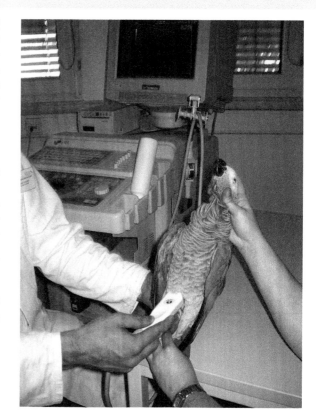

Fig 5.8 Sonographic examination of an African grey parrot (*Psittacus e. erithacus*), ventromedian approach. The bird should be held as upright as possible.

probes may lead to acceptable results. If there are insufficient coupling possibilities, a stand-off consisting of a semi-solid gel is useful. The same might be true for the examination of small birds, in order to obtain a clear image of the upper tissues.

Patient preparation

Depending on the size, the bird should be fasted for approximately 3 hours prior to the ultrasound examination. This period should be extended to 1–2 days for birds of prey. An anaesthetic is usually not necessary; the birds are either held by an assistant (Fig. 5.8) or placed on a Plexiglas® plate (see radiology section) in dorsal or lateral recumbency. Birds with severe circulatory problems should be examined in an upright position.

The area of contact is comparatively small in most pet birds, and is situated between the xiphoid process of the sternum and the pubic bone of the pelvis (in the ventromedian approach, Fig. 5.8) with lateral extension to the right- or left-hand caudal area of the last rib (in the parasternal approach). Preferably the feathers are just parted in this area. Depending on the species of bird, some plucking might be necessary. A water-soluble acoustic gel is then applied to ensure good contact between the scanner and the skin.

Ultrasonography of the liver

In many cases, the indications for sonography are similar in both birds and mammals. Any clinical symptom or laboratory result indicating abnormal liver function can be followed up and further clarified by a sonographic examination of the liver.

Enlargement of the liver is frequently visible on radiographs, and further clarification by means of radiography is not possible. Ultrasound provides more information, especially regarding the internal structure of the organ. A radiological evaluation of the internal organs (with the exception of the air-containing lungs) is not possible if the patient has ascites; however, this fluid provides an ideal contrast medium for sonography, and makes examination of the liver easy.

The physiological echotexture of the liver is homogeneous (Figs 5.9, 5.11), delicately granulated and of average reflex intensity. The inner structure is interrupted by blood vessels passing transversally and longitudinally. These are seen as anechoic channels.

Sonography is mainly used in suspected liver disease in order to demonstrate inflammatory processes and tumours, in the diagnosis of ascites or cysts, and to estimate the degree of alterations with regard to the prognosis. The sonographic image of a fatty liver degeneration shows a higher reflex intensity and hepatomegaly. Hepatic neoplasms may be seen as obviously non-homogeneous liver tissue; the parenchymal alterations can be focal or diffuse. Diffuse necrosis is typically seen as a spotted non-homogeneous pattern. Separate abscesses, granulomata or necroses are sharply separated from the normal liver tissue. Depending on their content, these areas may be hypoechoic (fluid) with corpuscular parts, or hyperechoic (tissue), sometimes separated into small cavernae. Haematomata are sometimes found in hypoechoic parts of the liver and tend to organize after several days. This is associated with an increase in the reflex intensity.

Ultrasonography of the gall bladder

Patients may have to fast for 1–2 days for examination of the gall bladder. A filled gall bladder in birds is easily recognized sonographically as a round-to-oval structure within the liver parenchyma (Fig. 5.9). (A gall bladder is absent in most Psittaciformes and Columbiformes.) It normally appears as a smooth, clearly defined organ, with thin, reflex-intense walls and echolucent contents. It causes acoustic enhancement, as do other fluid-filled structures. Some large vessels, such as the right portal vein and the right hepatic artery, may be seen adjacent to the gall bladder. Alterations of the gall bladder seem to be rare in birds; however, with the help of ultrasonography, neoplasia of the wall or the bile ducts as well as abnormal concrement content can be diagnosed.

Ultrasonography of the spleen

Alterations of the splenic parenchyma cannot be diagnosed radiographically. Although the normal spleen is also very difficult to identify in sonography, indications for a sonographic examination may consist of any case of supposed splenic disease where the radiological diagnosis is insufficient. For example, examination may be indicated in the case of splenomegaly in order to demonstrate inflammatory processes and tumours or post-traumatic reaction.

The parasternal approach is used for the examination. The identification of the normal spleen can be difficult, as mentioned before. The size and shape of the spleen varies greatly between the various species. The spleen is slightly more echogenic, compared to the relative hepatic echogenicity. The parenchyma is of fine and dense granularity, and is of even texture throughout.

The spleen is often markedly enlarged in pathological alterations. In these cases, the organ is also easily visualized from the ventrodorsal approach. Homogeneous enlargement is frequently seen due to infectious or traumatic causes. Post-traumatic bleeding can be seen as hypoechoic areas. Splenic tumours are usually of mixed echogenicity, and this may be seen as a marked focal or diffuse inhomogeneous echotexture.

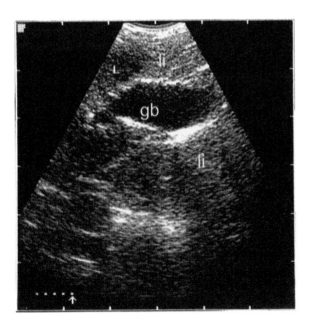

Fig 5.9 Goshawk (*Accipiter gentilis*), ventromedian approach, showing normal liver parenchyma (li) and gall bladder (gb).

Ultrasonography of the gastrointestinal tract

There are only a few indications for sonographic examination of the digestive tract. A survey radiograph and a radiographic contrast or double-contrast study of the gastrointestinal tract usually provides sufficient information on pathological alterations or functional disorders.

The ventriculus of seed-eaters is usually easily identified, from either the ventromedian or the parasternal approach. Grit content is readily visible as hyperechoic particles, usually surrounded by an area of lower echogenicity (depending on the type of food eaten). The wall of the ventriculus is seen as a round echogenic margin. The proventriculus and the intestinal loops, as well as the cloaca, can also be identified on the sonographic image (echogenic wall, hypoechoic content, typical shape in corn eaters; Fig. 5.10). The motility of the intestinal loops is clearly visible on the screen, and the duodenal loop is especially easy to identify by its position and shape. A stand-off is necessary for the examination of the pancreas. The cloaca is seen in the ventromedian approach by sweeping the scanner caudally. The wall of the gastrointestinal tract may be difficult to examine sonographically, but this is facilitated when the tract is nearly empty and is then filled with fluid for contrast purposes. With probe frequencies of 10 to 12 MHz, the demonstration of the wall layers is possible, and the wall thickness can be assessed. Food particles, especially bones in carnivorous species and gas content, make it impossible for the sound beam to penetrate, precluding an adequate evaluation of the gastrointestinal tract.

Ultrasonography of the heart

Echocardiography has much to offer in the cardiac evaluation of birds. It is an excellent diagnostic tool for obtaining information on the heart's function and on pathological alterations, e.g. pericardial effusion, hypertrophy and dilatation of the ventricles, and valvular insufficiency. Any clinical sign indicative of cardiac disease should be followed up by a sonographic examination. Another indication is radiographic evidence of heart disease, such as alterations in the heart's size, shape and radiographic density.

The B-mode technique can be used for sonographic examination of the heart. Due to anatomical peculiarities of the class Aves standard M-mode traces cannot be interpreted correctly in birds. Spectral Doppler function is useful for determining the velocity of the blood flow (inflow, outflow).

The chambers, valves and large vessels and the motility of the heart and the valves can all be identified sonographically (Fig. 5.11). A standardized schedule for routine echocardiography in birds has been established

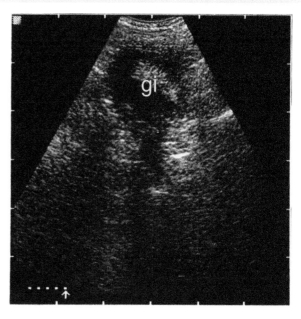

Fig 5.10 Sulphur-crested cockatoo (*Cacatua galerita*), ventromedian approach, showing the gizzard (gi).

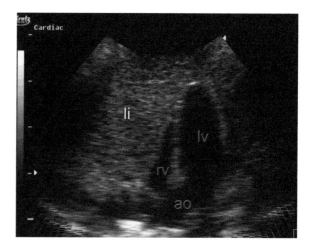

Fig 5.11 African grey parrot (*Psittacus e. erithacus*), ventromedian approach, showing the heart (lv = left ventricle, rv = right ventricle, ao = aorta), and the liver (li).

(Krautwald-Junghanns et al 1995, Pees et al 2004). The following views and approaches are recommended: with the ventromedian approach the apical horizontal (four-chamber) view and the apical vertical (two-chamber) view, and additional short axis views from the parasternal approach.

Alterations of the pericardium, especially pericardial effusion, can be diagnosed easily by sonographic examination. The fluid is recognized as an anechoic band separating the epicardium and the pericardium. Morphometric (B-mode) and functional (B-mode and spectral Doppler)

assessment of the heart is also possible, and reference values have been published (Tables 5.1 and 5.2). Besides pericardial effusion, the most frequent pathological findings are hypertrophy and/or dilatation of the right ventricle.

Ultrasonography of the urogenital tract

Ultrasonography can be used to differentiate renal tumours, inflammatory processes and cystic alterations of the kidneys. Sonography of the reproductive tract is indicated in suspected egg-binding, salpingitis, and ovarian or oviductal cysts or neoplasms. Both the ventromedian and the parasternal approach can be used.

At this time, it is not possible to demonstrate the normal kidneys in birds by transcutaneous sonography. The inactive testes and ovaries are also difficult to identify in birds; they cannot be visualized sonographically because the intestinal loops (ventromedian approach)

Table 5.1 2-D-Echocardiography, important measured and calculated parameters in birds (mean value ± standard deviation)

Parameter	Psittacus e. erithacus (Pees et al 2004)	Amazona spp. (Pees et al 2004)	Cacatua spp. (Pees et al 2004)	Diurnal raptors[a] (Boskovic et al 1999)	Pigeons (Schulz 1995)
Body mass (g)	493 ± 55	353 ± 42	426 ± 162	720 ± 197	434 ± 52
Left ventricle					
Length systole (mm)	22.5 ± 1.9	21.1 ± 2.3	19.0 ± 1.3	14.7 ± 2.8	17.9 ± 1.0
Length diastole (mm)	24.0 ± 1.9	22.1 ± 2.2	19.9 ± 1.6	16.4 ± 2.7	20.1 ± 1.4
Width systole (mm)	6.8 ± 1.0	6.7 ± 1.2	6.4 ± 1.7	6.3 ± 1.1	5.2 ± 0.4
Width diastole (mm)	8.6 ± 1.0	8.4 ± 1.0	8.3 ± 1.5	7.7 ± 1.2	7.4 ± 0.6
Width fractional shortening (%)	22.6 ± 4.4	22.8 ± 4.2	25.6 ± 7.0	Not given	27.2 ± 4.5
Right ventricle					
Length systole (mm)	9.2 ± 1.4	9.4 ± 1.8	10.3 ± 1.2	12.7 ± 2.7	Not given
Length diastole (mm)	11.5 ± 1.9	10.3 ± 1.3	11.3 ± 2.3	13.9 ± 2.5	9.9 ± 0.8
Width systole (mm)	2.8 ± 0.9	3.1 ± 0.7	2.3 ± 0.0	2.1 ± 0.6	Not given
Width diastole (mm)	4.8 ± 1.1	5.2 ± 1.3	3.5 ± 0.5	2.5 ± 0.8	4.0 ± 0.5
Width fractional shortening (%)	40.8 ± 11.9	34.1 ± 3.7	33.3 ± 10.3	Not givven	Not given
Interventricular septum					
Thickness systole (mm)	2.9 ± 0.5	2.2 ± 0.1	1.9 ± 0.3	1.9 ± 0.6	3.8 ± 0.1
Thickness diastole (mm)	2.5 ± 0.3	2.1 ± 0.4	1.7 ± 0.4	1.9 ± 0.5	3.3 ± 0.2

[a]Diurnal raptors including Buteo buteo, Accipiter nisus, Accipiter gentilis, Milvus milvus.

Table 5.2 Velocities of intracardial blood flow in some bird species (anaesthetized)

Parameter	Amazona spp. (Pees et al 2005)	Ara spp. (Carrani et al 2003)	Cacatua galerita (Carrani et al 2003)	Psittacus erithacus (Carrani et al 2003)	Falco spp. (Straub et al 2001)	Buteo buteo (Straub et al 2001)
Diastolic inflow left ventricle (m/s)	0.18 ± 0.03	0.54 ± 0.07	0.32 ± 0.15	0.39 ± 0.06	0.21 ± 0.03	0.14 ± 0.01
Diastolic inflow right ventricle (m/s)	0.22 ± 0.05	Not given	Not given	Not given	0.21 ± 0.04	0.14 ± 0.02
Systolic outflow aortic root (m/s)	0.83 ± 0.08	0.81 ± 0.16	0.78 ± 0.19	0.89 ± 0.13	0.95 ± 0.07	1.18 ± 0.05

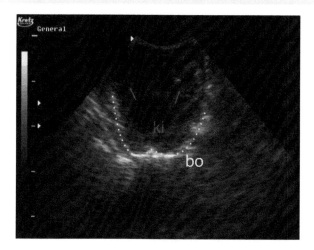

Fig 5.12 Budgerigar (*Melopsittacus undulatus*), ventromedian approach. Massive enlargement of the kidneys (ki, arrows) showing inhomogeneous echogenicities (focal necrosis). This bird suffered from a renal neoplasia (bo = bones of pelvis and spinal column, forming a typical W-shape).

and the abdominal air sacs (parasternal approach) prevent their examination. The determination of a bird's sex with the help of ultrasonography has been successful with the use of intracloacal transducers. Active gonads may also be demonstrated via transcutaneous ultrasonography.

Developing follicles can be seen as round areas with an echogenic content (the yolk). Later, the strongly echogenic shell is easily differentiated from the surrounding tissue; the egg content is divided into two parts of differing echogenicity (hyperechoic yolk, hypoechoic egg albumen).

Renal neoplasia (Fig. 5.12) is frequently accompanied by massive enlargement and parenchymal lesions. In these cases the kidneys are easily demonstrated by using the ventromedian approach to show round, non-homogeneous structures.

Cysts can also be diagnosed sonographically. The characteristic appearance of a cyst is a clearly defined, rounded, echolucent structure, with marked posterior acoustic enhancement.

Egg-binding is easily diagnosed if the egg has a shell. The demonstration of laminated eggs without a shell is also possible by sonographic means. They are easily differentiated from the surrounding tissue, and appear as oval or round areas with varying echogenicity.

Endoscopy

Endoscopes commonly used in companion birds are rigid and have a diameter of 1.7–2.7 mm. In avian medicine, the use of endoscopy is described for diagnostic procedures including tissue biopsies, for local treatments (e.g. aspergillosis), for surgical interventions, and above all, for sexing of monomorphic species.

Diagnostic procedures

The endoscope can be used for the visual examination of any body orifice large enough to allow the insertion of this instrument. Apart from laparoscopy, which will be discussed under surgical sexing, tracheoscopy is the most common endoscopic procedure in avian medicine. It is used as an additional diagnostic tool for the detection of inflammation, occlusion or other lesions.

Tracheoscopy

Tracheoscopy is indicated in birds showing clinical signs of dyspnoea presumably caused by an obstacle in the trachea or syrinx. Tracheoscopy is limited by the diameter of the patient's tracheal lumen and by the length of the patient's neck. In birds the size of cockatiels, the tracheal lumen does not allow the insertion of an endoscope. In birds with long necks, such as swans or storks, only the proximal portion of the trachea can be examined endoscopically. Because of the length of the neck, it is impossible to get a view of the syrinx with the rigid endoscope in these birds.

Tracheoscopy must be performed under anaesthesia. Most patients requiring this procedure show signs of dyspnoea, and trying to insert an endoscope into the trachea of a bird which is already having trouble breathing is difficult. In cases of severe dyspnoea, the patient's condition has to be stabilized with the aid of an abdominal air sac breathing tube before the endoscope can be inserted into the trachea. The bird is positioned in dorsal or vertical recumbency. Dorsal recumbency is better for establishing the bird's condition. The neck has to be extended, and the operator opens the beak, pulls the tongue forward and carefully inserts the endoscope through the glottis. Scraping the tracheal wall with the endoscope can cause lesions and stimulate coughing, and this is minimized if the tip of the endoscope is always directed towards the centre of the tracheal lumen while the instrument is gently pushed downwards. In most cases, reflexive coughing stops when the endoscope is in place.

The tracheal examination can be used to diagnose foreign bodies, parasites and any kind of plaques obstructing the tracheal airway. Parasites are rarely seen in pet birds. If diagnosed they have to be treated medically, as their presence must be assumed throughout the whole respiratory tract. Foreign bodies and plaques are seen particularly in the region of the tracheal bifurcation. Seed hulls or whole seeds are commonly aspirated as foreign bodies. Plaques can be caused by hypovitaminosis A, are composed of squamous material, and may provoke secondary infections. Bacterial or fungal infections of the respiratory tract can also lead to inflammatory reactions and cell debris in the form of plaques in the respiratory tract. At the beginning of such an infection the process may be limited to the area of the bifurcation, but these infections usually spread very quickly over the whole respiratory tract. The extent of this expansion determines the bird's prognosis and the veterinarian's chance of treating the problem.

Any plaques observed in the trachea should be removed and examined if possible. Ideally, biopsy forceps can be passed alongside the endoscope and reach the plaque. If this is impossible because of the limited size of the tracheal lumen, an attempt can be made to loosen the plaque with the tip of the endoscope and remove it by suction with the help of a small catheter. With this method there is the risk of losing pieces of plaque into the deeper parts of the trachea while exchanging the endoscope for the catheter, and the bird should therefore be positioned horizontally before loosening plaque material. If this method is also unsuccessful, surgical removal by opening the trachea is necessary.

Liver examination and biopsy

The endoscope has proved to be a useful tool for the examination and biopsy of the liver. This organ is involved in many infectious avian diseases. Although examination of the liver with the aid of radiographs, ultrasonograms and blood chemistries can provide information regarding the liver gross morphology and function, these methods are not always exact enough to diagnose the cause of changes; in these cases, a visual approach and a biopsy may be necessary.

The liver is approached from the ventral aspect of the patient. The bird is placed in dorsal recumbency and its legs are pulled caudally. Just behind the sternum, in the midline, a 1 cm skin incision is made, followed by a smaller incision or puncture of the abdominal musculature before the abdominal cavity is opened bluntly. Underneath the abdominal muscles, the ventral hepatic peritoneal cavity membrane appears; this is held up with forceps in order to avoid lesions of the liver, and then carefully punctured with a blade or scissors. The hole is extended by inserting forceps and spreading them.

Having opened the peritoneal cavity, the operator can insert the endoscope and examine the ventral surface of both liver lobes. For the liver biopsy, small spoon-shaped biopsy forceps originally designed for otolaryngological examination are used. The forceps are passed alongside the endoscope until the jaws are visible through the scope. When they reach the area that is to be sampled, the jaws of the forceps are opened and a small piece of the liver is grasped. The jaws are held closed in this position for about 30 seconds, to prevent excessive bleeding, and the forceps are then removed with the sample between the jaws. At the end of the procedure, muscles and skin are closed with separate sutures. The bird should be kept under recovery conditions for about 2 days to minimize the risk of haemorrhage.

Another method for taking a liver biopsy which is also less traumatic and therefore preferable if the equipment is available is the ultrasound-guided fine needle biopsy. Using a 20-gauge true-cut needle, hepatic material is obtained for a histological examination.

Oesophagus, crop and cloaca examination

The oesophagus, crop and cloaca are the parts of the alimentary tract that are accessible to endoscopic examination. Indications are palpable structures of unknown origin, supposed obstruction, and other conditions in which neither palpation nor radiographs lead to a conclusive diagnosis. Infectious agents such as *Trichomonas*, bacteria or fungi can be diagnosed with the aid of swabs taken from the crop or from the cloaca, and do not require endoscopic examination under anaesthesia.

For the endoscopic examination of the upper alimentary tract, the patient must be fasted until the crop is empty. The bird is then anaesthetized and held vertically with the neck extended. The beak is opened and the endoscope gently introduced from the left side to the right side into the crop like a crop cannula. Since the lumen of the oesophagus is normally closed, mucus will cover the lens of the endoscope and blur the view. The lens can be cleaned by wiping it against the oesophagus or crop wall. The view in the oesophagus is usually less blurred when the instrument is withdrawn rather than moved forward. Once the crop has been entered, an assistant can gently pull the skin over the thoracic inlet and upward in order to increase the view within the crop.

It is almost impossible to pass the endoscope into the proventriculus when entering from the oral cavity. If it is necessary, the crop can be surgically opened and the endoscope passed down the remainder of the oesophagus into the proventriculus. A small catheter can be inserted along with the endoscope and used to inflate the proventriculus. This makes operation easier, even when there are large amounts of secretions in the proventriculus.

Examination of the nares and ears

Depending on the size of the bird, the nares and ears can also be examined endoscopically, but deep penetration of these sites is not possible, even in large birds.

Surgical sexing

A laparoscopic examination with accentuation of the reproductive tract is performed for surgical sexing. This is the most common indication for endoscopy in avian medicine, and because of this laparoscopy and surgical sexing are not described separately.

Presurgical considerations and anaesthesia

Surgical sexing or laparoscopy should be performed under general anaesthesia. Performing this operation without general anaesthesia carries a high risk of puncturing organs within the abdominal cavity when the bird moves and struggles. The danger of shock due to hyperventilation and an excessively increased heartbeat is also greater without general anaesthesia. Also, it cannot be considered humane to puncture the abdominal wall of a conscious bird.

Surgical sexing is a routine operation, and appears to the owner to be very low risk – especially since the bird concerned is generally healthy. Therefore, if any complications arise, the owner is likely to believe that the veterinarian is at fault regardless of the actual cause. This means that the risks of the surgery must be explained to each owner, and that the veterinarian must examine every patient carefully to determine whether or not the bird is in fact healthy and a good surgical candidate. If the bird is in moult, there is an increased risk of bleeding in the area of the skin and feather follicles. In birds with adiposity, there is an increased risk of anaesthesia, and vizualization of the organs might be more difficult due to fat deposits.

The operator has to make sure that the bird's crop does not contain palpable amounts of water or food, because passive regurgitation into the oropharynx under general anaesthesia can cause aspiration and asphyxia. The bird should have fasted in order to guarantee that neither the proventriculus nor parts of the intestine are at increased risk of being punctured accidentally with the trocar or the endoscope. The duration of fasting depends on the species; for example, birds with a slow transit time of the alimentary tract, such as raptors, should fast longer than psittacines. Furthermore, it is advisable to examine the bird's skeleton for old fractures or other abnormalities, since these can cause injury when the bird is positioned for surgery. The abdomen should also be examined by palpation. A bird with ascites, severe adiposity or palpable abnormal tissue masses can have difficulties during the procedure.

The endoscope should be sterilized in a liquid disinfectant that not only inactivates fungi and bacteria in general, but is also effective against mycobacteria and viral agents. It must be rinsed in sterile water before contact with the bird's abdomen, since most disinfectants cause irritation.

Gas anaesthesia is the most comfortable method of anaesthetizing a bird for surgical sexing or laparoscopy, as it allows a very quick recovery of the patient. The anaesthetic gas of choice is isoflurane, and the patient is usually induced through a face mask. Since routine surgical sexing only takes a few minutes, assuming no

complications arise, the bird is usually not intubated for this procedure. The initial introduction is done with 5% isoflurane, and anaesthesia is maintained at 1–2% with an oxygen flow rate of 1–2 L/min.

Surgical procedure

Three different entry sites can be recommended for sexing procedures or laparoscopy, and it is important to position the bird correctly for each approach used for surgical sexing. Improper positioning of the patient can lead to a different anatomical arrangement of the organs within the abdominal cavity, which not only increases the risk of puncturing organs but can also prevent an adequate view of the gonads.

All three entry sites are on the left side of the patient. This is important because females only have a functional left ovary, and when this is inactive it is small and difficult to find from the right side. The bird is placed in right lateral recumbency. Its head is grasped from behind and held in position by supporting the mandibular joints with the thumb and the index finger of the right hand. The position of the legs depends on the entry site preferred for the procedure. The feet are held with the left hand; the right leg can be left unsecured. The wings are pulled dorsally over the body and held down in this position, with the forearm of the hand restraining the head.

In the most commonly used approach, the legs are extended caudally. This position reveals the entry site in a depression between the ribs cranially, the synsacrum dorsally and the greater trochanter with the femur caudally (Fig. 5.13). In psittacines, the insertion site is located directly anterior to the proximal one-third to one-quarter of the imaginary line between the greater trochanter and the knee. In mynah birds the kidneys are found in a more ventral position than in psittacines, and this means the entry site must be moved more ventrally in order to avoid a contusion of the kidney. The second possible

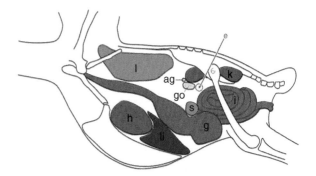

Fig 5.13 Correct position of the endoscope (red arrow, e) in the most commonly used entry site for surgical sexing: ag = adrenal gland; e = endoscope; g = gizzard; go = gonad; i = intestine; k = kidney; l = lung; li = liver; s = spleen; h = heart.

approach is made just caudal to the pubis and ventral to the ischium. The leg must be pulled slightly forward.

The bird's position for the third entry site is the same as for the second, but the left leg is pulled forward more strongly. The lateral pelvic apterium is located, and the last rib is palpated. At this point, an inverted V-shaped landmark is seen where the semitendinosus muscle (flexor cruris medialis) passes over the rib. The skin incision is made just caudal to this point. The fascial attachment of the semitendinosus is bluntly separated to reflect the muscle dorsally; the lateral body wall then becomes visible and allows the operator direct access with either a trocar or blunt dissection.

After disinfecting the skin, an incision of 3–5 mm is made without injuring the underlying muscle in order to avoid diffuse bleeding, which could disturb the view later on. Then a probe, a trocar or fine closed mosquito forceps can be used to puncture the abdominal wall. A trocar should not be used in birds that weigh less than 100 g because it increases the diameter of the endoscope by at least 1 mm, which can make a large difference in the narrow abdominal cavity of a small bird.

A growing resistance is felt when attempting to penetrate the abdominal wall, and a characteristic 'pop' can usually be heard when penetration occurs. The probe is directed downward and has to pierce the abdominal air sac membrane gently so that the abdominal air sac cavity can be entered. Its medial membrane is then penetrated and the intestinal peritoneal cavity is reached. Since it is not easy to introduce the endoscope through the punctured hole, it can be inserted alongside the probe, allowing the end of the probe to guide the endoscope. The operator can then examine the area in which the abdomen has been penetrated and ensure that no damage has occurred during the process.

The probe is then removed so that the visual examination can begin. It may take a few moments to get a clear view through the endoscope. Sometimes the lens may be in direct contact with the air sac membrane or an organ, and in this case the position of the endoscope has to be corrected by gently withdrawing the instrument. If viscera are clearly visible, the endoscope has entered the intestinal peritoneal cavity. If only air sac membranes are seen, the tip of the endoscope is inside the abdominal air sac cavity. In this case, the lens of the endoscope is pushed gently against the air sac membrane until it is punctured.

With a clear view of the viscera, the operator first becomes orientated. In most cases the left kidney is easily recognizable; it is reddish-brown in colour and is located in the dorsal part of the visual field (Fig. 5.14). Following the kidney to the left, its cranial pole becomes visible through the endoscope. Physiologically it has a rounded and smooth surface, and is generally larger than either the adrenal gland or the gonad. The adrenal glands are located anterior to the cranial poles of the kidneys, and are yellowish-orange in colour and highly vascular (Fig. 5.14). In the most cranial part of the field of vision, the pink tissue of the lung is visible.

Gonads, adrenal glands, spleen, intestines and the dorsal portion of the proventriculus are situated within the intestinal peritoneal cavity that runs along the midline from the cranial pole of the kidney to the cloaca. The kidneys are located retroperitoneal to this cavity (Fig. 5.13).

In the male, the testes are located slightly ventrally to the cranial pole of the kidneys and the adrenal glands. In the female, the ovary's position is similar to that of the left testis. In the adult female, the active ovary may completely or partially cover the left adrenal gland (Fig. 5.14).

When the examination is over, muscle and skin are sutured together and the bird is put in a quiet place for recovery. Antibiotics are not routinely administered after this surgery. When several birds from one owner are surgically sexed, they are often put together

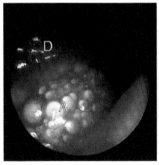 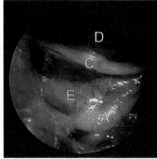 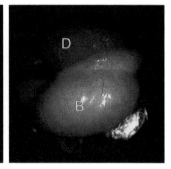

Fig 5.14 Endoscopic imaging of the gonads. Left: adult ovary; middle: juvenile ovary; right: adult testis (A = ovary, B = testis, C = ovarial ligament, D = kidney, E = adrenal gland).

in a single box during recovery. However, this should be avoided since the most heavily sedated bird is often bitten by the others.

The gonads

The testes have a bean-shaped or cylindrical appearance, a smooth surface, and are creamy-white in colour (Fig. 5.14) although they can be melanistic in some species. In psittacine birds, white cockatoos and many of the Australian parakeet species have melanistic testes. Sometimes a black gonad will be seen in a species that does not normally have melanistic gonads, but this should not be interpreted as a pathological finding.

The testes can vary in size, depending on the age of the bird and the stage of the reproductive cycle. In immature individuals they are very small and usually avascular. Testes that are just becoming active may appear pink due to the superficial vessels, which increase in diameter in this functional stage. In a mature bird the testes can vary in size, and may be as much as 500 times their normal size during the breeding season. In general, they are larger than the adjacent adrenal gland and more vascular on the surface. Under physiological conditions, both the testes are almost the same size. In the mature male they atrophy after a period of sexual stimulation, but never become as small as they were in the immature stage.

Like the testes, the ovary is usually creamy-white but may be pigmented. In the immature bird it is comma-shaped and dorsoventrally flattened, and it may resemble a piece of fat (Fig. 5.14). The inactive ovary of a mature bird has many small follicles; the active ovary has a grape-like cluster of small but prominent follicles that are easy to identify.

Ovarian cysts are common, and they appear in the form of clear vesicles that can be larger than the rest of the ovary. When they occur, they usually represent the only follicular activity detectable. These patients should not be mistaken for successfully breeding birds.

Sometimes the testes appear to have a rough surface. This is caused by the development of testicular cysts, which are less than 1 mm in diameter and do not appear to enlarge. They do not seem to affect the function of the organ. Small or misshapen testes can sometimes be seen in successfully breeding birds.

Shrunken, fibrotic gonads can be found in both sexes, and seem to affect the function of the gonads, since these birds generally show poor breeding results.

Hermaphrodites are very rarely encountered in birds. The author has seen one bird with one testicle and an ovary which showed constant feather picking and self-mutilation.

Some pathological findings are not directly associated with the gonads but can nevertheless affect breeding results – for example, opaque air sac membranes with or without plaques, and the presence of plaques on the surface of non-gonadal structures. These findings are not always significant for breeding, especially when no adhesions are visible. However, if the plaques or granulomata are large and adhere to the gonads or surrounding structures, the female's ability to ovulate may be disturbed. The oocyst may be hindered in entering the infundibulum of the oviduct because the opening is physically closed by adhesions. Similar lesions are not believed to affect the ability of males to breed.

Another abnormality frequently seen is the enlargement of the spleen. This organ is normally no more than 1 cm in diameter in large psittacine birds, and is bright red in colour. An obvious enlargement in size or change in colour to an intense red can be caused by a systemic infection. Psittacosis should always be considered as a differential diagnosis in such cases, especially in a newly imported bird. Multiple white urate deposits of about 1 mm in diameter may be detected in the kidney. In most cases these are not linked with clinical or functional pathological symptoms.

Complications and errors

Haemorrhage is the most frequently encountered problem, preventing adequate viewing of the viscera. When a small amount of blood covers the lens of the endoscope, it can be cleaned by blotting the tip gently against an intra-abdominal organ or by withdrawing the instrument and rinsing the tip with sterile water. If bleeding persists, the procedure should be discontinued and repeated another day.

Fat or air sacculitis can also restrict the view. Obese birds frequently have large amounts of abdominal fat that can partially cover the gonads or other organs or limit the space in which to manoeuvre the endoscope. Tachypnoea occurs from time to time in extremely excited birds, during initial anaesthetic induction or throughout the entire laparoscopy. Excessive ventilation through the air sacs causes the loosely attached digestive organs to move rapidly, making it difficult to position the endoscope properly. Altered anatomy, as found in neoplastic diseases of the kidneys, liver or spleen, can cause lesions during the procedure as well as obstructing the operator's view.

As well as the risk of complications originating from the bird, possible iatrogenic errors should also be considered. One of the most common errors is to confuse an immature female with a male. The young female ovary looks more like a piece of fat and is flattened with indistinct edges. It usually has sulci on its surface. A testicle is smooth with rounded ends. In the female, the supporting ligament of the infundibulum of the oviduct crosses the cranial portion of the kidney (Fig. 5.14). This structure is absent in males. Furthermore, only one ovary but two testicles can be found. Therefore in young birds, if two gonads are visible, even though their shape may be relatively indistinct, the bird is most probably a male. Nevertheless, the operator should bear in mind that in young psittacines the remnant of the right ovary may be visible for at least several months after weaning. It sometimes appears cylindrical and smooth like a testicle.

Another mistake is to confuse a section of intestine with a testicle. A loop of intestine can appear round, smooth and white or yellow, and may lie directly at the cranial pole of the left kidney. Its extent may not be initially apparent.

References

Boskovic M, Krautwald-Junghanns M E, Failing K et al 1999 Möglichkeiten und Grenzen echokardiographischer Untersuchungen bei Tag- und Nachtgreifvögeln (Accipitriformes, Falconiformes, Strigiformes). Tieraerztliche Praxis 27:334–341

Bush M, Montali R I, Novak R G et al 1976 The healing of avian fractures – a histological xero-radiographic study. American Animal Hospital Association Journal 12(6):768

Carrani F, Gelli D, Salvadori M et al 2003 A preliminary echocardiographic initial approach to diastolic and systolic function in medium and large parrots. European Association of Avian Veterinarians, Proceedings, p 145–149

Krautwald-Junghanns M E, Schulz M, Hagner D et al 1995 Transcoelomic two-dimensional echocardiography in the avian patient. Journal of Avian Medicine and Surgery 9(1):19–31

Pees M, Straub J, Krautwald-Junghanns M E 2004 Echocardiographic examinations of 60 African grey parrots and 30 other psittacine birds. Veterinary Record 155:73–76

Pees M, Straub J, Schumacher J et al 2005 Pilotstudie zu echokardiographischen Untersuchungen mittels Farb- und pulsed-wave-Spektraldoppler an Blaukronenamazonen (*Amazona ventralis*) und Blaustirnamazonen (*Amazona a. aestiva*). Deutsche Tierärztliche Wochenschrift 112:39–43

Schulz M 1995 Morphologische und funktionelle Messungen am Herzen von Brieftauben (*Columbia livia* forma *domestica*) mit Hilfe der Schnittbildechokardiographie. Doctoral thesis, Giessen

Straub J, Pees M, Schumacher J et al 2001 Doppler-echocardiography in birds. European Association of Avian Veterinarians, Proceedings, p 92–94

Suggested reading

Bennett R A, Harrison G J 1994 Soft tissue surgery. In: Ritchie B W, Harrison G J, Harrison L R (eds) Avian medicine: principles and application. Wingers, Lake Worth, FL, p 1096–1136

Krautwald-Junghanns M-E, Enders F 1997 Ultrasonography. In: Altman R, Dorrestein G, Quesenberry K (eds) Avian medicine and surgery. W B Saunders, Philadelphia, PA, p 200–211

Krautwald-Junghanns M E, Tellhelm B, Hummel G et al 1992 Atlas of radiographic anatomy and diagnosis of cage birds. Paul Parey, Berlin

Lierz M 2006 Diagnostic value of endoscopy and biopsy. In: Harrison G J, Lightfoot T (eds) Clinical avian medicine. Spix Publishing, Palm Beach, FL, p 631–652

McDonald S E 1996 Endoscopy. In: Rosskopf W, Woerpel R (eds) Diseases of cage and aviary birds. Williams & Wilkins, Baltimore, MD, p 699–717

McMillan M 1994 Imaging techniques. In: Ritchie B W, Harrison G J, Harrison L R (eds) Avian medicine: principles and application. Wingers, Lake Worth, FL, p 246–261

Taylor M 1994 Endoscopic examination and biopsy techniques. In: Ritchie B W, Harrison G J, Harrison L R (eds) Avian medicine: principles and application. Wingers, Lake Worth, FL, p 327–347

Nursing the sick bird

Gerry M. Dorrestein

6

Introduction

The interest in avian medicine grows every year, and the degree of successful diagnosis and treatment in our avian patients has increased tremendously over the last two decades (Nemetz 2005). Many avian patients require emergency treatment and critical care. They accept our care and love, or tolerate it, and may welcome us into their lives. At the same time, companion birds are reluctant to reveal their frailties, 'hiding' their ailments until they are unable to compensate any longer. If veterinarians are to care for these patients, they must be prepared for emergency and critical cases (Jenkins 1994).

Live birds are generally presented to a veterinary practice in one of three conditions: healthy (or apparently so), injured or ill. Often the injured bird can be specifically treated with emphasis on the injury while supportive measures are initiated. **The sick patient requires an approach that addresses immediate medical needs and will lead to stabilization and at the same time investigates the nature of the illness; therein lies the greatest challenge in avian medicine (Fig. 6.1) (Harris 1994).** The advances in medical equipment and diagnostics have allowed the avian veterinarian greater opportunities to treat the critical avian patient properly (Loudis & Sutherland-Smith 1994). There is no master list of equipment that every avian practitioner must own. Needs must be catered to the species seen and the individual interest of the practitioner. The author implores interested veterinarians to investigate the great learning experiences before casually deciding to add avian patients to a general companion animal practice (Nemetz 2005). Continuing education courses are now offered throughout the country on various aspects of avian medicine. The Association of Avian Veterinarians provides a journal, yearly conference, website, and a wide range of support materials.

All drugs, supplies and equipment should be preassembled at a central location to facilitate their application (Murray 1994, Raftery 2005).

Environmental requirements

Much of the equipment needed to accommodate sick birds is available in the average companion animal practice. Several publications go into detail about practice equipment (Raftery 2005, Harrison & Flinchum 2006). In order to transform a traditional small animal clinic into an 'avian friendly' clinic, a number of modifications

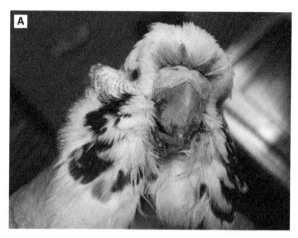

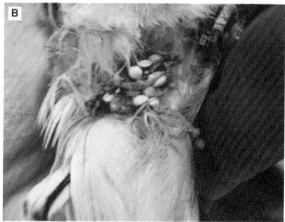

Fig 6.1 A severely ill budgerigar **A** exhibiting signs of ocular, nasal discharge and regurgitation with **B** a pasty vent.

should be considered. A separate avian waiting room would be ideal, but if that is not possible an area that is not in direct contact with dogs, cats and children should be designated for bulky bird enclosures and carriers (Johnson-Delaney 1994).

Admitting a sick bird to the veterinary hospital for intensive care has many advantages and few disadvantages (Coles 1996a).

Advantages of hospitalization include the following:

1. The bird is under the direct observation of the veterinary surgeon and his/her experienced staff, and its condition can be monitored.

2. The bird receives regular therapy if necessary.

3. Immediate action can be taken if the bird's condition deteriorates.

4. The veterinary surgeon has time to think about the case, to carry out any necessary laboratory tests, etc., and to reconsider the differential diagnosis list.

5. The bird can be kept in a controlled microclimate under optimal conditions during its recovery.

6. Birds are usually by nature members of a flock, and the sight of other hospitalized birds often has a beneficial psychological effect.

7. Many owners are totally unable to medicate their birds or give the supplementary feeding required.

Disadvantages of hospitalization include the following:

1. The bird is in unfamiliar surroundings with an unfamiliar routine; this may increase stress and the bird may be less willing to eat.

2. There may be a strong bond between the owner and the bird; this is broken and may increase stress.

3. The owner is often prepared to give the bird 24-hour tender loving care; however, an over-anxious owner may cause more stress to an already sick bird.

4. There is a risk of infection to other patients and to members of staff (zoonosis).

Housing of the sick bird

Appropriate enclosures for avian patients are a necessity. Severely ill birds or those requiring more intensive treatment, including tube feeding, fluid therapy, nebulization therapy, oxygen supplementation or monitoring, are hospitalized (Fig. 6.2) (Rupley 1997).

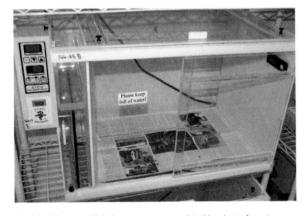

Fig 6.2 A low-cost digital temperature-regulated incubator for avian patients.

The success of treating a critical avian patient relies very heavily on the environment in which the bird must recover. Sick birds are often hypothermic and should be placed in heated enclosures in a quiet environment (Loudis & Sutherland-Smith 1994, Lichtenberger 2005, 2006, Harrison et al 2006). A separate avian housing area that can be maintained at 25–30°C is preferable but not essential. Avian enclosures should be easily viewed from across the room or through a window, thereby minimizing the need to approach the enclosure in order to evaluate a patient. The staff member who feeds, cleans and interacts with the birds should preferably be different from the person who provides 'threatening' medical treatment. The bird is less likely to be defensive around a non-threatening person, and a more accurate assessment of changes in its daily condition can be made (Johnson-Delaney 1994).

A simple warming cage can be made using a glass aquarium with a screened cover, a heating pad and a 60 W bulb in a utility fixture. Aquariums are relatively inexpensive and easy to clean and disinfect. Screen-covered tops provide good ventilation, while the aquariums themselves hold heat and reduce hospital contamination from discarded food and droppings. They offer complete visibility and easy access to the patient (Johnson-Delaney 1994, Jenkins 1997a). Instead of the light bulb, an Elstein infrared element can be used. The main advantage with this is that there is no light, only heat. A 24-hour visible light may interfere with the day–night rhythm of the bird, inducing a hormonal disturbance that can result in moulting and/or influence other hormones in many bird species.

Both the floor and air temperature should be monitored to ensure that the patient is not burned or overheated. A simple indoor/outdoor thermometer placed inside the cage will provide both readings and, when equipped with a maximum/minimum reading, a permanent record of the temperature range during the day and night will be available. Clean towels or surgical drapes can be used to cover portions of the aquarium in order to reduce heat loss and allow the bird a more private convalescent area. The temperature of the floor of the aquarium may be further modified by layering towels between the heating pad and the glass.

Avian isolation units, as seen in more specialized hospitals, are easily built, complete with separate heat and ventilation for each 'cage'. When the inside floor area is at least 50×50 cm, the average parrot cage (without the bottom part) can easily be fitted inside. **Underpressured ventilation prevents spread of airborne diseases inside the hospital area.** A heating system (e.g. Elstein bulbs of 100 W) can be mounted under a stainless steel bottom plate that supports the inside cage, with a removable perch (PVC) placed over newspaper or brown wrapping paper as bottom cover (Fig. 6.3).

Keeping the patient in a cage inside the 'hospital unit' has the advantage that cleaning the enclosure and transporting the bird is possible without catching the

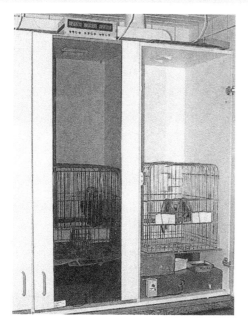

Fig 6.3 A parrot hospitalization unit with under-pressure air system on top, heating unit with thermostat in the bottom, and grey glass doors for quietness and observation.

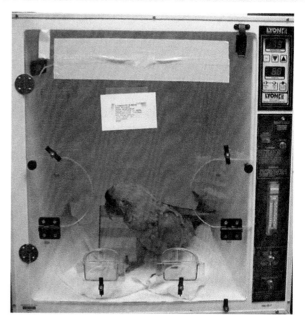

Fig 6.4 A more expensive intensive care unit in which oxygen therapy can be administered as well as nebulization treatment.

bird; also, most of the companion birds are used to being housed in such cages. Food and water can be provided in hard plastic containers fitted at perch height, so there is easy access to the container for the bird.

For extremely ill birds, low perches can be constructed from PVC pipe. This material is easy to clean and disinfect. To prevent foot and leg problems from long-term perching (longer than 2 weeks), the diameter of the perch should be modified to fit the grasp of the patient's foot. The perch should be wrapped with a layer of self-adherent bandage material to improve traction. The bandage material is changed when dirty and between patients.

Existing small animal kennels can be converted by installing a removable perch and covering the bottom of the kennel with paper. Heating pads or clamp-lamps provide supplemental heat, and towels, plastic wrap, acryl or Plexiglas® sheets can be placed over the front of the enclosure to retain heat. Enclosure doors should be removed, scrubbed and soaked in disinfectant after each bird. Spraying a light coat of Pam® cooking oil or silicone on the bars will facilitate the removal of excrement (Johnson-Delaney 1994).

Intensive care units are essential for critically ill patients or birds recovering from severe surgery. Many commercial intensive care units are available, and each has advantages and disadvantages. These units ideally can supply controllable heat, humidity and oxygen (Fig. 6.4). A dehydrated bird cannot regulate hypothermic and hyperthermic challenges, due to lack of control of evaporative heat loss and poor tissue perfusion. The incubator must also provide moisture because dry heat

will increase fluid loss in the avian patient. Many commercial units are designed to provide heat and oxygen, without regard to humidity. Although the exact levels have not been researched, it is suggested that a relatively humid environment (50–80% humidity) within the intensive care unit is beneficial. In the dyspnoeic bird presenting with open-mouthed breathing, uncontrolled water loss can contribute greatly to further dehydration and hypovolaemia (Dawson & Whittow 2000). A simple and practical method of providing heat and humidity is to place a pan of hot water covered by a rubber grill inside the intensive care unit. The bird is placed on the grill, allowing the mild steam to envelop its body (Harris 1994). The patient should be visible through a door or wall of the incubator, and there should be a port through which oxygen and fluids can be administered.

Preventing the spread of diseases

Many avian pathogens can spread though aerosol and feather particulates, and an efficient ventilation system of laminar flow design will minimize hospital contamination. Air filtration systems (purifiers) designed to decrease particulates and pathogens to the 0.1–1.0 μm range are recommended for use in the housing area as well as in the reception, examination and treatment areas (Fig. 6.5). In initial hospital design, areas with separate airflow systems should be incorporated to allow for separation of patients requiring routine care from those that may have infectious diseases. Hospital suites for housing sick birds should be divided into small, easily cleaned areas that also have separate ventilation systems.

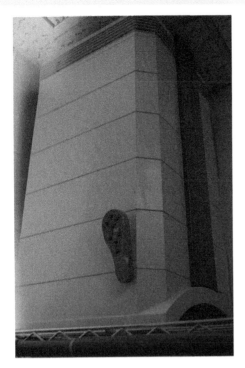

Fig 6.5 An air filtration unit within the avian hospital ward.

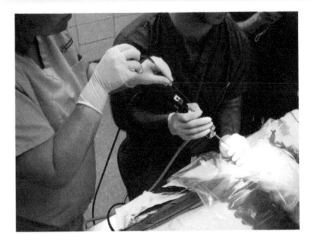

Fig 6.6 Utilizing a 2.7 mm diameter endoscopic unit to explore the coelomic cavity of an avian patient.

All materials used on avian patients should be thoroughly cleaned and disinfected between patients. It should be stressed that all disinfectants are toxic and must be handled with care to prevent problems both in the hospital premises and in patients. Birds, in most cases, are more sensitive to environmental toxins than are dogs or cats. Good ventilation is important when using any disinfectant, and instruments, utensils and surfaces must be thoroughly rinsed and dried before coming in contact with patients again.

The order in which hospitalized avian patients should be maintained follows the same pattern as with other animals: clean, feed and treat; beginning with the healthiest and ending with the most highly contagious and critically ill. Any bird within the hospital that is sick for an unconfirmed reason should be considered highly contagious until proven otherwise. **When working with a patient with a highly contagious disease or a suspected zoonosis, it is advisable for the attendant to wear a mask and hospital gown that can readily be changed.** In these cases, attendants should also use a disinfectant spray on their clothing and hair between birds. Hospital counters, shelves and tables should be wiped down with disinfectant after each use (Johnson-Delaney 1994).

Equipment

Special equipment needed to practise avian medicine is minimal. Many small animal practices already have

isoflurane anaesthesia capabilities (mandatory for an avian practice), ophthalmic-sized surgical instruments and suture materials, an endoscope (2.7 mm diameter or less), a binocular microscope with oil immersion capability, a radiosurgery unit and radiographic equipment (Figs 6.6, 6.7).

Laboratory equipment, such as a centrifuge, a haemocytometer and a biochemistry testing system, must be present, or the clinician must have access to a quick laboratory service near the practice.

A gram scale with an accuracy of ±1 g is necessary to calculate correct dosages and monitor patients' weight changes (Fig. 6.8). Both mechanical and electronic scales work well, but electronic scales are recommended. Electronic units that have an automatic tare feature are easiest and quickest to use. Scales can be fitted with perches or a container for ease of weighing avian patients. A clear, transparent, lightweight plastic box (such as a bread bin) or a container (such as a weightbox) can be used to facilitate weighing and allows observation of the patient.

Additional equipment should include a variety of syringes (including low-dose insulin syringes – see Chapter 3), small hypodermic needles, spinal needles, small butterfly catheters, avian mouth specula, gavage needles, small cuffed and Cole endotracheal tubes, and a radiographic positioner (e.g. a Plexiglas® positioning board). A quick-staining kit for smears and cytology should be available in the outpatient laboratory. Bandaging and splinting supplies, protective collars and dental acrylics for orthopaedics and beak repair are also necessary in the general avian practice.

Other equipment required for patient maintenance includes heavy ceramic, stainless steel, hard plastic or crockery feeding and drinking containers that fit to the hospital cages, and a variety of perches that can easily be cleaned and disinfected. It is important that hospital

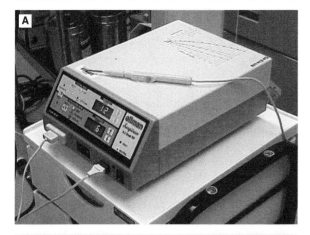

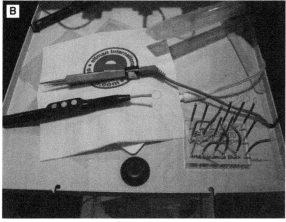

Fig 6.7 A radiosurgery unit is indispensable to an avian practice. **A** The digital 4.0 mHz unit provides state-of-the-art surgery technology for performing delicate procedures on critical patients. **B** There are multiple tips that can be used in the monopolar mode and multiple forceps that are available for the bipolar mode.

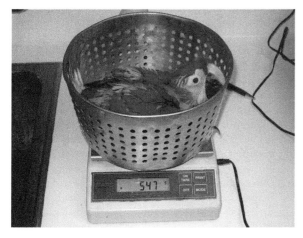

Fig 6.8 A digital gram scale is one of the most important pieces of equipment in an avian practice.

perches be made of non-porous material such as heavy plastic or PVC.

Mental support

The intelligence and attitude of avian patients demands special attention. The hospitalized patient undergoes changes due to stress, and these can delay healing and inhibit proper immunological response. Stress can involve many factors, and the following help in reducing it (Loudis & Sutherland-Smith 1994):

1. Avoid handling the bird more than is necessary.
2. If possible, allow recovery to continue at home or in familiar surroundings.
3. The cage mate of the patient may be brought to the hospital if the clinician can determine that the new bird will not be harmed or cause harm to the patient.
4. Avoid 'high traffic' areas, where the bird will be exposed to unfamiliar people, pets and possible predators such as snake and cat patients.
5. Respect the diurnal cycle of the patient and try to maintain a 12-hour light cycle.
6. Consider sounds and smell as well as sight; encourage clients to bring a familiar toy or perch to the hospital.
7. Barking, bird calls and predator odour can be distractions to the recovering patients.

Feeding

The success of emergency therapy is largely dependent on the long-term management of the recovered patient. Partial or complete anorexia is a prominent feature of many diseases, occurring at a time when the sick bird often has increased nutritional requirements and can least afford an inadequate feed intake. The nutritional management of debilitated avian patients can be the most frustrating component of a case (Loudis & Sutherland-Smith 1994). The route, composition and frequency of feeding must be considered, especially if the patient has primary gastrointestinal disease. For a quick overview, see Appendices 6.1 and 6.2 to this chapter. Iatrogenic complications can also occur, including trauma to the force-fed patient, bacterial and/or yeast ingluvitis and osmotic diarrhoea.

Provision of small quantities of highly palatable food at frequent intervals is often helpful in restoring the appetite of a sick or recovering bird. **Familiar foods should be offered, and clients encouraged to bring in the patient's regular food.** Clients will often help to feed the bird if it is hospitalized, because the patients are often more responsive to their owners.

Prevention or treatment of inappetence is an important facet of therapeutics that is often neglected. Several agents are commonly used to promote appetite in mammals, although no definitive evidence is available to prove their worth in either mammals or birds. Vitamin B supplementation, corticosteroids and anabolic steroids have been advocated as appetite stimulants, but they may simply make the animal feel better rather than having any specific action to stimulate the appetite. The use of corticosteroids in birds should be avoided because the long-term immunosuppression will often result in opportunistic fungal and bacterial infections.

In mammals, inappetence is a prominent and early feature of zinc deficiency; this element is necessary for normal taste acuity, and the response to zinc supplementation is often excellent (Jenkins 1997a).

During tube feeding, daily attempts should be made to help regain the normal eating habits of the patient. Familiar foods should be left with the patient, or offered by the staff or client on a regular basis.

Liquefied diets and force-feeding

Composition of supportive formulae is a matter of individual preference. Different bird species require different food types. Psittacine patients will fare well on a number of commercial avian dietary and paediatric formulae. Human diets used for enteral feeding can also be used, and have good caloric value and appreciable fat content (Quesenberry et al 1991). Maintaining or increasing body weight during recovery is the main supportive goal after the first emergency is over (Appendices 6.2 and 6.3). A safe volume of formula for feeding directly into the crop is roughly 3–5% of the bird's normal body weight (Quesenberry & Hillyer 1994).

A variety of commercial products have been developed in an attempt to provide an easy-to-use diet for sick birds (Fig. 6.9). These products, as well as home-made

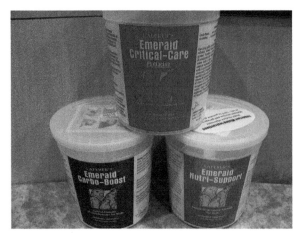

Fig 6.9 Critical care nutritional supplementation is commercially available for avian patients.

diets, must be evaluated for use in a given situation. The calorific value of foods can be estimated by calculating 4.49 kcal/g of protein, 4.09 kcal/g of carbohydrate and 9.29 kcal/g of fat. Not all of this energy will be used; the actual amount available for metabolism is influenced by the digestibility of the specific ingredients, the amount lost through urination and defecation, and the temperature of the environment (Quesenberry et al 1991).

Once an efficient diet has been selected, the caloric requirement of the patient – basal metabolic rate (BMR) plus maintenance requirement (MER) – may be calculated through allometric scaling (Appendices 6.2 and 6.4). The MER may be 1.3–7.2 times the BMR, while ill birds may require up to 1.5 times the MER. All situations where force-feeding is necessary require a diet that is easy to administer, highly digestible and contains sufficient energy.

Birds that do not drink must have fluid supplementation (Appendix 6.5), and the maximum suggested volumes and frequencies are presented in Appendices 6.3 and 6.6. However, even when a bird does not drink, fresh water (without additives) must always be available. For an illustrative case, see Box 6.1.

The following therapeutic agents can be added to the semi-liquid diet used for crop feeding (Coles 1996a):

1. Methylcellulose or ispaghula husk may help to slow down the gastrointestinal transit time. Also, this product may absorb enterotoxins.
2. Lactulose is another product that may help to absorb enterotoxins, but it has a mild laxative action.

Various foodstuffs can also be homogenized with a blender. For parrots, blending fruits and vegetables with peanut butter for calories will facilitate gavage. Bottled pureed baby food can be used, but keeping these products fresh may be a problem (Coles 1996a). Pelleted diets can be fine-ground and mixed with water or electrolyte solutions, and Columbiformes, Gruiformes and Galliformes will do well with blended pelleted feeds. Water should be added to provide the desired consistency. Ratites can be fed a gruel of pellets or blended dog food (Honnas et al 1993). Carnivorous water birds can be force-fed whole prey, and if regurgitation occurs a liquefied fish formula can be prepared. Raptors can often be force-fed parts of whole prey, and canned feline diet and raptor meat products can be made into a liquid diet although delicacy items such as skinned young mice and chicks may be preferred. Insectivores can be fed cereal or insect gruels or dog food for a short period of time. Nectivores should be fed a 15–20% dextrose solution if found down (less active), and switched to their regular nectar substitute when hospitalized. Nectivores generally do not handle large volumes well, so a fine needle feeding tube should be used for gavage or the bird offered the food on the end of a small syringe.

Box 6.1 Case with gavage treatment

A 400 g African grey parrot, 23 years old, easy to handle, is debilitated, eating very little and approximately 5% dehydrated because of diarrhoea.

Faecal smear:	Gram-negative rods (+++) and yeasts (+)			
Blood results:	Ht	0.39	TP	15 g/L
	WBC	14.0	A/G ratio	0.87
	Lympho's	16%	Ca	1.91 mmol/L
	Leuco's	84%	P	2.05 mmol/L

Preliminary diagnosis:

Multideficient bird with secondary intestinal bacterial and yeast infection (hypoproteinemia, hypocalcaemia, slight anaemia, elevated WBC with left shift).

Treatment:

- Starting directly after blood collection: 0.3 mL i.m. multivitamins (vitamin A = 15 000 IU/kg)
- Gavage feeding with antibiotic, antimycotic and protein supplementation
- Amoxicillin–clavulanic acid 50 mg/kg p.o.   0.4 mL   q8h
  q8h (Synulox® (Pfizer) oral suspension: amoxicillin 40 mg/mL, clav acid 10 mg/mL)
- Amphotericin B 5–10 mg/kg p.o. q8h   1 gtt   q8h
  (Fungizone® (Bristol-Myers Squibb) oral suspension 100 mg/mL)
- *Fluid requirement*

  50 mL/kg/day = 20 mL/day
  + 5% dehydration = 20 mL

D1	20 mL + 10 mL = 30 mL	10.0 mL	q8h
D2/3	20 mL + 5 mL = 25 mL	12.5 mL	q12h

- Fluids as extra amino acids: Aminoplasmol 10%® 400 kcal/L caloric value

D1	30.0 × 0.4 = 12.9 kcal/day plus 3.0 g protein
D2/3	25.0 × 0.4 = 10.0 kcal/day plus 2.5 g protein

- Caloric requirement

  MER = (1.5) BMR = 1.5 × 39.2 = 58.8 kcal/day

  Nutrilon Soya® (5.1 kcal/g)

D1	(58.8 − 12.9)/5.1 = 9.1 g/day	3.0 g	q8h
D2/3	(58.8 − 10.0)/5.1 = 9.6 g/day	4.8 g	q12h
R/D1	Nutrilon Soya® (approximately 3/4 measure spoon)	3.0 g	
	Aminoplasmol 10%®	10.0 mL	

	Synulox® oral suspension	0.4 mL
	Fungizone® oral suspension	1 gtt
S:	As gavage q8h for 1 day	

- After the blood results indicated a hypocalcaemia, the gavage was supplemented q24h with calcitriologum 0.025 μg/kg (Rocaltrol® (Roche)) and CA²⁺ 50 mg/kg (Calcium-Sandoz® forte) for 5 days.

Frequency of feeding is variable depending on each case, and the total daily requirement is divided into an equal number of daily feedings (Loudis & Sutherland-Smith 1994).

Gavage or tube feeding (oral alimentation)

Nutritional support is most commonly provided via tube feeding. Contraindications to tube feeding include crop stasis, ileus, gastrointestinal impaction, or other gastrointestinal abnormalities that do not allow the passage of ingesta or nutrient absorption (Rupley 1997).

For gavage feeding, curved ball-tipped metal feeding tubes are good choices for psittacine patients (see also Chapter 3) (Fig. 6.10). **The tube should be inserted near the left commissure of the beak,** sliding the tube over the tongue toward the right side of the bird's neck and gently into the crop without causing beak trauma. The crop should be palpated to verify that the tube or the feeding needle is in the correct place (Fig. 6.11). The neck is maintained in extension while the food is injected to deter regurgitation.

For waterfowl and passerines, plastic or size 14 French red rubber feeding tubes are recommended, and metal specula are rarely needed. The relative absence of the crop in many passerines demands using smaller, softer feeding tubes.

When crop gavage is not desirable due to stasis or trauma, a red rubber feeding tube can be passed directly into the proventriculus and small boluses of supplement administered. Extreme caution should be taken with this procedure because the distal oesophagus and proventriculus are thin-walled and rupture will occur with overfeeding or improper tube placement.

Before fluids or food are administered via oral gavage the crop should be palpated, and if food is present in the crop, tube feeding should be deferred (Rupley 1997). Tube feeds are preferably fed warmed to prevent delayed crop emptying. The bird should be weighed before tube feeding, and any other procedures performed at this stage because restraint after tube feeding may result in regurgitation and aspiration. If food refluxes into the oral cavity during the procedure, the bird should be released and allowed to clear its mouth on its own.

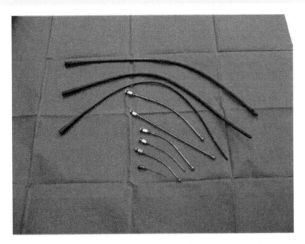

Fig 6.10 Red rubber tubes and stainless steel gavage needles that can be used to provide nutritional supplementation to the critically ill avian patient.

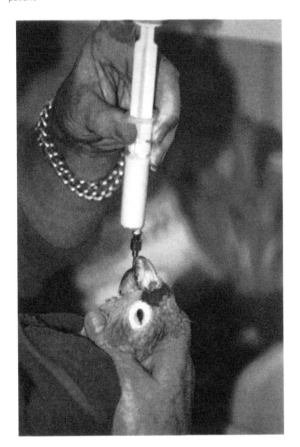

Fig 6.11 An Amazon parrot being fed using a gavage feeding tube.

Oesophagostomy

Tube placement is required in situations where the mouth, proximal or distal oesophagus or crop needs to be bypassed and food deposited directly into the proventriculus or beyond. This can be done with a tube via the mouth into the proventriculus. However, babies suffering from crop burns or those with refractory crop dysfunction, and birds with severe beak injuries, benefit greatly from an indwelling proventricular feeding tube installed via the oesophagus (Bennett & Harrison 1994, Altman 1997, Forbes 2005). To perform this procedure, an appropriately sized rubber or plastic feeding tube is passed down the oesophagus of an anaesthetized bird, manipulated through the crop and into the thoracic oesophagus and inserted to the proventriculus, where resistance is felt. A 2–3 cm longitudinal incision is then made on the right side of the neck over the feeding tube, which can be identified within the oesophagus (Fig. 6.12). The tube is isolated through the incision and transected, the oral end is removed completely, and the proventricular end is extracted 2–3 cm from the incision. Another possibility is first to place a metal feeding tube and this tube is tented up in an appropriate position in the cervical oesophagus (cranial to the crop). A small incision is than made over the end of the feeding tube. The rubber or plastic tube is than passed via the incision into the oesophagus and via the crop into the proventriculus (Forbes 2005).

A 1 × 5 cm strip of Elastikon® is then wrapped around the protruding end of the feeding tube, and it is sutured in place on the neck. If the incision is large it may be sutured, but suturing is not generally necessary. A male adapter plug can be used to cap the tube between the feedings. Such a device has been left in place for as long as 7 weeks without complications, and removal is accomplished simply by cutting the stay sutures and extracting the tube. Debridement and surgical closure of the wound is not necessary (Harris 1997).

Duodenostomy

In cases where it is desirable to bypass the entire upper gastrointestinal tract, an indwelling feeding tube can be installed directly into the ascending limb of the duodenum. For a more detailed description, the reader is referred to specialized books (Bennett & Harrison 1994, Altman 1997, Harris 1997).

Monitoring

It is essential to monitor a patient to follow progress and assess the effects of treatment; monitoring also provides information regarding adapting the treatment if necessary. Record keeping is essential for evaluation, and also for future reference. **Progress may be assessed by observation and clinical signs but, when the status of the patient allows, serial monitoring of the packed cell volume (PCV), total protein (TP) and urine output, along with short-term evaluation of weight gain or loss, will provide more reliable data.**

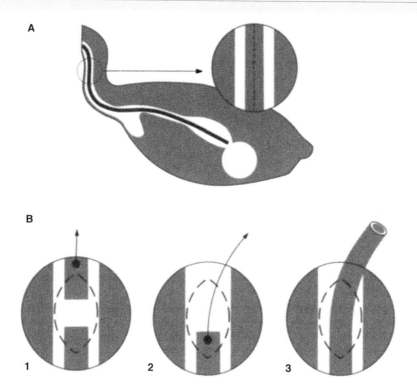

Fig 6.12 Schematic diagram of an oesophagostomy. (**A**) Insertion of the tube. (**B1**) After making the incision the tupe is cut, (**B2**) the cranial part of the tube removed and (**B3**) the caudal part extracted for 2 cm through the incision and fixed to the skin.

Record keeping

The (computerized) medical record system used in most small animal hospitals can be modified for avian patients. An admission form should be produced for each hospitalized bird, for daily assessment, containing the following information:

1. name of the responsible veterinarian, the record code, date of hospitalization and reason for hospitalization
2. the name of the bird and of the owner
3. identification of the patient – species, breed, colour, gender, weight on admission, age, ring number or transponder
4. information regarding the owner – address, telephone number, fax number, etc. (means of contact)
5. information about the referring veterinarian – name, address and phone number
6. special remarks or warnings related to the patient
7. a summary of the history, initial examination, laboratory results and initial treatment
8. estimate of the costs
9. (preliminary) diagnosis and medical plan.

For daily assessment of the hospitalized bird's condition, the following information should be recorded on this admission form along with the staff member's signature and the date:

1. food and water intake, dietary support
2. droppings – quantity and appearance
3. clinical observations
4. medication – quantities and administration route
5. medical operations.

During hospitalization, all findings and treatments should be added to the patient's record to keep track of progress, for future reference, and for preparing the bill.

A label or sticker should be attached to the hospital cage, with information identifying the patient, client and referring veterinarian. All items in use for the patient (such as drugs, special food, feeding tubes, etc.) are best kept in a separate container marked with the patient's details. **All personal belongings of the patient that do not go home and that have to be kept until the bird is discharged from the hospital should also be labelled with the owner's name.**

Preliminary evaluation

To ascertain the patient's stability, meaningful information should be obtained from the owner and the bird observed on presentation. Although it may seem that a chronically ill bird might be closer to death than an acutely ill patient, the opposite is often true. Birds that display signs of illness for several days to weeks often compensate for their disease and consequently become stable. Those that develop serious clinical signs acutely may be seriously affected by the disease process (Harris 1994).

Whatever the background information provided by the client, the clinician must observe the patient before attempting to handle it (see also Chapter 3). This may seem straightforward, but it cannot be overemphasized that the bird's life may depend on this 'hands off' assessment. A thorough step-by-step visual examination provides preliminary information that minimizes the chances of unexpected deaths (Harris 1994).

Observation

When possible, the hospitalized bird should be observed from a distance. A bird will often appear more alert and responsive when approached, giving the illusion of wellness. Observations made from a distance reveal the bird's condition and its clinical developments more accurately. **A resting bird that displays open-mouth breathing, tail-bobbing, closed eyes and ruffling of the feathers will tolerate little (if any) stress.** The same bird may perk up and seem less critical when examined closely. The patient's behaviour when noted from a distance may warn the clinician to proceed with caution. The bird that brightens when approached may be stronger than the one that continues to show significant signs, but a false sense of security may exist when an examiner fails to realize the ability of many avian species to mask signs of clinical illness (Harris 1994).

After the bird is visually examined, it may be removed from the original cage or carrier for further evaluation. Any evidence of distress should prompt immediate release of the bird into a suitable intensive care unit. The physical examination, at this point, should focus on indicators of the patient's hydration, thermal condition, acute clinical signs, etc. In many situations it will be necessary to treat dehydration and hypothermia prior to further manipulations. Care must be taken not to over-handle the bird (Harris 1994).

Once fluids have been administered, the patient may be placed in an intensive care unit that ideally supplies heat, humidity and oxygen.

A critically ill bird handled in the proper manner will often show clinical improvement within a short period of time – sometimes in less than an hour. At this time, the clinician may choose to examine the bird further, collect diagnostic samples, or implement further therapy.

After a bird has been observed from a distance, it may be examined more closely. Attention should be paid to the bird's response upon approach, the feed and water intake, the droppings and other (ab)normal signs such as blood, feather loss, etc.

All signs found at the initial physical examination, as well as new observations, must be assessed and recorded on the patient's hospitalization form. Based on the information that has been collected from physical examination, the clinician must decide whether to continue, adapt or modify the treatment protocol. It is also necessary to decide whether to:

- place the bird in (or release it from) a supportive intensive care chamber
- administer basic supportive treatment before proceeding further
- perform additional physical examinations, with or without collecting diagnostic samples
- discharge the patient as healthy or for further treatment at home.

Experience will fine-tune the clinician's ability to determine which route to follow.

Laboratory monitoring

A blood sample should be taken from every sick hospitalized bird, preferably immediately after hospitalization and before taking any other tests or starting treatment. Using a heparinized syringe, a sample of 0.5% of the body weight (or 2 mL from a parrot heavier than 400 g) will be sufficient for most routine tests. The surplus of plasma should be frozen and stored for additional biochemical tests or future reference. A white blood cell count (WBC) is useful for monitoring the patient's progress and response during therapy. When treating a metabolic acidosis, blood bicarbonate should be tested.

The progress or improvement of critical initial blood values should be monitored regularly after beginning treatment.

Monitoring the patient's faecal material may aid in assessing treatment response. Faecal examination includes gross evaluation and direct and faecal parasite evaluations. Microscopic examination of a stained smear (cytology) is an easy and valuable technique for following the progress of lesions and the bacterial status of the intestines. In species without functional caeca (e.g. psittacines, pigeons and doves, and passerines), only a very small number of microorganisms visible by staining are acceptable. Large numbers indicate poor hygiene, impaired gastric secretion, immunosuppression or bacterial enteritis. The effect of antibiotic treatments can easily be evaluated by looking at follow-up smears.

To help determine caloric intake, examination of droppings for faecal material will alert the clinician to the anorectic bird. Anorectic birds commonly have scant, slimy, dark green faeces. Birds exhibiting these signs may require supplemental gavage feeding.

The urine in the droppings of normal birds is clear, and the urates white. An increase or decrease of urine or a change of colour is abnormal and should be assessed.

Physical monitoring

Body temperature

The average adult bird has a core body temperature of 38–42.5°C. Regulation of internal body temperature relies upon many factors – feather condition, adipose and muscle condition, hydration, food intake and respiration (Dawson & Whittow 2000). Wet, oil-fouled, destroyed or plucked feathers will cause greater heat loss through the skin. Poor body condition also hinders effective heat regulation. Dehydration will interfere with the evaporative heat loss system in birds, from the respiratory tract as well as from the skin. If capable, overheated birds will pant to help cool themselves.

Monitoring the body temperature directly is stressful and even dangerous if the patient is fractious or if a rigid thermometer is not handled carefully. A flexible temperature probe inserted in the cloaca in comatose birds allows a permanent monitoring of the body temperature, which at this location is mostly 2–3°C lower than the internal core temperature. Although measuring the body temperature using a cloacal probe is relatively easy and less stressful to an avian patient, an oesophageal body temperature measurement is more accurate. Overheating (as evidenced by panting) can become a problem if the patient is not monitored while in the intensive care unit.

Body weight

Monitoring the body weight is a major concern in ill birds. Sick birds are often malnourished, anorectic and dehydrated. Avian patients should be weighed daily if possible, especially when tube feeding. Weights should be recorded at the same time every day, preferably in the morning or evening before feeding.

Surgical nursing

The staff should make sure that all hospitalized birds have a clean cloaca if they are passing abnormal fluid droppings or have cloacitis. Some birds will irritate wounds or tear sutures, so patients should be monitored during hospitalization. A restraining collar (e.g. Elizabethan collar) may need to be fitted (Fig. 6.13). A bird with an oesophagostomy tube or an auxiliary airway tube inserted should have the tubes kept clean and unblocked. If splints have been applied to a leg or wing, a careful watch should be made that the foot or wing tip does not become swollen. Birds should be kept on clean perches to prevent foot problems. The technicians should make a habit of examining the bird's droppings rather than just clearing them away, and should look for signs of blood, undigested seed or the occasional tapeworm segment, and note any changes in the normal colour or character of the droppings (Coles 1996a).

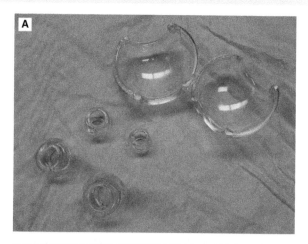

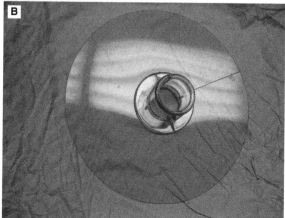

Fig 6.13 Special avian Elizabethan collars: (**A**) spherical; (**B**) disc.

Fluid therapy

Fluid therapy is extremely important in the critical avian patient. Parenteral fluids will restore effective blood volume, normalize cardiac output and optimize tissue oxygenation. Most metabolic imbalances can be corrected with proper fluid therapy (Redig 1984). An additional benefit is enhanced diuresis, which facilitates the elimination of toxic by-products and metabolites (e.g. urates). Deciding the route of administration depends on patient status and cooperation, fluid type and cost (Loudis & Sutherland-Smith 1994). Oral and subcutaneous routes are inappropriate when dealing with critically ill patients. The routes of choice for a patient in shock are intravenous and intraosseous. Intraosseous catheters are less stressful than repeated venepuncture, and are the favoured route in cases of shock (Hernandez & Aguilar 1994, Lichtenberger 2005, 2006). Close monitoring of the avian patient is required during fluid administration to ensure tolerance of the process. Heart rate, respiration rate and overall condition must to be monitored during the procedure (Redig 1984).

Anaemia and hypoproteinaemia are common sequelae of aggressive fluid therapy (Redig 1984). **If the PCV falls to less than 10–20%, a whole blood transfusion should be considered.** When total plasma protein values fall below 15 g/L, the decreased plasma osmotic pressure will allow fluids into the interstitial space and pulmonary oedema and compromised organ function may follow (Hernandez & Aguilar 1994). For calculation of the fluid requirement, see Dehydration and Appendix 6.5.

Choice of fluids

Crystalloids are the initial fluids of choice in avian shock or dehydration because they are effective, easy to administer and inexpensive. In birds, only one-quarter of the total fluids administered remain in the vascular compartment 30 minutes after treatment. The circulatory benefits obtained from fluid therapy are transient, and additional fluid therapy is required (Appendix 6.5).

Lactated Ringer's solution (Hartmann's) is the favoured fluid because metabolic acidosis is present in most situations. Lactate is metabolized to bicarbonate by the liver. In severe acidotic states, lactated Ringer's solution should be supplemented with bicarbonate. Bicarbonate supplementation may be estimated by subtracting the blood bicarbonate value obtained from the 'normal' avian bicarbonate value as follows:

Bicarbonate deficit = 20 mmol/L
(mmol/L)   − blood bicarbonate (mmol/L)
Bicarbonate dose   = deficit × body
(mmol/L)   weight (kg) × 0.4

Alternatively, when no means are available for determining blood bicarbonate, a dose of 1 mmol/kg can be given every 15–30 minutes to a maximum of 4 mmol/kg/day (Hernandez & Aguilar 1994). The first dose should be given intravenously, followed by the remainder subcutaneously (Redig 1984). Commercially available bicarbonate solutions include an 8.4% solution containing 1 mmol/mL and a 1.4% solution containing 0.17 mmol/mL. Calcium gluconate (50–100 mg/kg, administered slowly) as a cardioprotectant and glucose to facilitate the movement of potassium across cell membranes are advisable in cases of severe tissue injury, extreme catabolic state or severe renal impairment (hyperkalaemia). Lactated Ringer's solution does not contain enough potassium to aggravate such a situation (Redig 1984).

Potassium chloride can be added to lactated Ringer's solution in cases of aggressive fluid therapy or persistent vomiting. The fluid therapy can be supplemented with a potassium chloride solution (0.1–0.3 mmol/kg), to a maximum of 11 mmol/day.

Hypertonic saline (7.5%) solution can be used as an adjunct to therapy to re-establish circulatory function. Its use should be followed by the administration of isotonic fluids. In mammals, a small volume (4–5 mL/kg) induces a rapid improvement in cardiovascular function as a result of osmotic expansion of the vasculature. Hypertonic saline is particularly useful in cases of hydropericardium, pulmonary oedema or increased intracranial pressure. Its use is contraindicated in dehydration, hypernatraemia and head trauma, because of the possibility of an intracranial haemorrhage.

Colloids

Dextrans are polysaccharides of high molecular weight with a size similar to that of albumin. Their effect is similar to that of hypertonic saline, but with a longer half-life (approximately 24 hours). **A dramatic improvement in birds in shock using 6% dextran, administered at a rate of 10–20 mL/kg (Redig 1984) or 10-20 mg/kg (Carpenter 2005), has been reported.** Adverse effects include hypervolaemia, haemorrhagic diathesis and anaphylaxis.

Blood transfusions appear to be beneficial for birds with chronic anaemia for the purpose of stabilizing the bird while the cause of the anaemia is being pursued (Rupley 1997). Birds with a PCV less than 20% as a result of acute blood loss may benefit from a homologous blood transfusion (Dorrestein 1997). Approximately 1% of the donor bird's body weight in blood volume can be safely collected using a small-gauge butterfly catheter (anticoagulant citrate dextrose, 0.15 mL/mL blood). Following collection, the donor should be given an amount of saline or Ringer's solution, or an equivalent amount of colloid fluids, equal to one to three times the quantity of blood donated (Jenkins 1997a). Transfusion of approximately 10–20% of the calculated total blood volume of the recipient is usually ideal.

There is evidence that heterologous transfusion may be of no benefit (red blood survival is approximately 12 hours in some species), and homologous transfusions (with a red blood survival in pigeons of 7.1 days) may be of only limited benefit (Murray 1994).

Antibiotics

Antibiotics or steroids may be added to the fluids if indicated. If bacterial sepsis is suspected, antibiotics such as cefotaxime (40–80 mg/kg) or sodium amoxicillin (50–100 mg/kg) may be given directly either i.v. or via i.v. fluids. When adding drugs to the fluids, incompatibilities (precipitation of the solution) should be avoided. Amikacin or other aminoglycosides should be avoided in dehydrated birds. Laboratory samples for culturing should be collected before administration of antibiotics and antifungals whenever possible.

Corticosteroids

In situations where the patient is possibly in shock, steroids may be indicated. Despite conflicting opinions concerning the efficacy of steroids in critical situations, they remain a viable choice in cases involving trauma, lead poisoning and central nervous system compromise (Hernandez & Aguilar 1994). Their use in shock caused by haemorrhage and hypovolaemia is not currently recommended (Lichtenberger 2005). In emergencies, steroids with a rapid effect and a short half-life are preferred. Non-steroidal anti-inflammatory drugs (NSAIDs) may also be of benefit to the critical patient.

In a dose–response study in pigeons, dexamethasone proved to be the most potent glucocorticoid, resulting in the longest suppression of plasma corticosterone concentration. Following the highest dose of dexamethasone that was tested (0.5 mg/kg), plasma corticosterone concentrations were restored within 5 days, and within 48 hours following the highest doses of cortisol (15 mg/kg) and prednisolone (3.5 mg/kg). The lowest doses that resulted in suppression of the plasma corticosterone concentrations were 0.5 μg dexamethasone/kg, 15 μg cortisol/kg and 0.7 μg prednisolone/kg. Following these doses, plasma corticosterone concentrations were restored within 24 hours (Westerhof et al 1994). It took 30–60 minutes before the onset of suppression of plasma cortisone concentration following 1 μg dexamethasone/kg, 30 μg cortisol/kg or 7 μg prednisolone/kg.

Of the non-steroidal anti-inflammatory drugs, ketoprofen, flunixin and carprofen can all be used at a dose rate of 2 mg/kg. However, they are all contraindicated when renal disease, hypotension or dehydration is suspected, and they may occasionally cause vomiting. Carprofen probably has the fewest side effects of the NSAIDs previously mentioned (Coles 1996a).

Adverse effects of glucocorticosteroids include severe immunosuppression, water and salt retention, delayed wound healing, adrenal insufficiency, hypertension, weakness, retarded growth and a decrease in the intestinal absorption of calcium. However, in most critical avian patients the benefits of administering glucocorticosteroids far outweigh the adverse effects.

Intravenous approach

For any patient requiring moderate to heavy fluid supplementation (see Dehydration) or serious cardiovascular support, intravenous fluid support is necessary. Fluids containing glucose may be of great benefit in anorectic patients. Long-term catheterization or short-term bolusing can be performed, but bolus therapy is not recommended for long-term support due to the fragility of avian veins.

The basilic (wing) vein is easy to access in all species, but it is fragile and injection usually results in the formation of a large haematoma at the administration site (Fig. 6.14) (Harris 1997). This can be minimized by removing the needle from the vein but not the skin after fluid administration, and injecting a large volume of fluid subcutaneously. The fluid compression then lessens vascular leakage.

The medial metatarsal vein can be used most easily in long-legged species. The jugular vein can be accessed in most birds, but not easily in pigeons and doves (see also Figs 3.41 and 3.42).

Intravenous fluids may be administered in birds as a bolus at the fastest rate the needle will allow. The syringe and fluids should be warmed to approximately body temperature (37–39°C) prior to administration (Harris 1994). Devices are available to keep fluids warm while they are being administered. Heating pads may be used to wrap the syringe on a syringe pump (Jenkins 1997b).

Syringe and infusion pumps

The ability to administer intravenous or intraosseous fluids to a small patient over an extended period of time depends on equipment that allows a very low rate of administration along with a high degree of safety and accuracy. Intravenous infusion pumps work well for infusion rates higher than 60–100 mL/hour. Syringe pumps allow infusion rates much lower than those of infusion pumps – it is possible to use a syringe pump to administer maintenance fluids to a budgerigar at 0.006–0.10 mL/hour via an intraosseous catheter (Fig. 6.15) (Jenkins 1997b).

Appendix 6.5 advises how to calculate the fluid requirement in birds. Appendix 6.6 gives the maximum suggested volumes of fluids to be administered to psittacines as an initial i.v. bolus.

Contraindications

Contraindications to intravenous fluid support include diagnosis or history of coagulopathy, lack of equipment

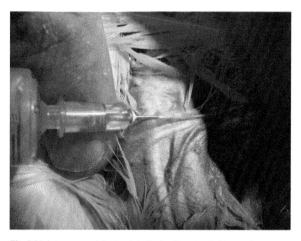

Fig 6.14 Intravenous injection into the basilic vein of a blue and gold macaw.

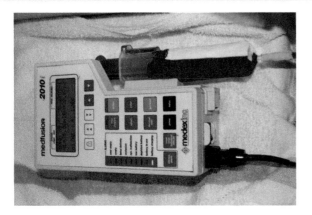

Fig 6.15 Syringe pumps are useful in allowing infusion rates in amounts that small avian patients will tolerate.

and technical skill, and self-inflicted trauma by the patient resulting in loss of catheter patency.

Technique of intravenous jugular placement

A 20-gauge, 25 mm Teflon over-the-needle i.v. catheter is required. The patient is placed in left lateral recumbency and the feathers over the right jugular vein parted. The skin is cleansed with a gentle surgical scrub and, in some species, feathers may have to be plucked. The head is grasped and the catheter threaded into the jugular vein; the vein may have to be held off proximally to aid in venous distension. It is important to place the catheter as near to the thoracic inlet as possible to avoid kinking when the neck is in normal flexion. Once blood is seen in the hub, the catheter is advanced fully into the vein. A male T-port adapter that has been filled with saline flush is applied, and the catheter is checked for patency and gently flushed. The catheter may be sutured to the neck or held in place by a non-constricting bandage.

Intraosseous approach

The intraosseous route has proved to be a very effective and stable method of accessing the avian circulatory system. A 20–22-gauge, 35 mm spinal needle with a stylet (Monoject spinal needle) is often used. If these are unavailable, 28–30-gauge wire may be placed inside the cannula to avoid occlusion of the needle by bone. For smaller birds, a 25-gauge needle may be used. Indications are the same as for intravenous therapy. The patient is usually anaesthetized, but the procedure can be performed with restraint and local anaesthesia. Aseptic technique is essential. The fluids should be administered slowly in order to avoid leakage (which will be minimal with careful technique) and pain (which can be significant with high pressure).

Intraosseous catheterization of the ulna and tibiotarsus (Fig. 6.16)

For catheterization of the distal ulna, the bird is placed in dorsal recumbency – although ventral recumbency or the standing position may be more beneficial in the severely compromised patient. The feathers over the carpus are plucked, and the area over the distal ulna is sterilized. The ulna is grasped in one hand as the needle is placed over the distal bony protuberance of the ulna, and the needle is directed parallel to the median plane of the ulna. The spinal needle is gently rotated to help facilitate its passage through the cortex, and once the needle penetrates the cortex the needle can be directed further with less force. Resistance after entering the medullary cavity can indicate contact with cortical bone; if this happens, reposition the needle (Rupley 1997). A taped butterfly can be used to help secure the catheter with a suture to the soft tissue of the distal ulna. A pre-flushed male T-port adapter is applied, and the wing wrapped in a figure-of-eight bandage. Care must be taken to avoid the ligaments of the carpus, which pass near the insertion point. These can often be visualized through the thin skin of the bird.

For catheterization of the proximal tibiotarsus, the patient is placed in dorsal recumbency. The area around the cnemial crest is plucked and prepped for asepsis, and towelling off the area helps to prevent contamination. The cranial cnemial crest is located and the tibiotarsus grasped with the other hand. The needle is directed parallel to the plane of the tibiotarsus, and slightly rotated with moderate pressure; it will slide in easily once the cortex is penetrated (Fig. 6.16C). A taped butterfly is applied and the pre-filled T-port connector is attached. Suture stabilization and light bandaging are warranted if the catheter is to remain in situ after surgery (Loudis & Sutherland-Smith 1994).

Subcutaneous approach

Subcutaneous fluid administration should be used only in cases of mild dehydration. Patients with circulatory compromise and under adverse environmental conditions will have reduced circulation through the vessels of the skin. Due to the paucity of vessels in bird skin, large volumes may not be readily absorbed from sites that include the propatagium (wing-web), dorsally between the wings, the axilla and the inguinal fold (groin). Close association of the cervicocephalic air sac system warrants avoidance of fluid administration to the neck area. Only isotonic fluids heated to body temperature should be used, in small increments (5–10 mL/kg/site) and via small needles (23–27-gauge).

Abdominal approach

Warm, isotonic fluids can be given within the abdominal coelom. Unfortunately because of the close anatomical

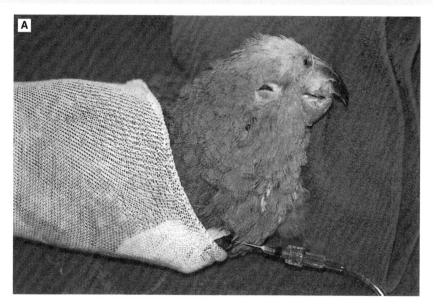

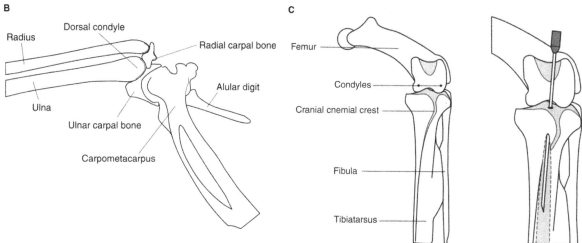

Fig 6.16 (**A**) Intraosseous catheters are useful in providing an effective and stable access to the avian circulatory system. The distal ulna (**B**) and proximal tibiotarsus (**C**) are recommended sites for placing an intraosseous catheter.

association of the air sacs, this technique is not recommended. A ventral midline approach with a small (25–27) gauge catheter is used.

Oral approach

If the patient is alert and active, oral alimentation is the route of choice. It is safe, effective and causes minimal stress. Contraindications include primary gastrointestinal disease (diseases causing vomiting or stasis), poor patient reflexes or recumbency (to avoid regurgitation and aspiration), and oral and upper gastrointestinal trauma. Offering unlimited water and foodstuffs high in water content is important. Oral fluid therapy can be accomplished with gavage tubes. Appendix 6.5

advises on calculating the fluid requirement in birds. In Appendices 6.3 and 6.6, the maximum suggested volumes of fluids and the frequency of gavage feeding are presented.

Medication

Medication may be administered to birds orally (medicated water or food); by injection (intramuscular, intravenous, subcutaneous, intraosseous, intratracheal); topically; by nebulization; and as sinus and nasal flushes. Selection of the route of administration is based on the severity of infection, the number of birds to be treated, the ability of the owner to administer the medication, and the formulation available. Parenteral administration of medication is suggested for critically ill birds. Birds maintained in flocks or aviaries are often treated with medicated food or water, but therapeutic drug concentrations are seldom achieved in companion and aviary birds (Rupley 1997). Availability and absorption after oral administration are influenced by crop, crop flora, crop pH, gizzard function and morphology, the presence of grit, the form and function of the intestines, the presence of functional caeca, and the indigenous microflora (Dorrestein 1997).

Individual oral medication

Direct oral administration is difficult in psittacines because it is difficult to get them to open their mouths and some birds refuse to swallow medication, but this method is commonly used in pigeons, waterfowl and gallinaceous birds. Oral medication should not be used in critically ill birds.

Tablets and capsules

Many birds have a crop, which acts as a storage organ. The unpredictable emptying time of the crop, the lack of a large volume of fluid and the relatively high pH mean that the crop cannot be compared with the mammalian stomach, resulting in unpredictable pharmacokinetic behaviour of the drug. However, administration into an empty crop improves the uniformity of the pharmacokinetics. The problem can be overcome by grinding the tablet, making a suspension and feeding it by crop cannula (Fig. 6.17).

Coated tablets are of no use in birds with a muscular gizzard, which will destroy the coating and give hydrochloric acid and pepsin full access to the drug.

Capsules are good alternative dosage forms to tablets, and again are best administered into an empty crop. Capsules are especially useful for the treatment of individual birds. In psittacines this dosage form will be difficult to deliver because of the beak anatomy.

Solutions and suspensions

Solutions and suspensions can be used for direct administration to individual birds. A disadvantage of all liquid drug forms is that direct administration may result in regurgitation or inhalation, and part of the dose may be lost or aspiration pneumonia may occur. These preparations can be mixed with food or administered by gavage, especially in hand-fed baby birds or in sick birds requiring oral fluids and nutrients.

Medication of feed or water

The major method of administering drugs to poultry and many other birds is via feed and water. This is largely for convenience and because of the difficulties associated with individual administration to large numbers of birds. However, for the majority of drugs water medication is unreliable for psittacines, passerines, pigeons and most other birds, and it should not be used except under specific circumstances.

Feed medication is a reliable way of administering drugs to companion birds, as long as the birds are still eating normally. The total intake of the drug with the food during the day should be equal to the desired daily dose calculated on an individual base. Crushed tablets, oral suspensions and powders can be mixed with moist foods. However, the interactions between a drug and food cannot be entirely predicted, and the energy content and palatability of the diet affect the amount consumed and therefore the dose of medicine ingested. The only proof of bioavailability is a pharmacokinetic study in various species. Because of the negative influence of calcium and magnesium on the bioavailability of tetracycline, grit-mineral administration has to be stopped during treatment. During egg production and breeding this can lead to nutrient deficiencies, resulting in soft-shelled eggs and rickets in the chicks.

A practical method of adding drugs to a grain mixture is by coating a moist food that is then added to the mixture. This method is often used for pigeons and backyard poultry. Pharmacologically, food medication can simulate a slow-release system, which provides decreased fluctuations in drug concentrations in tissues.

Medication in water is controversial in companion avian medicine, but is often considered the only practical means of drug administration. It is the least stressful method for medicating birds, especially using drugs that are palatable. Theoretically, the bird will frequently self-dose during the day. However, studies in parrots, pigeons and chickens show that therapeutic blood levels for many drugs were not attained via the drinking water because of factors such as lack of acceptance, poor

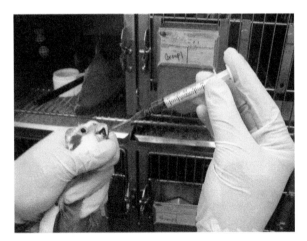

Fig 6.17 Medicating a cockatiel with a crop cannula.

solubility and day length. Many birds refuse to drink water with an abnormal taste, and this may result in dehydration. As a guide, the volume of water consumed by the bird needs to contain the calculated daily dose in mg/kg body weight. Many drugs are stable for only a short time in water, which necessitates frequent changes.

While therapeutic blood levels may not be achieved with many drugs, levels in the intestine may be sufficient to control enteric infections. The use of medicated water can be valuable for reducing the spread of diseases that have arisen through contaminated water.

Parenteral dosage forms

Parenteral administration is the most exact and effective method for administering drugs to companion birds. This route is used mainly in individual birds that are difficult to handle (like many psittacines), critically ill birds, or birds that are unconscious.

Intramuscular injection, especially in many psittacines, is often easier than oral administration (Rupley 1997). A problem with intramuscular antibiotic usage on parrot patients is the short dosing intervals required with many products. An exception to this statement is treatment for chlamydiosis using doxycycline or long-acting oxytetracycline, because an injection will provide blood levels for almost 1 week. The parenteral preparations are most commonly administered into the pectoral or leg muscles. The venous plexus, which lies between the superficial and deep pectoral muscle, should not be punctured. A disadvantage is the relatively large volume that may have to be injected, and individual birds should therefore be carefully weighed and appropriate dilutions and syringes used for accurate dosing. General guidelines for maximum injection volumes in psittacines and small passerines include: macaw and cockatoo, 1 mL; Amazon and African grey, 0.8 mL; cockatiel and small conures, 0.2 mL; and budgerigars, canaries and finches, 0.1 mL (Rupley 1997). **Repeated injections in the same side of the breast or the use of irritating drugs i.m. may result in muscle necrosis or atrophy.** The i.m. injection of irritating formulations increases the creatine phosphokinase (CK) activity, the activity of alanine aminotransferase (ALAT), and aspartate aminotransferase (ASAT). Drugs administered in the posterior pectoral muscle or legs may pass through the renal portal system prior to entering the general circulation. Sympathetic stimulation tends to open the valves in the renal portal system, resulting in a direct flow of the blood from the caudal part of the bird to the vena cava caudalis.

Subcutaneous injections in the axillary area are often a preferable alternative when 'large' volumes are injected (Appendix 6.6). However, because of the minimal amounts of dermis and the low elasticity of the skin, part of the fluid may flow out and irritating drugs may cause skin necrosis and ulceration.

Intravenous injections should be reserved for emergencies and single dose drug administration. Haematomas are common when administering therapeutic agents i.v., and veins may also be needed for blood withdrawal for diagnostic tests. Intraosseous administration allows stable access to the intravascular space if repeated 'i.v.' drug administration is required.

Other injection sites

Air spaces may effectively be reached by intratracheal or air sac injections. Joint injections, nasal flushes and infraorbital sinus flushes and injections are other areas where direct application of drugs may be useful.

Intratracheal or air sac injections

Intratracheal injections are a route for delivery of drugs to the lungs and airways of birds (Jenkins 1997a). Volumes up to 2 mL/kg of water-soluble medication may be administered safely. A small-diameter metal feeding needle is used to administer the drug. The bird is restrained in a towel and the beak held open using a speculum or gauze loops. The medication is injected into the trachea with some force, and the bird is then released and allowed to cough and clear its throat.

Nasal and sinus flushes

A nasal flush is often important in the successful treatment of infraorbital sinus infections. Antibiotics or antifungals can be used in a lower dose than recommended for nebulization (Appendix 6.7). The bird is restrained and the head held lower than the body; the syringe is pressed against the nostril and the fluid is flushed into the sinuses, and the fluid exits via the opposite nostril and through the choana and mouth. Isotonic solutions and minimal pressure should be used. The amounts of fluids for nasal flushing are 1–3 mL for a budgerigar and up to 10–15 mL for a large macaw or cockatoo (Rupley 1997, Jenkins 1997a).

A sinus flush is used to deliver medication directly into the infraorbital sinus for treatment of sinusitis. A sinus flush can also be used to dislodge exudate and foreign bodies from the sinuses, or to obtain samples for cytology, culture and sensitivity testing. The bird is restrained with the head secured, and a needle inserted midway between the commissure of the beak and the medial canthus of the eye (Fig. 6.18). The needle is directed under the zygomatic arch at a 45° angle to the side of the head. The sinus is more easily entered if the mouth is held open. Once the sinus has been entered, sterile water and an antibiotic or antifungal solution may be used for treatment of sinusitis. The same concentration can be used as recommended for a nasal flush (Appendix 6.7). Only non-irritating solutions

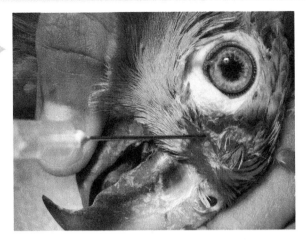

Fig 6.18 A sinus flush or aspirate can be performed by entering the infraorbital sinus between the medial canthus and nares.

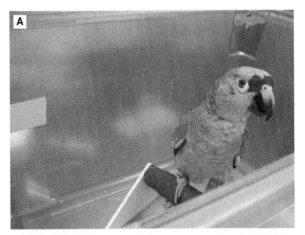

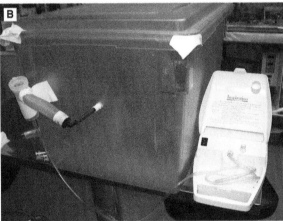

should be injected (Rupley 1997). To effectively treat avian sinus and nasal infections the medication must reach the affected tissue. **Significant amounts of serous and mucoid nasal discharge fl uid may be removed using a human infant nasal suction bulb.** One or two squeezes of the bulb once the hole is placed over a nasal opening will effectively clear large amounts of fluid within the infraorbital sinus caused by infection and inflammation.

Topical medication

Topical medications include skin applications, eye drops and ointments. External applications should be careful and sparing, because they will stick the feathers together and may be ingested when the bird preens, leading to toxicity. Topical corticosteroid ointments or combination ointments with antibiotics should never be used on avian patients. There have been numerous reports of avian patient death after application of a topical steroid ointment. **It is recommended to have owners apply only enough topical medication on skin wounds that will make the affected area look moist.** There should be no excess ointment on the applicator before treatment to reduce the chances of feather damage or ingestion.

Nebulization

Nebulization can be an important adjunct to the management of respiratory disease (Fig. 6.19) (Jenkins 1997a). A particle size of less than 3μm is required in order to have a local effect in the lungs and air sacs. Several inexpensive nebulization units are available (Acorn II nebulizer, Marquest Medical) that produce

Fig 6.19 A Nebulization therapy is required for many respiratory conditions diagnosed in avian patients. **B** Equipment used for nebulization therapy includes the container in which the bird perches, the air pump and container from which the therapeutic agent is aerosolized.

suspended particles in the size range of 0.5–6μm. Many commercial humidifiers and vaporizers do not produce particles this small. The parabronchi of birds range in size between 0.5 and 2mm, and the air capillaries vary in size from 3 to 10μm in diameter. Because the avian lung differs from that of mammals in that the air capillaries are not dead-end saccules, nebulization therapy can be an effective treatment (Loudis & Sutherland-Smith 1994). However, if there is considerable airway congestion or lack of flow, this form of treatment may not reach the tissues needing it the most.

Most intravenous antibiotics and some antifungal medications can be mixed with saline for nebulization. Nebulization should be initiated before culture and sensitivity tests are known, using a broad-spectrum antibiotic (Appendix 6.7), but the selection of antibiotics can be altered based on sensitivity testing. The patient should be nebulized for 10–30 minutes, two to four times daily, in conjunction with systemic therapy (Rupley 1997).

Basic emergency treatment

In non-emergency situations, laboratory and ancillary diagnostics are essential for establishing a diagnosis and determining appropriate treatment. Unfortunately, the delicate condition of a critically ill bird may prohibit the use of usual diagnostic protocols. Often the stress of sample collection or the time needed to process the samples is more than the patient can endure. Managing the case becomes a matter of careful, precise and efficient use of therapeutic and diagnostic options in order simultaneously to stabilize the patient and diagnose the disorder. Successful management depends on an accurate assessment of the severity of the patient's condition and the degree to which the patient will tolerate handling (Harris 1994).

The goal of supportive therapy is to stabilize the patient until specifi c therapy can be established. Initially, therapy concentrates on correcting fluid deficits and hypothermia. As the diagnosis is delineated, treatment becomes more focused. Supportive care may be withdrawn after the patient demonstrates a satisfactory degree of self-suffi ciency. Successful management means providing aggressive support carefully, one step at a time.

Medical management of the critically ill patient

Because it is frequently difficult to establish an accurate diagnosis, supportive care is an essential component of companion bird medicine. A checklist of supportive care is given in Appendix 6.1. Not all of the steps should be applied at once or in the given sequence; it is better to move step by step, giving the bird time to react to each action and evaluating the effects! It is the practitioner's primary responsibility to assess 'how much is too much' with regard to critical patients.

A critically ill bird is defined as a patient that requires immediate medical attention (Harris 1994). Such patients must be provided with some form of medical support either before or after diagnostic procedures, but definitely cannot wait days or even hours for test results prior to receiving crucial medical attention.

Before handling the bird for any reason, a detailed plan based on the fi ndings of preliminary observations must be formulated. This plan must account for all the diagnostic and therapeutic actions warranted by the patient's condition while identifying the degree to which the bird is expected to tolerate handling. More delicate patients require greater care in handling. These birds, however, are the ones that need the most support. A diffi cult situation then exists, in which the patient needing most help is the one least capable of tolerating stress. The key to managing these birds is conservative

progression – gently performing one manoeuvre at a time, prioritizing relative to estimated needs, then waiting for the clinical effect before proceeding. It is imperative that every detail of the diagnostic/therapeutic plan is anticipated and accounted for in advance. It could be fatal to remember a necessary item after the process has begun (Harris 1994, Raftery 2005).

Specific supportive measures depend on actual needs; these may be estimated in critically ill patients without background clinical data (see also Appendix 6.1).

Birds that are collapsed on the bottom of the cage, and/or have been ill for a long period of time, are probably severely dehydrated and hypothermic. A bird that collapsed within the previous hour or so may not suffer from either condition.

Dehydration

Dehydration can be assessed by closely observing the eyes and skin of the face and keel. The eyes may appear dull and dry, and the skin of the lower legs and feet may appear discoloured, withered and wrinkled. PCV, TP and WBC are useful tools in determining the patient's degree of dehydration and clinical status (Appendix 6.8).

In general, any bird presenting in critical condition due to illness (as opposed to injury) can be presumed to be at least 7–10% dehydrated and acidotic; those that have been regurgitating may be alkalotic. The following signs will give an indication of the grade of dehydration:

1. A bird that is 5% dehydrated will demonstrate brief tenting of the skin over the tarsometatarsus, face, or between the shoulders, dryness of the eyes and a dullness to the skin.
2. At 10% dehydration, the patient will show persistent tenting, mild hypothermia and thick oral secretions.
3. At 15% dehydration, the above signs will be seen plus profound weakness, tachycardia and collapse.

Fluids (at 37–39°C) may be administered via the jugular, basilic or medial metatarsal veins, or through an intraosseous catheter. If the patient is significantly dehydrated, the oral or subcutaneous approach may not be beneficial. Intraperitoneal approaches are not advised, and may be hazardous due to the risk of fluids entering the air sac system (Harris 1994).

Hypothermia

A bird that is fluffed and trembling on the perch or huddled on the cage bottom can be presumed to be

hypothermic. This includes most avian patients in critical condition. A hypothermic bird will have cold beak and feet, and often feels noticeably cool when handled.

Use of warmed i.v. fluids and a heated intensive care unit (25–30°C) will simultaneously elevate the core and peripheral body temperatures effectively. Overheating, especially with severe hypotension, may cause peripheral vasodilation; this may exacerbate the hypovolaemia, further lowering body core temperature, and may aggravate metabolic acidosis. It is important that the hypothermia is not attended to without recognition of the fluid needs (Harris 1994).

Warm, moist air in an intensive care unit appears to reverse hypothermia safely and effectively, possibly because of its effect of reducing evaporation from the extensive internal respiratory surface area. Also, the drying tendency of oxygen (when used) is nullified. Monitoring hypothermia is a matter of clinical perception. The use of convective air warming units will also aid in raising the body temperature of a critically ill bird or surgical patient (Fig. 6.20).

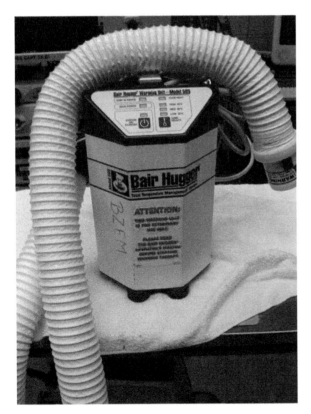

Fig 6.20 The Bair hugger convective heat unit can be used to warm a critically ill patient as well as an avian patient during a surgical procedure.

Circulatory condition

The circulatory condition can be assessed by evaluating the turgidity of the basilic (median ulnar) vein as it crosses the ventral elbow. Circulatory collapse will be indicated by slower refilling of this vein after digital compression (it normally takes less than 0.5 seconds). A circulatory collapse needs direct attention (see 'Shock' and Appendix 6.9).

Oxygen

The administration of oxygen is often beneficial and is rarely contraindicated. A critical patient, especially one in shock, may suffer from diminished cardiac output. Providing oxygen maximizes the efficiency of the cardiorespiratory system. If the bird is dyspnoeic for any reason, oxygen is recommended. Over-oxygenating the patient prior to handling may also decrease the risk of handling (Harris 1994).

When possible, it is best to humidify and warm the oxygen before delivery to the patient. This is best accomplished by bubbling the gas through warmed isotonic or half-strength saline solution (Harris 1997). Methods of oxygen supplementation include using an oxygen chamber (Fig. 6.4)/cage or direct delivery via a face mask. A 30–40% oxygen saturation is recommended when using an oxygen cage for prolonged oxygen therapy. A flow rate of 50 mL/kg/min will provide the same oxygen saturation with a face mask (Hernandez & Aguilar 1994). One hundred per cent oxygen may be used for periods up to 12 hours, but this has been shown to be toxic within 3–4 days. Additionally, carbon dioxide levels should be maintained at a level less than 1.5% by the use of a CO_2 absorber or maintained adequate gas flow rates to flush out accumulating carbon dioxide (Murray 1994).

Continued care

Once the patient has begun to stabilize, it may be possible to use routine handling methods. Supportive care should never be abruptly stopped, but diagnostic procedures may be initiated to establish a diagnosis for instituting more specific therapy. Fluid therapy should be continued (or hydration monitored) for 3–4 days to be sure that the deficit is fully corrected and the patient has re-established a normal maintenance intake. Supplemental heat is usually not necessary for adult birds once they have stabilized, and oxygen is only needed where specifically indicated. Caloric and nutritional support is a major consideration once the bird has stabilized. It is not practical in avian medicine to supply a bird's total nutritional needs parenterally, and oral alimentation is therefore necessary as soon as the patient's status allows if spontaneous food intake is absent.

Specific conditions and treatments

Hypocalcaemia syndrome in African grey parrots

Hypocalcaemia is most common in African grey parrots, but it may also occur in other psittacines and raptors. The aetiology is uncertain; however, affected birds are often on diets deficient in calcium, phosphorus or vitamin D_3 or with an inappropriate Ca:P ratio (all-seed diets). In African grey parrots, skeletal mineralization often appears normal with hypocalcaemia. Clinical signs include seizures, ataxia, opisthotonus, weakness or tetany.

Diagnosis is based on history, clinical signs, low blood calcium levels and response to calcium therapy. Blood calcium levels below 1.8 mmol/L (normal range = 2.1–2.9 mmol/L) may result in clinical signs. It is generally considered more useful to measure serum ionized calcium levels (normal range for African grey parrots 0.96–1.22 mmol/L) in parrots rather than total calcium levels when investigating disorders of calcium metabolism (Stanford 2003). Other studies give reference values of the African grey determined in Pico syringes ranging from 1.35 to 1.68 mmol/L (Westerhof et al 2007). The protein-bound calcium fraction is physiologically inactive. It is mainly bound to albumin and so any physiological or pathological condition affecting serum albumin will affect total calcium concentration, giving an imprecise result. It will also be affected by the acid–base balance, without affecting the total calcium level.

After an initial blood sample has been submitted, parenteral administration of 10% calcium gluconate, 0.5–2.0 mL/kg (50–200 mg/kg calcium), preferably slowly and intravenously, will control seizures. This enables the diagnosis to be confirmed retrospectively, and facilitates subsequent monitoring of any dietary changes and supplementation. Diazepam (0.6–1.5 mg/kg i.m.) will help to control the convulsions (Coles 1996a, Jenkins 1997b). Hydration must be maintained and corticosteroids should not be used in these patients. The bird should be given a proper diet, and calcium and vitamin D_3 supplementation provided (see Box 6.1). Exposure to increased UV light also has a significant effect on calcium metabolism in this species. In African grey parrots fed a seed- or pellet-based diet, there was a significant increase in the concentration of ionized calcium in the plasma of both groups, independent of the calcium and vitamin D_3 content of the diets fed, and a significant increase in the plasma concentration of 25-hydroxycholecalciferol in only the seed-fed group (Stanford 2006).

Cardiopulmonary arrest

The prognosis following respiratory and cardiac arrest varies according to the cause. Patients that arrest due to an isoflurane anaesthetic overdose or acute illness (e.g. acute tracheal obstruction) often respond well to cardiopulmonary resuscitation (CPR), but those that arrest during a chronic illness rarely do so (Rupley 1997).

The same basic rules of resuscitation apply to birds as to mammals. Most birds can be easily intubated. A speculum may be needed to hold the beak open if the bird arouses. If an obvious upper airway obstruction is found or there is tracheal damage, air sac intubation should be performed (see below). An open anaesthesia circuit should be used to deliver 100% oxygen, and the anaesthesia system designed to allow the operator good control in delivery of positive pressure ventilation (a rate of once every 4–5 seconds). Care must be taken not to overinflate the bird, as rupturing of air sacs can occur. Respiratory assistance via the operator's mouth to the endotracheal tube is not recommended due to the zoonotic potential of some avian diseases (e.g. *Campylobacter*, psittacosis, tuberculosis). If needed, unidirectional respiration can be attempted by increasing the air flow through the trachea and allowing the gas to escape through an air sac breathing tube, or vice versa (Fig. 6.21).

Cardiac and pulmonary auscultation can be performed during assisted respiration. If time permits, an electrocardiogram can be established; however, measurements are difficult to obtain if the patient is small or moving. In critical cases, quick access to the circulatory system should be made (see 'Fluid therapy'). If there is no heart beat or peripheral pulse, firm and rapid compressions of the sternum should be started, ventilation continued and adrenaline (epinephrine) (0.5–1.0 mg/kg i.m., i.v., i.o.) and atropine (0.5 mg/kg i.m., s.c., i.v., i.o., i.t.) administered. Adrenaline and atropine can be given intravenously, followed by a bolus of saline or sterile water to encourage transport of the drugs to the heart. Intratracheal administration, through the tracheal wall into the lumen, is often the easiest route in arrested birds (Rupley 1997). Doxapram (20 mg/kg i.m., i.v., i.o. or dropped on the tongue) and sodium bicarbonate (5 mmol/kg i.v., i.o., once) are also used in birds in situations of cardiopulmonary resuscitation (see Appendix 6.10) (Carpenter 2005). Although it is not likely that direct pressure has an effect on the heart itself, changes in the blood pressure and cardiac output can be made by altering the intrapulmonic and abdominal pressures (Loudis & Sutherland-Smith 1994).

Respiratory disease

The majority of critical avian patients present with respiratory disease resulting in acute respiratory distress (ARD). Resuscitative intervention is required most often prior to aggressive diagnostics to minimize stress (Lichtenberger 2006). After administering oxygen (mask or cage) or establishing an airway and providing

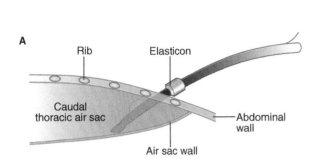

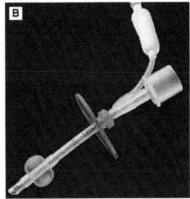

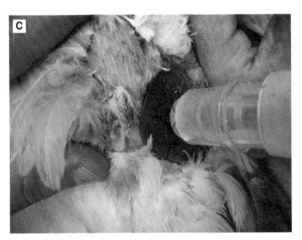

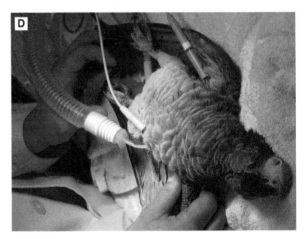

Fig 6.21 An air sac breathing tube (**A**) can be put in place if the trachea is compromised or oral surgery is being performed. (**B**) Commercially available avian air sac breathing tubes are easy to apply. (**C**) Commercial and (**D**) a modified endotracheal tube in place for coelomic respiration.

adequate ventilation, the bird's respiratory tract must be evaluated (Jenkins 1997b). It is important to differentiate between upper airway, pulmonary and air sac disease.

The differential diagnosis includes (Lichtenberger 2006):

1. Causes of large airway disease include obstruction by foreign body (i.e. seed in cockatiel), mass, *Aspergillus* granuloma or oropharynx granulomas.
2. Causes of parenchymal disease include cardiogenic pulmonary oedema; smoke inhalation; pneumonia; *Aspergillus* species, *Chlamydophila* species, Gram-negative bacteria, poxvirus, etc.
3. Causes of coelom space disease include heart disease; hypovolaemia; liver disease; egg-related peritonitis; organomegaly.
4. Small airway disease includes inhalant respiratory irritants such as smoke, Teflon toxicity, aerosols and candles.

A thorough oral examination is necessary to ensure that the oral cavity and larynx are clear of debris, abscesses or other discharges. The rate and pattern of breathing as well as the patient's stance and character of breathing (tail pumping, etc.) can help to differentiate. Auscultation of many areas can also help; the head and neck should be auscultated as well as the trachea. Lung sounds can best be heard on the dorsal aspect of the body beneath the wing, and abdominal placement of the stethoscope may help in the localization of air sac disease.

Pulmonary disease can be difficult to differentiate from air sac and tracheal disease. If the condition of the patient permits, auscultation and radiology may be helpful to localize the pathology. Laparoscopy is a useful procedure for the culture and biopsy of respiratory disease. Oxygen and humidity are important factors, as mentioned before. Therapeutic strategies for respiratory disease related to parenchymal disease or with a history of regurgitation or vomiting include systemic treatment and/or aerosol therapy (nebulization) of bronchodilators and antibiotics. When a cardiogenic oedema is suspected, furosemide (2–4 mg/kg i.v.) and nitroglycerine ointment on the tongue are administered and the bird is allowed to stabilize prior to further diagnostics (Lichtenberger 2006).

Air sac breathing tube

The physiology of avian respiration is complex, and the unique respiratory anatomy of birds has allowed us to treat airway disease with unique methods. **The placement of the air sac breathing tube is extremely helpful in the management of upper airway obstructions and surgery.** It is very important to have a definite diagnosis of upper airway obstruction; pulmonary parenchymal disease can resemble airway obstruction, and air sac cannulation has little effect with parenchymal disease.

The procedure can be performed in the conscious bird, but anaesthesia is highly recommended when time permits (Fig. 6.21).

The patient is placed in right lateral recumbency, and the tube is most often inserted into the left abdominal or caudal thoracic air sac because of its relatively greater size (Jenkins 1997a). Feathers are removed from the stifle to the vent, and from the ventral midline to the ischium. The independent leg is gently stretched cranially (Loudis & Sutherland-Smith 1994), or is flexed and abducted to expose the last rib (Harris 1997). After cleaning and disinfecting the skin, a small incision is made caudal to the tight muscle, midway down the thigh. Using a sterile haemostat, blunt dissection is directed medially and cranially into the coelom. The breathing tube can be installed into the caudal thoracic air sac, just dorsal to the caudal edge of the pectoral muscle. The breathing tube can be fashioned from a red rubber feeding tube and a tape butterfly, or a strip of Elastikon may be used to help facilitate attachment. Small (3 mm inside diameter) cuffed endotracheal tubes can be adjusted (Harris 1997). The tube is guided gently through the incision, and airflow should be felt and heard at this time. Patency can be tested by holding a microscope slide at the tube opening to observe for breathing-induced fogging (Harris 1997). If the tube is inserted too deeply, it may press against the lung or an abdominal organ. The tube is anchored to the skin with small non-absorbable sutures (Loudis & Sutherland-Smith 1994).

If inhalation anaesthesia is used, the air sac tube should be attached to the circuit so the bird will remain anaesthetized. Careful attention should be paid to the flow rate, because air sac and pulmonary damage may occur if the bird is overinflated. The oxygen flow should be started at 0.5–1.0 L/kg body weight per minute, and the patient's breathing and appearance of the anaesthesia rebreathing bag closely observed.

Air sac cannulae have been left in place for more than 7 days, but the clinician should be aware of complications arising from this procedure, including abdominal

organ damage, secondary bacterial infections and inadvertent occlusion of the breathing tube. The normal filtration devices of the nasal passage are absent, and a direct pathway to the pulmonary tissue is present. The incubator should be kept clean and free of faeces and debris. During normal respiration, a large amount of water loss is regained in the nasal conchae; therefore, a high amount of fluid replenishment should be administered while the cannula is in place.

On removal of the cannula, the abdominal muscles and the skin are surgically closed; in some cases, these have been left to heal by second intention.

Shock

Although shock has not been clearly defined in birds, several debilitated birds in a shock-like state are often seen in practice. **Shock is defined as a state in which, regardless of the cause, inadequate distribution of systemic blood flow causes diminished delivery of oxygen and nutrients to tissues (Hernandez & Aguilar 1994).** The classification of shock by aetiology includes haemorrhagic, cardiogenic, traumatic, septic and anaphylactic syndromes. Because the ultimate result of these states is circulatory comprise, shock is more aptly classified functionally, according to its haemodynamic effects, as hypovolaemic, cardiogenic or vasogenic.

Hypovolaemic shock is caused by a decrease of circulating blood volume due to haemorrhage, including trauma, coagulopathy, gastrointestinal bleeding, surgical mishaps, or a ruptured neoplasia (absolute hypovolaemia) or, indirectly, severe dehydration secondary to vomiting, diarrhoea or polyuria, or loss in a third-body space such as coelomic cavity (relative hypovolaemia) (Lichtenberger 2005, 2006). There is evidence to support the statement that blood loss is better tolerated in birds than in mammals (Sturkie & Griminger 1986, Murray 1994, Lichtenberger 2005, 2006).

Cardiogenic shock is the result of impaired cardiac function and a decrease in cardiac output. This is often associated with the administration of certain anaesthetics and drugs.

Vasogenic shock is more often associated with sepsis, endotoxaemia and toxicosis.

Regardless of the cause, the ultimate result of shock is a circulatory compromise resulting in a lower tissue perfusion and interstitial dehydration. This may be evidenced as follows:

1. Perfusion. The effects of perfusion are demonstrated on physical examination by perfusion parameters, which include mucous membrane colour, capillary refill time, resting heart rate, as well as blood pressure (Lichenberger 2005, 2006). Poor capillary refill time in a weak, depressed bird with a rapid, weak peripheral

pulse (Murray 1994). The normal refill time for the basilic vein is less than 0.5 seconds (Quesenberry & Hillyer 1994).

2. Dehydration. Clinical parameters evaluated during assessment of interstitial dehydration include mucous membrane moisture, position of the ocular globe, and eyelid turgor (Lichtenberger 2005, 2006). The degree of dehydration is estimated based on these clinical signs and baseline blood samples – PCV, TP and WBC (Appendix 6.8). The buffy coat can give a rough quick estimate of the total leucocyte count.

3. Metabolic acidosis. The measurement of plasma bicarbonate is the most practical means of characterizing metabolic acidosis in birds (Redig 1984). 'Normal' avian bicarbonate is 20 mmol/L.

4. High uric acid values, which are common in severely ill patients. Hyperuricaemia occurs as a result of either renal failure or accelerated tissue metabolism.

5. Plasma glucose levels, which may vary on a case-by-case basis.

6. Hyperkalaemia (a common cause of bradycardia and cardial arrhythmias) or hypokalaemia and hyponatraemia (in cases of profuse vomiting or diarrhoea).

The recommended steps for treating birds with shock are given in Appendix 6.9. Because hypotension and hypoxaemia are detrimental, restoring effective blood volume and pressure and improving tissue oxygenation are immediate therapeutic requirements in the treatment of shock.

Trauma

The avian practitioner may encounter a variety of clinical presentations associated with the avian trauma patient. An understanding of the physiological response to trauma and the therapeutic means necessary to control inappropriate compensatory mechanisms is critically important in successful management of trauma cases (Murray 1994). As with all animals (including humans), it is important to initiate therapy of the traumatized avian patient within the 'golden period'. This is defined as the period of time following the injury during which appropriate therapy will result in the most satisfactory outcome (Jenkins 1997b).

Central to the concept of trauma management is hospital preparedness. All drugs, supplies and equipment should be preassembled in a central area such as the anaesthetic induction area (Appendix 6.10). Generic drug dosage charts for the most commonly encountered species should be prepared and readily accessible. Such charts should contain precalculated volumes of drugs to

be administered, including fluids, corticosteroids, diuretics, analeptics and antibiotics. Effective and complete hospital and staff preparation before the presentation of the avian trauma case is important in the management of the patient during the first few hours following injury.

In the trauma patient, despite the condition of the bird presented, a thorough and complete physical examination is critically important (Murray 1994, Riggs & Tully 2004). Before handling the injured bird, the attitude and posture should be noted. Injuries to the appendicular skeleton are often more readily identified with the bird in its cage or standing on the examination table. The exact order and technique of examination is a matter of clinical preference, but the clinician should not overlook a complete ophthalmic examination. Cases of suspected head trauma should be subjected to a thorough neurological examination (Bennett 1994, Williams 1994). The diagnosis of shock is often difficult. Clinical evidence of shock mandates immediate and aggressive therapy (Appendix 6.9). Although the clinician is encouraged to perform a complete and thorough examination on all trauma cases presented, such examination should, of course, be accomplished within the limits of the patient. Additionally, clinicians must be aware of the possibility of pretrauma disease in these patients (Murray 1994, Ritzman 2004).

Control of haemorrhage

One of the first priorities in the therapeutic management of the trauma patient is the control of haemorrhage (Murray 1994):

1. Damage to developing feathers can result in active haemorrhage. The feather should be removed, taking care to hold the surrounding skin, and direct pressure applied. Should the haemorrhage continue, judicious surgical glue (Superglue®) should be applied to the distal part of the follicle. Chemical or electrocautery should not be used, as they can result in permanent follicle damage.

2. Haemorrhage from horny structures, such as the beak and claws, is typically controlled with chemical cautery using such as ferric chloride, ferric subsulphate or silver nitrate, talc or wound powder, or even flour or radiosurgery (Coles 1996a).

3. For soft tissue wounds with haemorrhage, direct pressure is the treatment of choice. In refractory cases, the use of bipolar radiosurgery on individual vessels or the use of tissue glue may be required. Chemical cautery agents should be avoided because of tremendous local tissue necrosis and a subsequent inflammatory reaction.

Quantification of the degree of blood loss may be quite difficult. In general, a bird can easily tolerate a loss of 30% of its blood volume, which is approximately equivalent to 2% of its body weight. As a result of the rapid movement of the interstitial fluid into the vascular compartment, the PCV tends not to stabilize for 24 hours (Quesenberry & Hillyer 1994). Therefore, this parameter should not be used for diagnosis or prognosis until 24–48 hours after the blood loss.

Blood transfusions, either heterologous or homologous, may be required in cases of severe blood loss. However, generally the bird benefits most from the volume expansion accomplished with fluid therapy (Appendices 6.5, 6.9 and 6.11). Of particular importance is the delivery of the fluid directly into the vascular network via the intravenous or intraosseous route (Lichtenberger 2006). Oral or subcutaneous routes are of limited value in the traumatized patient (Murray 1994). In cases of respiratory compromise, physical restraint should be limited and oxygen used during handling.

The trauma patient should be housed in quiet and warm surroundings within the veterinary facility. Antimicrobials may be indicated in infected wounds or in those cases where the clinician anticipates a secondary immunosuppression resulting from the stress associated with prolonged hospitalization.

Blood loss

Blood volume (cells and plasma) in birds ranges from 4.5% of the body weight in ostriches to 9.2% in pigeons (Jenkins 1997b). In response to blood loss, baroreceptor and catecholamine-induced arteriolar vasoconstriction tends to maintain normal blood pressure and adequate perfusion of vital organs, and this process is aided by movement of interstitial fluid into vascular spaces. The efficiency of these processes makes birds substantially more tolerant of blood loss than mammals (Murray 1994, Lichtenberger 2006).

Stress

Trauma is obviously quite stressful to the bird, and this stress results in the release of catecholamines (noradrenaline and dopamine). There are documented differences between birds and mammals in their response to catecholamines; however, the catecholamine release has several profound effects, all of which are directed at the patient's preservation. These include:

1. Elevation of the heart rate and peripheral arteriolar vasoconstriction to maintain adequate perfusion of the heart, brains and lungs.
2. A hyperglycaemic effect – therefore, most traumatized birds will have normal to elevated blood glucose levels, alleviating the need for supplemental glucose administration (Quesenberry & Hillyer 1994).

3. Raising the pain threshold, which may cause complications in relatively simple injuries during the struggle associated with the 'fight or flight' response.

Pain and analgesia

Pain is almost certainly a physiological response to trauma. **Unfortunately, the typically stoical nature of most avian patients precludes clinical recognition of pain or distress in all but the most serious injuries.** The issue is therefore not whether birds feel pain, but whether their response to pain is recognized by humans (Paul-Murphy & Ludders 2001). Other than the previously mentioned effects of catecholamines on the pain threshold, most of the changes associated with pain are probably associated with recovery and rehabilitation from the traumatic injury. During the recovery phase, pain may preclude normal food and water consumption. Additionally, pain may prevent normal function of injured regions of the body, thus delaying recovery and return to normal use.

Most analgesic drugs and dosages have been extrapolated from non-avian species, but increasing amounts of research is being done. There are two group of importance:

1. Opioids
   - Butorphanol tartrate, an opioid, 1–3 mg/kg i.m. has shown much clinical promise (Paul-Murphy & Ludders 2001). Other authors have recommended a dose of 0.5–2.0 mg/kg i.m. (Jenkins 1997b). It has little effect on the cardiovascular function of budgerigars, but may result in slight motor deficits.
   - Buprenorphine hydrochloride, also an opioid, at a dose of 0.1–0.5 mg/kg i.m. was considered ineffective (Paul-Murphy 1997, Paul-Murphy & Ludders 2001, van Engelen et al 2005). One study showed a good analgesic effect at a dose of 0.5 mg/kg q.i.d. in pigeons (Gaggermeir et al 2000).

2. Non-steroidal anti-inflammatory drugs (NSAIDs)
   - Phenylbutazone p.o. 20 mg/kg t.i.d in raptors and 3.5–7.0 mg/kg in psittacines
   - Acetylsalicylic acid p.o. 5.0 mg/kg t.i.d. and 325 mg per 250 mL drinking water. Change water t.i.d. It alters the taste/smell of water and may not be well accepted.
   - Flunixin meglumine appears to be safe at 1–5 (10) mg/kg i.m. (Jenkins 1997b); however, its analgesic effects are, at this point, uncertain. Flunixin may cause regurgitation following administration. The recommended dose is 1.0 mg/kg s.i.d. Hydration is essential. Use only for short

duration; it is potentially nephrotoxic (Paul-Murphy & Ludders 2001).

- Ibuprofen p.o. in a dose of 5–10 mg/kg b.i.d.–t.i.d. Use the paediatric suspension for small birds.
- Ketoprofen i.m. or s.c. 2.0 mg/kg s.i.d.–t.i.d.
- Carprofen p.o. 2.0–4.0 mg/kg b.i.d.–t.i.d. Higher doses are sometimes needed for oral route.
- Piroxicam p.o. 0.5 mg/kg is used for chronic osteoarthritis.
- Meloxicam p.o. 0.1–0.5 mg/kg s.i.d. (Wilson et al 2004).

Commonly encountered traumatic injuries

Beak injury

Beak injuries are generally caused as a result of aggressive bird-to-bird interaction. The primary goals of the repair are to restore the beak to normal function and appearance and to preserve and protect the soft tissue and osteoid underlying structures present in both the rhinotheca and gnathotheca. To do this, the clinician should be familiar with the normal anatomy and growth patterns of the beak of the species involved.

During the initial examination of a traumatized beak, the extent and severity of the beak injury should be determined as well as the effect on function of the various articulations between the beak and the skull (Fig. 6.22). The age of the injury is important, because older wounds are likely to be contaminated. Under no circumstances should definitive repair be attempted in infected traumatic beak injuries (Murray 1994). Following examination and the patient's stabilization, repair of the beak injury may be initiated. In most cases judicious use of general anaesthesia is indicated, using an air sac tube, to facilitate the repair process. Bulky face masks and endotracheal tubes are difficult to work around at the operative site. Basic wound treatment should be applied, cleansing and debriding the wound. Heavily infected wounds should be allowed to heal by second intention prior to applying a semi-permanent cyanoacrylate patch.

A modified 'wet-to-dry' bandage has proved quite beneficial in infected beak injuries. The wound should be gently flushed with a sterile saline solution, and sterile gauze sponges of an appropriate size used to pack the defect. Following moistening with sterile saline or diluted chlorhexidine (0.05%), the wound is then covered with a semi-occlusive dressing (Tegaderm®, 3M) which is changed every 12–24 hours as indicated by the discharge and debris that adheres to the gauze.

Systemic antibiotics are indicated to protect the surrounding vascular network and dermis from bacterial infection. Wounds treated in this manner tend to granulate quickly, allowing definitive treatment with a cyanoacrylate patch (Murray 1994). The manufacturer's

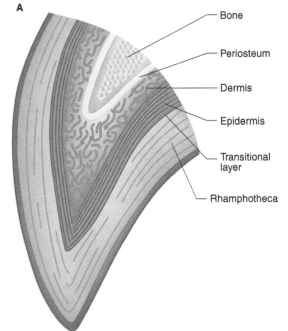

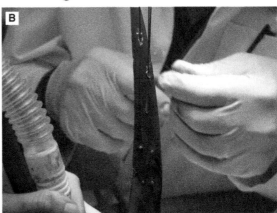

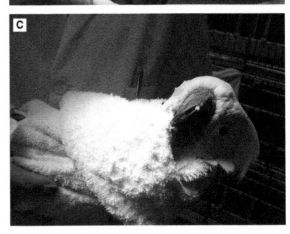

Fig 6.22 (**A**) The anatomy of the avian beak is complex and requires an understanding of the anatomy in order to develop a proper treatment plan when injured. Beak injuries can occur due to trauma (**B**) or disease (**C**).

instructions should be followed when applying a cyanoacrylate patch.

If not avulsed, beak injuries can heal, with a return to normal function. During the rehabilitation period, birds should be monitored closely to ensure adequate caloric intake.

Lacerations

Treatment of lacerations depends upon the site and age of the injury. As in all animals, infected or contaminated injuries should not be closed until these aspects have been addressed. Radical surgical debridement is not practical in most avian wounds. In most cases the use of a series of wet-to-dry bandages, as previously described, facilitates granulation tissue formation. Wounds may then be allowed to heal by secondary intention, or a delayed secondary closure may be used. An exception to this conservative approach may be necessary when vital structures are exposed by the laceration. If at all possible, an early attempt at closure should be made to protect viscera, large vessels, tendons and joints. If primary closure is not practical, bandaging techniques that preclude tissue desiccation and infection should be used (Murray 1994).

Suture selection is generally dependent upon clinicians' preferences. Surprisingly, most birds are very tolerant of skin sutures, and restraint devices are generally not required.

Any injury or suspected injury that occurs as the result of an interaction between a bird and a dog or cat should be addressed as an emergency. Not only are these predators capable of inducing serious crushing and internal injuries, but the presence of *Pasteurella multocida* within the oral cavity may contaminate wounds. The use of betalactams is always indicated, and is typically continued for 14 days post-injury.

Contusions

Serious muscle contusions frequently occur as a result of wall or window crashing. Such injuries may result in skeletal, central nervous system (CNS) or visceral damage. Affected birds should be treated as for any bird suffering blood loss – i.e. fluids, heat and, potentially, corticosteroids.

Another frequent contusion presented to the avian practitioner is that suffered by a bird during a 'panic attack' within its cage. Affected appendages are swollen, painful, and contain various amounts of subcutaneous blood. Following the administration of appropriate supportive care, such injuries should be addressed to protect the skin and soft tissues of the wings. A self-adhering semi-occlusive bandage should applied in a sandwich fashion with the wing in between two layers of material, and the dressings changed daily for 5–7 days and then as needed.

Fractures of the appendicular skeleton

Birds presented with fractures of either the pectoral or pelvic limb should receive appropriate therapy in a timely fashion. Several considerations in the management of fractures warrant discussion:

1. Fractured bones may potentially result in significant blood loss into the surrounding soft tissue. Therefore, fluid replacement is indicated to aid the maintenance of circulatory blood volume.
2. Most of the appendicular skeleton has little regional soft tissue support, and this predisposes the avian patient to the development of open fractures. Many initially closed fractures are complicated by bone penetrating the skin during the bird's inappropriate movements and anxiety.
3. The lack of extensive soft tissue support results in a close anatomical relationship between fracture fragments and regional arteries, veins and nerves. Preservation of these structures is critically important to the eventual recovery of the fracture patient.

To prevent the above-mentioned complications, as well as the degree of pain associated with the movement of fractured fragments, some form of temporary external fixation may be necessary. This should be applied as soon as possible and left in place until radiography and a proper evaluation can be carried out. However, it is often wiser to do nothing at this stage unless a wing is trailing badly, in which case a temporary figure-of-eight bandage using Vetrap® or similar material may be used (Coles 1996b).

As with any trauma patient, supportive care should include an appropriate hospital environment and the administration of fluids and drugs. Should the use of intraosseous fluids be contemplated, the fractured bone and the contralateral limb should not be used as sites of catheter placement.

Orthopaedic techniques need skill, practice and experience. Therefore, after temporary external fixation and stabilization to the point of tolerance of orthopaedic intervention, an orthopaedic surgeon should be consulted or specific literature studied (Degernes 1994, Coles 1996b, Bennett 1997, Rupley 1997, Harcourt-Brown 2005). Regardless of the type of fixation or splint used, the affected limb requires close monitoring. Bandages may need to be replaced within 48 hours, because they tend to loosen as local swelling is reduced. Generally, analgesia is not recommended in fracture cases because elimination of the pain associated with excessive use of the affected limb predisposes the limb to additional stress and subsequent injury (Murray 1994).

Head trauma

Head trauma is common. Window, ceiling fan, wall and mirror crashing are the most common incidents resulting

in significant cranial trauma. Affected birds are typically depressed, there may be haemorrhages, and clinical evidence of CNS trauma may be present. Birds with CNS trauma should be treated aggressively to prevent irreversible damage. They should be kept relatively cool (for the treatment protocol, see Appendix 6.11). Long-standing injuries or those that fail to respond within 48 hours carry a poor prognosis, and neurological deficiencies may be permanent (Murray 1994).

Burns

Most burns are due to contact with hot liquids such as water or cooking oil, hot formula fed to unweaned birds, or electrical causes such as chewing on electric wires (Jenkins 1997b). Burns may be classified according to their severity as superficial, partial thickness or full thickness.

There is likely to be smoke exposure in situations where smoke accompanied the burn, especially in enclosed spaces or involving materials likely to produce toxic fumes (fat, Teflon®).

If more than 50% of the body surface is affected by partial or full thickness burns, the prognosis is grave and the client may consider euthanasia.

Birds with severe or extensive burns need emergency treatment. **Dyspnoeic birds often have laryngeal oedema and accumulation of upper airway secretions, and may benefit from an air sac tube and oxygen.** Other treatments include an intraosseous catheter and treatment for shock. Systemic bactericidal antibiotics should be started in birds with severe burns, to prevent sepsis. Renal function should be monitored by the quantity of droppings and the urine volume, uric acid concentration and serum electrolytes. Fluids and diuretics (furosemide at 2–4 mg/kg) should be continued, and analgesics are indicated for birds that appear to be in pain. The burns should be cleansed gently, debrided daily and treated with a water-soluble antibiotic dressing. This procedure can be very painful and may be done under general anaesthesia.

Complications most likely to occur include circulatory collapse, oliguria, renal failure (most likely to occur within the first 24–48 hours) and sepsis (in birds surviving the initial injury).

Crop burns in young birds and chemical burns in adult birds are similar to other burns (Fig. 6.23). Many partial thickness burns result in the formation of an eschar that will later open to form a fistula. These fistulae should be closed surgically as soon as the patient's condition allows.

Foreign body in the upper alimentary canal

Owners are notoriously careless with regard to the objects they let their birds play with. Larger psittacines can chew

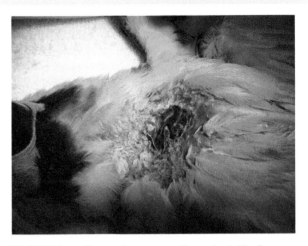

Fig 6.23 A thermal burn to the crop caused by overheated feeding formula. Crop thermal burns are a common presentation to the avian veterinary practice.

up and splinter wood, metal (especially aluminium) and bone (particularly poultry bones). They may also play with cotton or wool attached to needles, and with large cactus houseplants. In waterfowl, impacted hooks and/or line may be found in the oesophagus. Foreign bodies can become lodged in the tongue, oesophagus or crop. Metal or plastic crop feeding tubes can be lost down the upper alimentary canal unless care is taken.

In many cases, it will be known what type of foreign body has been swallowed. The bird may be presented trying to regurgitate the offending object, which can sometimes be palpated in the oesophagus or crop or demonstrated on radiography.

In some cases, e.g. a swallowed metal or plastic catheter, the foreign body can be gently 'milked' back out of the oesophagus with the bird conscious. However, general anaesthesia or deep narcosis and forceps removal is easier. Ingluviotomy (crop surgery) may be required in some cases. If the foreign body has been present for some time, ulceration and fistula of the crop may occur (Coles 1996a).

Discharge and follow-up

Before a bird is discharged from the hospital the client should be instructed on how to administer medication and provide the recommended care, including provision for keeping the bird warm on the way home. It is usually advisable that written home care instructions, the hospital bill and the recheck appointment are discussed prior to reuniting the bird and the client, to prevent the client from being distracted by the bird (Johnson-Delaney 1994).

Maintaining a good line of communication with the client is very important because the status of the patient

can quickly change. The client should be informed of the unpredictable outcome of the critical avian patient. Telephoning the client the day after discharge allows the veterinarian to evaluate the patient's condition and gives the client an opportunity to ask questions.

In multi-bird households and aviaries, the diagnosis of many avian diseases must be made rapidly. The best diagnostic approach is often by post-mortem examination and histopathology. Organ cytology can often help to lead the clinician in the right direction.

References

Altman R B 1997 Soft tissue surgical procedures. In: Altman R B, Clubb S L, Dorrestein G M, Quesenberry K E (eds) Avian medicine and surgery. W B Saunders, Philadelphia, PA, p 713–715

Bennett A 1994 Neurology. In: Ritchie B W, Harrison G J, Harrison L R (eds) Avian medicine: principles and application. Wingers, Lake Worth, FL, p 723–747

Bennett A 1997 Orthopedic surgery. In: Altman R B, Clubb S L, Dorrestein G M, Quesenberry K E (eds) Avian medicine and surgery. W B Saunders, Philadelphia, PA, p 933–966

Bennett A, Harrison G H 1994 Soft tissue surgery. In: Ritchie B W, Harrison G J, Harrison L R (eds) Avian medicine: principles and application. Wingers, Lake Worth, FL, p 1124–1125

Carpenter J W 2005 Exotic animal formulary, 3rd edn. Elsevier Saunders, St Louis, MO

Coles B H 1996a Nursing the sick bird. In: Beynon P H, Forbes N A, Lawton M P C (eds) Manual of psittacine birds. BSAVA, Cheltenham, p 87–95

Coles B H 1996b Wing problems. In: Beynon P H, Forbes N A, Lawton M P C (eds) Manual of psittacine birds. BSAVA, Cheltenham, p 134–146

Dawson W R, Whittow G C 2000 Regulation of the body temperature. In: Whittow G C (ed) Sturkie's Avian physiology, 5th edn. Academic Press, San Diego, CA, p 343–390

Degernes L A 1994 Trauma medicine. In: Ritchie B W, Harrison G J, Harrison L R (eds) Avian medicine: principles and application. Wingers, Lake Worth, FL, p 417–433

Dorrestein G M 1997 Metabolism, pharmacology and therapy. In: Altman R B, Clubb S L, Dorrestein G M, Quesenberry K E (eds) Avian medicine and surgery. W B Saunders, Philadelphia, PA, p 661–670

Forbes N A 2005 Avian soft tissue surgery. In: Harcourt-Brown N, Chitty J (eds) BSAVA Manual of psittacine birds, 2nd edn. BSAVA, Cheltenham, p 107–119

Gaggermeier B, Henke J, Schatzmann H et al 2000 Lihtersachunjen en Schmerzlinderung unit Buprenorphin bei Hanstauben *Columba livia*, Gurel, 1739, var. *domestica*. Proceedings XII Conference on Avian Disease, Munich, p 21

Harcourt-Brown N H 2005 Orthopaedic and beak surgery. In: Harcourt-Brown N, Chitty J (eds) BSAVA Manual of psittacine birds, 2nd edn. BSAVA, Cheltenham, p 120–135

Harris D J 1994 Care of the critically ill patient. Seminars in Avian and Exotic Pet Medicine 3:175–179

Harris D J 1997 Therapeutic avian techniques. Seminars in Avian and Exotic Pet Medicine 6:55–62

Harrison G J, Flinchum G B 2006 Clinical practice. In: Harrison G J, Lightfoot T L (eds) Clinical avian medicine, Vol. I. Spix Publishing, Palm Beach, FL, p 1–28

Harrison G J, Lightfoot T L, Flinchum G B 2006 Emergency and critical care. In: Harrison G J, Lightfoot T L (eds) Clinical avian medicine, Vol. I. Spix Publishing, Palm Beach, p 213–232

Hernandez M, Aguilar R F 1994 Steroid and fluid therapy for treatment of shock in the critical avian patient. Seminars in Avian and Exotic Pet Medicine 3:190–199

Honnas C M, Jensen J, Cornick J L et al 1993 Proventriculotomy to relieve foreign body impaction in ostriches. Journal of the American Veterinary Medical Association 202:1989–1992

Jenkins J R 1994 Critical care, introduction. Seminars in Avian and Exotic Pet Medicine 3:176–178

Jenkins J R 1997a Hospital techniques and supportive care. In: Altman R B, Clubb S L, Dorrestein G M, Quesenberry K E (eds) Avian medicine and surgery. W B Saunders, Philadelphia, PA, p 232–252

Jenkins J R 1997b Avian critical care and emergency medicine. In: Altman R B, Clubb S L, Dorrestein G M, Quesenberry K E (eds) Avian medicine and surgery. W B Saunders, Philadelphia, PA, p 839–863

Johnson-Delaney C 1994 Practice dynamics. In: Ritchie B W, Harrison G J, Harrison L R (eds) Avian medicine: principles and application. Wingers, Lake Worth, FL, p 131–143

Kollias G V 1993 Nutritional support for captive wild birds. In: Proceedings of the Annual Conference of the Association of Avian Veterinarians, p 23–4. Association of Avian Veterinarians

Lichtenberger M 2005 Shock, fluid therapy and CPCR for the avian patient. Proceedings of the 6th Scientific ECAMS meeting, Arles, p 374–387

Lichtenberger M 2006 Emergency case approach to hypotension, hypertension, and acute respiratory distress. Proceedings of the Annual Conference of the Association of Avian Veterinarians, p 281–290. Association of Avian Veterinarians

Loudis G, Sutherland-Smith M 1994 Methods used in the critical care of avian patients. Seminars in Avian and Exotic Pet Medicine 3:180–189

Murray M J 1994 Management of the avian trauma case. Seminars in Avian and Exotic Pet Medicine 3:200–209

Nemetz L 2005 Equipping the avian practice. Veterinary Clinics of North America: Exotic Animal Practice 8(3):427–435

Paul-Murphy J 1997 Evaluation of analgesic properties of butorphanol and buprenorphine for the psittacine bird. In: Proceedings of the Association of Avian Veterinarians, p 125–7.

Paul-Murphy J, Ludders J W 2001 Avian analgesia. Veterinary Clinics of North America. Exotic Animal Practice 4:35–45

Quesenberry K E, Hillyer E 1994 Supportive care and emergency therapy. In: Ritchie B W, Harrison G J, Harrison L R (eds) Avian medicine: principles and application. Wingers, Lake Worth, FL, p 382–416

Quesenberry K E, Mauldin G, Hillyer E 1991 Review of methods of nutritional support in hospitalized birds. In: First Conference of the European Committee of the Association of Avian Veterinarians, p 243–54. European Association of Avian Veterinarians.

Raftery A 2005 The initial presentation: triage and critical care. In: Harcourt-Brown N, Chitty J (eds) BSAVA Manual of psittacine birds, 2nd edn. BSAVA, Cheltenham, p 35–49

Redig P T (1984). Fluid therapy and acid-base balance in the critically ill avian patient. In: Proceedings of the Annual Conference of the Association of Avian Veterinarians. European Association of Avian Veterinarians, p 59–74

Riggs S M, Tully T N 2004 Wound management in nonpsittacine birds. Veterinary Clinics of North America. Exotic Animal Practice 7:19–36

Ritzman T K 2004 Wound healing and management in psittacine birds. Veterinary Clinics of North America. Exotic Animal Practice 7:87–104

Rupley A E 1997 Manual of avian practice. W B Saunders, Philadelphia, PA

Sedgewick C, Pokras M, Kaufman G 1990 Metabolic scaling using estimated energy costs to extrapolate drug doses between different species and different individuals of diverse body size. Proceedings of the Annual Conference of the American Association of Zoo Veterinarians, p 249–54. American Association of Zoo Veterinarians

Stanford M D 2003 Measurement of 25-hydroxycholecalciferol in captive grey parrots (*Psittacus e. erithacus*). Veterinary Record 153:58–59

Stanford M D 2006 Effects of UVB radiation on calcium metabolism in psittacine birds. Veterinary Record 159:236–241

Sturkie P D, Griminger P 1986 Body fluids; blood. In: Sturkie P D (ed) Avian physiology, 4th edn. Springer-Verlag, New York, p 102–129

van Engelen J, Akkerdaas I, Schoemaker N J 2005 A study into the analgetic efficacy of buprenorphine and butorphanol in pigeons (*Columba livia domestica*). Proceedings 6th Scientific ECAMS meeting, Arles, p 19–20

Westerhof I, van der Brom W E, Mol J A et al 1994 Sensitivity of the hypothalamic–pituitary–adrenal system of pigeons (*Columba livia domestica*) to suppression by dexamethasone, cortisol and prednisolone. Avian Diseases 38:435–445

Westerhof I, Haaksema F, Lumeij J T 2007 Influence of blood sample containers on calcium and protein values in birds. Proceedings of the 7th ECAMS Scientific Meeting, Zurich, p 3–4

Williams D 1994 Ophthalmology. In: Ritchie B W, Harrison G J, Harrison L R (eds) Avian medicine: principles and application. Wingers, Lake Worth, FL, p 673–694

Wilson G H, Hernandez-Divers S, Budsberg S T et al 2004 Pharmocokinetics and use of meloxicam in psittacine birds. Proceedings of the Annual Conference of the Associations of Avian Veterinarians, p 7–9, Association of Avian Veterinarians; or Proceedings of 6th Scientific ECAMS meeting, Arles, p 230–237

Appendix 6.1: Checklist of supportive care used in companion bird medicine (after Carpenter 2005)

Because it is frequently difficult to establish an accurate diagnosis, supportive and stabilization care are essential components of companion bird medicine. Supportive care includes:

1. Minimizing handling and other stressors.
2. Hospitalization
   a. Patient should be placed in a warm, quiet, well-ventilated environment with minimal to no disturbance
   b. Heating should be supplementing (30–32°C) because debilitated birds are often hypothermic.
3. Administration of fluid therapy (see Appendices 6.5, 6.6).
4. Use of corticosteroids (with caution, because of their immunosuppressive effects, etc.) in cases of:
   a. Shock and poor vascular perfusion
   b. Extreme stress
   c. CNS trauma
   d. Selected toxaemias and intoxications.
5. Vitamin therapy
   a. Multiple vitamins (including vitamin A) as needed
   b. B complex in selected cases of injury, anorexia, cachexia, CNS disorders or blood loss.
6. Use of antibiotics and/or antimycotics to control primary infections and for injured or debilitated birds where secondary infections may result (use stained faecal smears for evaluation).
7. Iron dextran (6% iron dextran 20 mL/kg i.m.) (Redig 1984)
   a. In cases of iron deficiency or following haemorrhage
   b. Care must be taken with mynahs, toucans and toucanettes, because of iron storage disease.
8. Normal photoperiod (or subdued lighting if needed).
9. Oxygen (for dyspnoea, hypoxia, or severe pneumonia and aerosacculitis).
10. Maintenance of body weight
    a. Bird should be weighed daily if possible
    b. A variety of favourite foods should be offered; the bird's diet should not be changed when it is ill.
11. Gavage when necessary
    a. In cases of malnourishment, anorexia, cachexia and dehydration
    b. A high carbohydrate formula is initially recommended

c. High protein/high caloric formulae may be used to increase body weight during recovery.

Appendix 6.2: Calculation of enteral feeding requirements for birds (after Carpenter 2005)

This appendix will aid the practitioner in calculating caloric requirements for birds (see Appendix 6.4 regarding calculation of basal metabolic rate and maintenance requirements; Appendix 6.5 regarding calculation of the fluid requirement; Appendices 6.3 and 6.6 regarding the maximum suggested volumes of fluids and frequency of gavage feeding).

Caloric values for the three food types are:

Protein	4.29 kcal/g
Carbohydrate	4.09 kcal/g
Fat	9.29 kcal/g

Animals are unable to fully use all the calories in these nutrients, but efficiency is estimated at between 80 and 90%, depending on the type of nutrient. Commercially available enteral solutions are estimated to have a high digestibility of 95%. Some commercially available enteral products are listed below. Each product has varying levels of fat, carbohydrate, protein and water. Other food sources can be used, as long as nutrient levels and digestibility can be determined. The following is an example of a calculation of nutrient requirements based on BMR.

Example

A 250 g lilac-crowned Amazon is debilitated and not eating because of a bacterial infection.

$$\text{BMR (kcal/day)} = k\text{W}^{0.75}$$

$$\text{MER (kcal/day)} = (1.5 \times \text{BMR})$$

where k = kcal/kg/day constant (non-passerines = 78; passerines = 129; placental mammals = 70; marsupials = 49; reptiles at 37°C = 10).

First calculate MER:

$$\text{MER (kcal/day)} = (1.5)(78 \text{ kcal/kg/day})(0.250 \text{ kg})^{0.75}$$
$$= 41.4 \text{ kcal/day}$$

An adjustment for sepsis is made by multiplying by 1.5 (see BMR, Appendix 6.4):

$$\text{Sepsis} = 1.5 \times \text{MER} = (1.5)(41.4 \text{ kcal/day})$$
$$= 62.1 \text{ kcal/day}$$

Isocal® HCN (2 kcal/mL) is selected as the nutrient source:

$$\text{Volume of Isocal®} = (62.1 \text{ kcal/day})/(2 \text{ kcal/mL})$$
$$= 31 \text{ mL/day}$$

The average Amazon parrot can be gavaged 2.5% of its body weight, so:

$$\text{Volume that can be gavaged} = (0.025)(250 \text{ g})$$
$$= 6.25 \text{ mL}$$

Therefore, 31 mL/day of Isocal® HCN can be administered via gavage feeding of 6.25 mL every 5 hours.

However, this volume may need to be reduced initially depending on the bird's degree of debilitation.

(Refer to Appendix 6.3 for suggested volumes and frequencies of gavage feeding anorectic birds.)

Nutrient values for selected nutritional products (Kollias 1993)

Product	Protein (g)[a]	Fat (g)[a]	Carbohydrate (g)[a]	Water (mL/L)	kcal/mL
Isocal® (Mead Johnson)	3.4	4.4	13.3	840	1.0
Traumacal® (Mead Johnson)	5.5	4.5	9.5	520	1.5
Pulmocare® (Ross)	4.2	6.1	7.0	520	1.5
Isocal® HCN (Mead Johnson)	3.8	5.1	10.0	355	2.0
Nutrilon soya® (Nutricia)[b]	10.2	20.3	37.8	667	3.7
Emeraid-II® (Lafeber)[c]	10.8	2.25	28.1	450	1.53

[a]Nutrients per 100 kcal energy.
[b]72 g + 67 mL H_2O = 100 mL (1 spoon (4.3 g) + 4 mL H_2O = 6 mL ~22 kcal) = 5.1 kcal/g.
[c]45 g + 45 mL H_2O = 100 mL.

Product	Protein (%)	Fat (%)	Fibre (%)	Moisture (%)	kcal/mL
a/d Hill's Prescription Diet	8.5	6.6	0.5	78	1.3
CliniCare Canine/ Feline Liquid Diet (Abbott)	8.2	5.1	–	81	0.92
Emeraid Critical Care (Lafeber's)	20	9.2	0.5	9	–
Exact Baby Bird Hand Feeding Formula (Kaytee)	22	9	5	10	3.89
Exact Macaw Hand Feeding Formula (Kaytee)	19	13	5	–	4.09
Maximum-Calorie Nutritional Stress/Weight Gain Formula	14	12	11	66	2.1

Appendix 6.3: Suggested initial to maximum volumes and frequency of gavage feeding[a] in anorectic birds (after Carpenter 2005)

Species	Volume (mL)[b]	Frequency
Finch	0.1–0.5	q4h
Budgerigar	0.5–3.0	q6h
Lovebird	1–3	q6h
Cockatiel	1–8	q6h
Small conure	3–12	q6h
Large conure	7–24	q6h–q8h
Amazon parrot	5–35	q8h
African grey parrot	5–40	q8h
Cockatoo	10–40	q8h–q12h
Macaw	20–60	q8h–q12h

[a]Adjust volume and frequency as crop accommodates larger volumes.
[b]Generally 3–5% of body weight.

Appendix 6.4: Determining the basal metabolic rate of animals (after Carpenter 2005)

The following information is provided so the drugs can be allometrically scaled for different species, and to assist in calculating metabolic needs for nutritional requirements and fluid therapy.

BMR (basal metabolic rate)

BMR differs between species.

The general equation to calculate BMR is (Sedgewick et al 1990):

$$BMR = kW^{0.75}$$

where BMR = kcal/kg/day, k = kcal/kg constant (non-passerines = 78; passerines = 129; placental mammals = 70; marsupials = 49; reptiles at 37°C = 10) and W = weight in kg.

Other equations have been determined for passerine and non-passerine birds in relation to the daylight cycle. These cycles are termed 'active phase' and 'rest phase'. However, results are similar to the above formula.

Phase	Passerine	Non-passerine
Active phase	BMR = (140.7)W$^{0.704}$	BMR = (91)W$^{0.729}$
Rest phase	BMR = (113.8)W$^{0.726}$	BMR = (72)W$^{0.734}$

Maintenance energy requirement (MER)

The maintenance energy requirement (MER) = (kcal/day) = (1.5 × BMR). In birds, the MER can then be adjusted for health status as follows (Quesenberry & Hillyer 1994):

Physical inactivity	0.7–0.9 × MER
Starvation	0.5–0.7 × MER
Hypometabolism	0.5–0.9 × MER
Elective surgery	1.0–1.2 × MER
Mild trauma	1.0–1.2 × MER
Severe trauma	1.1–2.0 × MER
Growth	1.5–3.0 × MER
Sepsis	1.2–1.5 × MER
Burns	1.2–2.0 × MER
Head injuries	1.0–2.0 × MER

Appendix 6.5: Fluid therapy recommendations for birds (after Carpenter 2005)

1. Ideally, when evaluating a patient for fluid therapy, the following factors should be considered:
   - hydration status
   - electrolyte balance
   - acid–base status
   - haematological and biochemical values
   - caloric balance.
2. Warm fluids to 38–39°C to help prevent or correct hypothermia.
3. Use caution when giving dextrose parenterally; 5% dextrose is a good choice for simple dehydration. However, it can exacerbate problems significantly if used concurrently with significant electrolyte loss.
4. When given orally, dextrose is rapidly absorbed from the intestinal tract without creating an influx of fluid into the intestinal lumen and secondary dehydration.
5. Potassium chloride can be diluted in fluids to correct for potassium depletion based on electrolyte analysis (0.1–0.3 mEq/kg).
6. Hetastarch at 10–15 mL/kg i.v. q8h for up to four treatments or dextrans may be effective for hypoproteinaemia. Synthetic colloids should be used with caution in patients with congestive heart failure of renal failure.

Total parenteral nutrition may also be considered.

Maintenance and deficit replacement

Determine fluid deficit:

Fluid deficit (mL) = body weight (g) × per cent dehydration

Determine daily maintenance:

Daily maintenance = 50 mL (range: 40–60 mL/kg/day) in many avian species (the smallest passerines drink 250–300 mL/kg daily).

If possible, replace 50% of the deficit in the first 12–24 h and the remainder over the next 24–48 h; some clinicians recommend replacing 20–25% of the deficit in the first 4–6 h and the remaining volume during the next 24–72 h. If the volume has been acutely lost, the rate of administration is given over 6 hours or divided into two administrations over 6 hours.

Example

A 250 g lilac-crowned Amazon is 10% dehydrated.

Weight	250 g
10% dehydration	25 mL
Maintenance at 5% body weight/day	12.5 mL

$$1\text{st day fluid requirements} = (\text{maintenance} + 0.5 \text{ of deficit})$$
$$= (12.5 + 12.5)$$
$$= 25 \text{ mL/day}.$$

$$2\text{nd day fluid requirements} = (\text{maintenance} + 0.25 \text{ of deficit})$$
$$= (12.5 + 6.25)$$
$$= 18.75 \text{ mL/day}.$$

$$3\text{rd day fluid requirements} = (\text{maintenance} + 0.25 \text{ of deficit})$$
$$= (12.5 + 6.25)$$
$$= 18.75 \text{ mL/day}.$$

Total amount of fluid administered after 3 days is 62.5 mL.

Appendix 6.6: Routes of administration and maximum suggested volumes of fluid that can be administered to psittacines (after Carpenter 2005)

Route	Maximum suggested volume of fluid[a]
Gavage	Administer up to 5 mL/100 g bird[b]
	Initial volume should be much less in critically ill and anorectic patients (begin with half to one-third of estimated crop volume)
	Crop volume may be up to 10% body weight in neonatal birds
i.v. or i.o. bolus	Administer up to 10 mL/kg (ideally over a 5–10 min period)
Subcutaneous	50 mL/kg[c,d]

[a]Combinations of routes (p.o., s.c., i.o./i.v.) are recommended if large fluid volumes are administered.
[b]Crop volume may be estimated at 5% BW.
[c]Volumes of 10–15 mL/kg may be comfortably given per subcutaneous injection site, although up to 25 mL/kg per site may be given. Overdistension of the area may compromise blood supply to the area and reduce absorption.
[d]Hyaluronidase (150 IU/L fluids) may be used in most species to increase the absorption rate of fluids.

Appendix 6.7: Nebulization agents used in birds (after Carpenter 2005)

Agent	Dosage	Species/Comments
N-acetyl-L-cysteine 10–20%	–	See amikacin, aminophylline, gentamicin, for combinations
	22 mg/mL sterile water until dissipated	Most species/Mucolytic agent; tracheal irritation and reflex bronchoconstriction reported in mammals; use is preceded by bronchodilators in mammals
Amikacin sulphate	5–6 mg/mL sterile water or saline × 15 min q8–12h	Most species/Discontinue if polyuria develops
	6 mg/mL sterile water and 1 mL acetylcysteine (20%) until dissipated q8h	Most species
Aminophylline	3 mg/mL sterile water or saline × 15 min	Most species/Bronchodilator; allergic pulmonary disease; can mix with dexamethasone, aminoglycosides and acetylcysteine
Amphotericin B	0.1–1.0 mg/mL sterile water × 15 min	Raptor/Antifungal
	0.25 mg/mL saline × 15 min q12h	Hummingbirds/Low efficacy; may cause weight loss
	1 mg/mL sterile water or saline × 15 min q12h	Most species/Antifungal
	7–10 mg/mL saline	Most species
Carbenicillin	20 mg/mL saline × 15 min q12h	Psittacines/Pseudomonas pneumonia; use in combination with parenteral aminoglycosides
Cefotaxime	10 mg/mL saline × 10–30 min q6–12h	Most species

Ceftriaxone	40 mg/mL sterile water	Poultry/PD[a]
	40 mg/mL sterile water and DMSO	Poultry/PD; 1 ceftriaxone in 10 mL sterile water. Plus 15 mL DMSO
	200 mg/mL sterile water and DMSO	Poultry/PD; 4 g ceftriaxone in 10 mL sterile water; plus 10 mL DMSO
Chloramphenicol	13 mg/mL saline	Most species/Human health concerns
Clotrimazol (1%)	10 mg/mL propylene glycol or polyethylene glycol × 30–45 min q24h × 3 days, off 2 days, repeat prn for up to 4 months	Treatment of aspergillosis for stable patients without respiratory distress; can be toxic to psittacines at this dose
	10 mg/mL polyethylene glycol (PEG 300) × 30–60 min	Raptors, psittacines/Used in combination with systemic amphotericin B, flucytosine and itraconazole
Doxycycline hyclate	13 mg/mL saline	Psittacines
Enilconazole	10 mg/mL sterile water	Most species/Antifungal
	11 mg/mL saline	Falcons/Aspergillosis
	0.2 mg/5 mL saline q12h × 21 days	Most species including raptors, psittacines
Enrofloxacin	10 mg/mL saline	Most species
Erythromycin	5–20 mg/mL saline × 15 min q8h	Most species
Gentamicin	5 mg/mL saline × 15 min q8h	Most species
	3–6 mg/mL saline or sterile water and 1–2 mL acetylcysteine (20%) × 20 min q8h	Most species, including cranes
Lincospectin	250 mg/mL water	Most species
	250 mg aerosolized drug/m³ chamber × 15–30 min	Chickens/PD; antibiotic; therapeutic concentrations in blood, lungs, and trachea for up to 24 hours
Miconazole	Nebulize 15 min q8h × 10 days	Raptors/aspergillosis
Oxytetracycline	2 mg/mL × 60 min q4–6h	Parakeets/PD
Piperacillin	10 mg/mL saline × 10–30 min q6–12h	Most species
Polymyxin B sulphate	66 000 IU/mL saline	Psittacines/Poorly absorbed from respiratory epithelium
Sodium chloride	–	Viscosity of respiratory secretions may be decreased by hydration
Spectinomycin	13 mg/mL saline	Most species
Sterile water	–	Viscosity of respiratory secretions may be decreased by hydration
Sulfadimethoxine	13 mg/mL saline	
Tylosin	100 mg/mL saline	10–60 min b.i.d.

[a]Pharmacological data.

Appendix 6.8: Interpretation of changes in the avian packed cell volume (PCV) (after Hernandez & Aguilar 1994)

PCV changes			Interpretation
PCV	TP	WBC	
Decreased	Normal	Normal	Anaemia
	Decreased	Normal	Recent blood loss
	Increased	Increased	Anaemia of chronic disease
Normal	Normal	Normal	Healthy
	Normal	Increased	Acute infection
	Increased	Increased	Dehydration; masked anaemia; acute infection
Increased	Normal	Normal	Polycythaemia
	Increased	Normal	Dehydration and leucopenia
	Increased	Increased	Dehydration

Appendix 6.9: Recommended steps for treating birds with shock (after Hernandez & Aguilar 1994 and Lichtenberger 2005, 2006)

1. Presumptively diagnose shock. Place in a warm incubator (30–32°C) with oxygen supplementation for 2–4 hours. Active haemorrhages must be stopped immediately. Most birds benefit from the administration of warmed crystalloids at 3 mL/100 g body weight i.v., i.o. or s.c. to restore perfusion Birds should be offered water and food during this time.

When the bird appears stable (alert, responsive) and can be safely anaesthetized with mask isoflurane or sevoflurane, the diagnostics and treatment for hypovolaemia and dehydration can be performed. Blood pressure monitoring using Doppler and an ECG should be used during these procedures (Lichtenberger 2006).

2. Take baseline blood sample for packed cell volume, total protein and bicarbonate. Record weight. Additional glucose determination may be performed. Other laboratory tests can be postponed.
3. Place an intraosseous or intravenous catheter, when possible.
4. Calculate degree of interstitial dehydration and fluid requirements (Appendix 6.5).
5. Initiate lactated Ringer's solution at half of the fluid deficit over the first 12 hours and give as bolus.
6. Give vitamin B complex (10 mg/kg thiamine), steroids (2–6 mg/kg i.m, i.v. q12–24h) or non-steroidal anti-inflammatory drugs (ketoprofen, flunixin and carprofen 2 mg/kg) and iron dextran (20 mL/kg 6% i.m.). Provide parenteral nutritional support if necessary.
7. Initiate antibiotics if fractures, open wounds or soft tissue injuries are found, or if (bacterial) infectious disease is suspected (cytology faecal smear).
8. Monitor PCV, TP, bicarbonate, and urine output.
9. Obtain a complete history and initiate diagnostic testing.
10. Begin maintenance fluids and start force-feeding (Appendices 6.2, 6.3, 6.5, 6.6).
11. Monitor weight until bird is able to self-feed.

Appendix 6.10: Agents used in emergencies in birds (after Carpenter 2005)

Agent	Dosage	Species/comments
Adrenaline (1:1000)	0.5–1.0 mL/kg i.m., i.v., i.o., i.t.	CPR; bradycardia
Atropine	0.2 mg/kg i.m., i.v., i.o.	Bradycardia
	0.5 mg/kg i.m., i.v., i.o. i.t.	CPR
Aminophylline	4 mg/kg p.o. q6–12h	Can give orally after initial response
	10 mg/kg i.v. q3h	Use for pulmonary oedema
Calcium gluconate	50–100 mg/kg i.v. slowly, i.m. diluted	Hypocalcaemia; dilute 50 mg/mL; hyperkalaemia; facilitates potassium movement across cell membranes

Dexamethasone sodium phosphate	2-6 mg/kg i.m, i.v. q12–24h	Head trauma (until signs abate); shock (one dose); hyperthermia (until stable)
Dextrose (50%)	50–100 mg/kg i.v. (slow bolus to effect)	Hypoglycaemia; can dilute with fluids
Dextran 70	10-20 mg/kg	Most species / hypovolaemic shock
Diazepam	0.5–1.5 mg/kg i.m., i.v. prn	Seizures
Doxapram	5–10 mg/kg i.m., i.v. once	Raptors/respiratory depression or arrest
	20 mg/kg i.m., i.v., i.o.	CPR; respiratory depression
Fluids	10-25 mL/kg i.v., i.o.	Bolus over 5–7 min
	50–90 mL/kg fluids i.v., i.o., s.c.[a]	See 'Fluid therapy'
Haemoglobin glutamer-200	–	Haemoglobin replacement product
	3–10 mL/kg i.v. slowly	Most species
	5 mL/kg i.v.	Mallard ducks
	10 mL/kg i.v.	Raptors
	15 mL/mL i.v.	Chickens/PD[b]; haemoglobin levels fell near zero by 50 min after administration
Hetastarch (HES)	10–15 mL/kg i.v. (slow) q8h × 1–4 treatments	Most species, including raptors/hypoproteinemia; hypovolaemia
Mannitol	0.2–2.0 mg/kg i.v. (slow) q24h	Raptors/cerebral oedema; anuric renal failure
Oxyglobin	–	See haemoglobin glutamer-200
Prednisolone Na succinate	10–20 mg/kg i.v., i.m., q15min prn	Head trauma, CPR
	15–30 mg/kg i.v.	Raptors
Sodium bicarbonate	1 mEq/kg q15–30 min to maximum of 4 mEq/kg total dose	Metabolic acidosis
	5 mEq/kg i.v., i.o. once	CPR

[a]*Because of the presence of peripheral vasoconstriction, subcutaneous administration is not adequate for patients in shock.*
[b]*Pharmacological data.*

Appendix 6.11: Recommended treatment protocol for the avian head trauma patient (after Hernandez & Aguilar 1994)

1. Diagnose head trauma; check pedal reflex and cloacal tone.
2. Place an intraosseous or intravenous catheter.
3. Start oxygenation via oxygen cage (40% oxygen) or face mask at 50 mL/kg/min. Check ventilation rate.
4. Check PCV, TP and bicarbonate.
5. Start emergency fluid therapy. Hypertonic saline (7.5%) 4–5 mL/kg and iron dextran (6%) at 20 mL/kg may be used if no dehydration exists. If critically dehydrated, initiate lactated Ringer's solution administered at 30 mL/kg as bolus.
6. Give dexamethasone at 2–6 mg/kg i.m, i.v. initially, followed by gradually tapering doses q12–24h (Appendix 6.10).
7. Give vitamin B complex (10 mL/kg thiamine), antibiotics and nutritional support if required.
8. If the situation deteriorates, use mannitol (25%) at a dose of 0.25–2.0 mg/kg and furosemide at a dose of 2–5 mg/kg.

Psittacine birds

7

Nigel H. Harcourt-Brown

Introduction

The order Psittaciformes contains parrots, macaws, cockatoos and lories. This order is extremely well reviewed and illustrated by Rowley (1997) and Collar (1997). Rowley suggests 6 genera of Cacatuidae (cockatoos) with 21 species, Collar describes 78 genera of Psittacidae (parrots, macaws, lories) with 332 species; Sibley & Ahlquist (1990) suggest 358 species in 80 genera; other authorities suggest minor variations to these numbers.

Parrots may be defined by their distinctive, well-developed, hooked rostrum (upper beak) with a prominent cere (the featherless area dorsal to the upper beak); the rostrum is hinged to the skull by a synovial joint in large birds (e.g. macaws) and an elastic zone in small birds (e.g. budgerigars); this feature is unique amongst birds, and there are some unique muscles associated with the jaw; the prehensile feet are zygodactyl, having digits I and IV directed caudally and digits II and III cranially; there is a well-developed crop, proventriculus and gizzard, but there are no caeca; the gall bladder is usually absent; the preen (uropygial) gland is tufted or in some genera absent, e.g. *Amazona* and *Pionus*; the furcula (united clavicles) is weak or absent; the syrinx has three pairs of intrinsic muscles, is tracheal and well developed, having a syringeal valve at its entrance.

Parrots nest in holes, lay white eggs and have nidicolous (stay in the nest for a long time) young, which are ptilopaedic (covered with down when hatched). Adult parrots have patches of powder down; these are areas of down feathers which fragment at their ends and cover the bird and its plumage with a soft, usually white, powder (Fig. 7.1). The other more esoteric anatomical characteristics that define the order are covered more comprehensively by Sibley & Ahlquist (1990), who also conclude that parrots have no close living relatives.

Psittaciformes are commonly referred to using the all-embracing term 'psittacine birds' (or psittacids) and are very popular as either caged pet birds or aviary birds. Psittacine birds range in size from the hyacinth macaw (*Anodorhynchus hyacinthinus*), which measures 100 cm and weighs 1500 g (although the kakapo (*Strigops habroptilis*), a flightless parrot, is even heavier at 2060 g), down to pygmy parrots, e.g. the buff-faced pygmy parrot (*Micropsitta pusio*) at slightly less than 10 cm and weighing 11 g. The numbers within a species vary

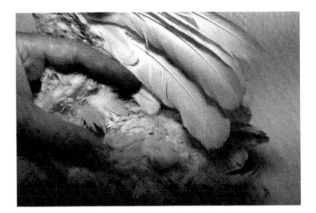

Fig 7.1 Powder down feathers on the flank of a cockatoo.

from 37 individuals for the Spix's macaw (*Cyanopsitta spixii*), to being very numerous and considered a pest species, e.g. some cockatoos (*Cacatua* spp.) in Australia. The family is mainly vegetarian; some of its members are specialized feeders, such as the lories and lorikeets that eat only pollen and nectar.

The attraction of parrots as companion animals is in their intelligence and potential for taming and training, their ability to mimic vocally, and their rounded faces which most people find an attractive feature in any animal. Not every species of parrot can be kept in captivity, either because of rarity, or more usually dietary requirements, e.g. pygmy parrots (*Micropsitta* spp.) which eat mostly lichens and fungus. A few psittaciform families provide the general public with many of their pet birds. The following concentrates on species that may usually be encountered in captivity.

Macaws

Macaws range in size from the hyacinth(ine) macaw (*A. hyacinthinus*) at 100 cm to the noble macaw (*Ara nobilis*) at 30 cm. They are characterized by large beaks and long tails. They are South American in origin and eat nuts, seed, berries and fruit. The immensely strong beaks of the larger birds, such as the green-winged macaw (*Ara chloroptera*), are able easily to break open Brazil nuts. Macaws are very strong and potentially destructive; they require large cages or stands, but are best kept in aviaries.

Parrots

Parrots are short-tailed, large-beaked, stocky birds. There are several African parrots, the commonest in captivity being the grey parrot *(Psittacus erithacus* – and known commonly as the 'African grey parrot'). It is the familiar black-beaked, red-tailed, grey parrot. There is a subspecies, the Timneh grey parrot (*P. e. timneh*), which is smaller and darker, with a horn-coloured beak and a dark maroon tail. Both come from West and Central Africa. They live in woodland and eat seeds, nuts and berries; they are particularly fond of palm oil nuts and will raid maize crops, causing much damage.

Another commonly encountered family of parrots is known as Amazons (*Amazona* spp.). Out of nearly 30 species in the family, three are commonly kept: the blue-fronted Amazon (*A. aestiva*), which is mainly green with a blue and yellow face, a red carpal edge – easily visible when the bird is perching normally – and a red wing spectacle on five or more secondary feathers; the orange-winged Amazon (*A. amazonica*), which is also green with blue and yellow feathers around its face but an orange wing spectacle and no red on its carpal edge; and finally the yellow-crowned Amazon (*A. ochrocephala*), which is green with a green face and a yellow patch somewhere on its head or neck, with a red wing spectacle and a red carpal edge. These birds come from Central and South America, where they live in forests and eat fruit, berries, nuts, blossoms and leaf buds.

There are many smaller parrots that are popular as aviary subjects. These include *Pionus* spp. and *Brotogeris* spp. from South America, and lovebirds (*Agapornis* spp.), Senegal parrots (*Poicephalus senegalus*), Meyer's (brown) parrots (*P. meyeri*) and brown-headed parrots (*P. cryptoxanthus*) from Africa. Lovebirds are very popular, several species being completely captive bred with a huge variety of colour mutations.

Cockatoos

Cockatoos (Cacatuidae) are medium- to large-sized birds, usually white, and nearly all have an erectile crest that can be raised when alarmed or excited. The popular pet cockatoos are the sulphur-crested cockatoo (*Cacatua galerita*), lesser sulphur-crested cockatoo (*C. sulphurea*) and the Moluccan cockatoo (*C. moluccensis*), which is a pale pink colour. There are other species of various colours, including black, white, pink or even nearly red. Cockatiels (*Nymphicus hollandicus*) are also cockatoos. All are very gregarious birds and are Australo-Pacific in origin.

Cockatoos are very noisy, even by parrot standards! They eat a varied diet of fruit, berries, nuts, flowers, leaf buds, roots and also insects and their larvae which they may dig out of the ground or from trees. Black cockatoos are seldom kept as pets in Europe.

Parakeets

Parakeet is a term restricted to small parrots with long graduated tails. There are many genera and they are mostly Pacific and Asian in distribution. Australia will not currently export any birds, but its parakeets have been popular in captivity for generations, due to their size and muted voices (compared with other Psittaciformes!); they are also less destructive in the aviary and are prettily coloured. In Europe most parakeets are cheap to buy. They are not usually kept as pets, except for the budgerigar (*Melopsittacus undulatus*). Other Australian species including grass parakeets (*Neophema* spp.) and rosellas (*Platycercus* spp.) are frequently kept as aviary birds. New Zealand has provided the aviculturalist with the kakariki (*Cyanoramphus novaezelandiae*). Asian parakeets are all very similar and are from the genus *Psittacula*; they include the rose-ringed or ring-necked parakeet (*P. krameri*), the Alexandrine parakeet (*P. eupatria*), the plum-headed parakeet (*P. cyanocephala*), the blossom-headed parakeet (*P. roseata*), etc.

Conures

Conures are South American parakeets, and range from the small and quiet *Pyrrhura* spp. to the medium-sized, noisy and destructive *Aratinga* spp. Many *Aratinga* conures are similar in form and habits to the small macaws, to which they are closely related.

Lories and lorikeets

Lories tend to be larger (approx. 30 cm, and lorikeets smaller (approx. 15 cm), but all are from the same family: Loriidae. They are typified by their brilliant colours and Australo-Pacific origin, and they have a modified brush-tipped tongue which they use to collect and compress pollen into a pellet so they can swallow it. Pollen is their main protein source, but they also eat nectar when available plus occasional insects and fruit. They are very popular amongst aviculturalists and their dietary requirements can now easily be met by supplying proprietary 'nectar' mixtures.

Pet parrots

The earliest known captive pet birds were from the parrot family. There are records of Alexander the Great bringing ring-necked parakeets with him from India to Europe. Budgerigars (*Melopsittacus undulatus*) were first seen alive in Europe in 1840, and over the next 40 years many tens of thousands were imported from Australia. From the naturally found, predominantly green-coloured, yellow-faced bird a huge variety of colours has been produced, although a red budgerigar has yet to be bred! Adult male birds of most colours (but not lutinos, which have yellow feathers and pink eyes, or albinos, with white feathers and pink eyes) have a blue cere; adult females have a brown cere.

The best time to obtain a pet budgie is when it first leaves the nest, at around 6 weeks old. At that time the bird has feathers edged with black or brown, that give a barred appearance to the frontal region (forehead) above the cere (Fig. 7.2). These barred feathers are moulted at the first partial moult about 2 months later, leaving the forehead a plain colour. Male 'barheads' have a pinkish cere with a blue tinge; however, this is not a reliable guide to gender. Also, females bite far harder than males, even when still babies in the nest! It is unfortunate that budgerigar breeders have developed what is known as a buff plumage for their show birds. The buff feathers are very large and appear to have deformed barbules as they do not unite to form a normal contour feather shape. Buff feathers have a hairy appearance. Breeders' budgerigars also tend to live only about 4 years. 'Mongrel' pet budgerigars seem to live far longer, and 8 years is average, although the author has seen a budgerigar, with a dated closed- ring, of 21 years.

The cockatiel was named by a bird-fancier, Mr Jamrach, being an English adaptation of a Dutch/Portuguese word for little cockatoo (Newton 1896). By the end of the nineteenth century the cockatiel was already a popular pet caged bird and has remained so ever since. The general grey colour, with orange cheeks and a distinct head crest, is present in males and females. However, the male has a yellow face and crest while the female is grey; the male's orange cheeks are brighter; the tail and wing feathers are solid grey in the male, whereas they are mottled grey and white (especially underneath), in females. Cockatiels of this coloration are termed 'normals', but there are many colour

variants – lutino (yellow), white, fallow (with a brownish tint), etc. Immature birds resemble females.

The cockatiel is a peaceful, active, cheerful bird that mimics well; it deserves its popularity and would be the author's first choice for anyone wanting a pet bird. It is also relatively cheap to purchase, house and keep.

Grey parrots are very popular pets, and are hardy, medium-sized (450–500 g) birds. The reason for this parrot's popularity is its talking and mimicking ability; *erithacus* means mimetic. Unlike the popular 'mynah birds' (which are not in fact mynahs but grackles, *Gracula religiosa*), these parrots will learn new words and noises throughout their lives. They are usually friendly throughout their entire lives but hand-reared birds do often feather-pluck, especially when sexually mature. A large cage or small indoor aviary is required to keep them happy. Like all parrots, when kept on their own they need to fly around and have a lot of human contact, but are destructive and should not be left unattended. They tend not to like water, either as a bath or when sprayed. However, it is still necessary to spray them or let them bathe at least weekly to keep their plumage in good condition. Grey parrots also tend very quickly to become 'hooked' on a seed-only diet.

The Timneh grey parrot is smaller and more subdued in colour. It is, however, as satisfactory as a pet as its close relative. Its treatment should be the same.

To some extent the age of many species of parrot can be deduced from the iris. This structure is important to the bird as its movement is effected by skeletal muscle and is therefore under conscious control. The bird can use the iris to signal to other birds (owners and vets) by expanding the iris to cause a flash of colour. During the first year of life of parrots such as greys, Amazons and macaws the colour of their iris slowly changes. Newly weaned birds have blue/brown irises, which change to yellow in greys and large macaws, or orange in Amazons. (See also Chapter 3, Figs 3.7–3.10.) Some species of cockatoo have a brown iris if female and a black iris if male, while in the juvenile it is a neutral hazel colour. As parrots become sexually mature the iris brightens, while in later life the iris becomes thinner and less pigmented, and in old age there are often degenerative eye changes such as cataracts (Clubb & Karpinski 1993). Old age is considered to be 45 to 50 years in macaws, and 35 years in greys and Amazons. Reports of a life expectancy of 100 years are rarely true.

The orange-winged Amazon is imported in large numbers and not usually bred in captivity, unlike the blue-fronted Amazon; a number of ingenuous owners have been sold the cheaper orange-winged Amazon as a more expensive blue-fronted Amazon. Amazon parrots like fruit and vegetables as well as a seed diet.

Blue-fronted, orange-winged and yellow-fronted Amazons are all popular as pets, although various other species are also kept. In the main they are not as talented

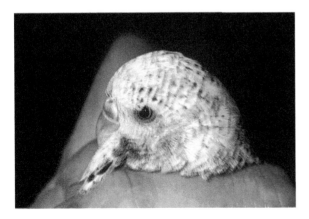

Fig 7.2 A young budgerigar. The barred feathers extend to the cere, which is turning blue showing that the bird is male. The barred feathers are lost from the forehead at about 12 weeks old; this bird is known as an opaline and its head will have no barred feathers. Most adult budgerigars, known as 'normal' have bars from the middle of their head.

as the grey parrots at talking, but are considerably more attractive. Amazons (and *Pionus* spp.) all enjoy being sprayed and will hang from the bars of their cages and fan their tails and wings to get as saturated as possible when being sprayed. They enjoy being outside in the rain and in the UK acclimatized parrots living in aviaries can be seen bathing happily in sleet or even snow! They much prefer to be sprayed in the morning, and seem unhappy about going to roost wet. Amazons are much less likely than greys to feather-pluck as they get older, but often change temperament in the breeding season and single pet birds can become quite dangerous, attacking and biting humans that they think are rivals. This behaviour is not apparent outside the breeding season. Also in Amazons, behaviour initiated in stressful situations is manifested by apparent irritation to the skin and feathers.

Amongst the macaws, it is only the larger birds that are popular as pets, because of their size and colour; they are very striking. The green-winged macaw is very gentle and pleasant and probably makes the best pet; the blue and yellow (gold) macaw is also popular. The scarlet macaw looks very attractive and is a reasonable pet bird when young, but it becomes very spiteful and even aggressive when adult, especially when sexually active. All the macaws have loud voices and will use them, especially at first light. The macaws may have their wings clipped to prevent them flying, but they still need a very large cage or indoor aviary to exercise in. A large freestanding cage can be made quite economically by cutting 5 cm security mesh into panels and wiring them together. These birds tolerate being sprayed and some even like it. They can all mimic and talk to a reasonable degree.

Cockatoos are kept by some people, but they are the most prone to psychological disturbances and can become very unhappy on their own, even when attention is lavished on them by their owners. They are very noisy, more so even than the macaws. They can become very depressing pets and are the most likely parrot to self-mutilate, drawing blood when they chew through their skin into muscle. I have yet to see a pet Moluccan cockatoo that does not have some chewed feathers. Owing to the noise and psychotic behaviour, cockatoos frequently get passed on through a serious of owners, thus exacerbating their behavioural problems.

Housing

Most psittacine birds are better kept as individual pairs in aviaries made of stout wire mesh. There should be a space between pairs of parrots, or they will attack the toes of neighbouring birds and amputate them. A convenient method of aviary construction is to suspend the cage above the ground. The cage should be a reasonable size for the species being housed, and should allow the birds room to fly. Birds are happier being able to get

higher than their keeper and so a minimum height for the roof should be two metres, even if the cage is only one metre high and wide, which is suitable for lories, small parrots, conures, etc. Suspended aviaries minimize contact with old food, faeces, etc., and make cleaning very easy. Ideally the suspended aviaries should be enclosed in a large netted area to prevent escape if a bird gets out of the cage whilst being caught or fed, and also to minimize contact with wild birds and their diseases or parasites.

Aviaries should be made from wire ranging from a 19-gauge 2.5×0.5 cm mesh for small birds, to 16-gauge 5 cm mesh for macaws, etc. The wire should be galvanized. In some parts of the world (not the UK), this galvanization process seems to cause zinc toxicity to the birds when they are first housed, and it is recommended that new mesh is washed in dilute acid first.

Environmental enrichment

Corvidae (crows) and Psittaciformes (parrots) have, relatively, the largest avian cerebral hemispheres; Galliformes (fowl-like birds) and Columbiformes (doves and pigeons) the smallest. Psittacine birds (and crows) appear to be very 'intelligent'. However, the interaction between the ability to learn and the various related behavioural reflexes makes this statement contentious. Mentally normal parrots prefer to be kept with others of the same species and they must also have the facility to perform functions other than sitting, eating and sleeping. Cages must be large enough for flight, birds should have different-sized perches of varying materials and there must be a suitable environment for foraging, playing and other social interactions. Perches made of smooth hardwood will cause pressure problems on the plantar aspect of the birds' feet, similar to bumblefoot in birds of prey. To avoid this, perches of different shapes and diameters (preferably branches covered with bark) are very useful. The birds will chew and destroy these branches and they must be replaced regularly. The author has tried many different woods in his aviaries (sycamore, elm, ash, hawthorn, elderberry, pine, pine treated by tannalization, etc.), and has yet to find any wood that is toxic to the parrots. However, it would be prudent not to use woods known to be poisonous to mammals such as rhododendron or yew. Loops of hessian rope suspended from the roof of the cage also make good perches, as there is some 'give' as the bird lands. The same may be accomplished by anchoring one end of a branch with a hinge or hook and eye and suspending the other end from a piece of wire; again this allows the perch to move more naturally.

Nutrition

Although parrots eat a wide range of foodstuffs they are primarily vegetarian. Birds that live in tropical or subtropical forests and woodland eat a wide range of

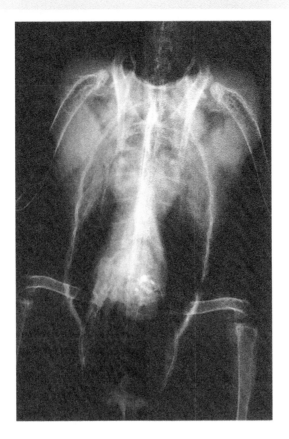

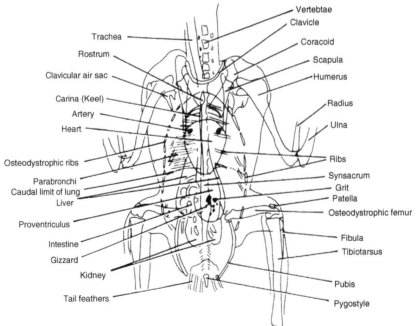

Fig 7.3A Ventrodorsal view of an adult grey parrot.

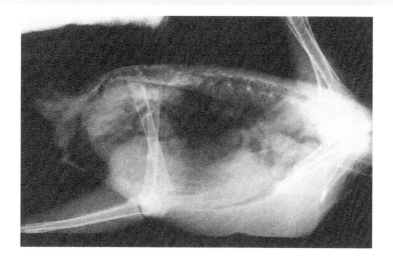

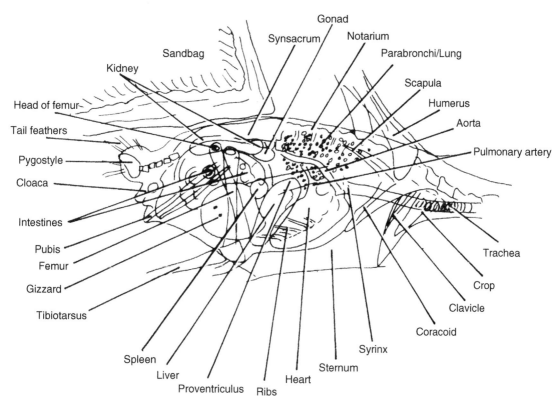

Fig 7.3B Lateral view of an adult grey parrot.

flowers, fruits and seeds; those living in drier conditions eat mainly seeds, especially xerophilic (adapted to dry conditions) birds such as cockatiels and budgerigars. There are some specialized feeders: lories and lorikeets (Loriidae) which eat pollen and nectar and have a specialized tongue with a border of brush-like projections to aid them; pygmy parrots (*Micropsitta* spp.) eat lichen and fungi as a staple part of their diet. Many parrots have been found with insects in their crops when examined by zoologists (Forshaw & Cooper 1973), and in a number of species insects and grubs form a significant part of their diet.

All animals require carbohydrate, protein and fat in their diet. Psittaciformes are no different and thought must be given to the food content of each part of the diet that is fed to a captive bird as well as its palatability.

Parrots require diets that contain about 20% protein, and vegetarian diets must be carefully balanced to avoid major deficiencies of important foodstuffs. Finally, and most importantly, parrots must NOT be allowed to feed selectively, or a well-balanced diet becomes a deficient diet. **Dietary deficiency in captive birds plays a huge part in determining the bird's general life-long health.**

Seeds

It must be borne in mind that many pet shops sell all-seed diets as 'parrot-food', 'parrot-mix' or 'cockatiel-food', and give this to owners asking for suitable food for their pets. Loose seed sold like this does not have a 'best before' date and could be several years old even before it arrives at the shop. Seeds such as sunflower, peanuts and pine nuts are low in calcium, vitamins A and D and protein; they are also very high in oil. Cereals and smaller seeds, such as millet, are similar but have less oil and more starch; they are similarly deficient. Seeds are variably deficient in iodine. In a survey of budgerigars (Blackmore 1963), 85% had dysplasia of the thyroid gland; this will still be the situation for budgerigars that are fed on loose seed from the pet shop.

When given the opportunity, many pet parrots (especially the greys) become habituated to eating only seed, especially sunflower seed, and appear to refuse to eat anything else; long term, this is a life-threatening situation.

Fruit and vegetables

Fruit and vegetables are useful in the diet but are often low in protein, calcium and vitamin D. They are high in fibre, contain vitamins A and C, and are low calorie compared with seeds. It is preferable to use non-sludging fruit and vegetables such as apples and carrots. Food pots must be kept clean, as a build-up of vegetable debris encourages the growth of *Aspergillus* spp. and various potentially pathogenic bacteria. This is especially common in warm, damp climates.

Pulses

The seeds of leguminous food plants are known as pulses. Peas, beans and maize (sweetcorn) are all very useful foods, as they contain good levels of protein (20–30%). However, be aware that they contain around 60% carbohydrate and are also low in calcium. Soya bean protein contains the most similar range of amino acids to those in animal protein. Soaking pulses and allowing them to germinate increases their digestibility, decreases the toxin content of some beans, and improves their taste. They should be prepared by soaking for 24 hours. Too warm a temperature allows fermentation; too cool prevents germination. The pulses should then be washed thoroughly in clean running water, which removes any noxious metabolic products and also any potentially fermentative bacteria. After initial soaking the pulses may be kept moist and cool in the fridge for several days, but they must be washed daily and before use. In warm climates it may be better to boil the pulses just prior to feeding rather than soak them; boiling reduces the risk of fermentation.

Minerals

Most seed-eating small parrots appreciate grit to aid their grinding gizzard, but there is discussion as to whether or not it is *essential* in larger species. Mineralized grit and oyster shell grit are used. Oyster shell grit does not last as long in the gizzard but is a good source of calcium. Care must be used not to over-use mineral grit, to avoid the risk of impaction, a quarter to half a teaspoonful once a week with the food is usually sufficient. Grit sold for pigeons is satisfactory for most medium and large parrots. Mineral blocks containing calcium or iodine are produced for small pet birds and can be useful, as is cuttlefish; again the bird has to eat this solid material and not all birds will.

Vitamin supplements

All parrots require a vitamin and mineral supplement with their food unless they are fed on an appropriate all-in-one commercial ration. There are a large number of supplements on the market. Water-soluble products seem not to contain the range of compounds found in powders. Mixing powder with seed works reasonably well but it is better to take the fruit and vegetable portion of the diet, chop it up and mix it with the seed. This gives a wet mixture, which is a very satisfactory vehicle in which to mix the powder. A specific avian vitamin and mineral supplement should be used, as this will contain a better balance of vitamins and minerals.

BEWARE: many owners will feed a vitamin and mineral supplement in too small a quantity, and often infrequently; occasionally owners will feed several different brands at once plus cod-liver oil and therefore give a completely unbalanced amount of vitamin D. In either case there can be disastrous consequences.

Commercial diets

All-in-one diets have become widely available and are theoretically a good idea. There is no doubt that an appropriate all-in-one pelleted diet is far better than a badly balanced diet; it also overcomes the problem of selective feeding. However, self-selection from a wide range of foodstuffs can be a good way of feeding a bird but small quantities of each food item and a sensible dietary balance must be struck if selective feeding and nutritional deficiency are to be avoided. Constraining the individual bird to eat one dietary mix long term is certainly boring for the bird and also may produce nutritional problems over the years. This is especially possible as so many parrot species have different and inadequately researched nutritional requirements. Very few, if any, diets have been fed unchanged to significant numbers of individual birds for even a decade. Manufacturers have relied on the fact that breeding birds show dietary deficiency much more quickly than pet, caged birds. As general advice to pet bird owners an all-in-one diet should take the place of a seed mix and a proportion of various types of fruit and vegetables should be included.

Pet grey parrots and cockatiels are the most frequently malnourished birds. Both of these will do well on pelleted diets, but there can be major problems changing many of these birds onto their new regimen. Amazons, pionus, macaws and cockatoos have a much greater liking for fruit and vegetables and appear less likely to become malnourished. However, selective feeding will cause problems even in these birds. Cage-confined Amazons and budgerigars particularly will over-eat and become obese.

Protocol for dietary change

Under veterinary or informed supervision the bird and its droppings should be observed for a few days to assess what is normal. The owner should be encouraged to regard parrot seed as sweets, cookies and crisps: treats that may be used as reward and positive reinforcement, but not a sensible staple diet. The bird should be weighed daily for a few days before the dietary change starts.

Once the new diet has been selected, this alone should be placed in the cage in the morning and the food intake monitored. If no food is eaten during the day, some of the previous (well-loved) diet in a *small* quantity may be mixed in for 15 minutes in the evening. Grey parrots can get enough calories for 24 hours from about a tablespoonful of sunflower seed, so if too much seed is provided they need not eat until the following night. Each morning give the new diet and provide less seed in the evening.

Alternatively the new diet can be mixed with the old diet and the ratio of the mixture altered over a period of time until the bird is provided with and eating 100% of the new diet and none of the old.

Throughout this time, the bird's weight should be monitored, daily if possible, and the droppings observed. A lack of faeces indicates that there is no food being eaten. Owners will always worry that their bird is likely to die of starvation; this is unlikely with the larger parrots but is a possibility with cockatiels, lovebirds and budgerigars. The author had one Amazon who did not eat for 8 days but whose weight dropped from (a too fat) 550 g to only (a still fat) 500 g over this period; on day 9 she ate the new diet well and continued to do so thereafter. However, this is not an ideal method of changing the diet and has potential dangers.

As the new diet is eaten, enzyme systems in the gut and liver will change to accommodate the new food intake. The faeces will also change and on a fruit and vegetable diet the faeces will enlarge and lighten in colour, there will also be more fluid voided. Overweight birds with fatty livers will adjust more slowly, and must be regarded as high-risk patients. In these cases fasting is a danger, and it is useful to feed these birds and birds with other subclinical illnesses with a hand-rearing formula twice daily using a crop tube. This provides the birds with a well-balanced diet and prevents 'starvation' whilst the birds acclimatize to their new diet. This is the preferred method for 'converting' the parrot that has refused to change its diet at home: invariably by the fifth day of crop-tube feeding the parrot starts to eat the all-in one diet. It requires the bird to be an inpatient.

Table 7.1 indicates average weights for various species. It can be seen from this table that although it is easy to produce a guide for an average weight it must not be relied upon as a weight for the individual. The weights in the table have mostly been taken from birds in the author's clinic that were anaesthetized after having endoscopic gender determination; they were not fat and were starved. In some cases there were too few birds to give an average weight. The weights for wild birds have been taken from Dunning (1993).

Breeding and determination of gender: 'sexing'

All parrots form a strong sexual bond. They mature sexually between 1 and 5 years of age depending on the species; smaller birds such as budgerigars are able to breed at 1 year old. A few parrot species are obviously sexually dimorphic, notably eclectus parrots where the males are predominantly green and females are red and purple. In others the differences require closer observation:

- many of the small lorikeets (*Charmosyna*) or cockatiels have obvious colour differences in their adult plumage although it is difficult to differentiate them when they are immature as they all tend to have the female coloration
- many species of white cockatoos, when adult, have a brown iris if female and a black one if male
- most adult male budgerigars have a blue cere and females a brown one (Figs 7.2 and 7.20B).

On casual inspection the majority of remaining Psittaciformes are sexually monomorphic; however, there are still subtle differences that may be seen by the experienced observer – for example:

- grey parrots are blacker if male and grey if female
- orange-winged male Amazons have very much broader heads than females

Table 7.1 Weight chart

Species	Average weight	Range of weights in grams (number of birds)
Blue and gold macaw		950–1175 (5)
Green-winged macaw	1200	1060–1365 (10)
Scarlet macaw		750–1000 (6)
Grey parrot	500	395–585 (26)
Timneh grey parrot	325	
Senegal parrot	120	92–160 (14)
Blue-fronted Amazon	350	
Orange-winged Amazon	400	
Yellow-crowned Amazon		500–550 (6)
Maximilian's pionus	230	200–242 (20)
White-capped pionus	187	166–210 (14)
Bronze-winged pionus	210	194–228 (9)
Blue-headed pionus	230	206–270 (11)
Lesser sulphur-crested cockatoo	450	
Greater sulphur-crested cockatoo	800	
Moluccan cockatoo	850	
Cockatiel	90–110	
Budgerigar (wild birds)	30	
Budgerigar (pet birds)		30–85
Peach-faced lovebird (wild birds)		46–63 (29)
Masked lovebird (wild birds)		m – 49 (8)
		f – 56 (9)
Maroon-bellied conure		75–80 (7)
White-eared conure		50–55 (5)
Blue-throated conure		90–100 (30)
Painted conure		55–65 (10)
Ring-necked parakeet		120–135 (20)

- most male pionus parrots have a larger eye than the females.

Individual variation makes these slight differences difficult to see in every individual and for many aviculturalists the birds' gender must be determined by endoscopic examination of the gonad or genetically from DNA. Parrots, like most birds, can see ultraviolet light. Reflection of light in the ultraviolet wavelength shows that some birds have sexual dichromatism based on colours that we cannot appreciate.

Nesting

Parrots nest in holes. A few species use nesting material; some lovebirds (*Agapornis* spp.) line the nest cavity with bark or twigs that they carry to the nest held under their feathers, but most chew up the wood inside the nest chamber to make a bed for the eggs. One species, the Quaker or monk parakeet (*Myiopsitta monachus*), makes a large communal nest of twigs. Parrots lay white eggs, usually on alternate days. Incubation commences immediately and this causes the young birds in the same nest to be different ages. Some of the smaller parrots lay six eggs, thus allowing 11 days between the first and last youngsters; there is therefore a dramatic difference in size between the nestlings, but this seldom seems to cause a problem. Large parrots lay only two or three eggs. Baby parrots are nidicolous (helpless when first hatched and remain in the nest) and ptilopaedic (covered in down when hatched). The parents regurgitate food directly into the mouths of their chicks. There is no evidence of the production of crop milk as found in pigeons (Columbiformes) but, when looking at the difference in growth rates between hand-reared and parent-reared parrots over the first few weeks of life, it is evident that there must be some factor that makes parent-reared babies grow so much more quickly and also gives them a greater level of immunity than hand-fed chicks.

Hand rearing

Many breeders take over the role of parent birds. Eggs may be removed for incubation as soon as they are laid, but the hatching rate increases if the parent incubates them for the first third of the incubation period. Correct incubation temperature, regular weight loss and turning are the important factors for successful incubation. Eggs that are incubated at too high a temperature will produce deformed chicks, while too much humidity will prevent hatching or cause oedematous chicks that do not survive. Too low a temperature or too dry an atmosphere will kill the chicks. Regular rotation of the eggs on their long axis (turning) is essential: eight times daily seems ideal. Failure to turn the eggs results in the embryo sticking to the shell membrane, hence causing difficulty in hatching. Artificial incubation has been fully discussed by Low (undated).

Hand rearing has been made much easier by the formulation of specific hand-rearing diets by some pet food manufacturers. All the well-known reputable brands seem to be satisfactory. Owner-made rearing diets may be very good, but there is the risk that they may be improperly balanced and have poor vitamin and mineral content: they are best viewed with suspicion. There are no excuses for the production of malformed parrots due to inadequate nutrition, but this is unfortunately still very common. In one study 36 'normal' hand-reared grey parrots from a variety of sources were examined radiographically; it was found that 44% of these birds had been affected by juvenile osteodystrophy as evidenced by deformed bones (Harcourt-Brown 2003). Baby birds are fed from a specially shaped spoon or via a syringe or a crop tube; each of these methods requires patience, dedication and an immense amount of time. Hand rearing should not be taken on lightly.

Birds that are being hand reared are usually more active than birds reared by their parents. Growing bones are not strong enough for the bird to be able to run around. Breeders often encourage the baby parrots to follow the feeding spoon quite actively or firmly restrain active baby birds whilst syringe feeding. Both these actions risk causing bony deformity.

Imprinting occurs in parrots as in all birds. Parrots that are hand reared without contact with their own species as siblings and parents become misimprinted. Misimprinting produces very appealing baby birds desired by the pet trade but may cause immeasurable difficulties over subsequent years. Weaning by the new pet owner, as encouraged by many pet shops, is to the benefit of the pet shop and not the bird. Hand-reared birds will often take twice as long to wean as parent-reared birds.

Clinical examination of the ill parrot

Detailed examination of the bird is covered in Chapter 3 and under each disease section. However, examination of the cage and cage floor is almost as important as examining the bird. Owners should be asked, if possible, to bring the bird in its cage, and the cage should not have been cleaned out for at least 24 hours. The cage size (which gives an idea of how much activity the bird gets), and the types of perches and their suitability should be noted; toys are a good guide to 'owner type'; and food remains will prove or disprove the veracity of the owner's assurance that the bird gets a good mixed diet. Finally, the droppings and regurgitated food on the floor of the cage tell a story to the clinician.

Post-mortem examination of psittacine birds has been covered comprehensively by Dorrestein & deWit (2005).

Droppings

Droppings consist of three portions:

1. Water and water-soluble products of excretion – these are initially excreted from the kidneys and refluxed into the terminal bowel, where complete or partial reabsorption takes place. The water content of the droppings can vary considerably in illness and health.

2. Urate – a white, pasty, colloidal solution from the kidneys. Uric acid is not water-soluble and is secreted by the renal tubule and not filtered through the glomerulus. The colour of the urate portion can vary for a number of reasons.

3. Faeces – black, brown or green in colour, usually having a solid worm-like appearance.

It is useful to become familiar with the normal droppings of the various genera, as droppings vary due to species as well as diet (Fig. 7.4). Budgerigars and cockatiels produce small, dry, comma-shaped droppings; macaws produce large moist droppings; lorikeets produce mostly liquid. Faecal consistency reflects the diet: fruit and vegetable diets give large wet droppings; seed diets give small dry droppings.

Abnormalities of droppings

1. *Watery droppings*. Normal birds pass watery droppings if they are on a diet with lots of soft fruit or nectar, or if they are scared and pass their droppings before the water has been removed. Ill birds with polydipsia or polyuria – e.g. renal or hepatic disease, diabetes or hyperadrenocorticism – pass very watery droppings. Neurogenic

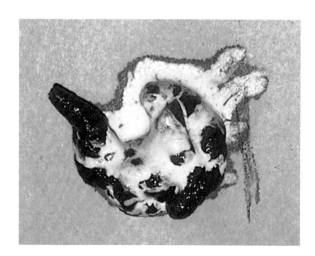

Fig 7.4 Normal faeces from a grey parrot that has been fed exclusively on pelleted food. There is a well-formed faecal mass (due to the high fibre content of the diet) covered in white urates with very little residual urine.

polydipsia or behavioural causes of polydipsia are rare. The watery portion should be tested with a (mammalian) dipstick test, the specific gravity should be measured, and it should also be examined microscopically. If the urine contains particles or is flocculent, it should be centrifuged before testing. Normal specific gravity is 1.005–1.020; pH is 6.5–8.0; and protein should be present as a trace in the urine but is present in larger amounts in the urates. Glucose is normally absent; blood, haemoglobin or myoglobin will cause a similar reaction on a dipstick and should be absent. The major bile pigment is biliverdin, which is much greener than (yellow) bilirubin.

2. *Discoloured urates* – usually green or yellow. Urates can be stained by faecal bile in normal birds, and this occurs especially in watery droppings. Discoloured urates can be caused by obstructive hepatitis of bacterial, chlamydial (Fig. 7.5) or viral origin; in these cases very green urates are due to biliverdin. Prehepatic overload from haemorrhage or bruising after surgery, trauma or large volume injections will cause the urates to be discoloured bronze, light green or yellow (Fig. 7.6).

3. *Diarrhoea.* This is a mixture of faeces, water and urates, and can be caused by worry, bacterial infections, papillomavirus or intestinal parasites. Diarrhoea on its own is rare in comparison with the condition in dogs and cats, and a diagnosis of diarrhoea must be differentiated from the polyuric bird and also the laying/incubating female. Birds laying or about to lay eggs store their droppings for longer than normal, and void a bulky, abnormal looking mass soon after leaving the nest site. This change starts a few days before laying the first egg.

4. *Presence of blood.* Blood may be mixed with faeces, and therefore from the bowel, or it may be in the urinary portion; it is usually difficult to tell. When seen, lead poisoning, an intestinal obstruction, e.g. intussusception, or possibly viral, bacterial or parasitic infestations should be suspected. 'Amazon haemorrhage syndrome' is often caused by lead poisoning. Blood that is not mixed with the droppings, but appears as drops or spots in or on the droppings, is usually cloacal in origin, and can be caused by an infected granuloma, urolith(s), viral papillomata, a prolapsed oviduct or large bowel and, very rarely, tumours.

5. *Presence of whole seed.* If seed is seen, mixed and coated with the faeces, the commonest cause is proventricular dilatation syndrome in parrots, macaws and cockatoos; however, it can also be caused by megabacteriosis (especially

in budgerigars), trichomoniasis, or other bowel irritants. If the seed is separate from the faeces it may be regurgitated.

6. *Lack of faeces but presence of urates.* This indicates starvation or an obstruction within the alimentary tract.

7. *Coloured faeces or urates.* Pigmented foods, such as beetroot, or medications – even topical medication – can change the colour of the faeces and/or urates (Fig. 7.7).

It is important to look at the faeces microscopically: smeared, fixed and stained for bacteria, yeasts and

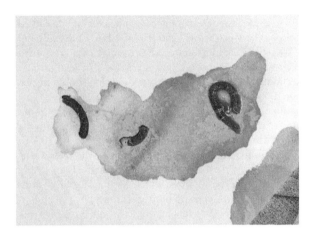

Fig 7.5 The faeces are reduced and wet, the urates contain some biliverdin and are therefore light green in colour. This parrot was very unwell; it had a reduced appetite and was polydipsic. The faeces were lighter in colour, there was copious urine and the urates were bright green, typical of a bird with severe obstructive jaundice. A lateral radiograph showed enlargement of the liver and spleen. A PCR test for *Chlamydophila* was positive.

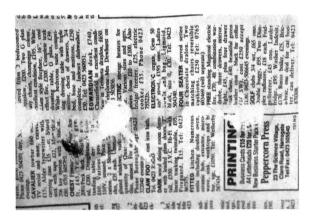

Fig 7.6 Although this is typical of birds with a mild hepatitis, this cockatoo had a severe haemorrhage in one lung and the green urates were caused by blood breakdown products causing a pre-hepatic 'jaundice'.

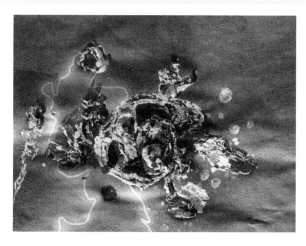

Fig 7.7 Dietary pigment in urates, caused by ingestion of beetroot.

parasites; as a wet preparation in warm (37°C) saline for protozoa; and as a flotation preparation using a saturated solution of salt (NaCl), sucrose or zinc sulphate for parasite eggs and cysts.

Regurgitation

As with vomiting in dogs and cats, regurgitation by birds can frequently be a cause for presentation at the surgery. It may be due to:

- fear
- travel sickness
- sexual or courtship behaviour – feeding a mate or young, mirror images (male budgerigars), owners
- drug induced – handling and injections, or oral administration of various drugs
- proventricular dilatation syndrome
- poisoning or consumption of a gut irritant
- obstruction – goitre in budgerigars, intussusception, tumours (e.g. papillomatosis) or foreign bodies
- inflammation of the crop/proventriculus/gizzard – trichomoniasis, candidiasis, megabacteriosis, fermented or hot food in hand-fed young birds.

Sampling

A clinical examination will usually require augmenting with various samples taken for further examination (see also Chapter 3).

Blood

Blood samples may be obtained from the following sites:

1. *The jugular vein* – the right jugular vein is usually the larger, and lies beneath a featherless area of skin on the neck of the bird close to the oesophagus and trachea (see Fig. 3.41).

2. *The brachial vein* caudoventral to the humerus, or the ulnar vein on the caudomedial aspect of the wing distal to the elbow. Both these sites usually require plucking of overlying feathers for adequate visualization of the vein (see Fig. 3.40).

3. *Claws* – small amounts of blood can be obtained by clipping a claw; a few drops are sufficient for a blood smear or DNA profile for sex determination. If this sample is to be used for biochemistry, make sure that there are no urates on the claw prior to collection.

Blood collected via a 25-gauge needle seems no more likely to be haemolysed than that obtained via a 23-gauge needle. Because of high venous pressure and a poorly developed dermis, haematomata are frequently formed at under-wing sites. These may be limited by collecting blood under general anaesthesia; by manual pressure on the vein distal to the venepuncture hole using dry cotton wool; or by using the jugular vein. If the bird is conscious and struggling violently, the bleeding will continue while the bird is restrained; replace the bird in its cage or box and the bleeding usually stops in a few minutes. Birds can safely have 1% of their body weight removed in the form of a blood sample. Using the jugular vein, budgerigars (*Melopsittacus undulatus*) can have up to 0.5 mL of blood collected; larger birds such as blue-fronted Amazons (*Amazona aestiva*), can have 1–2 mL collected from the ulnar or jugular veins. Very small birds can have a cleaned toenail clipped and blood can be collected, as it drips, into a heparinized capillary tube; one (unheparinized) drop may be used to make an air-dried smear. It should be assumed that the volume of subcutaneous bleeding will equal the amount removed for the sample; it rarely does. Vitamin K-deficient birds and those with lymphoma or severe liver disease can bleed to death after venepuncture.

Most commercial laboratories will perform haematology and biochemistry on a heparinized sample. Some authorities prefer it for biochemistry, providing the sample is centrifuged immediately and the plasma removed. A heparinized sample yields more plasma than a clotted sample yields serum; if only a small sample of blood can be taken then place it in heparin. If a heparinized sample only is collected then several air-dried smears should be made of whole blood, from the syringe, immediately after collection. However, whole heparinized blood is required by the laboratory to enable a cell count. Unfortunately whole blood degrades in the post: cellular components fragment and release enzymes and electrolytes into the serum. Therefore it is more satisfactory to obtain blood for haematology in EDTA and a gel heparin tube for the biochemistry. Gel tubes, which are centrifuged to separate the blood cells from plasma by a barrier of gel, are vital if the blood is to be posted to the laboratory as they prevent haemolysis and therefore distortion of the results.

Bacteriological samples

Faecal samples may be obtained from the floor of the cage, and defecation on new paper is the most satisfactory method of collection. A cloacal swab is too hit-or-miss; the swab may be collected from any of the three cloacal chambers, and as it is usually faeces that are required it is more satisfactory to obtain them after defecation. Because of rapid excretion of many drugs via the kidney and/or liver, faeces should be collected prior to any medication.

Samples for PCR tests in the live bird

Cotton buds or swabs on plastic are preferred to those on wood. For *Chlamydophila*, it is best to obtain three samples by swabbing the choana and the conjunctival sac and take a faecal sample. No transport medium is needed for these tests. If cost is an issue, swab the choana in upper respiratory tract cases, the conjunctiva in cases of conjunctivitis, and faeces collected from ill birds with urates discoloured green with biliverdin, or use the same swab and go from conjunctiva, to choana to cloaca – three for the price of one!

Psittacine beak and feather disease requires live feather pulp, from an erupting feather quill, to be milked out of the shaft into a container of transport medium. Whole blood can also be used: place a few drops into transport medium.

Polyomavirus tests are most reliable using a cloacal swab.

Diseases

Diseases of psittacine birds have been studied for many years, and there are comprehensive accounts of the diseases of parrots in early texts such as those of Zürn (1882) and Russ (1890). Many diseases were very accurately described, even though the causes and cures for many of them were obviously elusive and not understood by these early authors.

The dyspnoeic bird: diseases of the respiratory system

Parrots are frequently presented with a combination of respiratory signs: sneezing, nasal and/or ocular discharges, noisy breathing, changes in voice and dyspnoea. Some birds will learn to mimic human coughs and these birds do not have respiratory disease. Also, clinically normal pionus parrots will hyperventilate when they are upset or worried.

Examination (see also Chapter 3)

Observe the bird in its cage from some distance away, give the bird time to relax, and then note its degree of respiratory embarrassment. Birds with difficulty breathing 'bob' their tails up and down with each breath. Occasionally it is possible to see that the bird has a distended abdomen. Look for discharges from eyes and nose, and look at the droppings. Ask the owner about the duration and severity of any signs; the diet (with special reference to vitamin A sources); and any previous treatments and their outcome.

Before catching a bird in severe respiratory distress warn the owner that this may be a risky procedure but explain that the bird will never get better if left in the cage. Catch the bird as gently as possible and keep it upright; this avoids any fluid in the air sacs swamping the lungs and drowning the bird. Birds dislike mouth-breathing, and will attempt to breath through their nostrils even when these are obstructed. This means that it may be difficult to differentiate between upper and lower respiratory disease when the bird is in its cage.

To examine the upper respiratory tract, catch the bird, wrap it in a towel and look at its face. The nostrils should be cleared of discharge and checked for rhinolith masses. The nostril normally has a small piece of tissue protruding into its centre – the rostral concha. Observe the bird's face from dorsal and cranial aspects for subcutaneous masses or swellings in the infraorbital sinus. Press gently into the sinus and around the eye to see if exudates can be forced out of the nostril or lachrymal duct. Tempt the bird with your finger to make it open its mouth and examine around the tongue and also look at the choana; if necessary use a suitable gag. If the nostrils are not obstructed and there is no discharge, hold the beak shut and occlude first one nostril and then the other: listen for bubbling sounds, stertorous noises or lack of passage of air. All these indicate problems that need further investigation.

Some wheezing sounds can be from the larynx if this is involved in the pathological process. The entrance to the larynx can be seen with the bird's mouth held open by a gag.

Open-mouthed, apparently obstructed breathing and a change or loss of voice point to a syringeal or possibly a tracheal problem. Small birds can have their trachea transilluminated to examine for foreign bodies; part the feathers along a feather tract and damp them down prior to this examination. Larger birds can have their trachea and syrinx examined endoscopically, but this requires a general anaesthetic. In birds with tracheal obstruction a general anaesthetic can only be administered safely via an air sac tube (see Chapter 6).

Auscultation should always be attempted, even when the bird is making a lot of (vocal) noise; useful information can still be obtained that can confirm lower respiratory tract problems. Listen to the ventral, lateral and dorsal aspects of the body on both sides of the bird. Birds with lower respiratory infection often have 'crunchy' heart sounds, as if the beating heart is wrapped in crumpled cellophane. The air sacs should be auscultated ventrally and laterally. The lungs are best heard on the dorsal aspect of the bird, over the ribs.

Palpate the abdomen for abdominal distension with fluid or organ/tumour enlargements. This can cause dyspnoea by preventing the air sacs from circulating the air.

Many respiratory conditions require an anaesthetic for examination, diagnosis and treatment. Birds with apparently only upper respiratory disease frequently have a concomitant pneumonia which may not immediately be obvious. It is prudent to treat these birds for a few days with a broad-spectrum antibiotic, prior to an anaesthetic.

All birds with respiratory disease should be suspected of being vitamin A deficient, and their treatment should include vitamin supplementation. An oral multivitamin and mineral supplement specifically made for birds is preferred but changes will take up to a year to occur fully. Injections of multivitamins may have a short-term effect, but are occasionally fatal.

Specific problems
Rhinoliths

Rhinoliths are hard crusty lumps blocking the nostril and causing breathing difficulties. They are very common in African parrots (Fig. 7.8A) such as the grey and the red-fronted (Jardine's) parrot (*Poicephalus gulielmi*). Hook the rhinolith out of the nostril using a small dental osteotome, shaped like a tiny teaspoon about 1.5 to 2 mm in diameter. This instrument can be introduced behind the mass and used to lever it out (Fig. 7.8B). There is frequently mucopurulent discharge behind the rhinolith in the nasal cavity and occasionally the sinuses. Clean the discharge out and instil neomycin or gentamicin eye drops twice daily into the nostril, and re-examine after a week of treatment to clean out again. If the discharge does not respond to antibiotics, culture for *Aspergillus* spp. Medium to large rhinoliths will deform the bony structure of the nostril (Fig. 7.8C) and will often recur, requiring regular (about 3-monthly) removal. Vitamin A deficiency will play a significant part in this condition. Evening primrose oil will help prevent hard nasal secretions building up in the deformed nostril: instil one drop once or twice a week into the affected nostril(s).

Chlamydiosis

A watery conjunctivitis, which may give rise to a wet nasal discharge and occasional sneezing, is typical of *Chlamydophila* infection. This manifestation of chlamydiosis is most common in cockatiels and Australian parakeets including budgerigars. The birds are not usually

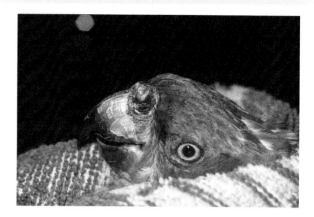

Fig 7.8A An 8-year-old pet Senegal parrot that lived on a diet mainly composed of seeds was presented for examination because it was sneezing and had a slight nasal discharge from its right nostril. A large rhinolith could be seen blocking its left nostril.

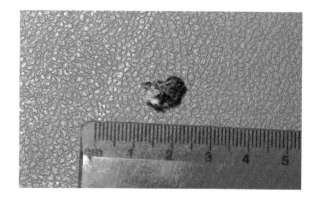

Fig 7.8B The rhinolith was easily removed from the conscious bird using a small dental probe.

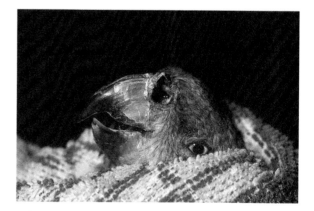

Fig 7.8C Rhinoliths slowly expand, causing a permanent deformity of the nasal passage. Although the entrance to the nostril will contract to half the size seen here, the bird will require treatment and permanent supervision. Treatment can be antibiotic drops (gentamicin eye drops) to remove infection, a drop of evening primrose oil once or twice weekly to prevent the nasal secretions from becoming too hard, and regular re-examination to remove secreted material before it blocks the nostril.

unwell, but they can infect other birds, which will die of the hepatic form of chlamydiosis and are potentially zoonotic. Confi mation with a PCR test on a conjunctival or choanal swab is required. Treatment with chlortetracycline eye ointment and oral or parenteral doxycycline is usually curative within a month.

Sinusitis

Sinusitis is typified by swellings of the infraorbital area. Nasal and ocular discharges are also possible signs. Culture of mucopurulent material obtained by aspiration of the sinus is vital for treatment. Many cases are colonized by Gram-negative organisms such as *Pseudomonas*. *Mycoplasma* spp. could be involved in moist sinusitis; enrofl oxadn or tylosin will kill this bacterium. Daily flushing by injecting into the sinus or flushing through the nostril (Fig. 7.9) is the best treatment for moist sinusitis. Some sinus deposits are inspissated, palpable and too hard to flush out and must be surgically removed.

Occasionally parrots (especially Amazons) are presented with sinusitis and/or sneezing. A caseous mass can be found in the nasal passages, usually by endoscopic examination through the choana. Culture often confirms the presence of aspergillosis. This must be treated by removal of all the pus and regular instillation of an antifungal drug for some weeks.

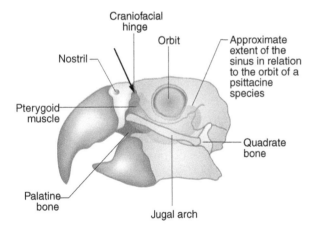

Fig 7.9 A lateral view of the skull of a blue and gold macaw (*Ara araraunɑ*) showing the approximate extent of the infraorbital sinus (broken line), the site of insertion of a hypodermic needle for sampling or flushing the sinus (arrow), and the position of the pterygoid muscle. The pterygoid muscle has an overlying artery and vein (and nerve) which are easily punctured if the needle is inserted too deep. This will cause a profuse haemorrhage.
For injection, the nostril and eye should be noted and midway between them it is possible to palpate a bone-free depression, bordered ventrally by the jugal arch. This space is increased by opening the bird's mouth. A needle is inserted here (arrow) directed slightly caudoventrally to enter the infraorbital sinus. Using a syringe it is possible to aspirate the contents of the sinus, which should normally be air. In this macaw the needle should be inserted no more than 5 mm as the sinus is subcutaneous at this point.

Choanal abscesses

Choanal abscesses will cause nasal discharge and difficulty breathing through the nostrils. They are best seen in an anaesthetized bird. It is usually wise to give a course of enrofloxacin for 4 or 5 days before anaesthesia and surgical removal of the abscess. The abscess is sometimes seated on the dorsal aspect of the choana and the edge of the structure must be rolled back to reveal the abscess. A 21-gauge hypodermic needle is useful as a stylet to open the epithelium, and a small blunt probe, such as an arthroscopy hook, is needed to push the inspissated pus out. Again attention to diet and the addition of vitamin A are paramount.

Foreign bodies

Tracheal foreign bodies will cause severe dyspnoea. A millet seed is a common foreign body in a cockatiel that is having difficulty breathing, and transillumination will show its presence. An air sac tube and general anaesthesia give a chance of removal. Stop the seed slipping down the trachea with a 25-gauge needle through the trachea distal to the seed, then partially open the trachea with a cut between the rings and remove the seed. Repair the trachea with fine suture material.

Aspergillosis

Laryngeal aspergillosis has, in the author's experience, been a cause of dyspnoea in imported *Pionus* spp. Removal of the purulent material from the rima glottidis and treatment with itraconazole or topical clotrimazole can be successful, but this condition carries a surprisingly poor prognosis.

Aspergillus spp. infection of the distal trachea, syrinx or primary bronchus is a common cause of dyspnoea; it will also affect lungs and air sacs. This condition should be suspected in a dyspnoeic bird that is wheezing and has a change of voice. Diagnosis requires an anaesthetic and endoscopy. A 2.7 mm 0° endoscope should be used to examine this area in Amazons, cockatoos, large macaws and large grey parrots. A parrot's trachea tapers distally, and smaller birds prove impossible to examine without a smaller endoscope. A general anaesthetic using an air sac tube will allow suction through a catheter placed down the trachea and into the syrinx. This technique can suck out most of the lesion. Treatment with enilconazole topically and itraconazole orally can be effective. Clotrimazole by nebulization may be used as well. The bird should be re-examined a few days later as the fungus and caseation can regrow. This condition is common in grey parrots and carries a poor prognosis; these birds should be referred to an avian veterinarian.

Birds with generalized aspergillosis can be either acutely affected, in which case they are presented either dead or with sudden onset of severe dyspnoea; or they can be chronically affected, in which case they will present as being unwell (to greater or lesser extent), underweight (in spite of eating reasonably well) and dyspnoeic; again the degree varies and is usually worsened by stress and exercise. There is little change in voice, but examination with a stethoscope reveals an increase in audible respiratory sounds. Diagnosis is by clinical examination, and a blood sample will reveal a very elevated heterophil count (15 000–40 000 cells/dL) and radiography will typically show a locular pattern in the lung and/or air sac region. Treatment using itraconazole orally and clotrimazole by nebulization can be successful in producing a cure.

Syringitis

Syringitis can be seen in some birds that have a voice change and/or an 'asthma' attack. Endoscopy will reveal an irritated syrinx with moist swollen edges to the syringeal valve and no sign of aspergillosis. This condition can be brought on by bacterial infection or some irritant trigger such as cooking fumes. A spasm of the syrinx can be induced during anaesthesia in some birds causing fatal asphyxia which may not be noticed in time to place an air sac tube.

PTFE poisoning

Polytetrafluoroethane (PTFE) poisoning from over-heated non-stick Teflon®-coated cooking utensils is a common cause of severe, rapid, terminal pneumonia. Over-heating is not difficult if the pan is empty, and it causes the coating to depolymerize to form a lethal vapour; birds in the same air-space will drop off their perches, dead, within half an hour of inhaling the vapour. Some self-cleaning ovens and some spotlight bulbs are also coated with Teflon®. Examination of the lungs at post-mortem shows oedematous bloody tissue throughout both lungs. Over-heated, smoking cooking oil can have a similar effect, as will bonfire or barbecue smoke.

Air sac worms

Air sac worms can be seen in recently imported birds as an incidental finding at post-mortem examination or during endoscopic gender determination. These worms do not seem to cause disease and can usually be safely ignored. Treatment with ivermectin should be successful, but could cause problems by producing dead worms in the air sacs.

Abdominal distension

Abdominal distension produced by tumours, hepatic or proventricular enlargement, ascites or egg-production will prevent the air sacs functioning and cause dyspnoea: all should be differentiated on radiography, with the use of contrast and other techniques if required (see Chapter 5). Serositis will also cause the abdominal and hepatic peritoneal cavities to fill with fluid and will cause dyspnoea. This condition appears to be a sequel to a viral infection.

Diseases of the digestive system

Probably the most common presenting sign for any clinician is the bird that is eating less food than usual and has loose droppings. It may have lost weight and may also be regurgitating. Some birds may die suddenly; other birds may be more chronically affected.

Examination

The owner should be encouraged to bring the bird in its uncleaned cage: half the clinical signs are found on the cage floor. Examine the bird from a distance looking for signs of illness, dyspnoea, general condition, soiled feathers around the vent, etc. Then examine the droppings on the cage floor. It is uncommon for birds to have diarrhoea and common for them to be polydipsic. Normal faecal shape varies between species (see earlier).

The presence of soft, swollen, undigested hulled seeds with no mixing of faeces is a sign of regurgitation.

The dropping (faecal/urinary mass) may be well formed if the bird is eating, but will be small, dark green and watery with white urates if the bird is not. It may be poorly formed in birds with diarrhoea, but also in scared birds or birds with cloacal papillomatosis/granulation, or cloacoliths. It may be blood-stained, or coated or mixed with blood. Sometimes droppings contain whole undigested seeds; this is abnormal. Take a faecal portion for microscopy and possibly microbiological culture. Check for parasites, bacteria or yeasts.

Next, assess the urinary portion. In birds on a dry diet such as seed, the urates should be formed and white with little water. If there is a lot of water in the diet (fruit, vegetables, pulses, nectar) or if the bird is polydipsic, then there will be a quantity of water passed with the urates. Metabolites may be visible in the urates: light green to dark green urates indicate a hepatitis; green to bronze urates can occur after trauma and bruising and can also be caused by hepatitis (Figs 7.5 and 7.6); some topical medications and food colourings will be excreted in the urine (e.g. topical proflavine can give yellow urates or beetroot can give purple colouring – neither affect the bird) (Fig. 7.7). If the faeces contain a lot of water use a dipstick test to check for glucose, blood and protein content. It is usually possible to avoid faecal contamination.

Next, examine the bird: catch it, look in its mouth and at the tongue; palpate the crop, thoracic inlet, and abdomen; examine the cloaca. If the crop is distended, then pass a crop tube and obtain a sample of crop contents. Smear this on a slide and stain it; look for bacteria, yeasts and protozoa; also look at a wet preparation. Carry out a microscopical faeces examination – wet and fixed stained preparations as well as a worm egg count.

In the author's opinion, the commonest cause of an illness of sudden onset in a single bird with watery droppings is a bacterial hepatitis or enteritis. Heart blood taken at post-mortem examination within 20 minutes of death has invariably produced a pure growth of a coliform, usually *Escherichia coli* (but also *Klebsiella* spp. or *Pseudomonas* spp., etc.).

Clinical signs are an ill bird with watery droppings containing some or no faeces and, often, light green urates. Some birds will regurgitate food, especially after travelling or following intramuscular injection. The bird should be assessed for hydration (crinkly skin around the eyes or a skin pinch that remains tented); weight loss, assessed on pectoral mass and weighing; crop palpation and abdominal palpation should be unremarkable. The vent should be clean.

Faecal examination tests for birds with watery droppings (in order of preference) include:

- faecal flotation for parasites
- microscopy for protozoa: dilute faeces with warm isotonic saline and watch for jerky swimming movements of single cell parasites – but note that particles smaller than a single cell can exhibit Brownian motion and may be mistaken for parasites
- Gram's stain, which may reveal lots of Gram-negative coliforms rather than Gram-positive cocci, indicating abnormal gut bacteria
- bacteriology: this may be useful, but hopefully results will arrive after the bird has recovered. Check for *Salmonella* spp.; *Salmonella enterica* serovar Typhimurium is common, especially in imported grey parrots, but can be seen in any birds.

If a diagnosis of bacterial hepatitis seems likely, then inject with a broad-spectrum antibiotic, use a crop tube to give the bird some fluids and place the bird in a warm, darkened cage. If the bird starts to improve, then it must be fed four times a day with some easily digestible food by crop tube and injected twice daily with antibiotic. If the bird worsens, then a change of antibiotic is indicated; adequate fluid must also be given.

Further investigation is required in birds that are not responding to treatment. It can be useful to combine the following procedures and possibly carry them out under anaesthetic, as it is less stressful to the bird. Take a blood sample for haematology and biochemistry: with a bacterial hepatitis there will be an elevated white blood cell count with increased heterophils and a left shift; elevated gamma glutamyl transferase and bile acids but normal uric acid, urea and glucose. A low albumin level is useful as a guide to chronic ill health, and a high PCV and high urea are indicators of dehydration.

After taking the blood sample, slowly inject an intravenous bolus of N/5 glucose saline, 5 mL to an Amazon or grey parrot and up to 10 mL to a large macaw. Indwelling intravenous or intraosseous catheters giving continuous fluids are useful but more complicated (see Chapter 6). Intravenous catheters can be placed in the basilic vein on the ventral aspect of the wing, by the humerus. The bird must be restrained from pulling out an indwelling catheter, so a collar and/or wing strapping is usually necessary. If i.v. fluids are to be used, be very careful to avoid over-perfusion; use a burette or a slow injection system. Do not attach a 500 mL bag of fluid, as it is only too easy to administer the whole bag, with fatal results.

Radiography should also be carried out at this time, and in cases of bacterial hepatitis there will be a normal or enlarged liver and kidneys (septicaemia/bacteraemia) or a normal liver and large spleen (enteritis). Note that green urates and a large spleen along with an enlarged liver usually indicate chlamydiosis, therefore perform a PCR test.

The gizzard often contains grit, but check for lead, glass or metallic foreign bodies, all of which can contribute to conditions resulting in hepatitis/enteritis.

Specific problems
Proventriculard ilatationd isease

Larger parrots, such as grey parrots, macaws and cockatoos, may be presented with signs of weight loss and regurgitation or weight loss and the passage of whole seeds; they may also exhibit neurological signs such as trembling and incoordination; many birds will appear to be hungry and make pathetic begging-for-food noises. Most of these cases have proventricular dilatation disease (PDD). This is an infectious disease, almost certainly of viral origin. PDD may be seen in birds of any age. Diagnosis in the live bird is aided by radiography. Lateral and ventrodorsal views often show a dilated proventriculus and gizzard. A barium meal may be needed to demonstrate this or to show a slowed passage of ingesta. Fluoroscopy will reveal that the normal movement of the gut has been compromised and instead of peristalsis the wall of the proventriculus and gizzard 'flutters' (Storm & Greenwood 1993).

Confirmation of the diagnosis in a live bird may be obtained in many cases from histopathology on a biopsy of the crop; this is relatively easy to perform. Under general anaesthesia (intubation of the trachea is vital), removal of a portion of full-thickness crop wall to include at least one large blood vessel will allow histological examination of the autonomic nerves and associated ganglia as they are found adjacent to the arterial supply to the gastrointestinal tract. Approximately 75% of cases can be confirmed with this test (Gregory et al 1996). A full-thickness proventricular biopsy is probably better but much more invasive, and carries a grave risk of peritonitis.

Post-mortem examination can be used to confirm the diagnosis in most outbreaks of this disease, as there is a high mortality rate. The crop, proventriculus and gizzard can be variously thin-walled, dilated and impacted with seed (Fig. 7.10); surrounding tissues often exhibit peritonitis. The duodenum can also be dilated in some birds, especially cockatoos. Occasionally there is ulceration at the proventricular/ventricular junction; this ulcer can perforate with fatal results. The lungs often show acute aspiration bronchitis and pneumonia. Histopathology is required to confirm the suspicion of this disease by the presence of lymphocytic, plasmacytic ganglioneuritis involving the autonomic ganglia at various levels in the gut wall. The brain shows similar changes.

Treatment of this disease is possible, and some individuals recover. Treatment is empirical: a high fibre, moist diet, with little seed; broad-spectrum antibiotics to prevent peritonitis and pneumonia (trimethoprim/sulphonamide is the author's first choice); and a prokinetic, cisapride (Prepulsid, Janssen), can be very helpful. Celecoxib (Celebrex, Pfizer) and meloxicam (Metacam, Boehringer Ingelheim), both NSAIDs, are also said to be very useful. The recovered bird could be a carrier. However, as apparently normal birds can also appear to be carriers, and as there is no reliable test developed that can detect the carrier state, treatment seems a reasonable option.

Papillomatosis

Weight loss, regurgitation and a soiled vent may be caused by papillomatosis. This disease usually affects the upper alimentary tract and cloaca of birds that have been imported from Central America. Hawk-headed parrots, macaws and some Amazons are those most commonly affected, and affected birds appear to have diarrhoea and their vents are soiled with faeces sticking to the feathers in lumps. (NB: Budgerigars that exhibit these signs are usually too fat to clean their vents; they do not have papillomatosis.) On cleaning the vent, a protruding mass of tissue may be seen (Fig. 7.11). Check the oral cavity – papillomata are frequently found around the choana and the rima glottidis, and these growths can extend through the alimentary tract. Removal of the papillomata that are causing problems is helpful. Histopathology will confirm the typical appearance of the lesions. Mild cautery of the lesions around the vent will often be sufficient. The disease will make the birds unwell, but this condition alternates with periods of good health in a cyclical manner; the periodicity in one closely observed case was around 4 months. Therefore, any and all treatments seem to work well for a time. Autogenous vaccines do not cure the disease. A papillomavirus has never been isolated from these cases, but a link has been made with a herpesvirus as a cause of this condition (Phalen et al 1998). In the long term, many of these birds become affected with malignant tumours of the pancreas or gall bladder and related structures (Graham 1991).

Salmonellosis

Salmonella spp. can affect parrots, especially newly imported birds. The usual isolate is *Salmonella* Typhimurium. Affected birds may die suddenly, but many cases are ill for a period with signs of general septicaemia: profuse watery diarrhoea; polydipsia/polyuria; dyspnoea/pneumonia; depression; inappetence and occasionally, neurological signs. Confirmation is on bacteriology. Treatment with a broad-spectrum antibiotic, with supportive nursing and feeding, will often allow the bird to recover, but a number of cases remain carriers and

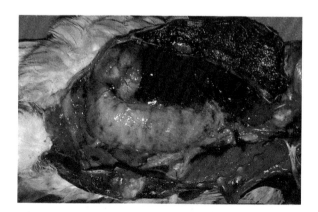

Fig 7.10 A lateral view of a female grey parrot that died because of proventricular dilatation syndrome. The lateral body wall has been removed exposing the massively enlarged proventriculus distended by whole seeds. The seed can be seen filling the proventriculus and gizzard as well as filling the oesophagus and crop.

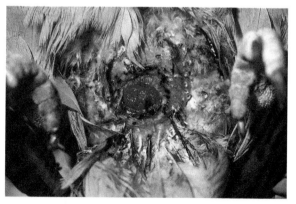

Fig 7.11 This Amazon parrot had a dirty vent and was unwell. General anaesthesia allowed the mass of feathers and soiled feathers to be removed revealing a protruding mass that is typical of 'papillomatosis'. Biopsies were taken and the masses were trimmed back to the fibrous layer of lamina propria; this layer must not be penetrated.

these individuals may or may not be chronically unwell. Three samples of faeces must be found to be clear of *Salmonella* spp. to rule out the carrier state; one sample is not sufficient. Carriers may be cleared by the use of an autogenous, inactivated vaccine. Two doses of vaccine, 2 weeks apart, have been found to clear carriers; each dose should be given orally (1 mL) and as a subcutaneous injection (0.5 mL). This regimen gives a significant rise in antibody titre (Harcourt-Brown 1986). Salmonellosis is a zoonosis, and appropriate measures must be taken. Other coliforms will produce similar, but usually less dramatic, signs of illness.

Pseudotuberculosis

Yersinia pseudotuberculosis is a common cause of outbreaks of acute illness and mortality, usually in aviary parakeets. It is transmitted via faeces from infected rodents and wild birds. The majority of affected birds die within a few days, having shown signs of pneumonia, enteritis with wet diarrhoeic droppings, and general ill health. At post-mortem examination the most acute cases have an enlarged, patchily discoloured liver, and more chronic cases have miliary white spots throughout the liver. Similar changes are found in the kidneys and spleen. Confirmation by bacteriology is needed (culture requirements are specialized so warn the laboratory that this pathogen is suspected), and antibiotic treatment is required. The drinking water must be kept uncontaminated and the flock will recover more quickly if the water contains either the appropriate antibiotic or a disinfectant such as 5–6 mg/L of free iodine or chlorhexidine. Prompt treatment will limit but not completely prevent deaths in the affected birds; the organ damage in some individuals will cause their death even in the absence of the organism.

Digestive problems in budgerigars

Budgerigars are often presented because they are regurgitating their seed or a white pasty substance. In many cases the birds are well and the regurgitation is onto their mirror or other reflective surface, or onto their owner. These birds are in breeding condition, and it is a normal part of their behaviour to try to feed their 'mate'. Budgerigars that are on an unsupplemented, shop-bought, loose-seed diet will usually be iodine deficient (Blackmore 1963), and the goitres that form can block the thoracic inlet sufficiently to cause regurgitation. Goitres may also affect the action of the syrinx and cause a wheezing respiration and an altered (or lost) voice. The enlarged thyroid may occasionally be palpable at the thoracic inlet. Supplementation with iodine will quickly alleviate the problem: a stock solution of 2 mL of strong Lugol's iodine solution is added to 30 mL of water, and 1 drop of this is added to 250 mL of drinking water, daily for treatment and 2–3 times weekly for prevention. Most proprietary multivitamin and mineral powders contain sufficient iodine.

In other cases birds are unwell, losing weight, and regurgitating sporadically. An ill budgerigar will have yellowish staining on the feathers around the beak; is thin; its crop often feels thickened and may be distended with fluid; the vent is frequently soiled; and the bird's droppings are enlarged and wetter than normal. After some time with these signs many budgerigars will die. Crop contents should be examined. It is possible to obtain crop fluid in some birds by milking the crop contents up the oesophagus, and the birds will spit out some of the viscous fluid. If this is not possible, passing a crop tube and introducing about 1 mL of isotonic saline and then aspirating will give a sufficient sample for examination. Warmed wet preparations will reveal *Trichomonas* parasites. The other cause of these signs, megabacteria (*Macrorhabdus*), will show on a dried and stained smear. Some birds have both problems. Occasionally yeasts (*Candida* spp.) are seen in the smears as well. Treatment with a mixture of amphotericin B (which will kill both yeasts and megabacteria) and metronidazole (which kills trichomonads) given via a crop tube or by mouth as a drop, twice daily for a week, will resolve the signs. These conditions are very common in budgerigar breeders' aviaries and in these cases treatment of the entire flock is needed. Faecal examination may reveal megabacteria, but only very fresh faeces will contain recognizable trichomonads. In all cases negative results do not rule out these diseases. Megabacteria are in greatest numbers in the proventriculus; trichomonads perish and disintegrate very rapidly. Post-mortem examination of a recently dead bird will allow samples to be taken from the oesophagus, gizzard and crop and examined by the hanging drop technique and as smears stained with Gram's method or Diff Quik. This will give a reliable diagnosis. The diseases caused by megabacteria, *Trichomonas* and *Candida* can be seen in other psittacine birds.

Parasitism

Examination of faeces from psittacine birds will, on occasions, reveal various intestinal parasites. However, some species of birds are more susceptible than others. *Giardia* spp. are an infrequent cause of diarrhoea (also causing feather-plucking in cockatiels) and may be difficult to demonstrate in the live bird as they are found in the upper small intestine; organisms should be looked for at post-mortem examination of a fresh carcass, using the hanging-drop technique. Australian parakeets are frequently affected by roundworms; the birds look ill and this disease will cause sufficient weight loss for the birds to die. The worms may not be laying eggs, so a negative faecal examination should not be trusted. It is vital that every ill Australian parakeet is wormed with a

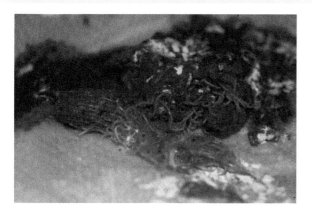

Fig 7.12 Roundworms in droppings from a parakeet.

dose of fenbendazole (Panacur 2.5% Hoechst, at a single dose of 50 mg/kg) give by crop tube. If possible the bird should be kept separately so that the droppings may be examined over the next 2 days for dead worms. A small parakeet may contain up to 50 large worms (Fig. 7.12). Roundworms, in this author's experience, are the commonest cause of death in this group of parakeets.

Macaws (*Ara* spp.) with low-grade ill health may be seen passing large wet droppings. Examination of the faeces by flotation in saturated salt solution will reveal the typical eggs (small with bipolar plugs) of *Capillaria* spp. In-contact birds may also be infested, and faecal samples should be checked. Affected birds must be dosed regularly with fenbendazole and great attention must be paid to hygiene or re-infestation will result. Outdoor cages, suspended in a sunny position, with frequent showering/hosing of the birds and cage, and with 2-weekly dosing with fenbendazole on an individual basis is required to remove this problem.

Chlamydiosis

The disease caused by the organism *Chlamydophila psittaci* may be known variously by the names chlamydophilosis or chlamydiosis, ornithosis, or – most commonly – psittacosis, since it is always linked with parrots. It was first reported in humans and psittacine birds in 1895 (Morange 1895). However, it has been found in many species of birds, especially domestic ducks and pigeons.

In parrots it can give rise to several syndromes. Firstly, there can be symptom-free carriers that can shed the organism intermittently and may remain carriers for many years. The carrier state is commonest in Amazon parrots and in commercially bred cockatiels and budgerigars. Secondly, some birds become extremely ill with a severe hepatitis: they are depressed, lose weight, may have respiratory signs and have droppings in which the urate portion is often a vivid green colour due to biliverdin levels in the blood rising above the renal threshold (owing to obstructive liver disease) (Fig. 7.5). These birds have been previously uninfected, and have then contracted the disease. In the author's experience, grey parrots seem to be uncommon as carriers but very susceptible to the disease, which is frequently caught from a symptom-free carrier such as a cockatiel. Thirdly, some birds, especially Australian parakeets, are presented with a unilateral or sometimes bilateral conjunctivitis; occasionally these birds are also unwell. Finally, some birds become chronically ill as a result of chlamydiosis and may even develop immunocomplex-linked glomerulonephritis.

Birds with chlamydiosis should be treated (provided the zoonotic potential is not significant), as many will make a complete recovery and – with adequate treatment – will not be carriers.

Diagnosis is best attempted using a PCR test to detect the organism. Blood samples for antibody levels and ELISA tests are less easily interpreted and less reliable. Ideally, three samples should be taken: a swab from the conjunctiva, a swab from the choana and a faeces sample. The test result will take some time, so presumptive treatment should be instituted immediately. Two drugs kill *Chlamydophila* in vivo: enrofloxacin and doxycycline. It is now considered that doxycycline is the more effective drug, and this can be given by injection, in food or in the drinking water. Doxycycline must be administered for 45 days to cure the bird in most circumstances. All birds should be checked after they are 'better', and providing that three samples taken at different times give a negative PCR result the bird can be considered 'cured'.

Avian tuberculosis

Occasionally, parrots are presented with weight loss and/or slowly growing lumps. These birds may have *Mycobacterium avium*. Smears from strange-looking masses may frequently reveal acid-fast organisms. Many of these birds are excreting the bacillus and it is possible to identify this using a PCR test for *M. avium*. Although some cases have been treated there is a zoonotic potential (for immunosuppressed people only) as well as the health of other birds to consider. Birds suffering from avian tuberculosis should be euthanized.

Diseases of the urinary system

The truly polydipsic bird is often presented, although owners often confuse polyuria with diarrhoea. Budgerigars, cockatiels and grey parrots seem most commonly affected, but perhaps because they are the most frequently kept pets.

Examination should include looking at the bird in the cage for signs of general illness, dehydration, abdominal distension, dyspnoea or leg weakness. The droppings should then be checked for consistency of faecal portion,

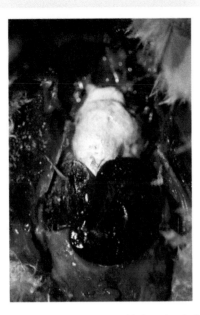

Fig 7.13 Visceral gout with urate deposits thickly coating the heart.

quantity of water and colour of the urates. Finally, the bird should be removed from the cage and examined in a routine manner. Many of these birds will be on a deficient diet, so this should be borne in mind.

An important point is that birds are uricotelic. They produce uric acid in the liver as an end product of protein catabolism. The uric acid is excreted via the kidney as a colloidal solution from which all the water can be reclaimed, either within the renal tubule or by the terminal bowel. Uric acid is excreted by the tubule; urea and other water-soluble products are filtered via the glomerulus. After excretion via the ureter, the urine is carried by retroperistalsis from the urodeum into the terminal intestine, where water is reabsorbed leaving only urates. By producing uric acid (insoluble) and not urea (water-soluble) a uricotelic animal can develop in a shelled-egg without being poisoned by the waste products of protein catabolism. In embryonic birds the uric acid is deposited within the fetal membranes, i.e. outside the fetus.

Renal disease can be very difficult to diagnose. Uric acid levels tend to remain unaltered even when there is chronic disease because the uric acid is laid down within the body cavities. Radiography may show enlarged kidneys; an intravenous pyelogram, using iohexol (Omnipaque, Nyomed) is useful to enhance their outline and show the presence of tumours. Endoscopy is useful, and an approach between the last two ribs allows visualization of the pericardium, the surface of the liver and the air sacs – all common sites for deposition of uric acid (visceral gout). (Fig. 7.13). Puncturing the oblique septum allows the kidneys to be seen and biopsied. All these tests may be helpful but not necessarily diagnostic

in early cases of renal disease. Later stages of the disease may show elevation of phosphorus and a change in the calcium/phosphorus ratio. **A blood sample in which the plasma has been separated from the cellular component within 30 minutes should be used for this assessment; delay in separation from blood cells will increase the phosphorus levels in the plasma.**

Hepatitis (see earlier) and diabetes will both cause polyuria. In cases of diabetes a urine 'dipstick' will show glucose in urine. Normal urine will contain no glucose. The pancreas of birds contains little insulin and this hormone appears to have a lesser role in glucose metabolism than in mammals. Injections of mammalian insulin have little effect and dietary change is the most sensible method of control. Cockatiels are very commonly affected with this condition and they tend to eat a seed diet that is rich in carbohydrate. Changing to an all-in-one diet is very useful in these cases and frequently makes the bird much better. Some of these birds have pituitary tumours and are Cushingoid.

Renal tumours are common and often palpable within the abdomen. Because the lumbosacral plexus is sandwiched between the kidney and the pelvis, renal tumours often cause paralysis of a leg rather than polydipsia. A unilateral lameness in a budgerigar should always be investigated for renal (or gonadal) enlargement.

Visceral and articular gout

These syndromes are commonly seen in parrots. The birds are often unwell, and pasty white uric acid deposits may be visible under the scaly skin of the legs and feet (Fig. 7.14). The uric acid will also be deposited around the viscera in the various peritoneal cavities (hepatic, pericardial, etc.) (Fig. 7.13). Affected birds seldom recover. Allopurinol has been suggested as a treatment because it works in humans (a 100 mg tablet crushed in 10 mL of water; 1 mL of this solution added to 30 mL of drinking water). However, its efficacy in birds has been questioned as it has been shown to *cause* gout in some birds.

Diseases of the reproductive system

The most frequently presented reproductive problem is egg binding. Female birds that may or may not have laid previously are presented as unwell, slightly dyspnoeic and usually with a palpable abdominal mass. The bird may also have difficulty standing and appear very weak. The most frequent cause is a lack of calcium. The egg-bound bird is usually on a poorly supplemented diet and may, as is the case with many pet cockatiels, be laying her 10th or even 20th egg that year. The diagnosis should be confirmed radiographically, when an egg should be visible. The egg has usually started to form a shell, but this demand on calcium cannot be sustained.

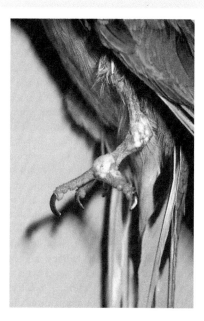

Fig 7.14 The typical appearance of urate deposits under the skin on the leg of an Australian parakeet. These parakeets are often affected by 'gout'. This bird was euthanized and internal examination found substantial urate deposits within its pericardium and on its liver.

Parrots lay an egg every other day. The egg takes nearly 48 hours to form and spends 80% of this time in the shell gland. The shell gland (uterus) is a part of the distal oviduct, and when it contains a shelled egg this is often palpable through the abdominal wall. It is useful to know when the last egg was laid. Oral supplementation with calcium and a little vitamin D_3 may be used; a bolus of a high-calcium powder (Nutrobal, VetArk in the UK), containing 200 mg calcium in 1 g of powder, is mixed with a small amount of cereal-based baby food and given into the crop with a crop tube. A dose of 100 to 500 mg of calcium (depending on the bird's size) is usually sufficient to allow the bird to be able to stand, and the egg is usually passed. If the egg is not passed after calcium administration, oxytocin and various other treatments have been suggested. Oxytocin has profound effects on blood pressure in birds and should be used with caution in small incremental doses. It has been suggested that dinoprost (Lutalyse, Upjohn) is a better choice, but neither of these drugs is favoured by the author. If the egg can be seen radiographically or palpated, an anaesthetic followed by gentle pressure on the egg will force it through the vagina and out of the cloaca. Another method of removing thin-shelled eggs is to introduce a hypodermic needle through the abdominal wall into the egg and to aspirate the contents. This allows the shell to collapse, and the egg is easily expelled. Occasionally eggs are not passed out of the oviduct and torsion of the oviduct should be suspected; this requires a laparotomy for egg removal. In cases such as this ecbolics are contraindicated.

Birds that have been egg-bound need to have their diet and husbandry fully reviewed. Vitamin D_3 deficiency is just as important as calcium deficiency.

Diseases of the central nervous system (CNS): the wobbly and/or convulsing parrot

Parrots are frequently presented unable to stand on their perches, and the clinician must differentiate those birds that are very ill from those with CNS problems.

The commonest presenting neurological sign is of a bird that is exhibiting incoordination, to the point of falling off its perch and having some degree of unsteady or jittery movement. Nystagmus is sometimes seen, but anisocoria is rare. Some birds convulse and some even spin around and around continually until they die. Clinical examination is usually unrewarding.

There are many causes of neurological signs, including the following:

- Parrots eat or chew any new object; poisoning is therefore a common cause of neurological problems. Lead from paint, solder, lead shot, etc. are all common causes of lead poisoning.
- The next most common neurological problem is calcium/vitamin D_3 deficiency. This is more frequent in grey parrots. An all-seed diet, no supplementation, and sunlight that is filtered through glass (which removes ultraviolet light), must all be contributory factors.
- Zinc toxicity will give neurological signs, and is usually seen in aviary birds in aviaries made with new galvanized mesh, or in caged birds with cheap galvanized clips and links on toys.
- Paramyxovirus will also cause irreversible neurological signs, and in the UK is usually seen in Australian parakeets. These birds will convulse, but are usually affected by torticollis and exhibit very abnormal movement which is often permanent.
- Proventricular dilatation disease will cause neurological signs (tremors and muscular weakness), especially in young macaws which are making 'baby-bird' noises and are also off their food, regurgitating and looking unwell.
- Some birds with advanced renal and/or hepatic disease can exhibit neurological signs.
- Hypoglycaemia will cause collapse and brief convulsions before the bird dies.
- Old parrots are increasingly seen by clinicians, and some of them develop neurological signs. Some of these birds are suffering from atherosclerosis of the arteries in the brain; others have non-specific cellular degeneration; rarely they have brain tumours.

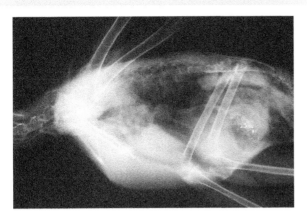

Fig 7.15 A lateral radiograph of a cockatoo that was regurgitating and unwell. The bird can be seen to have a dilated proventriculus and radiodense particles within its gizzard. The bird was treated with sodium di-calcium edetate by alternate day injections. The bird recovered within 2 days, treatment was continued for five injections and by day 10, radiography showed that all the particles of lead were gone from the gizzard. A lithium heparin whole-blood sample could have been used to confirm the diagnosis but the owners found the source of lead in their house: an antique chandelier that the bird had been roosting on!

If a bird is presented suffering from seizures or other neurological problems, the first step (as always) is to get a good history, with poisoning and dietary deficiency in mind. If lead poisoning seems to be likely, then radiography will usually reveal very radiodense particles in the gizzard (Fig. 7.15). These particles are denser than grit, which may also be seen on the radiograph. A blood sample must be taken for lead (lithium heparin blood is used for this estimation) and calcium (heparin or clotted blood) estimation. It is important to measure *ionized* calcium as this gives a true picture of available calcium. Normal levels in grey parrots are between 0.96 and 1.22 mmol/L; any results below 0.75 mmol/L should be considered suspicious and the parrot treated.

If lead poisoning is suspected, then treatment should be undertaken whilst waiting for the result. Sodium di-calcium edetate may be injected safely as an undiluted intramuscular bolus; this seems to work as rapidly as a diluted intravenous bolus and is very safe. Improvement will be seen within 24 hours. The intestinal tract will have been inactive prior to treatment but quickly recovers, and the lead is often ground down by the grit in the gizzard over a 2-week period, providing that the antidote is given every other day. Treatment should continue for a week after the lead is seen to have gone on follow-up radiographs.

If the lead is not being removed by normal digestion it is possible to remove it in parrots by flushing it out of the gizzard. The bird should be anaesthetized, intubated, and suspended upside down at an angle of about 45°; a wide bore tube (the sheath from a 4 mm endoscope is ideal, or a 5 mm wide inflexible tube of some sort) is then introduced through the mouth and into the distal proventriculus. A small catheter is threaded through this tube until it is in the gizzard, and water from a syringe connected to the catheter is then used to flush the gizzard clear of grit and lead. Water at less than body temperature will rapidly cool the bird to a dangerous level of hypothermia. Peanut butter has been suggested as a gastrointestinal lubricant, but it is difficult to see how this works in vegetarian parrots that easily digest vegetable oils.

Calcium deficiency should also be corrected without waiting for the laboratory result if this will take some time. An oral bolus of calcium-rich vitamin and mineral supplement (Nutrobal, VetArk contains 200 mg of calcium per gram of powder) should be mixed with a small amount of food such as human baby cereal or parrot hand-rearing formula. Calcium-rich solutions usually contain far less calcium than powders, and hypertonic calcium solutions are unpalatable and will also cause the bird to regurgitate. An injection of multivitamins is not necessary and may even be contraindicated: excess vitamin D can remove calcium from already depleted bones and, being fat soluble, it will last longer than the oral calcium. Most hypocalcaemia cases are suffering from other dietary deficiencies, so twice daily crop tubing with hand-rearing formula and a calcium supplement is usually required for about 7 days for optimum results. Needless to say, correction of the diet is required long term.

If paramyxovirus (PMV) is suspected then a sample of serum should be sent to a laboratory for antibody levels. Paired samples may be necessary; 1 mL of clotted blood is usually sufficient, but if the birds are small then advice should be sought as to the most appropriate serotypes to test as it may not be possible to take 1 mL of blood safely.

Paralysis

Birds are frequently presented with weakness or even paralysis of their limb(s). This has usually developed over days to weeks and is rarely acute. Budgerigars seem frequently to be affected.

Firstly examine the bird in its cage and ascertain which leg is involved. Catch the bird and check the limb for swelling, crepitus or muscle wastage. Examine any closed ring to make sure that it has not become too tight and trapped the limb; this will cause gangrene. If the ring is too tight then it must be cut off. This will frequently require an anaesthetic, especially in larger birds. If there is crepitus, the leg must be examined radiographically and any fracture stabilized by internal or external fixation. If there is muscle wastage, the limb and also the whole body should be radiographed in two views.

Nerve injuries are quite a common cause of paralysis. In budgerigars the cause is often a tumour of the gonad or kidney; this may be seen radiographically, and can often be palpated through the abdominal wall. If the radiograph shows an amorphous visceral mass the tumour may be delineated by giving a barium meal, which will show the displacement of the intestines. Such tumours are invariably inoperable. Kidney infections can also cause a unilateral or bilateral paralysis. The lumbosacral plexus runs between the kidney and the pelvis and is therefore easily compressed by enlargement of the kidneys. Infection can spread from the kidney to the nerves, causing a neuritis and subsequent paresis. Most of these cases seem to be due to a coliform infection and respond to broad-spectrum antibiotic therapy.

Deficiency syndromes

Invariably, birds that have signs of a single nutritional deficiency will have more than one deficiency problem. Treatment of a single deficiency will allow the other deficiencies to show at a later date.

Calcium and phosphorus in the diet should be in 1.5–2.0 : 1 ratio. Seed diets have low calcium and may contain phytates, which further reduce the available calcium and phosphorus levels. Vitamin D precursors are present in vegetarian diets but require metabolism by ultraviolet light to be converted to the usable form: vitamin D_3.

Calcium and vitamin D_3 deficiencies will lead to egg-binding and osteoporosis in breeding birds and osteo-dystrophy in growing birds. Unobstructed egg-binding may be relieved by injecting calcium solution or administering it orally. Oxytocin may or may not be useful in these cases as the bird is more likely to be calcium deficient than oxytocin deficient. Osteodystrophy may result in fractures of long bones in adult laying birds as well as growing babies. Although only one limb may be fractured, the whole bird should be radiographed because other bones will be affected. Badly affected birds should be euthanized. Some cases may be repaired surgically.

Fits due to hypocalcaemia most commonly affect adult pet grey parrots that have had a seed diet and no access to sunshine except through glass windows (see earlier).

Vitamin A is essential for growth, optimum vision and maintaining the integrity of mucous membranes. Vitamin A deficiency predisposes to upper respiratory diseases and alimentary tract diseases by causing the mucous membrane's simple epithelium to become stratified, squamous, keratinized epithelium. The keratin plugs the ducts of the mucus-secreting and salivary glands, causing pustule formation and even salivary gland abscesses. In breeding birds there is decreased egg hatchability and in (poultry) chicks it prevents the kidneys from excreting uric acid which remains visible in the kidney and ureters (this is commonly seen in post-mortem examination of grey parrots, the species most frequently seen with hypovitaminosis A).

Vitamin E deficiency should be considered in pet, caged birds that have muscular weakness, and also in birds that are failing to come into breeding condition. It is especially common in cockatiels.

Iodine deficiency causes delayed moulting and feather disorders, as it is the usual cause of thyroid deficiency. The thyroid will become enlarged and may cause dyspnoea with 'squeaking' breathing and a change in vocalization.

Lack of sulphur-containing amino acids (commonly deficient in all seed diets) and polyunsaturated fatty acids affects the plumage. The feathers appear dry and brittle. Their feather barbs fail to interlock, and the feathers look hairy rather than intact. Dirty feathers can look similar: spray the bird daily with warm water.

Hyperglycaemia and fatty liver occur in a high percentage of cockatiels, Amazons, and many grey parrots on all-seed diets. All-in-one diets are the best way of overcoming this problem.

Infectious viral diseases

Avian influenza

Influenza viruses come in three groups; B and C affect humans and rarely birds; influenza type A affects birds and rarely humans. Avian influenza has affected parrots causing anything from no illness to sudden death; or death after depression, diarrhoea and neurological signs. However this is a virus that is rarely seen in parrots and most psittacine infections have occurred either in quarantine stations where it was caught from other birds in the quarantine station, or it has been caused experimentally. Avian influenza virus varies considerably in its pathogenicity, and the serotypes that affect poultry are not usually a great risk to parrots and vice versa.

Paramyxovirus

Newcastle disease (PMV-1) and several other paramyxovirus strains have caused disease in Psittaciformes. The signs can be peracute death; respiratory disease or gastrointestinal disease or a combination of both; chronic central nervous system disease (sudden onset and incurable opisthotonus, torticollis, tremors or paralysis). It is an uncommon disease in parrots, and is not seen in single pet birds. The disease is diagnosed on virus isolation from the trachea, lung and brain. This range of viruses will cross the species barrier very readily and is highly contagious.

Herpesvirus

This is the cause of Pacheco's parrot disease: a sudden-onset, usually overwhelming, hepatitis. Many birds that are ill will die. Some that recover and some that are subclinically infected will become lifelong symptom-free carriers. In stressed or low-grade unwell birds, e.g. imported birds in quarantine, the morbidity and mortality are high. In healthy birds that are well fed the morbidity seems to be much lower, but mortality is the same. Post-mortem signs include a very enlarged liver and some enlargement and darkening of spleen and kidneys. Histopathology reveals intranuclear inclusion bodies, and it is possible to isolate the virus. Treatment with aciclovir may work, but it is not known how this affects the carrier status of recovered birds. Vaccination with a dead vaccine is available in the USA, but not legally obtainable in Europe.

The virus is *not* the same as those affecting owls, hawks and pigeons, and there is no cross-infection from these species.

Psittacine beak and feather disease

This common disease is caused by a circovirus that occurs in wild Australian cockatoos but is known to be able to infect nearly all species of Psittaciformes. It has an affinity for growing cells and will therefore affect growing feathers, causing the feathers to drop out before maturation. The virus typically causes signs in younger birds. Contact with the virus during the growth period is the common method of infection, and feather dust from affected birds is highly infective; faeces less so. The bird becomes unwell, and the virus affects rapidly growing cells and will cause feather loss by preventing further feather growth in the fledging birds. The feathers lose their blood supply, pinch off at the base and fall out of the follicle; the quill will have a small, sharp, pinched-off appearance at its tip. The quantity of feather loss varies with the individual (Fig. 7.16). The virus will affect the rest of the skin and powder down, giving a dirty plumage and a black shiny beak, which is particularly evident in cockatoos. It will reduce horn production in the beak, and can also affect the bone marrow and cause a rapid and almost complete reduction in the heterophil count. Birds infected later in life have less obvious clinical signs, but as the disease progresses the bird becomes unwell with various secondary infections exacerbated by the suppression of the immune system. Growing feathers fall out and fail to regrow, and feather colouring can be affected: grey parrot feathers become pink (Fig. 7.17; see also Fig. 3.36), vasa parrot feathers become white instead of black (Fig. 7.18), and the beak and claws degenerate as the keratin is not formed at the base of the claw, allowing infection to cause a slough. The course of the disease is magnified by its immunosuppressive nature, but even when treated, affected birds always die, usually of secondary infections or organ failure. It is possible for adult birds to carry the disease, especially cockatoos. Young birds are most frequently seen infected, especially when hand reared. The earlier that they are infected, the more

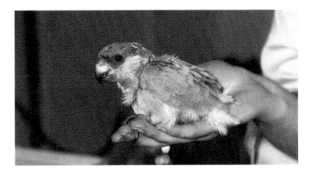

Fig 7.16 This young hand-reared Senegal parrot was brought for examination because its large wing and tail feathers were falling out. The breeders had a mixed collection of parrots, including 'healthy' cockatoos, none of which were tested for circovirus. The bird appeared very healthy but it had no powder down: its beak was clean and shiny and feathers were not dusty. A blood smear showed very few white blood cells and almost no heterophils. There were no actively growing feathers so a 23-gauge needle was used to obtain a small sample of bone marrow and blood using a proximal tibial approach. This was positive for circovirus using a PCR test.

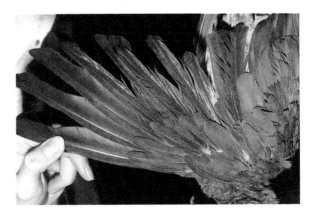

Fig 7.17 This 2-year-old Timneh grey parrot was unwell. It had been kept in the presence of pet cockatiels and other parakeets by its owner since acquiring it at 10 weeks old. The bird was anaesthetized for radiography. Its newly growing primary and secondary feathers were deformed and instead of being uniform grey they were pale in some areas and pink in others. Feather pulp from this bird was positive for circovirus on a PCR test.

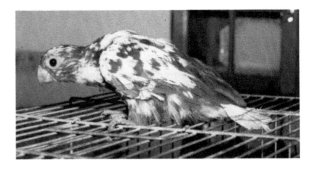

Fig 7.18 Vasa parrot with PBFD, showing white feathers instead of dark grey.

rapid and dramatic is the disease. Haematology in many cases, especially from grey parrots, Senegal parrots and other African parrots, will show severe depression of the heterophil numbers and, on occasions, anaemia and a general leucopenia. These birds may not necessarily show beak deformity or much feather loss. Definitive diagnosis is by a PCR test using a DNA probe produced by the University of Georgia, which is available in Europe and America via commercial veterinary laboratories. This test will confirm the presence of the virus in live feather pulp, which is the best method for clinical cases. Symptom-free carriers should be detected by a PCR test on a sample of blood (or better still, bone marrow) as well as feather pulp.

This infection is a common subclinical problem in many captive budgerigars. It is one of the causes of 'French moult' where the budgerigar fails to grow its major feathers and is doomed to run around the floor of the cage. Subclinically infected budgerigars in pet shops shed the virus and this commonly infects baby parrots that are being sold from the shop as well. The virus survives in feather dust for long periods.

Polyomavirus

This is a widespread infection in Psittaciformes, but was first called budgerigar fledgling disease (BFD). Budgerigars have BFDV-1, the rest of the parrots BFDV-3 (polyomavirus will also affect finches). Budgerigar chicks can die in the first few weeks of life – either suddenly, or with abdominal distension, subcutaneous haemorrhages and ataxia. Some cases are more chronic and develop dystrophic primary and secondary wing feathers and tail feathers but do not die; this form is more commonly seen in the UK. These cases resemble PBFD. Other species of psittacine birds, when affected by polyomavirus, can be very ill at weaning with non-specific weight loss, anorexia, partial paralysis of the gut, polyuria and watery droppings. They have a tendency to haemorrhage easily, and may have CNS signs. Not all the birds get the disease and not all of those affected die; some (especially the older birds) recover to become symptom-free carriers. Diagnosis using a PCR test can be made using cloacal swabs or tissues from post-mortem examination. A vaccine has become available in the USA.

Fungal diseases

Candida

This yeast infection is more commonly seen in birds kept in high humidity and warm temperatures. It is more common in birds being hand reared and kept in brooders and in birds in tropical climates – it is a common pathogen in Florida but less common in Yorkshire. Affected birds develop caseous lesions in the commissure of the beak, around the tongue and palate (Fig. 7.19) and the lining of the crop has the gross appearance likened to a Turkish towel. Because the yeast invades below the surface, ketoconazole and itraconazole are more effective treatments than nystatin and amphotericin B.

Aspergillosis

This fungus invades the lungs and air sacs, and it is a common cause of dyspnoea and weight loss in parrots. It is more common in birds that are stressed, on a poor diet, or in contact with large numbers of spores due to a damp and dirty environment. It is frequently seen in imported birds. Old and dirty travelling boxes are also a source of this disease. Occasionally it invades the syrinx and causes dyspnoea and a loss of (or change in) voice. Diagnosis is by radiography, which will show a loculated appearance of the air sacs as well as densities in the lung tissue. Confirmation using endoscopy and

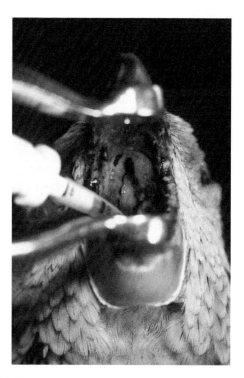

Fig 7.19 The typical appearance of a parrot whose oral cavity is infected with *Candida*. A smear made from the material coating the palate showed masses of Gram-positive yeasts. The injury to the commissures of the mouth is also typical of this disease. The bird has been anaesthetized and intubated for this examination and for endoscopy of the upper alimentary tract.

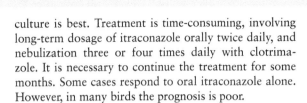

culture is best. Treatment is time-consuming, involving long-term dosage of itraconazole orally twice daily, and nebulization three or four times daily with clotrimazole. It is necessary to continue the treatment for some months. Some cases respond to oral itraconazole alone. However, in many birds the prognosis is poor.

Syringeal aspergillosis cases should be referred to an avian veterinary specialist; they are difficult to treat because the blockage in the trachea has to be removed. These cases also have a poor prognosis.

Some parrots, especially Amazons, develop *Aspergillus* abscesses in the nasal passages; see 'Sinusitis'.

Poisons

Lead

This is a very common poison in parrots. The bird becomes unwell, goes off its food, becomes unsteady on its legs and finally starts to convulse. Sources include old (usually white) painted wood; soldered joints in old, repaired cages; lead from windows and other sources. Hard core (quarry-waste) used as a base for outside aviaries may contain lead ores and has been seen as a source of lead in Yorkshire parrots! The lead particles are often seen on a radiograph (Fig. 7.15); grit is less radiodense. Some cases are not obvious, and a blood sample should be submitted to a laboratory. Much of the lead is in the erythrocytes, so 0.5 mL of whole unclotted blood should be sent in lithium heparin, *not* in EDTA. Intramuscular injection of undiluted di-calcium sodium edetate, is a low-risk, effective treatment (0.25 to 0.75 mL). An intramuscular injection works as well as an intravenous dose. Treatment should be given to all cases where lead poisoning is suspected, even prior to confirmation in doubtful cases. The dose should be administered after taking the blood sample.

Teflon®

Over-heating non-stick pans, even for a short time, causes the PTFE coating to depolymerize and form highly toxic, volatile fumes. Birds in the same airspace invariably die quickly after exposure with a dramatic pneumonia. Beware – some heat lamps are also Teflon®-coated. There is no treatment.

Zinc

'New wire disease' is sometimes seen in birds that are placed in newly meshed aviaries, and zinc toxicity may be suspected in birds that become chronically unwell in new cages. The diagnosis may be confirmed on blood samples, but the blood tubes must not have rubber stoppers or gaskets as some of these compounds contain enough zinc to provide a false-positive result (this should be checked with the laboratory in advance).

The source of zinc is either the white powdery coating found on the new wire (known as white rust), or lumps of zinc galvanizing that are chewed off the wire. Both cause zinc toxicity (Howard 1992). Zinc does not remain in the body and is quickly removed once ingestion has stopped; there is no evidence that EDTA treatment is useful. Lumps of metal in the gizzard should be removed by endoscopic retrieval, by flushing the gizzard under anaesthetic, or by surgical exploration of the gizzard through an incision in the proventriculus – these cases should be referred! Washing the white rust off the new wire with dilute acetic acid before introducing the birds into a new aviary is preventative.

Diseases of the integument

As with dogs and cats the range of signs of skin disease is limited, but the aetiologies for a particular set of signs may be diverse.

Standard examination procedures apply: the bird and its cage are observed. Is the patient the only inmate or is there more than one bird? What signs is the bird showing of skin disease? Is it pruritic; if so where and how often is it irritated? Is there feather loss, if so have the owners brought a feather? Is the bird bald because of feather loss or failure to regrow feathers, or both? Are there other signs of general illness: lethargy, inappetence, PU/PD, etc.? Once this inspection is complete, remove the bird from the cage and examine it conscious.

The head, beak and eyes should be examined first, including a check inside the beak. Note any abscesses, etc. (see vitamin A deficiency). Is the beak smooth and shiny (usually abnormal) or is it covered with a fine white powder (normal for most psittacine species)?

Each wing should be examined: spread the wing fully and inspect it both dorsally and ventrally. Examine feather stubs if they are chewed or cut short. Hold the wing open and look through the feathers towards a light: note any pinprick holes in the feathers through which the light shines. Examine the down feathers on the body under the wing: these are 'powder down' feathers (Fig. 7.1). Powder down is produced by the tips of these feathers breaking free and forming a fine white dust that is a feature of healthy parrot integument. Pigeons, toucans, storks and herons also have powder down, most other birds do not. Examine the feathers and skin over the rest of the body, as well as the feet and claws. The scaly skin should be supple and not be crusty; the claws should be smooth, dry and sharply pointed at their tips and there should be no discharge from their base. The toes should flex and extend normally. Look at the entire integument, including the preen gland. This is situated on the dorsal surface at the base of the tail. It is poorly developed in parrots and is totally absent in some families (such as Amazons and pionus parrots). The function of the preen gland can be checked by wiping a finger over the papilla; a normal gland will leave a greasy streak on the digit: underactivity is common and these glands leave nothing at all on your finger. Any enlargement should be viewed with suspicion.

In many case it is rewarding to examine the bird under anaesthetic. Look for external parasites: these are very uncommon in parrots, and even less commonly cause irritation or skin disease. If found, they can be identified from the website www.federmilben.de – look in the gallery. Examine broken or chewed feathers, especially at the base where they enter the skin as this can reveal pyoderma. Pluck a growing feather or two for PBFD testing (full details under specific virus diseases). Skin scrapings can be taken and are a useful way of looking for fungi, yeasts, bacteria, etc. using cytology and culture.

Some parrots get infection in their growing feathers. This can be identified by a darker colour and abnormal appearance of the follicles. It is useful to remove the contents aseptically and confirm the presence of infection by cytology and culture of the contents.

Skin biopsies are not as useful as in cats and dogs, since the integument is very fine, and even competent dermatopathologists can fail to find signs of disease in apparently grossly affected skin. However, if a biopsy is needed, a full thickness of skin (NB: with no preoperative preparation) should be taken with scissors and should include some normal and abnormal feather follicles. Multiple biopsies should be obtained and spread on paper or pinned to a wooden tongue depressor with 25-gauge hypodermic needles; then fixed in formol saline by floating the paper/wood with the skin immersed in the fixative Usually the skin deficit is sutured using fine soluble suture material. Biopsies should be taken from specific lesions or skin on the trunk of the body, remembering that the feathers grow from specific areas (feather tracts) separated by areas of skin with no feathers. Do not remove any major feather follicles from the wing or tail, as these feathers cannot regrow.

Lateral and ventrodorsal radiographs are useful to rule out internal disease such as air sacculitis, abscesses, liver disease, etc. A blood sample may do the same. Internal disease may cause birds to chew the area of their body over the internal lesion; these areas are not bilaterally symmetrical, see below.

Bald birds

Feather loss on the head is rarely self-inflicted. Some birds can be made bald by over-zealous head preening by a 'loving' mate (common in *Pionus* spp.). Occasionally birds become bald by fighting with other birds, but other lesions are usually evident in such cases. Soft food may become matted to the facial feathers in adults or youngsters being reared, and this will cause a skin infection.

The mat and feathers will be shed, leaving patches of feather loss around the face.

It is important at the outset to rule out circovirus as a cause of feather loss. Cases where there is a loss of powder down, low white blood cell count (especially in grey parrots), feathers that have died during growth, birds with beak abnormalities, and birds that have had contact with potential or known carriers of circovirus should be tested.

Feather picking or plucking is a common problem in parrots, especially grey parrots, cockatoos, cockatiels and macaws. These are nearly always hand-reared birds, even when imported, and they are usually socially deprived (kept on their own) and hormonally active (more often presented at the start of the breeding season). The birds are first presented appearing to be irritable with parts of their integument, pulling violently at their claws or feathers. They may start chewing at the cut base of their clipped wing feathers, or even chew off normal tail and wing feathers. They may decide to pull contour feathers out completely; common sites are around the neck and over the shoulders, under the wings on the body, and down the back. The feather-plucking bird often produces bilaterally symmetrical lesions. Some birds, especially cockatoos and lovebirds, will mutilate themselves so badly that they will chew through the skin into the subcutis and even into muscle. These birds should be checked for circovirus as this may be an underlying factor that will prevent recovery. Some birds, such as conures, will pull out or chew off their feathers when stressed by an environmental change; this may happen when the bird is admitted as an inpatient, which is embarrassing for the veterinarian.

Many feather-plucking birds have higher levels of (faecal) corticosterone than normal; this is an indication of increased levels of stress (Owen & Lane 2006).

Occasionally unilateral bald areas are produced. These should be investigated as they may be indicative of internal disease in that area. Amazon and pionus parrots can be affected by behavioural problems too, but seldom pluck their feathers right out. They will 'scissor' off parts of feathers, or appear much more irritated with their integument and will chew the skin on their legs violently; use their feet to scratch violently at their flanks; hang on their cage bars and rub their bodies on the cage as if very irritated by some skin problem. Again this is seen in birds that are hormonally active and socially deprived and it is more common in hand-reared birds. As with grey parrots, mites are exceedingly rare and are unlikely to be the cause of these signs.

Many cases where parrots are feather plucking are incurable, but some respond well. Treatment for feather pluckers should include dietary advice and environmental enrichment with toys and tree branches, etc. Companionship may be very useful if the patient is able to recognize and therefore respond to another bird.

In many cases the bird is so strongly imprinted on humans that it fails to recognize other parrots. The owner should be discouraged from too much sensual physical contact with the bird (e.g. stroking of neck or rump), as this reinforces the problem. It is very difficult to replace the social interaction seen in a flock of parrots within a captive pet environment.

Hormonal suppression can work in some cases, but progestogens will cause polyphagia and polydipsia and may well exacerbate occult metabolic problems. Drugs used for behavioural problems in humans can be useful. Diazepam in the drinking water (3 drops in 30 mL of water), haloperidol (0.4 mg/kg) or fluoxetine (Prozac) (1 mg/kg) have all been suggested. In some cases the medication is required at times of maximum hormonal influence and in other cases it is for life. However, prescribing these drugs should *not* be a first line of treatment for every plucking bird: all cases should be thoroughly investigated for possible causes.

Pruritic birds

External parasites are very uncommon in parrots, except for *Cnemidocoptes pilae* that causes 'scaly face' in budgerigars. These mites live in tunnels in the epidermis and cause considerable skin thickening (Figs 7.20A and B). The mite can easily be killed with an injection or oral dose of ivermectin (200 µg/kg), repeated after 2 weeks. Red mites can cause problems in aviary birds and, occasionally, pet birds. The mites are only active at night, and the birds chew their legs. Mite control may be necessary on the birds, but the environment must also be treated. Fipronil (Frontline Spray, Merial) is very effective; a squirt under each wing usually removes external parasites such as mites and lice. Feather lice and mites in birds tend to be species-specific, and as such are uncommon on parrots in the UK – presumably when they have been removed there is no reservoir from which they can return.

Most pruritic parrots have some definable behavioural problem, a pyoderma, or internal disease such as hepatitis, air sacculitis or an internal abscess.

Pyoderma

Areas of thickened, sore and crusted skin may be due to a pyoderma. Bacteriology, cytology and skin biopsy are all required for a definitive diagnosis. Appropriate antimicrobial therapy is required, often for some weeks or occasionally months. Attention must be paid to selecting the correct antibiotic: drug sensitivity of the pathogen, method of drug administration and the pharmacodynamics of the drug must be integrated for successful results. If the lesion is not resolving in spite of adequate treatment, the bird may have a behavioural problem.

The beak may also become infected; this is more usually caused by poor nutrition and trauma than by a primary pathogen. The virus causing psittacine beak and feather disease is the exception, and degenerative lesions in the beak and claws are highly suspicious of this disease (Fig. 7.21). A PCR test should be performed to look for the virus in all birds showing degenerative beak lesions. Dermatophytes are also able to infect birds, and these usually give a very crusty appearance. Again a scraping (or cytology and culture) is required. It can be difficult to know if some fungi are a secondary problem or primary pathogens. *Aspergillus* and *Candida* should be viewed with suspicion as primary pathogens in the

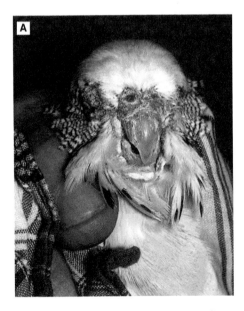

Fig 7.20A A budgerigar showing the typical appearance of cnemidocoptic mange. The bird was injected with ivermectin.

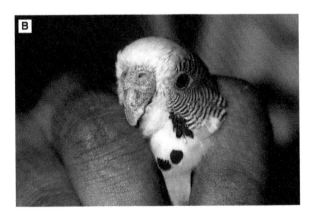

Fig 7.20B The same bird after 4 weeks. It had received two injections 2 weeks apart. This budgerigar has the typical feathers of an adult 'normal' bird; compare with Figure 7.2.

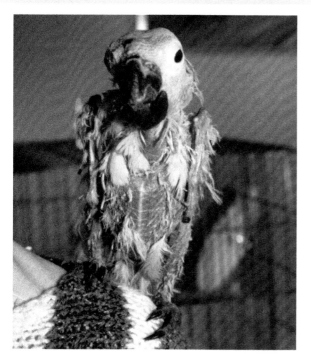

Fig 7.21 Degenerated beak in a cockatoo with advanced PBFD.

up in the feather's structure causing similar problems. Many birds on a poor diet become thyroid hormone deficient, and this results in failure to moult and grow new feathers. Always check with the owner when the bird moulted last – did it change all its feathers, have they grown in normally? A parrot should have a bloom, or fine covering of powder down.

Feathers may be found showing bands of differing colour. This is usually due to dietary change or ill health whilst the feather was growing, and may be mirrored by a line of changed keratin in the beak. Breaks in nutrition in growing feathers will cause lines of weakness (fret marks or stress bars). These are usually seen in young birds and occur in *all* the feathers that are growing, causing a line of weakness across all the tail or wing feathers. Fret marks can be found in isolation on feathers, and in these cases are usually formed by quill mites (*Syringophilus* spp.) which have eaten part of the growing feather when it was curled up in the erupting sheath. These mites are very difficult to demonstrate: look in a KOH-cleared squash preparation from the mid-third of the growing feather shaft of an affected feather. This mite seems to affect young birds more frequently than adults.

Beak and claw diseases

The beak can be injured by another bird. If the upper beak is bitten off completely then it is impossible to replace; the best that can be achieved is the production of a fibrous pad after granulation, and these birds manage surprisingly well. Small holes through the beak or injuries from flying into wire mesh will heal with antibiotic therapy and good husbandry. Macaws are prone to developing beak deformity whilst growing and young birds can be presented with the upper beak twisting to one side. Cockatoos become 'undershot' with the upper beak bending ventrally and going inside the lower beak, rather than outside. These cases should be corrected, and are easiest to do while the bird is still growing. There are several specialist techniques for doing this.

Loss or injury of a normal claw or the end of a digit is usually made good by the bird itself as it will often chew the digit back to healthy tissue. However, birds are sometimes seen with dry gangrene of the digit or a bitten, mangled toe. The bird should be anaesthetized, the digit amputated to healthy tissue, and the skin sutured with fine, soluble suture material. The surgical site should be kept clean, dry and open to the air and a 5-day course of antibiotic should be given.

The virus responsible for psittacine beak and feather disease is common; full details of its effects are given under 'Infectious viral diseases', but changes will be found in the beak and claws.

UK, as they are not encouraged to grow in our colder and less humid climate (unlike in most of the USA).

Xanthoma

Thickened yellow skin can occur in any permanently featherless area as a normal reaction of the body, but occasionally birds are presented with a massively swollen, thickened area of yellow skin (see Figs 3.31 and 3.32). This requires surgical intervention.

Feather damage and defects

The normal feather should be able to maintain its structure with routine preening from the bird. The barbules should all be interlocked, giving the feather a firm and unbroken appearance. The growing quills should emerge from the sheath and the sheath should fall away, allowing the feather to unfurl and form a normal shape; the colour of the feather should also be normal. Nutritional defects are a common cause of feather problems. Seed is deficient in sulphur-containing amino acids, and this will give very poor quality feathers, as will a lack of essential fatty acids: the feathers have poor colour, the barbules separate and the feather fails to lock into its correct shape. In birds that are not allowed to bathe or are not sprayed, dirt will build

References

Blackmore D K 1963 The incidence and aetiology of thyroid dysplasia in budgerigars. Veterinary Record 75:1068–1072

Clubb S L, Karpinski L 1993 Aging in macaws. Journal of the Association of Avian Veterinarians 7(1):31–33

Collar N J 1997 Psittacidae (parrots). In: Handbook of birds of the world, Vol IV, Sandgrouse to cuckoos. Lynx edicions, Barcelona, p 280–477

Dorrestein G, de Wit M 2005 Clinical pathology and necropsy. In: Harcourt-Brown N, Chitty J (eds) BSAVA Manual of psittacine birds, 2nd edn. BSAVA, Cheltenham, p 60–86

Dunning J B 1993 Handbook of avian body masses. CRC Press, London

Forshaw J M, Cooper W T 1973 Parrots of the world. Lansdowne Press, Melbourne

Graham D L 1991 Internal papillomatous disease – a pathologist's view. Proceedings of the Conference of the Association of Avian Veterinarians, p 141–143

Gregory C R, Latimer K S, Campagnoli R P, Ritchie B W 1996 Histologic evaluation of the crop for diagnosis of proventricular dilatation syndrome in psittacine bird. Journal of Veterinary Diagnostic Investigation 8:76–80

Harcourt-Brown N H 1986 Diseases of birds in quarantine, with special reference to the treatment of *Salmonella typhimurium* by vaccination: a novel technique. Proceedings of the British Veterinary Zoological Society, London

Harcourt-Brown N H 2003 The incidence of juvenile osteodystrophy in hand-reared grey parrots (*Psittacus e. erithacus*). Veterinary Record 152(14):438–439

Howard B R 1992 Health risks of housing small psittacines in galvanised wire mesh cages. Journal of the American Veterinary Medical Association 200(11):1667–1674

Low R, undated. Parrot breeding. Rob Harvey, Farnham

Morange A 1895 De la psittacose, ou infection speciale determine par des perruches. Thesis, Paris, 1895

Newton A 1896 Cockateel. In: A dictionary of birds. Black, London, p 92

Owen D J, Lane J M 2006 High levels of corticosterone in feather-plucking parrots (*Psittacus erithacus*). Veterinary Record 158:804

Phalen D N, Tomaszewski E, Wilson V G 1998 Internal papillomatosis: a herpesvirus connection? Proceedings of the Association of Avian Veterinarians, St Paul, MN, p 45–48

Rowley I 1997 Cacatuidae (cockatoos). In: Handbook of birds of the world, Vol IV, Sandgrouse to cuckoos. Lynx edicions, Barcelona, p 246–279

Russ K 1890 Diseases. In: The speaking parrots. Upcott Gill, London, p 52–76

Sibley C G, Ahlquist J E 1990 Parrots. In: Phylogeny and classification of birds. Yale University Press, New Haven, CT, p 380–390

Storm J, Greenwood A G 1993 Fluoroscopic investigation of the avian gastrointestinal tract. Proceedings of the European Conference of Avian Medicine and Surgery, p 170–177

Zürn F A 1882 Krankeiten des hausgeflügels (The diseases of household birds). Weimar

Further reading

Members of the parrot family:

Collar N J 1997 Psittacidae (parrots). In: Handbook of birds of the world, Vol IV, Sandgrouse to cuckoos. Lynx edicions, Barcelona, p 280–477

Rowley I 1997 Cacatuidae (cockatoos). In: Handbook of birds of the world, Vol IV, Sandgrouse to cuckoos. Lynx edicions, Barcelona, p 246–279

General husbandry and breeding:

Low R 1992 Parrots, their care and breeding. Blandford/Cassell, Poole, Dorset

Budgerigars:

Moizer S 1988 Budgerigars: a complete guide. Merehurst Press

Feeding birds and their responses:

Carey C (ed) 1996 Avian energetics and nutritional ecology. Chapman & Hall, New York

Stanford M 2005 Nutrition and nutritional disease. In: Harcourt-Brown N, Chitty J (eds) BSAVA Manual of psittacine birds, 2nd edn. BSAVA, Cheltenham, p 136–154

Passerines

Gerry M. Dorrestein

8

Introduction

Many veterinarians are relatively unfamiliar with the passerines. The aviculture, diagnostic procedures, and common diseases and their treatment will be discussed in this chapter, based on previous and recent publications (Dorrestein 1997a, Hawkins 2003, Sandmeier & Coutteel 2006).

Owners of passerines (songbirds) are utilizing veterinary care in increasing numbers as aviculturists recognize the advances in avian medical and surgical treatment of these patients.

The order Passeriformes contains between 5000 and 5700 different species (Sibley & Ahlquist 1990, Gill 1994), with body weights ranging from 4.8 to 1350 g. Toucans and mynahs are often grouped together, but are from different taxonomic orders. Toucans are members of the family Ramphastidae (order Piciformes); mynahs are members of the family Sturnidae (order Passeriformes). The toucans are described in Chapter 14 (Ramphastids). Relevant information related to mynahs will be discussed in this chapter.

Diseases in these avian species are often influenced by nutrition, housing and stress. For a complete understanding of diseases associated with problems of passerines, including diagnosis and treatment, clinicians must become familiar with the aviculture, housing and husbandry of their patients. Supportive care and measures to minimize stress are often needed to maintain the host's defence mechanisms.

Biology and husbandry

Passerines (perching or song birds) constitute more than half the species of birds in the world. They represent a diverse, species-rich, monophyletic order of mostly small land birds (Gill 1994). The most common representatives of the passerines in captivity are canaries, finches and mynahs.

Canaries

The canary (*Serinus canaria*) is the best-known representative of the songbirds. Canaries have been domesticated since 1400, and are bred and kept for different reasons: their song (e.g. the Roller canary, the Harzer, Waterslager, Timbrado or the American Singer); as coloured canaries, including the melanin (black, brown, agate, isabel) and lipochrome (red, yellow, white) groups; their build and shape like type canaries, including frilled canaries, e.g. North Dutch frill and Gibber Italico; type breeds, e.g. Japan Hoso, Yorkshire; shape breeds, e.g. Border Fancy and Norwich; crest and crest bred, e.g. Gloster; and feather pattern, e.g. Lizard, the oldest true breed canary (Coutteel 2003) (Fig. 8.1). The black-hooded red siskin (*Spinus cucullatus*) is the source of the red pigment that is added to the canary's genetic make-up, and is clearly in evidence in the red canary. The birds live approximately 6–16 years, are monomorphic and weigh 15–25 g. This longevity related to the small body size is typical for songbirds. Within the large songbird family Fringillidae (true finches), and especially the canary, mass-specific basal metabolic rates, longevity, longevity residuals and lifetime expenditure of energy are all positively correlated with the rate of cytochrome *b* evolution (Rottenberg 2007).

Finches

There are almost 1000 species of finches and other weaver relatives. They incorporate Old World granivorous and insectivorous birds, including weaver birds and estrildine finches; the ground-living wagtails, pipits, and accentors; the nectar-feeding sunbirds and flowerpeckers; sugarbirds and a few Australasian taxa; and

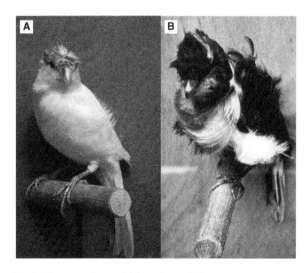

Fig 8.1 The North Dutch frill (**A**) and Gloster (**B**) canary.

the New World wood warblers, tanagers, and blackbirds, diagnosed by a strongly reduced tenth primary (Gill 1994).

The more domesticated species of finches and weavers have been bred in captivity for many decades, but many finches are still imported from Asia and Africa. There is a significant size disparity between the common finch pets (the smallest is the gold-breasted waxbill at 7 g, the largest is the Java rice sparrow at 20 g). Most common finches belong to the families Fringillidae and Estrildidae. Examples of commonly kept Fringillidae (true finches, approximately 150 species) are canaries (*Serinus canaria*), greenfinches (*Carduelis chloris*), goldfinches (*C. carduelis*), siskin (*C. spinus*), bullfinches (*Pyrrhula pyrrhula*) and chaffinches (*Fringilla coelebs*). Estrildidae (approximately 125 species) originating from Africa, Asia and Australia include waxbills, e.g. zebra finch (*Poephila guttata*) and Lady Gouldian or Gouldian finch (*Chloebia gouldiae*), nuns, e.g. spice finch (*Lonchura punctulata*), and parrot finches, e.g. the parrot finch (*Erythrura psittacea*). The finches are kept for breeding, but also as ornamental birds. Bengalese or society finches (*Lonchura striata domestica*) and zebra finches are used as foster parents for breeding Australian finches. This gives special problems, because they can be carriers of diseases that can kill the foster-fledglings – e.g. cochlosomosis and *Campylobacter* spp. infections. Conversely, using foster parents may prevent some infectious diseases that are transmitted from infected parent to offspring. For example, colonies of Gouldian finches that are air sac mite-free have been established by using society finches, which are not susceptible to air sac mites, as foster parents (Macwhirter 1994). One of the major disadvantages of fostered birds is that they imprint on the foster parents, and may therefore be less likely to breed with their own species. For species-specific imprinting to occur, a finch should be exposed to its own species from the fifteenth to the fortieth days of life.

Mynahs

Mynahs (*Gracula* spp.) and starlings are members of the Sturnidae (Passeriformes), a family of insect- and fruit/berry-eating songbirds consisting of over 110 species. They are commonly referred to as grackles. **The mynahs have the unique ability to mimic the human voice, and are often maintained as a single pet bird. The most common species is the hill mynah (*G. religiosa*), which has seven subspecies and originates from Southeast Asia.**

Africa, India and Southeast Asia comprise the native range of other mynah species. The veterinary approach of these pet birds is comparable to that for the psittacine birds. Other species commonly kept are the *Leucospar rothschildi* (Bali or Rothschild's mynah) and *Acridotheres* spp. (common mynahs). The Bali mynah

is a critically endangered species, and is involved in an intensive captive breeding and reintroduction programme (Norton et al 1995). The average body weight of the lesser Indian hill mynah (*G. r. indica*) is 110–130 g, that of the Java hill mynah (*G. r. intermedia*) is 150–200 g, and that of the greater hill mynah (*G. r. religiosa*) 210–270 g (Korbel & Kösters 1998).

Starlings

The starlings include the pagoda starling (*Temenuchus pagodarum*), the superb glossy starling (*Lamprospreo superbus*) and purple glossy starling (*Lamprotornis purpureus*). These birds are predominantly kept as aviary birds.

Basic anatomy and physiology

All birds have high basal metabolic rates (BMRs) and, for their various sizes, passerine birds have the highest rates of any group of vertebrate animals (Fig. 8.2). The average basal metabolic rate of a passerine bird (k = 129) is 50–60% higher than that of a non-passerine (k = 78) of the same body size (Walsberg 1983, Gill 1994; see also Appendices 6.5 and 6.6). The body temperature of passerines is about 2°C higher (about 42°C) than in non-passerines.

While some desert passerines (such as the zebra finch) have been known to survive months without drinking water, most small passerine birds drink 250–300 mL/kg body weight daily, and may eat up to 30% of their body weight daily (Macwhirter 1994).

Nestling estrildid finches normally have characteristic luminous mouth markings. Mucosal patterns are species-specific, and help to guide parents to their own chicks within the recesses of dark nests. Although most perching birds have anisodactyl feet, with three forward toes and one rear toe (the hallux or first digit), at least nine groups, including Piciformes (woodpeckers and toucans), most Psittaciformes, Strigiformes (owls) and Musophagiformes (turacos), have zygodactyl feet, with two forward (D2 and D3) and two rear toes (D1 and D4) (Gill 1994; Fig. 8.3).

The anatomy of the digestive tract varies depending on the species' feeding pattern. A bird's bill is its key adaptation for feeding, and the size, shape and strength of the beak prescribe the potential diet. Most passerines that specialize in seed-eating crack and shuck the seed husk with powerful bills. Finches extract seed kernels by either crushing or cutting the seed hull. These finches are called thick-bills, in contrast to the insect/berry-eating small-billed finches.

A crop and a large, strong, muscular gizzard (ventriculus), covered on the inside with a strongly polymerized koilin layer, is present in grain/seed-eating species

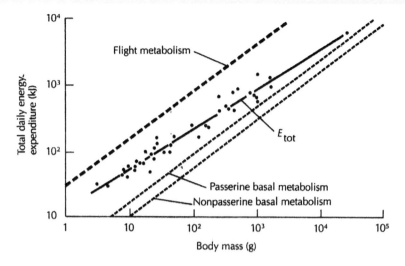

Fig 8.2 Passerine birds have higher metabolic rates than non-passerines (Gill 1994).

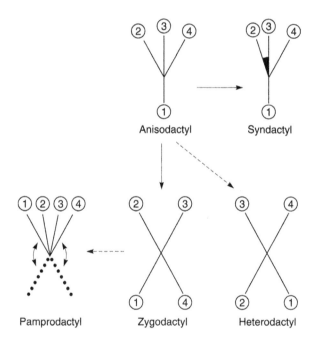

Fig 8.3 Schematic diagrams of differing foot structures of avian species.

such as finches, but not in species such as honey-eaters that consume nectar and soft foods. In birds that are insect-eaters in the summer, the gizzard becomes smaller and less muscular at that time. In the wintertime the food consists of dry seeds, and the weight of the gizzard can increase by 25–30%. In mynahs the crop is absent, and the ventriculus has (in contrast with seed-eaters) an obvious lumen with a moderately muscular wall.

If present, caeca are generally small and vestigial and play no role in digestion. None of the birds of these orders have an obvious permanent bacterial intestinal flora. However, in spite of a relatively short intestinal tract (in canaries it is approximately 31.1 cm) and a fast passage of chyme, seeds show high digestibility rates of starch (88–90%) and fat (97–99%). Research in canaries, rice finches and budgerigars has shown that maltase, saccharase, amylase and lipase are all present at much higher activity levels than in other species such as the dog, pig, horse and poultry (Wolf et al 1997). It also appears that the activity of the enzymes is markedly influenced by different foodstuffs (Martinez del Rio et al 1996, Wolf et al 1997).

The mynahs have no caecum and an intestinal tract that is shorter and wider than the seed-eating passerines, pigeons or psittacines. Passeriformes have gall bladders, in contrast to Columbiformes and Psittaciformes. The spleen in most passerines is long rather than spherical, as it is in Galliformes and Psittaciformes (Fig. 8.4).

In most Passeriformes, the right and left nasal sinuses do not communicate. In cases of bilateral nasal discharge, a sample for cytological examination should be taken from both the left and right sinuses.

Singing ability is highly developed in many passerine species, and is related to the complexity of the syringeal anatomy. Sounds result from the vibration of a thin membrane (membrana tympanica), the tension and position of which are controlled by syringeal muscles and air pressure in the interclavicular air sac. Many birds can stimulate each side of the syrinx independently, and thus can sing duets with themselves (Gill 1994). Roller canaries are specifically bred and trained for their singing ability.

Male canaries will usually sing best in the spring, in response to the endogenous testosterone 'surge'. If a bird becomes ill it may stop singing, and may not start vocalization until the following spring, even though the initial illness has resolved. In contrast, some canaries (even some females) sing all year round, and birds that stop singing because of illness begin singing as soon as their general condition improves. **Testosterone injections to induce singing should be discouraged, because testosterone has a negative feedback that causes shrinking of the testes and reduced fertility (Macwhirter 1994).**

The ability to mimic the human voice is well developed in some passerines, notably mynahs, starlings, mockingbirds and corvids. Fifteen to twenty per cent of the passerines in most regions of the world practise vocal mimicry (Gill 1994).

Like psittacines (but unlike ratites and penguins), passerines have a highly developed neopulmic and paleopulmonic parabronchi system. This allows for highly efficient oxygen exchange. In most passerines the cranial thoracic air sacs are fused to the single median clavicular sac, making a total of seven air sacs as opposed to the nine air sacs in psittacine species.

Housing

The small passeriform birds are kept in captivity both as individual pet birds and as flocks in two different types of aviaries: mixed ornamental and breeding aviaries. The former type is usually located outside and different species are kept together, mostly for ornamental purposes (Fig. 8.5). In the latter, large numbers of the same species are maintained, mostly indoors, for breeding and selecting. Breeders often go to shows and competitions, and there is frequently an exchange of birds (and possibly pathogens) (Fig. 8.6).

In mixed aviaries the bird population is less dense, and species-specific diseases are restricted to only a few

of the occupants. The birds are in the aviary all year, with a shed for shelter and a flight outside. Planted aviaries are popular for these passerines, because the vegetation provides observers with a more natural view of a bird's behaviour (Fig. 8.7). Planted aviaries can cause problems when trying to control microorganisms and medicate diseased birds (Macwhirter 1994). These plantings, however, are often necessary to get breeding results. For feather care in mixed ornamental aviaries, the birds should have access to water and/or sand-baths. In breeding aviaries, the housing depends on the season. Today, canaries are mostly bred indoors, and during the breeding season the birds are generally maintained as couples in small box-type cages approximately $50 \times 40 \times 40 \, cm$ (Fig. 8.8). Normally the fancier allows the birds to lay two to three clutches using artificial lighting (Fig. 8.9). The weanlings are housed in communal flights, with or

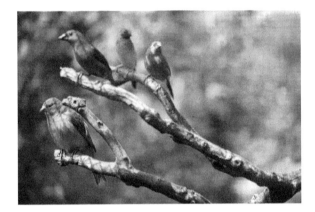

Fig 8.5 A mixed ornamental aviary. Left to right green canary (*Serinus canaria*), parrot finch (*Erythrura* sp.), star finch (*Neochmia ruficauda*) and blue waxbill (*Uraeginthus angolensis*).

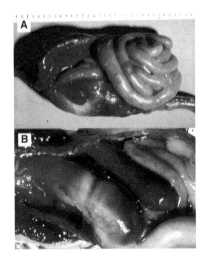

Fig 8.4 Normal spleen of a canary (**A**) compared to the splenomegaly as seen in atoxoplasmosis (**B**).

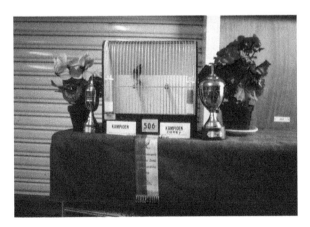

Fig 8.6 A Lady Gouldian finch (*Chloebia gouldii*) as champion of a bird show.

without outside quarters. In the winter season (resting season), the males and females are housed as separate groups in pens. Singing canaries are housed individually in small sing-cages (21 × 20 × 15 cm) for more than 5 months to be trained and enter singing competitions. The breeding aviaries are relatively easy to clean.

The mynahs should be kept in aviaries because of their size and need for exercise. Mynahs make a mess with their food and produce copious amounts of fluid droppings, which makes them less suitable as indoor house pets. The best form of indoor housing is a box-cage with an open ceiling and front; it should have a minimum floor area of 100 × 60–70 cm, and a height of at least 70 cm (Korbel & Kösters 1998). The cage and wooden nest boxes, which are used as sleeping boxes, need daily cleaning to prevent fungal growth.

In flights, where mynahs can be combined with other species such as the superb glossy starling and aracaris, an area should be created with plants or blinds for the birds to retreat or escape from sight. Also, mynahs are nest-robbers and hunt small birds.

The active, curious nature of the mynahs often leads them to pick up and consume inedible foreign bodies found in the enclosure (rocks, pieces of wood, screws, string, coins etc.). Resulting impactions from foreign body ingestion can cause perforation or stasis of the gastrointestinal tract, which may lead to death. These birds are capable of being extremely destructive, and can injure their beaks when biting on solid objects.

The floor of a mynah enclosure should be well drained and easy to clean. The large amount of moist foods that these birds consume results in the production of volumi-nous, malodorous excrement and uneaten food.

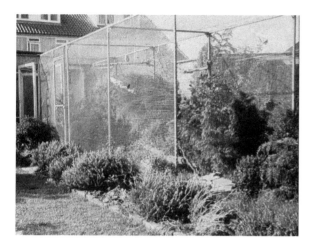

Fig 8.7 Plants should be used for environmentally enhancing free flight aviaries.

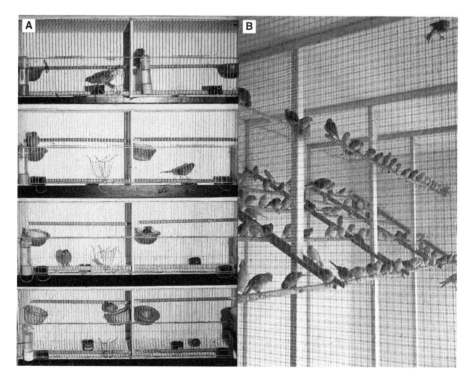

Fig 8.8 Canary breeding cages and indoor flight pen.

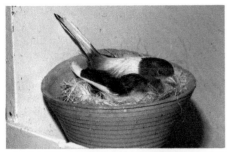

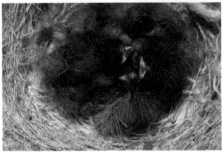

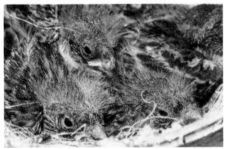

Fig 8.9 Female canary sitting on the eggs, hatchling of 3 days old and just before fledgling.

Diet and husbandry

Small passerines

Dietary and husbandry requirements are diverse. Most passerine species are primarily seed-eating or granivorous, while others are nectivorous, frugivorous, insectivorous, omnivorous or carnivorous. Most commercially available passerine diets are seed mixes, and may therefore be deficient in specific vitamins or minerals. The composition of the basic diet will be determined by the species of bird in question – some species adapt readily to commercially available diets, while others may require live food.

Common nutrient deficiencies from a seed-only diet include lysine, calcium, available phosphorus, sodium, manganese, zinc, iron, iodine, selenium, vitamins A, D_3, E and K, riboflavin, pantothenic acid, available niacin, vitamin B_{12} and choline. The nutrient deficiencies often found in seed diets affect the reproduction and health of adult birds.

It is commonly assumed that seed-eating birds need both soluble and insoluble grit in their diet. Although poultry studies have not yielded any conclusive results regarding the necessity of providing grit in the diet, investigations using canaries showed no significant differences in food intake between two groups (one with and one without soluble grit, but both with access to cuttlebone), and insoluble grit had no effect on digestibility values (Taylor 1996). The group of birds that were denied a source of soluble grit during the trial consumed a significantly higher amount of cuttlebone than the other birds (Taylor 1996).

When passerine birds are presented in wildlife rehabilitation with anorexia, many complicated food mixtures are advocated for nutritional supplementation. For insect-eating birds or nestling seed-eaters, a high quality puppy food soaked in water with a good vitamin and mineral supplement is recommended as a base diet (White 1997). The author has also good experience with soya-based products (see Chapter 6). Some insectivorous birds require insects as a substantial portion of their diet (30–60%). When mealworms make up a significant part of the diet, additional calcium must be added to bring the diet to the proper 2:1 calcium:phosphorus ratio. Starlings will not generally thrive on dog food unless additional fat is added.

Mynahs

Free-ranging mynahs eat a variety of fruits, small vertebrates such as lizards, rodents and small birds, various insects and spiders, and bird eggs.

Mynahs and softbills are extremely susceptible to diet-induced iron storage problems, or haemochromatosis; therefore the total diet should contain a low iron level – less than 40 ppm or, based on calculations referring to food intake per kg body weight, a maximum of 4–6 mg iron per kg per bird per day (Dorrestein et al 1992, Mete et al 2001).

In a field study, rainbow-billed toucans (*Ramphastos sulfuratos*) were observed to eat mainly five fruit items that had concentrations of less than 20–50 ppm iron (Otten et al 2001). Many dog and cat foods contain high levels of iron (up to 1500 ppm), and these high-iron diets should be avoided when feeding softbills (e.g. grapes, raisins). However, even the low-iron commercial diets with a stated maximum level of 100 ppm contained 210 ppm iron, and analysis often revealed levels five to six times higher than those stated (Otten et al 2001).

These birds may normally pass some undigested food. Undigested chitin and feather parts will be regurgitated as small pellets by mynahs. Large quantities of 'brown' mealworms have induced cloacal impactions in birds (Korbel & Kösters 1998). Birds that are losing weight and consistently excreting undigested food should be evaluated.

Breeding and sexing

Canaries

Breeding

The breeding season is the cornerstone of the canary fancier's hobby. Success or failure at this stage will determine the available birds for the autumn shows, and will also determine whether the breeder garners a position to advance a breeding programme the following year (Dodwell 1986). If the aviculturist does not produce enough home-bred birds he or she will have to purchase replacement stock. Although most fanciers work with pairs, it is a common practice to have breeding trios consisting of one cock bird mating with two hens. During the winter, hens and cocks are housed in separate groups.

Normally, canaries will start breeding when the following conditions are met (Coutteel 1995, 2003):

- maturity and good health
- an accepted partner
- a minimum daylight length
- the presence of a nest and nesting materials
- enough water and food
- a minimum temperature and photoperiodic stimulation.

The ultimate expression of readiness to breed, however, is when the hens crouch low upon the perch with tail raised, inviting the act of coition, whenever they hear the vigorous singing of a cock bird in a neighbouring cage. When these signs are noticed, no time should be lost in introducing the pair to each other. The breeding season will then proceed throughout the spring, and should finish by midsummer. During this period two or three clutches will have been raised, depending on breeding conditions. All young birds should be weaned and independent of their parents by the end of the summer.

After a period of long daylight hours, birds become refractory to photostimulation. Following the moult and period of decreasing daylight hours in the autumn, the breeding season starts again with the increasing daylight hours in the late winter and early spring.

Egg laying in canary breeding is the result of seasonal development of the left ovary, which is less stimulated by the increasing photoperiod than the testicles in the male. The female may require the presence of a male in breeding condition to trigger appropriate nesting and egg-laying responses.

Egg laying may be expected to start within about a week or 10 days of pairing the birds, although variations of some days either way can occur according to season and the condition of the breeding pair. During this period, the pair will have been building the nest.

Signs of the impending event are the hen roosting in (or near) the nest at night, and an increase in the consumption of water for approximately 48 hours. Eggs are laid singly and at 24-hour intervals, usually in the early hours of the morning.

Breeders remove the eggs as they are laid, and substitute them with dummies until the fourth egg has appeared, when they are returned to the nest for the hen to incubate for 13–14 days. The average number of eggs in a clutch is four, and breeders work on this assumption, but five is quite commonplace, and even larger clutches can sometimes occur.

The problems that are likely to present themselves at this period include (Dodwell 1986):

- hens that occasionally lay their eggs on the floor of the cage (a thick covering of sawdust will prevent breakage)
- hens suffering from egg-binding
- eggs sometimes being broken by an over-inquisitive cock bird.

The role of the length of daylight

Canaries need 14–16 hours of daylight to start breeding and to feed their nestlings and raise them properly. If the length of the daylight fluctuates, the birds will receive different hormonal signals (negative feedback), resulting in interruption of breeding and the beginning of an early moult. Artificial day lengths of 17–18 hours give less satisfactory results. If artificial light is produced for breeding birds, the kind of radiation produced by the lamps is an important factor, including such aspects as luminance, frequency and colour temperature (Coutteel 2003).

There are several ways to increase the length of the day (examples are given based on the northern hemisphere):

1. Following the natural increase in day length. These birds are called 'cold-temperature' breeders. The disadvantage is that the first chicks will hatch in April/June and that the time will be very short to mature for show season.

2. Gradually increasing the length of the day using artificial light, starting in November/December in a heated (15–16°C, 60–80% humidity) environment. It will take a period of 2–3 months to increase from an 8-hour natural day length to a 15-hour day, increasing at 2×15 minutes per week. A minimum luminance of 500–1000 lux is needed, preferably using a dimmer to simulate dawn and twilight.

3. Introducing an immediate full day length, extending it from 10 to 15 hours. In this case the birds will reach their breeding condition in 3–4 weeks, but they will often give bad fertilization of the first clutch and the birds are less able to give good results throughout the full breeding season (Coutteel 1995, 2003).

Sexing

Since canaries are monomorphic, it can be a problem sexing them, depending on the time of the year. As the breeding season approaches, the most obvious difference will become apparent; that of song. The cock sings, whereas the hen does not. Song also helps with the sexing of the juveniles; by the time they are 8–10 weeks old, most of the cocks will have started to twitter.

Apart from the song, there are two other methods of sexing: colour and general bearing, and the appearance of the sex organs during breeding.

Cocks are often more intense in colour than their counterparts. The difference will become apparent by comparison with a similar bird of known sex. It will also be observed that cock birds tend to have a bolder manner and more jaunty carriage than hens.

Birds have no distinctly different sex organs, but when in breeding condition, if the vent area is examined it will be seen that the cloaca of the cock bird is quite prominent and somewhat elongated due to swelling of the seminal glomerulus. In the hen, although the cloaca is raised above the general level of the abdomen, it is rounder and flatter.

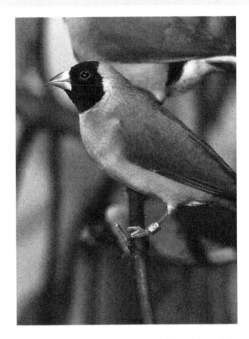

Fig 8.10 A male black-headed Gouldian finch (*Chloebia gouldii*).

Other finches

Breeding

Many varieties of domesticated finches bear little resemblance to their free-ranging ancestors, and are easy to care for and breed well in captivity. Java finches, zebra finches and Gouldian finches have a somewhat shorter history of domestication than canaries, but are also bred intensively in captivity, and many mutations have occurred (Fig. 8.10). Other passerines are directly imported from the wild, and need indoor, temperature-controlled rooms and sometimes artificial light for reproduction. Some passerines require special materials for nesting or to stimulate display behaviour. Any contact with fine synthetic fibres should be avoided, because these may become entangled around the bird's feet, toes or other body parts, causing damage, loss of limb or death (Fig. 8.11). Hessian cloth cut into small squares, cotton, torn strips of facial tissue, sheep's wool or coconut fibre make suitable, safe nesting materials.

In passerines indigenous to tropical or arid regions, seasonal changes related to daylight hours are less important to the reproductive cycle than the periodic available food and water (Gill 1994). Most successful breeders of these species mimic natural conditions by lowering the caloric, protein and fat content of diets and maximizing the bird's physical condition by allowing free flight in open aviaries during the non-breeding season. At the beginning of the breeding season the birds are 'flushed', or encouraged to come into breeding condition, by increasing the plane of nutrition.

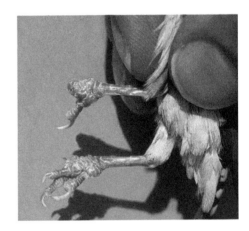

Fig 8.11 Zebra finch feet entangled in synthetic fibres.

Misting some species with water (to mimic rainfall) and providing green, fresh foods and foliage may stimulate breeding, particularly of those species from desert environments, such as the Australian grass finches. Birds must not become chilled during the misting process. Depending on the species, birds may be transferred in pairs to smaller breeding enclosures, or left in flights to colony breed (Macwhirter 1994).

Sexing

In some passerines, there are obvious or subtle morphological differences between the genders. Males are

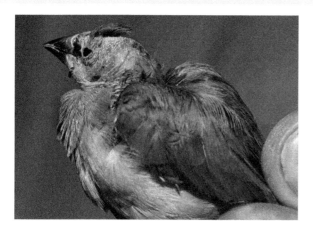

Fig 8.12 Gouldian finch (*Chloebia gouldii*) with feather loss and trauma due to cage mate aggression.

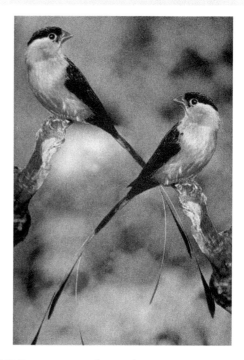

Fig 8.13 Two male whydahs (*Vidua* sp.) displaying their long tails.

generally brightly coloured or elaborately marked, particularly during the breeding season. As in canaries, differences in singing, courtship or nesting behaviour may also provide clues to gender. In many species, the male's seminal glomerulus will push the cloacal wall into a prominent projection (the cloacal promontory) during the breeding season.

DNA/PCR technology can be used to determine gender in monomorphic passerine birds. The cost of these procedures tends to limit their application to more expensive species.

Aggression

While passerine species may be small, some are quite territorial and others have well-developed pecking orders. Head trauma, feather picking, other injuries or death may occur in individuals that have been attacked by a companion (Fig. 8.12). Self-mutilation, poor body condition and increased susceptibility to disease are indirect results of such aggression in birds that are psychologically stressed because of their low social position (Macwhirter 1994). Aggression is more likely to occur if the birds are overcrowded in small, open enclosures, where less dominant birds have few opportunities to escape from more dominant ones. Aggression-related injuries can be particularly pronounced if new birds are introduced into collections where a social order has already been established.

Suggested measures to combat aggression include:

1. Prevent overcrowding; the fewer birds, the better.
2. Clip the wings or remove particularly aggressive individuals.
3. Provide extra vegetation or visual barriers (burlap sheets) to provide less dominant birds with an escape area.
4. Maintain subdued lighting in indoors areas.

5. Introduce all birds into a new environment simultaneously.
6. 'Tranquillizers' (haloperidol 0.02 mg/kg or sodium bromide 1–2 mg/L) may be useful in certain situations.

Parents that become aggressive towards their chicks are preparing to lay a second clutch of eggs, and the chicks should be removed (Macwhirter 1994).

Breeding parasitic species

Some finch enthusiasts enjoy the challenge of breeding parasitic species (birds that lay their eggs in the nests of other species) such as paradise whydahs (*Steganura* spp.), *Hypochera* spp., small-tail whydahs (*Tetraenura* spp.). Parasitic behaviour is found in only four waxbill genera of the Estrildidae: *Estrilda* spp., *Lagonosticta* spp., *Uraeginthus* spp. and *Pytilia* spp. Whydahs are generally bred in large planted aviaries, where the parasitized finch species has first been firmly established and is breeding freely. The parallels between the appearance and behaviour of the whydah chicks and the finch chicks that they mimic are striking, even though the adults of the two species are very different.

If male and female whydahs do not originate from the same geographic area, they may not enter breeding condition simultaneously, thus preventing successful reproduction. The male whydah develops a long, flowing tail during the breeding season (Fig. 8.13).

Mynahs

Breeding

Mynahs (Fig. 8.14) are difficult to breed in captivity. This may be due to their imprinting on humans at a young age, or to their need for a large aviary. In the wild, mynahs are associated with flocks and the birds only separate in pairs during the breeding period. Free-ranging mynahs nest in tree-holes, 10–17 m high, cliff areas, and some nesting boxes. In captivity, nesting boxes (or, better, natural hollowed logs), 20–30 cm wide and 30–45 cm high, should be used. The diameter of the entrance should be at least 8–10 cm, and the box should be suspended as high as possible. Nesting material consists of wood shavings, small twigs, straw, hay, moss and feathers. Flights with abundant foliage are recommended for breeding pairs.

The hen lays between two and five eggs per clutch; they are coloured turquoise with some red brown to black spots, and are usually laid 24–48 hours apart. Brooding starts after the second egg has been laid, and takes 14–15 days. The chicks are fully feathered at 22 days of age, and become independent or weaned at 4–5 weeks. The yellow feet, legs and fleshy wattles are absent in young birds. The youngsters can fly at 6–8 weeks, and sexual maturity is reached at 2–3 years of age.

During the breeding season, the diet should include an abundant amount of insects, baby rodents and lean meats. Young birds being hand-fed have been raised on rice, chopped fish and vegetables, and insect larvae such as mealworms. The diet should be supplemented with adequate amounts of calcium, vitamins and minerals. Softbill hand-feeding formulas can be used.

Adult mynahs have been known to crack their own eggs and even throw the young out of the nest (LaBonde 1996).

Sexing

Most hill mynah species are monomorphic and require surgical or genetic sexing.

Handling and restraint

Small passerines

Handling

A 'lights out/perching out' approach to capture is useful for small active birds. Birds will generally not move in a dark room, and can easily be removed from an enclosure; the bird can be restrained by placing the head between two fingers so that the body rests in the palm of the hand, or it can be restrained by holding the head gently between the thumb and first finger (Fig. 8.15). It is essential not to interfere with or restrict the movement of the sternum; this will kill the bird! The handling and restraint period should be as short as possible, and clinicians should be prepared to take samples and perform treatments in one handling session. A modified mask should be used to induce and maintain small passerines on the only general anaesthetic agent recommended, isoflurane.

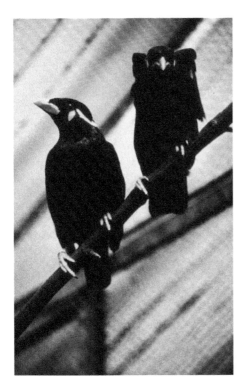

Fig 8.14 A pair of mynahs (*Gracula religiosa*).

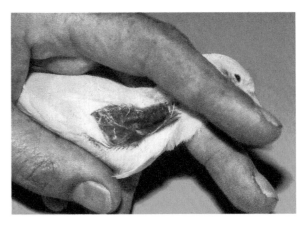

Fig 8.15 Proper handling technique for a small passerine.

Blood collection

The right jugular vein is generally the best site for collecting blood or giving intravenous fluids (see Figs 3.41 and 8.15) It is surprisingly large, even in very small finches. A nail clip is obsolete; the medial tarsal or cutaneous ulnar veins are alternative blood collection sites, but they frequently provide insufficient sample volumes. A skin-prick technique from these sites or from the external thoracic vein (which courses on either side of the ribcage just behind the shoulder) can be used. The blood is collected directly from the skin into a microcollection tube (Macwhirter 1994).

Injection sites

Although the right jugular vein can be used for administration of intravenous fluids, intraosseous catheterization using a 26-gauge needle is a practical means of fluid administration in a finch (Macwhirter 1994).

For intramuscular or subcutaneous injections, a 27-gauge needle is suggested; even this gauge of needle can cause significant haemorrhage if not used with caution. To minimize risk, the intramuscular injection site should be located in the caudal third of the breast muscle. Aspiration should be performed prior to injecting any drug to ensure that a blood vessel has not been cannulated. After the needle has been removed, the site should be observed for haemorrhage, and pressure applied digitally if bleeding does occur.

Drug dosing in small patients must be based on an exact body weight (as determined by a digital gram scale), and should be delivered with precise microlitre or insulin syringes to avoid overdose. There is little room for a dosing error in a small bird (Macwhirter 1994).

Mynahs

Handling

Mynahs can be loud, active and aggressive, particularly if untamed. Tame birds that are not given sufficient attention may also become very aggressive towards their keepers. The birds are best restrained by initially removing them from the enclosure with a net or large towel. A mynah can be controlled by holding the head gently between the thumb and first finger, with or without a towel.

Blood collection and injection sites

These are the same as described for the smaller passerines and for other birds (see Chapters 3 & 6).

Diagnostic procedures

Diagnostic and treatment options in small passerines may be limited by owners' financial constraints and by difficulties in collecting samples from small birds. However, in spite of their size, the medical management of passerine patients weighing less than 25 g is very similar to that of larger avian species. Special instrumentation allows veterinary practitioners to auscultate the heart, respiratory system and gastrointestinal tract of these birds. Low volume, preheparinized syringes can be used to collect enough blood to perform a complete blood cell count and abbreviated plasma chemistry analysis on birds less than 10 g in weight. Surgery can be performed using microsurgery instruments and operating microscopes or other forms of magnification (Massey 1996).

Veterinary care in these species is frequently directed toward appropriate preventive husbandry measures, and approaching medical problems from a flock perspective. The main clinical diagnostic procedures for these small birds are taking a history, examination of the cage, an external physical examination and limited clinical procedures. In many cases, especially in flocks, these procedures should be followed by a diagnostic necropsy.

The softbills are larger birds and more expensive. A sound medical work-up will lead to proper diagnosis and treatment.

Clinical diagnostics

The history should include information on the species, age, symptoms, diet and housing. A thorough history will provide much of the information needed to arrive at a diagnosis.

Examination of the cage or aviary can provide a great deal of useful information. Examination should include the droppings, the feed dishes and the floor. Most breeders of passerines bring their birds to veterinary clinics in transport boxes or cages, and birds should be put in an appropriate cage immediately, even before the history is taken. The birds will acclimatize to their new surroundings, and often a fresh stool will be produced for examination. Transport in their own cage is recommended whenever possible. 'Light out/perches out' catching techniques are almost mandatory, and strong lighting in combination with a magnification device will greatly facilitate any examination of the tiny birds. When handling the birds, keep the windows and doors closed!

The physical examination and clinical procedures are limited in the smaller passerines, but are nevertheless very important. Most digital gram scales can provide an accurate weight if the finch is contained in a paper box or bag, but the container must be weighed or tared. The usual physical examination is performed as for any other bird; the clinician should listen for respiratory sounds, and take care not interfere with the movements of the sternum, which could kill the patient. Special attention should be paid to the state of moult, the pectoral muscle mass (chronic or acute problem), the abdomen (by blowing the feathers apart and looking

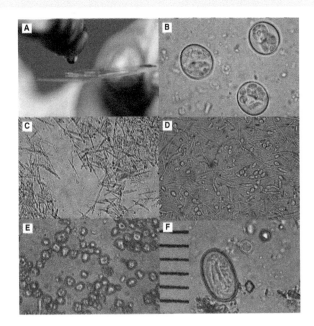

Fig 8.16 Wet mount with examples (**A**) technique using saline, (**B**) coccidia 48 hours after faeces production (black crow), (**C**) *Macrorhabdus ornithogaster* proventriculus canary, (**D**) yeasts intestines Lady Gouldian finch (*Chloebia gouldii*), (**E**) starch intestines in an orange-cheeked waxbill (*Estrilda melpoda*) and (**F**) *Dyspharinx nasuta* egg faeces, zebra finch.

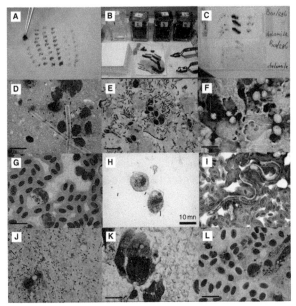

Fig 8.17 Impression smears, technique and examples. (**A**) Preparation of a tissue impression; (**B**) staining set (Hemacolor®); (**C**) the result before and after staining; (**D**) *Macrorhabdus* and *Atoxoplasma* stages, intestines canary; (**E**) yeast and bacteria intestines, Gouldian finch; (**F**) cryptosporidia on surface epithelial cells, bursa; (**G**) *Salmonella* sp. in macrophage liver, canary; (**H**) flagellates crop, canary; (**I**) Microfilaria lung bullfinch (*Pyrrhula pyrrhula*); (**J**) E. coli overgrowth intestine, canary; (**K**) *Salmonella* sp. intestine canary; (**L**) Atoxoplasmosis liver, bullfinch. (Bar = 10 µm.)

for an enlarged liver and dilatation of the gastrointestinal tract) and the skin (searching for pox lesions and parasites).

Routine diagnostic procedures also include the following:

1. Faecal examination (Figs 8.16 and 8.17). Helminth infections are very rare in small passerines, but are more often seen in wild-caught mynahs. Coccidia, which are common in small passerines, are excreted mainly between 2 p.m. and darkness. Yeasts and protozoal cysts (e.g. *Giardia* spp.) are found using direct wet preparations or flotation techniques. The diagnosis of cochlosomosis in society finches or Australian finches can only be made in direct wet mounts of fresh and warm stool without dilution. Passerine species are not considered to have a permanent gut flora, so minimal bacteria and/or other microorganisms should be found in stained faecal smears. Routine microbiological aerobic cultures should be negative. Microaerophylic strains (e.g. *Campylobacter jejuni*) can be found in stained faecal smears in many Estrildidae. In softbills, bacteria are commonly demonstrated in the stools of healthy birds and are considered as 'passage flora'.

2. Crop swabs. These are essential for the diagnosis of trichomoniasis, infections with other flagellates, and crop candidiasis.

3. Blood samples. For additional information in small individual passerine birds, blood can be collected in heparinized capillary tubes after puncturing the medial metatarsal vein. In softbills, blood normally is collected from the right jugular vein. One drop is used for a blood smear, which can be examined for blood parasites. The packed cell volume (PCV) normally ranges from 40% to 55%; a reading of less than 35% indicates anaemia. Total protein (TP) is a significant diagnostic measure. For the serological diagnosis of paramyxovirus infections or toxoplasmosis, 0.5–1.0 mL of blood can be collected from the right jugular vein. As with other avian species, no more than 1% of the body weight in blood volume should be collected at one time, less in a critically ill bird.

Normal haematological and serum biochemical references are presented in Table 8.1. The dosage regimens for passerines are listed in Table 8.2. Tables 8.3 and 8.4 contain the primary differential diagnoses and confirmations for canaries and finches.

The diagnostic necropsy

A necropsy should always be performed on birds that die from unknown causes, both so that flaws in management

Table 8.1 Some normal haematological and serum biochemical values in selected passerines (adapted from Carpenter 2005 and Altman et al 1997)

Measurement	Canary	Finch	Mynah
Haematology:			
PCV (%)	37–49	45–62	44–55
RBC (10^6/μL)	2.5–3.8	2.5–4.6	2.4–4.0
WBC (10^6/μL)	4–9	3–8	6–11
• Heterophils (%)	50–80	20–65	25–65
• Lymphocytes (%)	25–45	20–65	20–60
• Monocytes (%)	0–1	0–1	0–3
• Eosinophils (%)	0–2	0–1	0–3
• Basophils (%)	0–1	0–5	0–5
Chemistries:			
AP (IU/L)	20–135	–	–
AST = SGOT (IU/L)	145–345	150–350	130–350
LDH (IU/L)	120–450	–	(600–1000)
Ca (mmol/L)	1.28–3.35	–	2.25–3.25
P (mmol/L)	0.52–1.81	–	–
Glucose (mmol/L)	11–22	11–25	10.5–19.4
TP (g/L)	28–45	30–50	23–45
Creatinine (mmol/L)	8.8–88	–	8.8–53
Uric acid (mmol/L)	–	–	237–595
Potassium = K (mmol/L)	2.7–4.8	–	0.4–5.1
Sodium = Na (mmol/L)	135–165	–	136–152

Table 8.2 Dosage regimens for chemotherapeutics and antibiotics for canaries and small passerines

Drug	Conc. in drinking water (mg/L)	Conc. in soft food (mg/kg)
Amoxicillin	1000	300–500
Ampicillin	1000–2000	2000–3000
Chloramphenicol	100–150	200–300
Chlortetracycline[a]	1000–1500	1500
Dimetridazole	100	–
Doxycycline[a]	250–1000	1000
Enrofloxacin[b]	200–400	200
Erythromycin	125	200
Furazolidone	100–200	200
Ivermectin[c]	10[c]	
Lincospectin	100–200	200
Ketoconazole	1000	200
Metronidazole	200	100
Neomycin	80–100	100
Nystatin[d]	1000 000 IU	2000 000 IU
Polymyxin	500 000 IU	500 000 IU
Ronidazol	400	400
Spectinomycin	200–400	400
Spiramycin	200–400	400
Sulphachlorpyrazine	150–300	–
Sulphadimidine	150	–
Trim/sulpha[e]	150–400	200
Tylosin	250–400	400

[a] In case of ornithosis, 30 days.
[b] In case of ornithosis, 21 days.
[c] Alternatively by topical application, one drop of 1% solution.
[d] For the treatment of Candida albicans for 3–6 weeks.
[e] This dosage is for the trimethoprim part alone.

can be rectified and to protect against a possible epidemic. **The necropsy procedure may be considered the ultimate method of confiming a diagnosis (Dorrestein 1997b).** The following procedures can provide much additional information during the necropsy:

- direct wet preparations of the gut contents and of the coating of the serosae
- scrapings from the mucosa of the crop, proventriculus, duodenum and rectum
- contact or impression smears from a freshly cut surface of liver, spleen, lungs, and any altered tissues.

The smears are stained routinely with Romanowsky stains (e.g. Giemsa) or 'Quick' stains (e.g. Diff-Quick) and searched microscopically (cytology) under the oil immersion objective lens. Bacteriological, mycological, virological, serological and histopathological examinations and immunodiagnostic techniques are special techniques to help determine a diagnosis.

Metabolic and nutritional disorders

Nutritional problems, especially those resulting from an unbalanced diet, are often seen in mixed aviaries and individual pet finches. All granivorous birds need a certain amount of supplementation by an egg-food or 'soft-bill' food, as an unbalanced diet predisposes birds to health problems, especially with Enterobacteriaceae (e.g. *E. coli*, *Klebsiella* spp. and *Enterobacter* spp.) and yeast infections (especially *Candida albicans*). The breeding results are poor in birds with an unbalanced diet.

The primary cause of many problems in Australian and other tropical finches is an unbalanced diet; therefore, when treating disease problems in these birds, improvement of the diet has to be the first objective.

Table 8.3 Diagnostic table for canaries and finches

			Go to:
1	Species:		
	• Canary		2
	• Australian finch		12
	• Mixed aviary		7
2	Age:		
	• Nestling		3
	• Juvenile, under 1 year of age		4
	• Any age		5
3	• Interior of the nests are yellow stained by diarrhoea of the nestlings, the feathers sticky, the youngsters stunted, and there is greatly increased mortality between 1 and 3 days of age	*E.c oli* diarrhoea	
	• Very pale membranes visible by opening their beaks, and weak in stretching their necks. Females can be found dead sitting on the eggs	Blood-sucking mites	
	• Black spot on the right side of the abdomen, anorexia and mortality	Circovirus	
4	• The youngsters show huddling and ruffling of the feathers, debilitation, diarrhoea, sometimes neurological signs (20%) and death. Mortality can be as high as 80%	Atoxoplasmosis	
5	• Respiratory distress		6
	• Respiratory symptoms not main sign		7
6	• Dyspnoea, debilitation with scabs and pox-lesions, especially on eyelids, commissure of the beak and in feather follicles. Diphtheric lesions can be found in the mouth and larynx. Birds of all ages can be affected, and the mortality is between 20% and 100%; the infection spreads quickly	Avianp ox	
	• Severe respiratory signs, general illness and central nervous symptoms and iridocyclitis, which often results in blind birds after 3 months due to a panophthalmia	Toxoplasmosis	
	• Minor to severe respiratory symptoms with anaemia and sometimes a high mortality. The main complaint from the owner is usually a general depression in the bird	Blood-sucking mites	
	• Loss of voice, decline of physical condition, respiratory distress, wheezing, squeaking, coughing, sneezing, nasal discharge, head shaking and gasping. A low mortality	Sternostomosis	
	• Apathy, respiratory symptoms, regurgitation, blowing bubbles and emaciation, but seldom diarrhoea	Trichomoniasis	
	• Chronic tracheitis, pneumonia and air sac infections	*Enterococusf aecalis*	
7	• Diarrhoea		8
	• Diarrhoea not specific		9
8	• A general decline of the physical condition, huddling and ruffling of the feathers, debilitation, diarrhoea and emaciation. The mortality is low	Coccidiosis	
	• Several birds demonstrate a general malaise, with or without diarrhoea, and some birds show conjunctivitis and rhinitis. Some may die	Colibacillosis	
9	• Obvious wasting		10
	• Sudden death of several birds		11
10	• Most infections are seen in winter. The clinical signs are apathy, decline in food and water intake, debilitation, emaciation, diarrhoea, respiratory symptoms, ruffling of the feathers and high mortality	Pseudotuberculosis	
	• Especially in outdoor aviaries, clinically indistinguishable from pseudotuberculosis, more often chronic	Salmonellosis	
	• Many birds show signs including apathy, anorexia, regurgitation, and parts of or whole seeds in soft, watery, dark green to brown/black faeces	Macrorhabdiosis	
	• Apathy, diarrhoea, debilitation, nasal exudate and conjunctivitis. The mortality is usually less then 10%	Chlamydiosis	
11	• Not specific. CNS symptoms, often obvious salivation and dyspnoea or diarrhoea in apathetic birds	Toxicosis	
	• Often after a weekend when someone other than the owner fed the birds. Sometimes black-stained droppings or diarrhoea. Weakness is often interpreted as a CNS symptom	Starvation	
12	Age:		
	• Nestlings and fledglings under the age of 3 months		13
	• All ages affected		16

(continued)

Table 8.3 (*continued*)

13	• Bengalese or society finches as foster parents		14
	• Natural breed or foster parents		15
14	• From the age of 10 days until 6 weeks there is debilitation, shrivelling and yellow staining of the fledglings, difficulties with moulting, and parts of or whole seeds in the droppings. The foster parents show only watery droppings	Cochlosomosis	
15	• High losses of nestlings, adult Estrildidae can show apathy and yellow diarrhoea or yellow solid droppings due to large amounts of undigested amylum	Campylobacter	
	• In nestlings the crop is bloating, and a thickened crop wall is relatively common. In weanlings and adult birds, diarrhoea and moulting problems are more prominent	Candidiasis	
16	• Respiratory distress		17
	• Respiratory distress not the main symptom		18
17	• Respiratory distress, wheezing, squeaking, coughing, sneezing, nasal discharge, loss of voice, head shaking and gasping. The mortality is low	Sternostomosis	
	• Apathy, respiratory symptoms, regurgitation, blowing bubbles and emaciation, sometimes diarrhoea	Trichomoniasis	
	• Conjunctivitis and respiratory problems in Australian and African finches	Cytomegalovirus	
18	• CNS symptoms		19
	• CNS symptoms not a main symptom		7
19	• Torticollis is the main symptom. As long as these birds can still eat, mortality is low	Paramyxovirus	
	• Sudden death of several birds		11

Table 8.4 Special hints for further diagnostics

Atoxoplasmosis	A necropsy and demonstration of the parasites in imprints of several organs
Avian pox	Necropsy, virus isolation and PCR
Black-spot (circovirus)	Filled gall bladder. Circovirus demonstration in electron microscope and by PCR
Campylobacter	Demonstration in smears after staining with Diff-Quick. Cultivation only on special media
Candidiasis	A direct wet preparation and/or a stained smear. Culture
Chlamydiosis	Necropsy and demonstration of the agent by staining, IFT, PCR or ELISA
Coccidiosis	Parasitical examination of droppings collected between 2 and 6 p.m.
Cochlosomosis	Flagellates in a wet mount of fresh and body-warm faeces from the finches
Colibacillosis	Analysis of the situation for other factors in combination with the isolation
Cytomegalovirus	Cytology and histology of conjunctiva. EM and/or virus culture or PCR
Enterococcus faecalis	Culture from the trachea
Helminthic infestation	Not important in small passerines. *Syngamus* very occasionally
Intoxication	Detailed case history. A direct confirmation often impossible, when the toxin is not known
Macrorhabdus spp.	Faecal wet mount and cytology. At necropsy, smear from the mucosa of the proventricular-ventricular junction
Mites	Demonstration of mites in the nest or bird-room crevices
Paramyxovirus	Serological and virological screening. In the histology, a pancreatitis
Pseudotuberculosis	Necrotic foci at necropsy in liver and spleen and agent isolation
Salmonellosis	Necrotic foci at necropsy in liver and spleen and agent isolation
Starvation	Haemorrhagic diathesis (bleeding into the gut) at necropsy
Sweating disease	Demonstration and isolation of bacteria in the faeces
Sternostomosis	Diagnostic necropsy and demonstration of the parasite
Trichomoniasis	Demonstration of flagellates in crop-swab. Necropsy
Toxoplasmosis	Serology and demonstration of the parasite in brain smears, organ smears or histologically (immunohistochemical staining)

A good starting point is controlled feeding of three parts of a seed mix supplemented with one part soft food. It may be difficult, however, to make the birds eat the soft food. In some parts of the world pelleted foods for passerines are commercially available, and these are preferable rather than pure seeds.

Vitamin deficiencies

In small passerines, feeding rancid cod-liver oil or mixing oil through the seed may result in encephalomalacia

Box 8.1 The influences of nutrient supply on feathers' regrowth in small pet birds

The aim of this study was to quantitate feathering in several companion birds. Besides the ratio of feathers to whole body mass, feather length as well as featherweight were of interest. Furthermore, data on feather loss and growth rates were estimated. In general, it could be observed that the proportion of feathers relative to body mass varied between 14% (canaries) and 7.4% (lovebirds). Feather losses (outside the moult period) amounted to an average of 6.65 (canaries), 8.98 (budgerigars), and 8.43 (lovebirds) mg/bird/day respectively or 37 (canaries), 20 (budgerigars), and 17 (lovebirds) mg/100 g body weight/day (values of interest in calculating of protein requirements for maintenance). In canaries, the average growth rate of the developing feathers amounted to 2 mm/day. In contrast to the onset of feather regeneration, the growth rate of new feathers leaving the follicle was not influenced by the supplements used here. The regeneration period (first measurable feather growth) of a plucked pinion can be used as an indicator and objective parameter to test potential nutritional influences. Parallel to the improvement of nutrient supply the rates of feather losses and also replacement increased, whereas the rates decreased when seed mixtures without any addition of minerals, sulphurous amino acids, and vitamins were fed (Wolf et al 2003).

and fertility problems due to vitamin E deficiency. Vitamin B deficiency can cause CNS disturbances, reduced hatching, stunting, and moulting problems.

Vitamin A deficiency in recessive white canaries is caused by a genetic defect that prevents the absorption of carotenoids from the intestine (Table 8.5). The main signs associated with vitamin A deficiency in white canaries are general malaise, problems with Enterobacteriaceae and yeasts, and disappointing breeding results (Dorrestein & Schrijver 1982). Recessively white canaries are completely dependent on the presence of vitamin A in the food, and it is essential to increase the levels of vitamin A from approximately 15 000 IU/kg egg food for 'normal' canaries to approximately 20 000 IU/kg egg food, which will prevent deficiency problems.

Vitamin C is not normally needed as a dietary source, because most birds can synthesize sufficient amounts from glucose in the liver, kidney or both (Klasing 1998). Some species of Passeriformes completely lack the enzyme L-gulonolactone oxidase, and require a dietary source of vitamin C to prevent the quick onset of deficiency symptoms. All species that are unable to synthesize ascorbic acid are insectivorous or frugivorous, and receive a reliable dietary supply of this vitamin in their food source. Some Passeriformes that are able to synthesize ascorbic acid do so at rates two to ten times slower than those in species such as chickens, ducks and Japanese quail, which do not have a dietary requirement.

Even the high endogenous synthetic rate in other species may be inadequate during periods of severe stress, such as heat, physical trauma, infection, and the consumption of some types of purified diets. Ascorbic acid supplementation of seed- or grain-based diets has been reported to improve resistance to a variety of infectious diseases and to improve wound healing. Passerines depending on external sources for vitamin C (e.g. bulbuls,

Table 8.5 Mean values ($n = 5$) for vitamin A, total carotenoids, and β-carotene in liver and serum of different coloured canaries (adapted from Dorrestein & Schrijver 1982)

Colour	Egg food[a]		Serum (μmol/L)		Liver	
	Vitamin A (IU/kg)	Total carotenoids (mg/kg)	Vitamin A	Total carotenoids	Vitamin A (IU/g)	Total carotenoids (μg/g)
Red[b]	19 200	27.7	2.75	88.75	2552	72.45
Yellow	18 300	3.1	2.28	42.40	4154	9.83
Recessive white	18 300	3.1	2.88	2.25	3751	6.70
Recessive white	13 500	4.9	2.20	2.37	524	7.85
Brown	13 500	4.9	2.46	64.86	1428	21.22

[a] Egg food was given in a ratio of 1:4 with a canary seed mixture.
[b] Extra canthaxanthine for maintaining the red colour.

shrikes) develop clinical signs including weight loss, behavioural changes, lethargy, feather loss, and haemorrhages in the liver and leg joints within 15 days of being fed a deficient diet.

The daily requirement is not known, but beneficial responses have been observed at levels of between 50 and 150 L-gulonolactone oxidase mg/kg dry matter. Vitamin C is not widely distributed across avian foods, but certain fruits, vegetables, and many herbs are particularly rich while domestic grains are deficient.

The vitamin C content of avian foods decreases precipitously during storage. It is very susceptible to oxidation, especially in the presence of trace minerals. Food that has been stored for more than 4 months with unprotected vitamin C should be considered unsuitable for use. Vitamin D_3 and/or calcium deficiencies or problems with the Ca : P ratio, resulting in rickets and osteomalacia, are seen in small passerines. Mostly the problems are noticed during the breeding season and egg laying. Tetracycline may also cause problems if administered while the bird is breeding, because tetracycline binds serum calcium.

Haemochromatosis (see also Chapter 14)

Haemochromatosis, or iron storage disease, is the most common non-infectious disease in softbills. Clinically, dyspnoea, weight loss, abdominal distension (hydrops ascites), and weakness are seen with hepatic haemochromatosis. Clinical pathology results usually reveal a hypoproteinaemia and an elevated activity of liver enzymes. At necropsy, iron storage disease is detected primarily in the liver. In terminal cases, a liver fibrosis, concentric heart decompensation, lung oedema and hydrops ascites are noted. In some case presentations

iron will be found in other organs as well, especially in combination with an infectious disease. When iron is found in combination with an infectious disease, the iron is predominantly stored in macrophages, which can eventually form extensive focal granulomata.

Mynahs suffer from a primary haemochromatosis, which is a species-specific inherited metabolic disorder that causes a relative excess of iron to be absorbed from 'iron-balanced' diets (Dorrestein et al 1992, Mete et al 2001, 2003). In general, fructivorous, insectivorous and omnivorous birds accumulate more iron in their livers (Figs 8.18 and 8.19) than carnivorous, piscivorous and granivorous birds, even within the same order (Dierenfield & Sheppard 1989, Dorrestein 1997a). Figure 8.19 shows the distribution in hepatocytes and Kupffer cells in the livers of commonly affected avian orders. In Passeriformes, iron storage in hepatocytes is only noted in mynahs. In canaries and finches, the only iron found in the liver is related to an inflammatory reaction in Kupffer cells. These species/nutritional correlations are indicative of a species-specific genetic predisposition consistent with primary haemochromatosis.

In birds that are susceptible to iron storage in the liver, diets with 50–60 ppm can induce an iron liver storage (Cornelissen et al 1995). Therefore, diets with a total iron of less than 50 ppm should be fed to mynahs and toucans, or the daily intake of iron should be 4–6 mg/kg bird per day (Mete et al 2001).

Diets with 100 ppm iron or less have been recommended in order to reduce dietary sources. However, diets with less than 100 ppm iron are normally difficult to formulate. This observation may prove to be more in line with what is available to feed birds than what is needed to prevent excessive iron storage. Even diets with 100 ppm iron are in excess of the requirements for growth of poultry, which generally require 60–80 ppm.

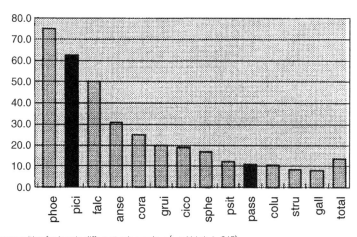

Fig 8.18 Percentage of livers positive for iron in different avian orders (total birds is 945).

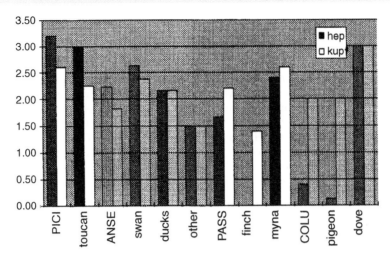

Fig 8.19 Average iron score (0 to 5) in hepatocytes and Kupffer cells with emphasis on Piciformes and Passeriformes. In the Passeriformes iron in hepatocytes is only found in mynahs, not in canaries or finches.

Box 8.2 A comparison of four regimens for treatment of iron storage disease using the European starling (*Sturnus vulgaris*) as a model

European starlings (*Sturnus vulgaris*) were fed an iron loading diet (3235 ppm) for 31 days to induce non-haem liver iron concentrations approaching those in birds that died with iron storage disease. All birds then were fed a low-iron diet (32–48 ppm) and assigned to four treatment groups: (1) low-iron diet only, (2) low-iron diet with phytate (inositol) and tannic acid, (3) low-iron diet and deferoxamine (100 mg/kg s.c. q24h), and (4) low-iron diet and phlebotomy (1% of body weight q7d). Starlings were treated for 16 weeks. In the groups treated with phlebotomy or with deferoxamine and a low-iron diet, non-haem liver iron concentrations decreased to safe levels after 16 weeks of treatment at similar rates (190 ppm/week and 163 ppm/week, respectively). The low-iron diet alone reduced stored liver iron levels at a slower rate (45 ppm/week). The addition of inositol and tannic acid to the low-iron diet had no impact on stored liver iron concentrations. These results suggest that both phlebotomy and treatment with deferoxamine are effective treatment options for birds with iron storage disease (Olsen et al 2006).

In cases of confirmed iron storage problems it is advisable to collect some food, especially when it is a 'low-iron' diet, and freeze it for future analysis.

Dietary ascorbic acid promotes the bioavailability of dietary iron in animals, and consequently decreases the iron requirements. Ferrous iron forms chelate with ascorbic acid that is soluble in the alkaline environment of the small intestine, and is relatively efficiently absorbed (Klasing 1998). In a comparative study in mynahs,

pigeons and rats, the author was not able to confirm this hypothesis (Dorrestein et al 1992). Moreover, haemochromatosis is a symptom of a vitamin C deficiency in mammals (Klasing 1998).

The presumptive diagnosis is made based on the diet, and on radiographs, which reveal an enlarged heart, liver and ascites; a liver biopsy confirms haemochromatosis.

Weekly phlebotomies to remove a blood volume equivalent to 1% of the body weight are an effective treatment, and these are usually performed in conjunction with low-iron diets. A less invasive treatment has been documented, using deferoxamine (100 mg/kg q24 h s.c.) combined with a low-iron diet (65 ppm) for up to 4 months, until the iron content in the liver of the toucan has normalized (Cornelissen et al 1995).

Amyloidosis

Amyloidosis is common in Gouldian finches, and is occasionally seen in other Passeriformes. Affected birds may be found dead, have a chronic non-specific history of illness or suffer from concurrent infections (polyomavirus, cryptosporidiosis). Social stress may play a role in the development of the disease. At necropsy the liver and kidney may appear grossly normal in some affected patients, but histologically the evidence of disease is severe. A hereditary predisposition is suspected in cases of amyloidosis in small passerines.

Fatty livers

Fatty livers (hepatic lipidosis) are occasionally seen in estrildid finches (zebra finch, parrot finch and star finch), and may be associated with inadequate exercise

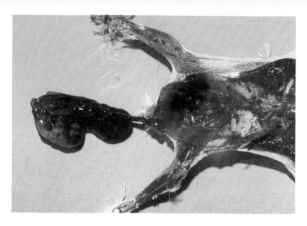

Fig 8.20 Canary haemorrhagic diathesis after 24 hours of fasting.

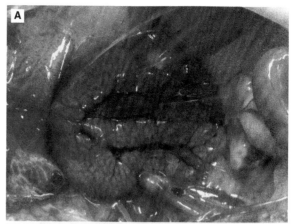

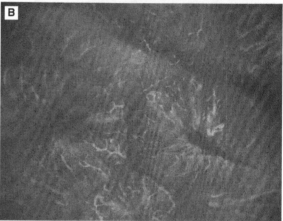

Fig 8.21 Bullfinch (*Pyrrhula pyrrhula*) kidney dehydration. **A** Kidney in situ; (**B**) close-up with visible urate congestion in the collecting tubuli.

and high-energy diets such as soft foods and mealworms. The liver is swollen, yellow or tan in colour, and may float in formalin. The use of some formulated diets may help to resolve or prevent hepatic lipidosis (Macwhirter 1994).

In canaries, lipogranulomata are commonly found in the liver. These lesions consist of foci formed by a variable number of vacuolated cells (probably macrophages), often mixed with lymphoid cells. In some cases heterophils have infiltrated as well. Lipogranulomata cannot generally be related to clinical problems, and the author has seen them in almost all canaries of all ages at necropsy. In other passerines or avian orders these lesions are only very rarely seen. Based on the fact that canaries are commonly fed with a large amount of rapeseed in their seed mixtures (up to 60%), the hypothesis is that some glycosides interfere with the fat metabolism, resulting in these lipogranulomata.

Haemorrhagic enteritis

'Haemorrhagic enteritis' is often diagnosed at necropsy, but this is not a 'true' enteritis and should be considered as a haemorrhagic diathesis (bleeding into the gut). This disease process is seen in small birds that are anorexic for over 24 hours (Fig. 8.20). Causes of anorexia in affected patients include being too ill to eat (e.g. because of an infection or intoxication), access to the wrong food or no food at all (e.g. if someone other than the owner is feeding the birds). A typical sign of haemorrhagic diathesis of the intestines at necropsy is an empty crop.

A similar interpretation should be given to swollen white kidneys, which are the result of uric acid precipitation in the collection tubules (Fig. 8.21). This occurs when birds do not drink and is often falsely called renal gout, although it should not be interpreted as either nephritis or gout. It should be differentiated from visceral gout caused by impaired renal function or a high-protein diet. Articular gout is a poorly understood chronic condition with no relation to renal function.

Toxicosis

1. Carbon monoxide exposure can be rapidly fatal. Canaries and finches are particularly susceptible to inhalant toxins because they breathe more air per gram of body weight than larger birds, and they have a highly efficient gas exchange system (Macwhirter 1994). There may be minimal changes at necropsy, or the lungs and blood may appear bright red.
2. Carbon dioxide poisoning may occur in crowded, poorly ventilated shipping boxes.
3. Polytetrafluoroethylene (Teflon®) released after overheating Teflon®-coated cooking utensils may be fatal to Passeriformes, as it is for psittacines. At necropsy, the extremely haemorrhagic, oedematous lungs are characteristic.

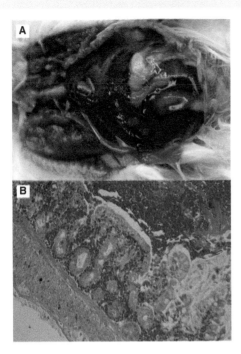

Fig 8.22 Canary haemorrhages after overdosing with
sulphachlorpyrazine (EsB3). (A) haemorrhages in situ; (B) histology
intestines; H&E.

4. Avocado, or at least certain varieties, may be
toxic to some passerines. Post-mortem findings in
intoxicated birds include hydropericardium and
subcutaneous oedema in the pectoral area (Hargis
1989).

5. Green almonds have been considered as a cause
of mortality in American goldfinches, presumably
from cyanide released by hydrolysis of amygdalin,
a cyanogenic glycoside.

6. Ethanol toxicity has been reported in free-ranging
passerines (especially cedar wax-wings) following
the ingestion of hawthorn apples or other fruits
that have frozen and then thawed, allowing
yeast fermentation of sugars to produce ethanol.
Birds are lethargic, ataxic, or may be in a stupor
('drunk'). Many intoxicated birds die from
accidents that occur while they are 'flying under
the influence'. The diagnosis is based on analysing
crop contents and liver for ethanol concentrations
(Fitzgerald et al 1990).

7. Heavy metal toxicosis caused by the direct
consumption of the metal is uncommon in
passerines, because they have limited capacity
to damage metal objects. Lead or zinc toxicosis
has occasionally occurred when galvanized wire
has been used in the construction or repair of
enclosures. Another source of zinc for passerine
species is galvanized containers for supplying
bath or drinking water. Removing the source of

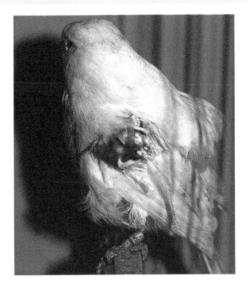

Fig 8.23 Canary with feather cysts (lumps).

heavy metals and the administration of chelation
therapy (Ca-EDTA 20–40 mg/kg i.v./i.m., followed
by 40–80 mg/kg p.o. b.i.d. until the lead has
disappeared) are recommended.

8. Overdosing of medicines, e.g. sulphonamides
causing clotting problems and haemorrhages
(Fig. 8.22).

Some non-infectious problems

Management and hygiene-related problems

Many problems in aviaries are management and hygiene-
related problems. These include location of the food and
water containers where large quantities of droppings
may collect; overcrowding, which leads to aggression;
and insufficient nesting sites, resulting in poor breeding
results. The control of ecto- and endoparasites is a matter
requiring constant attention.

Feather cysts

Feather cysts are common in canaries and are thought
to be more prevalent in certain breeds – e.g. Norwich
and 'intensive' type canaries (Fig. 8.23). Cysts may
occur individually or in clusters involving an entire
feather tract. Contents of the cysts may be gelatinous
in the early days, ranging to dry, keratinous material in
mature cysts. Treatment requires surgical removal of the
affected follicles.

Trauma

Picking is a common problem in aviaries, ranging from
a few feathers lost on the back of the head to cannibalism. Zebra finches are particularly prone to cage mate
trauma. Picking can also be the result of inappropriate

sexual behaviour of one or more dominant male birds. Hierarchical aggression occurs when aviaries are over-crowded and nesting site territories are being established. Sick birds may attract aggressive behaviour; the attacked bird should therefore be separated and the underlying problem addressed.

Trauma often results in fractures of the lower legs. Splinting in a flexed position using layered masking tape is sufficient to allow healing. Splints are well tolerated, and can usually be removed in 3 weeks.

Infectious diseases

Many infectious diseases are species-specific, although salmonellosis and pseudotuberculosis are exceptions. Coccidiosis is often diagnosed in finches, but most species appear to have their own coccidian species. These coccidia are often said to belong to the *Isospora lacazei* group.

Viral diseases

Avian pox

In captive passerines, avian pox as a septicaemic problem is almost exclusively seen in canaries and other *Serinus* spp. This disease predominates in the autumn and winter, with affected birds showing the cutaneous, diphtheric and septicaemic forms of the disease. The septicaemic or respiratory form causes a high mortality due to a severe tracheitis and, occasionally, pneumonic lesions around the bronchi (Fig. 8.24).

Birds of all ages can be affected, and the mortality ranges from 20% to 100%. The most alarming clinical signs are dyspnoea, debilitation and death. **The infection is primarily transmitted by insects (e.g. mosquitoes) and directly via blood from the lesions, and directly via the food and drinking water.** A presumptive diagnosis can be made on the clinical signs, the lesions and cytology. A positive diagnosis is made after isolation of the virus or histological demonstration of the eosinophilic intracytoplasmic inclusion bodies (Bollinger bodies) in the epithelial cells, followed by an electron microscopic examination.

As a differential diagnosis, *Staphylococcus* spp., *Candida* spp. infection and trichomonads must be considered.

Preventive vaccination is possible by the cutaneous wing-web method, preferable in early summer. The vaccination must be repeated once every year. In case of an epidemic, all birds must be caged individually or, if this is impossible, in small groups. All clinically healthy birds should be vaccinated; supportive treatment consists of the administration of antibiotics and multivitamin preparations. When there has been no mortality for 2 weeks, the birds can be housed in their flights again.

In masked bullfinches (*Pyrrhula erythaca*) a pox virus has been demonstrated, causing tumour-like lesions in

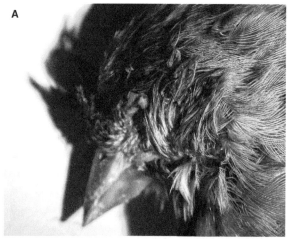

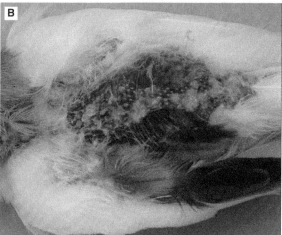

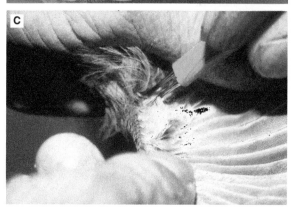

Fig 8.24 Avipox lesions. (**A**) Pox lesions near the beak, black-hooded red siskin (*Spinus cucullatus*); (**B**) skin lesions canary; (**C**) vaccination with the wing-web method.

the head region and inside the beak (Dorrestein et al 1993).

In young mynahs, keratitis, conjunctivitis and other eye problems have been identified in birds infected with avian pox virus. In other avian cases, pox lesions were located in the beak and commissure (Korbel & Kösters 1998).

Polyomavirus, polyoma-like and papilloma virus infections

These infections occur in finch aviaries across Australia, Europe and the United States, and are probably more common than the number of cases actually diagnosed. These infections are mainly reported in Estrildidae and Fringillidae (e.g. Gouldian finches, painted finches, canaries, goldfinches and green finches) and in Shama (*Copsychus malabaricus*) (Crosta et al 1997, Vereecken et al 1998). The disease causes young nestling mortality, a more chronic disease in which poor development and beak abnormalities predominate, and peracute death. Secondary infections appear to complicate the disease. Gross necropsy may reveal spleno/hepatomegaly, while the predominant histological lesions are hepatocellular necrosis, myocarditis, or lung adenomatosis showing karyomegaly with foamy, intranuclear inclusions. Myocarditis may be seen. The diagnosis is made by a specific fluorescent antibody test on liver and spleen impression smears. In an electron microscopic examination of the intranuclear inclusions, discrete round to icosahedral (20-sided) electron-dense particles, 45–50 nm in diameter, can be found.

Recently (Wittig et al 2007), using a newly developed polymerase chain reaction protocol, the DNA of the recently discovered finch polyomavirus (FPyV) was demonstrated in several affected birds. Between 2000 and 2004 a disease occurred in an aviary in Germany affecting various bird species belonging to the order Passeriformes including collared grosbeaks (*Mycerobas affinis*), Eurasian bullfinches (*Pyrrhula pyrrhula griseiventris*), brown bullfinches (*Pyrrhula nipalensis*), grey-headed bullfinches (*Pyrrhula erythaca*) and yellow-bellied tits (*Periparus venustulus*). The major clinical signs included increased mortality of fledglings and young birds, as well as feather disorders and feather loss in adult birds. In addition, adult Eurasian bullfinches showed in one year a disease course in which the major sign was inflammation of the skin beginning on the base of the beak and spreading over the head that occurred a few days before death.

Polyomavirus is also documented in wild passerines. Avian polyomavirus (APV) infection of recently imported Crimson's seedcrackers (*Pyrenestes sanguineus*) resulted in mortality in 56 of 70 (80%) birds in January 2000 (Rossi et al 2005). Viral infection in these birds was characterized by diarrhoea, anorexia, and lethargy, and death usually ensued within 48 to 72 hours of initial clinical signs. Bacteriological testing resulted in consistently negative results. Histological examination of tissues from dead birds revealed large

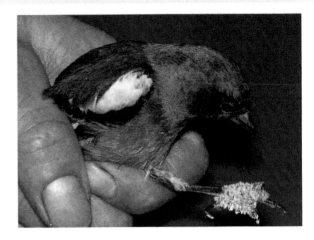

Fig 8.25 Finch with tassel foot.

intranuclear inclusion bodies, which at electron microscopy examination contained 42- to 49-nm viral particles. The diagnosis of APV infection was based on immunohistochemistry and immunoelectron microscopy, using a monoclonal antibody specific for VP-1 major capsidic APV protein (Rossi et al 2005).

Papilloma virus is found in European finches, and causes slow-growing, dry, wart-like epithelial proliferations of the skin of the feet and legs, 'tassel foot' (Fig. 8.25).

Paramyxovirus infection

Paramyxovirus (PMV) infection is commonly seen in many finches (e.g. African silverbills (*Lonchura malabarica cantans*), zebra finches and Gouldian finches) and canaries, and is mostly serotype 3 causing tremor, paralysis or torticollis in these birds. Depression and variable degrees of weight loss are other clinical signs often associated with this viral infection. The birds can be carriers for months before the clinical symptoms become manifest. The diagnosis is based on the signs, and can be confirmed by serology and virus isolation; necropsy is non-specific. A severe pancreatitis may be found on histological examination in some cases.

Antibiotic therapy produces no significant difference in survival rate or outcome. The disease must be differentiated from a vitamin E deficiency caused by feeding rancid cod-liver oil or mixing oil through the seed.

PMV-1 has been identified in recently imported mynahs (Korbel & Kösters 1998), and the clinical signs associated with these birds included central nervous signs, opisthotonus and greenish slimy diarrhoea which started 4 weeks after their introduction into a collection. The diagnosis of PMV is based on clinical signs, isolation and characterization of the virus. A preventive inactivated vaccine is available. PMV-1 and PMV-2 infections have been identified in weaver finches (*Parmoptila* sp.). In type 1 infections, clinical signs include conjunctivitis, pseudomembrane formation in the larynx, and death. Neurological signs are rare. Canaries rarely develop clinical signs: infected birds should be considered subclinical carriers. Type 2 infections occur commonly in African weaver finches and they are considered carriers of this virus. Many infected birds are subclinical carriers, but others may die following a period of emaciation and pneumonia (Ritchie 1995).

Herpesvirus and cytomegalovirus

These viruses cause conjunctivitis and respiratory problems in Australian and African finches (Macwhirter 1994). Lady Gouldian finches are very sensitive to this virus and can be infected by recently imported wild-caught finches from Africa. The diagnosis is confirmed by demonstration in cytology and histology of (basophilic) intranuclear inclusion bodies in the mucosal epithelial cells of the trachea and conjunctiva.

Circovirus infections

There have been confirmed or suspected circovirus infections in a variety of avian species other than psittacines and pigeons, including canaries (*Serinus canaria*), zebra finches (*Poephila guttata*), Gouldian finches (*Chloebia gouldiae*) and many other birds belonging to other orders (Sandmeier 2003, Shivaprasad et al 2004). Phylogenetic analysis provided evidence that canary circovirus (CaCV) is more closely related to pigeon circovirus (PiCV) and psittacine beak and feather disease virus (PBFDV) and more distantly related to goose circovirus (GCV) and the two porcine circovirus strains, PCV1 and PCV2 (Phenix et al 2001). A different circovirus was isolated from another passeriform species, the Australian raven (*Corvus coronoides*), with feather lesions similar to those that occur in psittacine beak and feather disease. Comparison with other members of the Circoviridae demonstrated that raven circovirus RaCV shares the greatest sequence homology with CaCV and PiCV and is more distantly related to the PBFDV, GCV, duck circovirus and the two porcine circoviruses (Steward et al 2006).

Although clinical signs vary the most common presentation is morbidity and mortality predominantly in young birds associated with immunosuppression caused by lymphoid necrosis and cellular depletion in the bursa of Fabricius and to a lesser extent in the spleen (Grifois et al 2005). Feather dystrophy has been described in some cases, but is not a classical symptom as it is in psittacine beak and feather disease. In canary nestlings showing the so-called 'black spot', which is a gall bladder congestion, a circovirus has been demonstrated at electron microscopy, but a cultivation and infection trial

were negative (Goldsmith 1995). In another report multiple cytoplasmic inclusion bodies were observed in the intestinal smooth muscle cells of an adult canary from an aviary with a history of high mortality (50%) both in adult and young birds. Grossly, a mild enteritis was the only lesion appreciable. Smears of the proventricular contents contained a few gastric yeasts (*Macrorhabdus ornithogaster*). The intestinal inclusions were found in very high numbers in all parts of the tract examined. Inclusions of the same type were occasionally detectable in the wall of a few splenic and pancreatic arteries. No inclusions or lesions were seen in the other organs examined. Transmission electron microscopy of the intestinal wall revealed circovirus-like particles either in paracrystalline arrays or loose arrangements, mostly within the cytoplasm of the intestinal muscle cells. Polymerase chain reaction amplification and sequence analysis confirmed infection with canary circovirus (Rampin et al 2006).

The Gouldian finches coming from an aviary that had housed about 100 Gouldian finches had nasal discharge, dyspnoea, anorexia, depression and a very high mortality (50%) in both adult and young birds. Gross and histopathology revealed moderate to severe lymphoid depletion in the bursa of Fabricius and thymus, and sinusitis/rhinitis, tracheitis, bronchopneumonia, myocarditis, nephritis and splenitis. Circovirus infection was diagnosed based on finding characteristic globular intracytoplasmic inclusion bodies in the mononuclear cells of the bursa of Fabricius, by transmission electron microscopy and by demonstrating circovirus DNA by in-situ hybridization (Shivaprasad et al 2004).

Emerging virus infections

Small Passeriformes play a minor role in the spreading of the emerging viral diseases West Nile virus (WNV) and avian influenza (AI).

The American crow (*Corvus brachyrhynchos*) plays the most obvious role as a reservoir of the mosquito-transmitted WNV in the US. The ability of the invading NY99 strain of WNV to elicit an elevated viraemia response in Californian passerine birds is critical for the effective infection of *Culex* mosquitoes. Of the bird species tested, Western scrub jays, *Aphelocoma coerulescens*, produced the highest viraemia response, followed by house finches, *Carpodacus mexicanus*, and house sparrows, *Passer domesticus*. Most likely, few mourning doves (*Zenaidura macroura*) or common ground doves (*Columbina passerine*) and no California quail, *Callipepla californica*, or chickens would infect blood-feeding *Culex* mosquitoes. All Western scrub jays and most house finches succumbed to infection (Reisen et al 2005). House finches and English sparrows are competent hosts for both West Nile and St Louis encephalitis viruses and frequently become infected during outbreaks.

Although mortality rates were high during initial infection with West Nile virus, prior infection with either virus prevented mortality upon challenge with West Nile virus (Fang & Reisen 2006).

Infections with influenza virus have been reported in finches and in imported mynahs. An avian influenza A virus of the subtype H7N1 was isolated in summer 1972 from a single free-living siskin (*Carduelis spinus* Linnaeus, 1758). Additional cases of morbidity or mortality were not observed in the area were the sick siskin was found. The virus induced following experimental inoculation of chicken embryos a high rate mortality (mean death time approximately 24 hours). This virus was considered as a highly pathogenic avian influenza A virus. Canaries that were housed in the same room with the siskin were accidentally exposed by contact to the sick siskin, which resulted in virus transmission followed by conjunctivitis, apathy, anorexia and a high rate mortality (Kaleta & Hönicke 2005). The role of passerines in the spread of avian influenza A is, however, negligible. A total of 543 migrating passerines were captured during their stopover on the island of Heligoland (North Sea) in spring and autumn 2001. They were sampled for the detection of avian influenza A viruses (AIV) subtypes H5 and H7, and for avian paramyxoviruses serotype 1 (APMV-1). For virus detection, samples were taken from (a) short-distance migrants such as chaffinches (*Fringilla coelebs*, $n = 131$) and song thrushes (*Turdus philomelos*, $n = 169$), and (b) long-distance migrants such as garden warbler (*Sylvia borin*, $n = 142$) and common redstarts (*Phoenicurus phoenicurus*, $n = 101$). Virus detection was done on conjunctival, choanal cleft and cloacal swabs. In none of the tested samples was AIV detected. Six out of 543 birds (1.1%) were found to carry non-pathogenic and lentogenic strains of APMV-1. This indicates that the passerine species examined in this study may play only a minor role as potential vectors of APMV-1 (Schnebel et al 2005). In another study 413 free-living migrating passerines from 37 different species were caught in the autumn of 2004 in Slovenia and cloacal swabs taken and processed by RT-PCR and virus isolation. Only one sample from a common starling (*Sturnus vulgaris*) by RT-PCR was positive for AIV, but negative for H5 and H7 (Račnik et al 2007).

Other viral infections

In a breeding flock of canaries, significant mortality of juvenile birds with neurological signs and nestling mortality has been associated with an adenovirus-like infection (Dorrestein et al 1996). Recently, a coronavirus has been demonstrated in the trachea of canaries with mild respiratory problems (Dorrestein et al 1998).

Suspected leukosis cases are sporadically found at necropsy in Passeriformes, especially in canaries. These birds historically show hepatomegaly and splenomegaly on gross necropsy. The histopathology is suggestive of leukosis. A virus aetiology is suspected, but this has never been confirmed.

A clinical syndrome similar to proventricular dilatation disease of psittacines, and characterized histologically by lymphoplasmatic infiltrates of the myenteric plexus of the gastrointestinal tract, is described in at least three species of passerines: a canary, a chaffinch and an Amazon umbrella bird (Perpinan et al 2005).

Box 8.3 Usutu virus activity is spreading in Europe

In 2001, Usutu virus (USUV), a member of the mosquito-borne-clade within the Flaviviridae family was responsible for mortality of blackbirds (*Turdus merula*) and great grey owls (*Strix nebulosa*) in the city of Vienna and surrounding villages. This was the first time that USUV had emerged outside Africa and caused fatalities in warm-blooded hosts. Although retrospective examination of blackbird tissues suggested introduction of USUV into Austria already 1 year earlier (in 2000), there were no reports of bird die-offs that year (Weissenböck et al 2002). In the following years there was an increase in the number of diagnosed cases with a maximum of 91 cases in 2003. In 2005 only 4 cases were diagnosed in Austria. The major macroscopic finding was hepatosplenomegaly; histologically, neuronal necrosis, myocardial lesions and coagulative necrosis of the liver and spleen were observed. The diagnosis is confirmed by immunohistochemistry (IHC) and in-situ hybridization (ISH) (Chvala et al 2004). Until 2006 the virus was only found in Austria (Bakonvi et al 2007).

In the summer of 2006 unusual bird mortalities were reported at Zurich Zoo, including wild blackbirds, wild sparrows (*Passer domesticus*) and captive Strigidae (more than 90 birds). Neuronal necrosis was the most prevalent finding in pathohistological examinations. In the same period a great grey owl (*Strix nebulosa*) originating from northern Italy, in the middle of a triangle formed by Milano, Como and Lecco, died and was histopathologically examined. The bird was captive bred and came from a large breeding collection of many different Strigiformes. The breeder was losing great grey owls and hawk owls (*Surnia ulula*) after a short period (a few days) of disease. The main pathological finding at necropsy was a hepatomegaly with congestion. By immunohistochemistry large amounts of USUV antigen were found in many different organs. This finding was confirmed by PCR and sequencing of amplification products (Dorrestein et al 2007).

Bacterial infections

E. coli *(and other Enterobacteriaceae)*

In normal healthy passerines, *E. coli* (and other Enterobacteriaceae) are absent in the intestines. However, these bacteria are very often demonstrated (by cytology) and isolated from the faeces or intestinal contents of diseased passerine birds both with and without diarrhoea.

E. coli septicaemia is suspected to be a major cause of epizootic mortality in newly arrived shipments of finches. *Citrobacter* spp. infection has also been reported as a cause of mortality in finches, and gross necropsy can, as with *E. coli*, be unrewarding. The Enterobacteriaceae present a secondary problem in finches more frequently than in canaries. The clinical signs and gross necropsy are not specific and include depression, conjunctivitis and rhinitis, and may be fatal in some birds. These are secondary pathogens, however, and should be considered as a sign of poor health or management conditions. Possible causes are an unbalanced diet, housing problems or husbandry problems. Other primary diseases may be present (e.g. atoxoplasmosis or coccidiosis). Cultures are necessary for diagnosis, and a sensitivity test is essential for treatment. Treatment temporarily improves this condition, but only by suppressing clinical signs. Clinicians must search for the primary underlying cause to prevent recurrence.

Enterobacteriaceae are regularly cultured from passerine nestlings with diarrhoea ('sweating disease'). The antibiotics of choice are neomycin or spectinomycin, because they are effective and not resorbed from the gut. The selected drug is administered via the soft food, while fledglings require extra water, chopped greens, and vegetables to prevent dehydration. As always, the clinician should remember that a specific culture and sensitivity is recommended to select the most effective antibiotic.

Yersiniosis (pseudotuberculosis)

Infection with *Yersinia pseudotuberculosis* is regularly seen in canaries and wild finches in the wintertime in Europe. The clinical signs are non-specific: ruffling of the feathers, debilitation and high mortality. At necropsy, a dark, swollen, congested liver and spleen with small, yellow, focal bacterial granulomata are often found, with an associated acute catarrhal pneumonia and typhlitis (Fig. 8.26). Many rod-shaped bacteria are seen in impression smears from all the organs, and diagnosis is confirmed after culturing the microorganisms. The treatment of choice is amoxicillin via drinking water and soft food. Once sensitivity test results have been obtained, the antibiotic might need to be changed. Cleaning and disinfection are essential to prevent a relapse after therapy has been completed.

Mynahs are very susceptible to yersiniosis, and mortality can be high due to a peracute pneumonia. Postmortem examination of affected birds demonstrates hepatomegaly, sometimes with small white foci, splenomegaly and an acute to peracute pneumonia. In Europe a formalin vaccine is available that appears to be clinically effective in reducing the prevalence of infections.

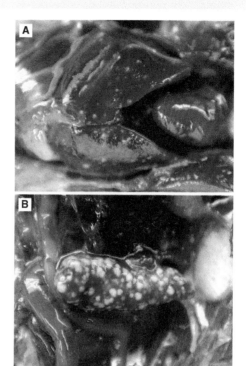

Fig 8.26 Canary pseudotuberculosis, liver (**A**) and spleen (**B**).

Salmonellosis (paratyphoid)

Infection with *Salmonella enterica*, serovar Typhimurium in small passerines appears identical with pseudotuberculosis, both clinically and at necropsy, although salmonellosis more often has a chronic course. Carriers are unknown in canaries. The diagnosis is confirmed after culturing the microorganism (Fig. 8.27). Fatal septicaemias are also reported in mynahs.

Antibiotics that are most effective are trimethoprim (with or without sulfa), amoxicillin or enrofloxacin, and must be combined with proper hygiene measures. A bacteriological examination of a pooled faecal sample in an enrichment medium should be performed 3–6 weeks after therapy to evaluate its success. The therapy and hygiene measures can be repeated until the bacteriological control remains negative.

Campylobacter fetus

Campylobacter fetus subsp. *jejuni* is often found in tropical finches, especially in Estrildidae (Fig. 8.28). Society finches are commonly identified as carriers without conspicuous clinical symptoms. Clinical signs include apathy, retarded moulting, yellow droppings and a high mortality, especially among fledglings. The yellow droppings are caused by large amounts of undigested suspension (amylum = starch) and occasionally parts of or whole seeds are found in the droppings.

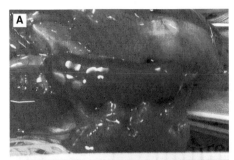

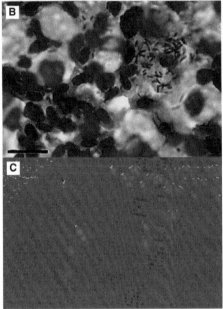

Fig 8.27 Canary salmonellosis splenomegaly (**A**), impression smear (**B**) and culture (**C**).

At necropsy the intestine is filled with a yellow amylum or whole seeds, resembling the beads of a rosary. Other necropsy findings are cachexia and a congested gastrointestinal tract. The diagnosis is confirmed by demonstrating the curved rods in stained smears from the droppings or gut contents, and cultivating the bacteria on special microaerophilic media. *Campylobacter* spp. have also been isolated from recently imported mynahs.

Treatment can be attempted with several antibiotics, but hygienic measurements are most important. Although campylobacteriosis is considered a potential zoonosis, there are no published reports of *Campylobacter* spp. transmission from passerines to humans.

Cocci infections

Streptococcus spp. and *Staphylococcus* spp. are often demonstrated in passerines. The clinical signs include abscesses, dermatitis, 'bumble foot', conjunctivitis, sinusitis, arthritis, pneumonia and death. In patients suffering

from these infections, cocci will be seen in the impression smears. The treatment of choice for cocci infections is local and systemic treatment with ampicillin or amoxicillin.

Enterococcus faecalis

Enterococcus faecalis has been associated with chronic tracheitis, pneumonia and air sac infections in canaries. Clinically affected birds have harsh respiratory sounds, voice changes and dyspnoea.

Pseudomonas *spp. and* aeromonas *spp. infections*

Improperly prepared sprouted or germinated seeds, dirty drinking vessels or baths, and water are often the source of *Pseudomonas* spp. or *Aeromonas* spp. bacteria. A polluted flower-spraying mister, used for spraying the birds, can cause a severe necropurulent pneumonia and aerosacculitis. *Pseudomonas* spp. are often found as the result of an improper antibiotic treatment. Proper treatment includes locating the source of the trouble and administration of an antibiotic (after performing a sensitivity test). Until the results are available, the first choice antibiotic in these infections is enrofloxacin. Painstaking hygiene is essential, because many strains are resistant to antibiotic treatment.

Avian tuberculosis

The classic tuberculosis with tubercles in the organs is seldom seen in small passerines. Tuberculosis (so-called atypical *Mycobacterium avium* or *Mycobacterium-avium-intracellulare* complex) is most commonly found accidentally at necropsy in canaries and finches (Estrildidae) (Fig. 8.29). A new species, *M. genavense*, is also associated with avian tuberculosis, and is mainly isolated from patients with AIDS (Hoop et al 1995, 1996). So far there is only one report of a canary with a tuberculous knot in the lung due to *M. tuberculosis*; it is the first description of *M. tuberculosis* in a non-psittacine bird species (Hoop 2002). Other mycobacteria from the *M. fortuitum* group are also documented in Gouldian finches, e.g. the so-called atypical form *Mycobacterium peregrinum* (Vitalli et al 2006).

Incidental infections with acid-fast bacilli are diagnosed relatively often. On histological examination, macrophages loaded with acid-fast bacilli can be found in many organs, especially in the liver or intestines. No signs are apparent at necropsy, except perhaps a dark, slightly swollen liver. In a flock of zebra finches with signs of a CNS disease, acid-fast bacteria were demonstrated in impression smears of brain, liver and intestines, and the bacterium was identified as *M. genavense* by using PCR (Sandmeier et al 1997).

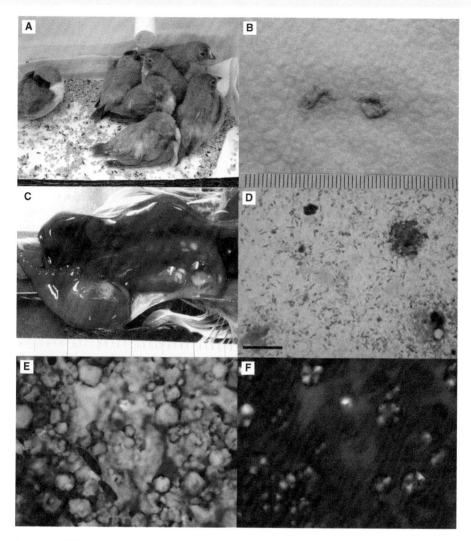

Fig 8.28 Campylobacteriosis. (**A**) Gouldian finches, sick fledglings; (**B**) typical faeces containing much starch; (**C**) intestines with undigested seeds; (**D**) intestinal smear with *Campylobacter* sp. (Hemacolor® = Hc, bar = 10 μm); (**E**) stained duodenal smear with starch (Hc); (**F**) the same smear showing the birefringent crystals (polarized light).

Infections with *Mycobacterium* spp. have also been reported in mynahs as a catarrhal enteritis, as well as classical tuberculosis (Korbel & Kösters 1998).

The diagnosis is confirmed by demonstrating the acid-fast bacteria in tissue smears, while differentiation is possible using PCR techniques.

Treatment is not often practised. There is a zoonosis aspect, mostly for people with an immunocompromised physiological status. The enclosures need to be cleaned and disinfected. In the infected soil, *Mycobacterium* spp. can survive for 2 years.

Avian chlamydiosis

This a relatively uncommon problem in passerines and softbills. The annual incidence of avian chlamydiosis in canaries at necropsy in the Netherlands is between 0% and 1.4%. *Chlamydophila psittaci* spp. have been isolated from the droppings of clinically normal finches in households in which clinical cases of chlamydiosis (psittacosis) occurred in psittacines (Macwhirter 1994). In a study in Israel, 26% of the Passeriformes tested by immunofluorescence test (IFT) were positive, ranging from 10% in zoo collections up to 41% in pet birds (Dublin et al 1995). Of these, 12% were found in the winter (December to February) and 41% in the summer (June to August). In a study of wild birds in Austria using an ELISA test, 5 of 29 passerines were positive for the antigen and 15 of 17 showed antibodies (Pohl 1995). Based on reviews, geographical areas and different test systems give large differences.

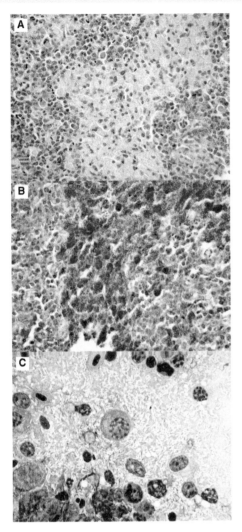

Fig 8.29 Bullfinch mycobacteriosis. (**A**) Spleen HE 40 × ; (**B**) the same spleen stained with acid-fast staining; (**C**) impression smear of the same spleen. Notice the non-stained ghost rod-shaped bacteria; Hc 100 ×.

The clinical signs associated with this disease are non-specific, and can include apathy, diarrhoea, debilitation, nasal exudate and conjunctivitis. The mortality is generally less then 10%. Avian chlamydiosis should be expected in passerines with recurrent respiratory disease, especially if they are exposed to psittacines.

The diagnosis is made at necropsy by the presence of the chlamydial organism in impression smears from the altered air sacs and organs, using special staining techniques, or an enzyme-linked immunosorbent assay (ELISA) from swabs.

In mynahs, shedding has been demonstrated in clinically healthy birds (Korbel & Kösters 1998).

Treatment with chlortetracycline (30 days) or doxycycline (30 days) via drinking water and soft food is clinically effective, but only when the birds continue to eat and drink the normal amount of food and water.

Mycoplasma *spp.*

Mycoplasma spp. have been isolated from canaries, and many cases of conjunctivitis and upper respiratory disease in canaries respond to tylosin; however, there has been no conclusive work proving that *Mycoplasma* spp. are associated with this syndrome. An epizootic of conjunctivitis in house finches (*Carpodacus mexicanus*) associated with *Mycoplasma gallisepticum* (MG) infection was reported in 1994 and 1995 from the United States and has been spreading from east to west in 10 years (Fischer & Converse 1995, Ley et al 2006). Ever since *Mycoplasma gallisepticum* emerged among house finches in North America, it has been suggested that bird aggregations at feeders are an important cause of the epidemic of mycoplasmal conjunctivitis because diseased birds could deposit droplets of pathogen onto the feeders and thereby promote indirect transmission by fomites. House finches infected via this route, however, developed only mild disease and recovered much more rapidly than birds infected from the same source birds but directly into the conjunctiva. While it is certainly probable that house finch aggregations at artificial feeders enhance pathogen transmission, to some degree transmission of *Mycoplasma gallisepticum* by fomites may serve to immunize birds against developing more severe infections. Sometimes such birds develop *Mycoplasma gallisepticum* antibodies, providing indication of an immune response, although no direct evidence of protection (Dhondt et al 2007). The clinical signs ranged from mildly swollen eyelids with clear ocular discharge to severe conjunctivitis and apparent blindness.

Tetracyclines and enrofloxacin are believed to be effective against many *Mycoplasma* spp. Clinical signs of conjunctivitis associated with MG infection in house finches resolved following oral tylosin (1 mg/mL drinking water for at least 21 days) as the sole source of drinking water, in conjunction with topical ciprofloxacin HCl ophthalmic solution for 5–7 days (Mashima et al 1997).

Other bacterial infections

Gram-negative oviduct infections, which if untreated can cause high mortality amongst canary hens sitting on their second round of eggs, are seen in epidemic proportions in canary breeding establishments in some years (Macwhirter 1994).

Erysipelothrix rhusiopathia, Listeria monocytogenes and *Pasteurella multocida* (cat-bite?!) are occasionally isolated from dead passerine and softbill birds.

Megabacteria were recently classified as yeast-like organisms (*Macrorhabdus ornithogaster*).

Mycotic infections

Candida and fungal infections are not a significant problem in canaries, but are much more common in tropical finches and mynahs. The most common mycotic infection in passerines is an infection with the yeast *Macrorhabdus ornithogaster*.

Candidiasis

Care should be taken in evaluating faecal smears from passerines for *Candida*. Many Passeriformes are fed yeast products, and yeast blastophores may pass through the gastrointestinal tract unchanged and appear in large numbers in the faeces. These organisms do not reflect disease, and do not grow on yeast culture media.

Cases of candidiasis are commonly seen in finches and can be related to an unbalanced diet, poor hygiene, crowded conditions, excessive moisture, spoilage of food, stress, and the uncontrolled use of antibiotics. In nestlings and fledgling, crop candidiasis (with gas formation caused by fermentation and a thickened, opaque crop wall whose mucosa is covered with a white coating) is relatively common (Fig. 8.30). In weanlings and adult birds, diarrhoea and moulting problems are more prominent. The typical signs in African finches with endoventricular mycoses were lethargy, weight loss, a 'fluffed' appearance, passage of whole seeds in the stool, and in many cases the bird 'tilted' forward, elevating the abdomen and tail (Suedmeyer 1997, Schmidt et al 2003) (Fig. 8.31).

It is not uncommon to identify the yeast *Candida albicans* in cultures of the gastrointestinal tract of softbills. Chicks that have poor daily weight gain or a poor feeding response should be examined for potential bacterial or yeast overgrowth. Cytology stain or cultures of the crop or cloaca should be performed to confirm the diagnosis.

The diagnosis is confirmed by finding the budding yeasts in crop swabs, faecal smears or skin scrapings. Intestinal candidiasis is treated with nystatin for 3–6 weeks, at a dose of 100 000 IU/L drinking water and 200 000 IU/kg soft food. The eye lesions and dermatitis can be treated with intravenous and topical amphotericin B. The predisposing factors should be addressed as well.

Fungi

Aspergillus spp. (Fig. 8.32) is an uncommon finding in small passerines. In captive mynahs, however, *Aspergillus* spp. infections can be a problem. **Clinically, chronic respiratory disease is a common clinical sign in birds associated with a mycotic infection.** In Munich, aspergillosis was diagnosed in 23.8% of 147 mynah necropsies (Korbel & Kösters 1998). In 92 necropsies of mynahs performed in Utrecht, seven cases showed a mycotic air sacculitis and pneumonia (Dorrestein & van der Hage 1988). Fungal infections are to be considered as opportunistic infections, and are generally the result

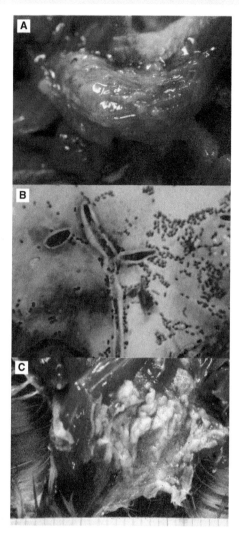

Fig 8.30 Crop candidiasis. (**A**) Crop nestling, orange-cheeked waxbill (*Estrilda melpoda*); (**B**) crop smear, Hc 100 ×; (**C**) severe crop changes, Gouldian finch.

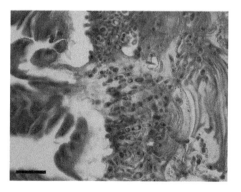

Fig 8.31 *Carduelis* sp., endoventricular mycosis; HE, bar is 20 μm.

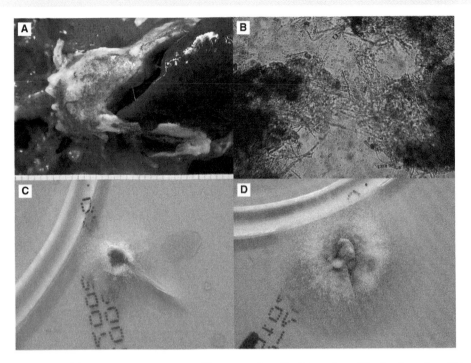

Fig 8.32 Bullfinch aspergillosis. (**A**) Bullfinch mycotic air sacculitis; (**B**) wet mount fungal hyphi from air sac; (**C**) culture from air sac 24 hours (malt); (**D**) culture 48 hours, *Aspergillus fumigatus*.

of an impaired immunosystem (e.g. due to haemochromatosis, hypovitaminosis A, misuse of antibiotics such as tetracyclines).

Clinical diagnosis involves culturing from tracheal swabs, radiographic examination and endoscopy. In some cases (e.g. syringeal aspergillomata or localized air sac involvement), surgery may be effective in treating the disease. In chronic cases, drug therapy has a poor prognosis. Preventive measures include adequate vitamin A supplementation and improvement of management techniques.

Dermatomycoses are occasionally reported in passerines, and generally cause alopecia of the head and neck, or hyperkeratosis. *Microsporium* spp. and *Trichophyton* spp. are the most common aetiological agents identified, but saprophytic fungi may also be involved. Zoonotic aspects should be considered. Also *Malassezia* sp. can be involved in skin problems (Fig. 8.33).

Treatment with ketoconazole and griseofulvin provides some improvement, but does not always eliminate the infection.

Other mycotic infections reported in passerines include *Cryptococcus neoformans*, but this is very rarely seen as a disease problem in these birds.

Zygomycosis (mucormycosis) has been reported as appearing as multiple granulomata in the lung, liver or brain of canaries and finches. The incidents are related to feeding damp, germinated seeds (Macwhirter 1994). In another publication three canaries showing feather loss on legs, dorsum, neck, and head, and hyperkeratosis

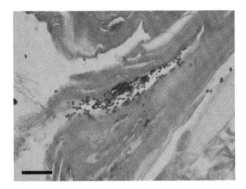

Fig 8.33 Finch with bald skin due to a *Malassezia* infection; PAS, bar is 20 µm.

on the feet revealed histologically, pronounced epidermal and follicular infundibular hyperplasia associated with orthokeratotic hyperkeratosis. Numerous fungal spores were observed on the stratum corneum of the epidermis and within feather follicles, associated with destruction of the feathers. This fungus was identified as *Mucor ramosissimus* (Quesada et al 2007).

Macrorhabdus ornithogaster

Macrorhabdus ornithogaster (formerly megabacterium or avian gastric yeast) is recently classified as yeast-like organisms (Tomaszewski et al 2003). *Macrorhabdus* spp. are large (20–50μm), Gram-positive, periodic acid–Schiff (PAS) positive, rod-shaped organisms that have fungal characteristics and have been found in the proventriculus or droppings of several avian species. Until recently it was not possible to culture the organism. In canaries, infection caused by these organisms in the proventriculus is common, and is predominantly found on the mucosal surface and in the ducts of the glands. *Macrorhabdus* colonization of the proventriculus in companion birds is not always associated with clinical signs or pathological lesions (De Herdt et al 1997). In one study, 22.9% of Psittaciformes (35.8% in budgerigars) and 19% of Passeriformes (only 16.7% in canaries) demonstrated a positive proventriculus at necropsy for these organisms (Ravelhofer et al 1998). In a more recent study in Belgium there was an increasing incidence of *Macrorhabdus* in canaries (Marlier et al 2006). At the time of death, macrorhabdiosis was diagnosed in 28% of canaries and 22.5% of budgerigars, but was not diagnosed in parrots. The incidence (or detection?) of macrorhabdiosis has significantly increased in recent years.

Clinical signs of birds suffering from *M. ornithogaster* infection can include apathy, anorexia, regurgitation, and the passing of part or whole seeds in soft, watery, dark green to brown/black faeces. These birds show a proventriculitis, and the pH in the lumen (originally 0.7–2.4) is increased to 8.0–8.4. These microorganisms can be seen in a smear (see Figs 8.16/8.17) taken from the thick, whitish mucus covering the mucosa, and sometimes in faecal smears. The birds are often debilitated; the morbidity is high, but the mortality is low.

Past diagnostic techniques were based on demonstrating the organism in wet-mount or stained microscopic smears since the organism was difficult to grow (Scanlan & Graham 1990). Recent research demonstrated that optimum growth conditions were found to be Basal Medium Eagle's, pH 3 to 4, containing 20% fetal bovine serum (FBS), and 5% glucose or sucrose under microaerophilic conditions at 42°C. Using these conditions, *M. ornithogaster* was repeatedly passaged without loss of viability (Hanafussa et al 2007).

At necropsy, the organism can be demonstrated in the mucus of the proventriculus. The proventriculus is mostly distended, and the mucosa is covered with a cloudy, thick, mucous layer, predominantly in the lower part of the organ. The wall of the proventriculus is thickened and often shows small haemorrhages. The koilin layer may appear soft and devitalized. In the Belgian study (Marlier et al 2006), the most common gross lesion seen at necropsy of the 59 macrorhabdiosis cases in the canaries was proventricular dilatation (86.1%). All the birds diagnosed as typical macrorhabdiosis cases were free of *Salmonella* spp. infections and of any parasitic infections. Four macrorhabdiosis cases (three canaries, one parakeet) were not included in statistical

analysis as salmonellosis, pseudotuberculosis, coccidiosis and chlamydophilosis were diagnosed concomitantly in these birds. With the exception of macrorhabdiosis, the most frequent causes of death were protozoan (e.g. coccidiosis, atoxoplasmosis) infections (18.4%) and salmonellosis (17.1%) in canaries.

Therapy aims at improvement of the management conditions, including provision of easily digestible food (egg food), and lowering the pH in the proventriculus (6 mL 0.1 N HCl/L or citric acid 1 g/L) to activate pepsin. Oral amphotericin B has proved effective in budgerigars, and oral nystatin in European finches (Filippich & Parker 1994, Phalen & Tomaszewski 2003, Scullion & Scullion 2004, Phalen 2005).

After 6 weeks the birds can be returned to a normal diet, which should include egg food as a regular supplement.

Parasitic infections

Protozoal infections

The most important protozoal infections in canaries are atoxoplasmosis, coccidiosis, toxoplasmosis and trichomoniasis. Atoxoplasma-like infections and cryptosporidiosis are found only occasionally in finches, starlings and mynahs, and are mostly restricted to individual birds; in those species of birds the infection is never seen as a flock problem. Coccidiosis, cochlosomosis and trichomoniasis are very common in finches. In softbills, *Giardia* spp. and coccidiosis are occasionally noted in faecal examination or post-mortem examination. There is one report of microsporidiosis in a flock of tricolor parrot finches (*Erythrura tricolor*). These birds showed a pale thickening of the serosal surfaces of the gastrointestinal tract, pancreas and air sacs (Gelis & Raidal 2006).

Atoxoplasmosis

Atoxoplasmosis (formerly *Lankesterella*) in canaries is caused by *Isospora serini*, a coccidium with an asexual life cycle in the organs and a sexual cycle in the intestinal mucosa. Atoxoplasmosis is a disease of young canaries ranging in age from 2 to 9 months. The clinical signs include huddling and ruffling of the feathers, debilitation, diarrhoea, neurological signs (20%) and death. Mortality can be as high as 80%. An enlarged liver may be observed as a blue spot on the right side of the abdomen caudal to the sternum, referred to by fanciers as 'thick liver disease' (Fig. 8.34). At necropsy, an enlarged and sometimes spotted liver (with necrosis in the acute phase) is noted, along with a huge, dark-red coloured spleen (see Fig. 8.4) and, often, an oedematous duodenum with vascularization. In the imprints of the liver, spleen and lungs, parasites are found in the cytoplasm of the monocytes. The nucleus of the host cell is crescent-shaped

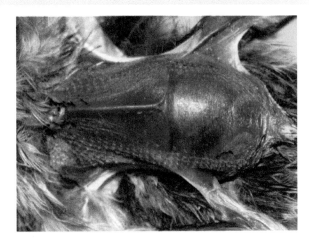

Fig 8.34 Canary in poor condition and hepatomegaly related to atoxoplasmosis.

(see Fig. 8.17). Coccidia are seldom found in the faeces or intestinal contents because, after the acute phase is passed, only a few coccidia (100–200/24 hours) are excreted. The therapeutic agent of choice is sulphachlorpyrazine (150 mg/L drinking water) until after moulting for 5 days a week. This treatment affects the production of oocysts, but does not influence the intracellular stages.

Other measures to improve health of young birds include feeding one part egg food and one part seed mixture until after moulting, prevention of crowding (e.g. stress reduction), and better hygiene (i.e. cleaning and changing the floor coating). These measures alone can prevent clinical outbreaks in infected canaries. This infection is also a common problem in other European finches kept in captivity (e.g. goldfinches, siskins, greenfinches, bullfinches).

Atoxoplasma-like infections

Atoxoplasma-like infections are seen in tropical finches, mynahs and other Sturnidae. Atoxoplasmosis and haemochromatosis are the primary medical problems in captive Bali mynahs. Atoxoplasma oocysts have been found in the faeces of wild Bali mynahs; however, it is unknown whether this disease is contributing to the birds' decline (Norton et al 1995).

Coccidiosis

Isospora spp. have been described in more than 50 species of passerines throughout the whole world. Although this species was formerly named *Isospora lacazei*, the author is convinced that there are many different species. A recent experimental infection supports this assumption. *Isospora michaelbakeri* is one of the *Isospora* species most commonly found in the wild, which can cause severe infection and mortality in young sparrows. This *Isospora* was orally inoculated to russet sparrows (*Passer rutilans*), spotted munia (*Lonchura punctulata*), canary (*Serinus canaria*), Java sparrows (*Padda oryzivora*), chicken (*Gallus domesticus*), ducks (*Anas platyrhynchos*) and BALB/c mice. The results indicated that *I. michaelbakeri* infected only russet sparrows and not any other species experimentally inoculated with *I. michaelbakeri* in that study (Tung et al 2007).

In canaries, *I. canaria* is identified as a specific intestinal coccidiosis, and can be a problem in canaries over 2 months of age. The primary clinical signs observed in *I. canaria* infected patients are diarrhoea and emaciation. At necropsy the duodenum is oedematous, often with extensive haemorrhages in the gut wall. Trophozoites of the parasite can be found in scrapings of the duodenal mucosa, and large amounts of oocysts are seen in wet preparations from the droppings. Therapy consists of strict hygiene measures and treatment with coccidiostatic drugs. Amprolium solution has been recommended for the treatment of coccidiosis at a dosage of 50–100 mg/L for 5 days, or sulphachlorpyrazine 300 mg/L drinking water, 5 days a week for 2–3 weeks.

Eimeria spp. are not common in passerines, but single cases are being reported, based on the morphology of sporulated oocysts (*Eimeria* spp. four sporocysts with two sporozoites, 4:2; *Isospora* spp. 2:4). In hill mynahs, *Eimeria* spp. are associated with a haemorrhagic enteritis (Korbel & Kösters 1998).

Other coccidia, e.g. *Dorisiella* spp. (2:8) and *Wendyonella* spp. (4:4), have also been identified in passerines.

Sarcocystis has been identified in skeletal muscle of many Passeriformes, especially in North America. Cowbirds, grackles and other Passeriformes have been shown to be intermediate hosts for *Sarcocystis falculata*, for which opossums are the definitive hosts. *Sarcocystis* is usually found incidentally when necropsy examinations are performed.

Toxoplasmosis

In the acute phase of toxoplasmosis, the birds (canaries and mynahs) may show severe respiratory signs. In canaries this phase is often not diagnosed, and the owner is only alarmed when several birds become blind many weeks after becoming infected. In a flock many birds were affected with blindness, which developed over a 3-month span, and two birds developed torticollis. The route of infection is not known, but it is likely that oocysts excreted in cat faeces get into the aviary. In the acute phase, hepatomegaly and splenomegaly, and mostly a severe catarrhal pneumonia and a myositis of the pectoral muscle, are found in canaries and mynahs at necropsy. The trophozoites are easily identified in impression smears. Microscopic alterations within the

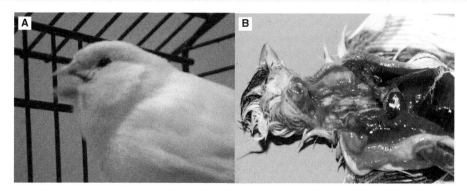

Fig 8.35A,B Canary with respiratory signs and diphtheric membranes in the crop with flagellates (*Trichomonas*-like).

eye consisted of a non-suppurative chorioretinitis with large numbers of macrophages that contained the tachyzoite form of *Toxoplasma gondii* in the subretinal space, and aggregates of tachyzoites were found in the nerve fibre layer of the retina with and without necrosis. Tissue cysts with bradyzoites were scattered throughout the meninges and neuropil of the cerebrum and cerebellum (Williams et al 2001). In histological slides from the brains, (pseudo)cysts are relatively easy to find. Serology, immunofluorescence on brain tissue slides, or infection of mice confirms the diagnosis. The Sabin–Feldman dye test will not detect *T. gondii* antibodies in the serum of birds (Patton 1996). No effective treatment is known, although some effect is claimed using trimethoprim 0.08 g/mL H$_2$O and sulfadiazine 0.04 g/mL in water for 2 weeks. A second treatment regimen was given for 3 weeks (Williams et al 2001).

Cryptosporidiosis

Cryptosporidiosis has been associated with acute onset, severe diarrhoea and death in a diamond firetail finch, but is not common in passerines. The case in the firetail finch showed focal cuboidal metaplasia of the glandular epithelium of the proventriculus and amyloid deposits in the proventriculus and kidneys. In another case, canaries were infected with cryptosporidia in the proventriculus and *Salmonella* spp. was concurrently isolated (Macwhirter 1994). Although they are generally opportunistic and secondary invaders, they have been reported as primary pathogens producing respiratory and/or intestinal disease in birds (Schmidt et al 2003).

Trichomoniasis

Trichomoniasis is commonly seen in many avian species. The protozoa are not very host-specific In canaries, infections with *Trichomonas* spp. are seen sporadically, and birds of all ages can be affected. Common clinical signs include respiratory symptoms, regurgitation, nasal discharge and emaciation (Fig. 8.35). The diagnosis can be made in a live bird, using a crop swab. At necropsy, trichomoniasis infections present as a thickened, opaque crop wall. The flagellates can be identified, even when the bird is not very fresh, in crop smears stained with Hemacolor® or another 'quick stain'. The treatment is the same as for cochlosomosis.

In mynahs, the lesions look like trichomoniasis in pigeons with typical lesions in the oral cavity.

Another flagellate is seen in the crop of canaries, causing the same clinical signs in full-grown birds and mortality in nestlings. The diagnosis can be made with a wet mount, but the flagellates are difficult to recognize. The parasite does not move about in the preparation, but 'waves' with its flagella (van der Hage & Dorrestein 1991). The same flagellate is held responsible for pruritus, feather loss and increased moulting time in individual kept canaries (Cornelissen & Dorrestein 2003).

Cochlosomosis

The flagellate *Cochlosoma* spp., living in the intestinal tract of society finches, can cause many deaths among Australian finches fostered by these carriers (Poelma et al 1978). It is a problem in young birds from 10 days until 6 weeks of age. Typical signs are debilitation, shivering due to dehydration, and difficulties with moulting.

The diagnosis of cochlosomosis is based on demonstrating the flagellates in fresh faeces. Treatment consists of ronidazole at 400 mg/kg egg food and 400 mg/L drinking water for 5 days. After a pause of 2 days, the regimen is repeated. This drug is relatively safe and no toxic signs have been seen. If dimetridazole is used, the concentration should not exceed 100 mg active drug per litre for 5 days. A sign of intoxication with dimetridazole is torticollis, and this will disappear after the medication is stopped. Metronidazole has also been reported to cause toxicity in finches.

Management should include disinfecting water containers, and the aviary should be kept clean and dry.

Giardia *spp.*

Giardia spp. have been reported to be associated with gastrointestinal tract infections in finches. Treatment for *Giardia* spp. is the same as for trichomonads.

Blood Parasites

Blood parasites may be detected on routine screening of apparently healthy passerines, but they are rarely implicated as the primary cause of disease or death. The most commonly encountered blood parasites include *Haemoproteus* spp., *Leucocytozoon* spp., *Trypanosoma* spp., *Plasmodium* spp. (malaria) and microfilaria.

Plasmodium spp., the cause of avian malaria, are mosquito-borne protozoa that occur worldwide. Sporogony occurs in the invertebrate host, schizogony occurs in the erythrocytes, and golden or black refractile pigment granules are formed from the host cell haemoglobin. *Plasmodium* spp. have been described in free-ranging passerines, including tits, finches, thrushes, starlings and sparrows. They are occasionally found in captive-bred birds such as canaries and other finches. The diagnosis is based on the demonstration of the parasite in erythrocytes, and is differentiated from *Haemoproteus* spp. by the demonstration of the schizont in malaria. Clinical and post-mortem signs include anaemia and splenomegaly. Molecular techniques (PCR) have also been developed and results of avian population surveys conducted with PCR assays suggest that prevalences of malarial infection are higher than previously documented, and that studies based on microscopic examination of blood smears may substantially underestimate the extent of parasitism by these apicomplexans. Nonetheless, because the published primers miss small numbers of infections detected by other methods, including inspection of smears, no assay now available for avian malaria is universally reliable (Fallon et al 2003).

Treatment with chloroquine (250 mg/120 mL drinking water for 1–2 weeks) or pyrimethamine is successful in some cases, but a lasting immunity does not occur. Controlling of mosquito vectors is necessary to prevent infection.

Haemoproteus spp. are also found worldwide, but cause only mild or non-apparent clinical symptoms. For most species of *Haemoproteus* the intermediate hosts are hippoboscid flies, biting midges or tabanids. Diagnosis is based on identification of typical pigment-containing gametocytes in erythrocytes; but schizonts are not found in blood cells. Treatment is seldom indicated, and will be identical to the treatment for avian malaria.

Leucocytozoon spp. occur worldwide, and can infect either erythrocytes or leucocytes. Parasitized cells are so distorted by the parasite that it may be difficult to determine their origin. Pigment is not produced by *Leucocytozoon*, and schizonts cannot be found in peripheral blood. Megaloschizonts can be found in brain, liver,

lung, kidney, intestinal, heart, muscle and lymphoid tissue. Most infections are subclinical, although vague signs and death are reported.

Trypanosoma spp. are also found worldwide, but their incidence is low and they are only found during summer months in temperate climates. Vectors are thought to include hippoboscid flies, red mites, simuliids and mosquitoes; treatment is not warranted.

Helminth parasitism

Helminth parasites are usually of no significance in small passerines. Acanthocephalans, cestodes and nematodes have mostly been reported in free-ranging and captive large passerines (e.g. thrushes, grackles and starlings). Insect-eating species in particular show more parasitic infections.

Nematodes

Two main types of roundworms affect passerines: *Ascaridia* spp., which have a direct life cycle, and *Porrocaecum* spp., which have an indirect life cycle,

with invertebrates such as earthworms as the intermediate host. Both types of roundworms may be associated with weight loss, diarrhoea, general debility and, sometimes, neurological signs. *Ascaridia* spp. are uncommon in small passerines. *Porrocaecum* spp. have been found in a variety of free-ranging passerines (e.g. pipits, thrush, blackbirds and corvids). Fenbendazole, piperazine, levamisole and ivermectin, all orally applied, are useful in treating ascarid infections.

Capillaria spp. are cosmopolitan in their distribution and affect a range of passerines, including mynahs. The life cycle is direct, or may involve earthworms as paratenic hosts. Susceptibility does not depend on dietary preferences, and the parasite has been found to cause disease in a variety of seed-eaters, insect-eaters, omnivorous species and honey-eaters.

High parasite loads may lead to weight loss, diarrhoea, general ill health and death. These worms may localize to a variety of sites in the gastrointestinal tract. They may be associated with white or creamy-coloured plaques in the buccal cavity or pharynx, and swelling of the crop, proventriculus, intestines or bowel. The typical *Capillaria* spp. egg has bipolar plugs and may be found by direct swabbing of lesions or faeces, or by faecal flotation.

Treatment may be more difficult than for ascarids. Aviary hygiene and removal of earthworms are important control measures. Anthelmintics may be effective in some cases. In a cleaned, dry environment, the eggs will lose their infectious capacity within 3 weeks without further disinfection (Korbel & Kösters 1998).

Syngamus trachea (gapeworm) are found in outdoor aviaries and are a serious problem in mynahs, corvids and starlings. Earthworms may act as a transport host. The signs include gasping for breath, and the small passerines often die from occlusion of the trachea by the worms and the mucus produced. The diagnosis is confirmed by demonstrating the worms in the trachea by using backlighting, or by finding the typical eggs in the droppings. The worms are easily identified in the trachea at necropsy. Ivermectin (injection 200 μg/kg) and levamisole or fenbendazole are effective in treating this parasite, but caution should be exercised when treating birds with heavy infections, because the dead worms can obstruct the trachea. In such a case with a heavy worm burden, treatment with a low dose of an anthelmintic (especially fenbendazole) over several days provides effective treatment.

Spiruroids

Geopetitia aspiculata is a parasite that lives in the proventriculus and has been reported in tropical birds housed at zoological gardens in Europe and North America (Kübber-Heiss & Juncker 1997, Tscherner et al 1997). Insects (e.g. cockroaches, crickets) serve as intermediate hosts. *Geopetitia aspiculata* are pathogenic, leading to perforation of the wall of the proventriculus, often resulting in death. The parasite is not host-specific and is demonstrated in six avian orders, including Passeriformes (e.g. Emberizidae, Estrildidae, Fringillidae, Icteridae, Sturnidae – including a hill mynah). The diagnosis is confirmed by finding the embryonated spiruroid eggs in the faeces (although this might not always be effective), followed by endoscopic demonstration of the proventricular lesions. At necropsy an enlarged abdomen is found, due to a mass of tightly coiled parasites attached to the serosa of the proventriculus, and worms are sometimes found in the liver. Infected birds can be successfully treated with ivermectin (300–400 μg/kg body weight s.c.) or fenbendazole (25 mg/kg body weight p.o. for 3 days). To interrupt the development cycle of the parasite, emphasis should be laid on eradication of the intermediate host.

The *Dispharynx nasuta* is a gastric worm and is also found in subtropical areas. Recently this parasite caused problems and mortality in tropical exhibits in a zoo (Dorrestein et al 2001). The diagnosis is mostly found at necropsy related to a proventriculitis with sometimes a very large number of worms attached to the surface (Fig. 8.36). Insects (e.g. wood lice/sow bugs/pill bugs) serve as intermediate hosts. All Passeriformes, but also Galliformes and some Columbiformes and Psittaciformes can become infected.

Acuaria skrjabini infections of the gizzard, with mucosal necrosis, have been reported in adult finches in Australia. The mortality rate was 4–5%, and oral treatment with 80 mg levamisole or 50 mg fenbendazole/L drinking water for 3 days was effective.

Feeding live food (such as maggots, mealworms or termites) or providing a compost heap in the aviary to attract insects for the birds to eat are both common management practices in Australia. These practices increase the likelihood of infection, as insects are the intermediate hosts for gizzardworms and tapeworms.

Tapeworm (*Cestoda*) infestations in softbills and insectivorous finches are common. They are not normally seen in canaries or exclusively seed-eating birds, except in situations where parents feed insects to their offspring or insects are accidentally consumed with the seeds (Macwhirter 1994). Some necropsies show small intestines literally packed with the tiny tapeworms. The typical hexacanth embryos are usually identified on faecal flotation. Effective treatment for passerines diagnosed with tapeworms include praziquantel and oxfenbendazole.

Trematodes have complicated life cycles that typically involve snails as initial intermediate hosts and other invertebrates as secondary intermediate hosts. Trematodes are seen occasionally in wild-caught passerines. *Schistozoma* spp. are trematodes that live in blood vessels and have been reported in North American goldfinches and cardinals. *Prosthogonimus* spp. are trematodes affecting the

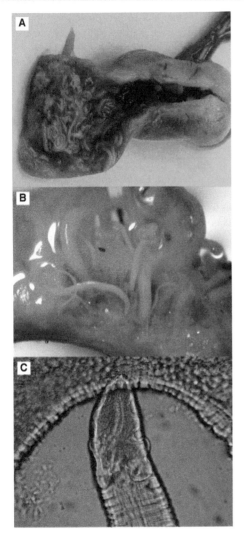

Fig 8.36 Proventriculus with large number of *Dispharynx nasuta* worms; (**A**) in a Northern cardinal (*Cardinalis cardinalis*); (**B**) transverse section of the stomach of a blue bishop (*Euplectes* sp.); (**C**) a close-up of a male worm.

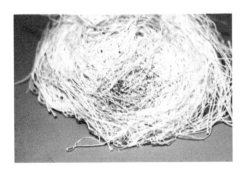

Fig 8.37 Nesting material with *Dermanysus gallinae*.

intestinal tract, cloaca, bursa of Fabricius or oviduct. These parasites been found worldwide in passerines, and are not particularly pathogenic. Dragonflies and snails are intermediate hosts. Praziquantel (10 mg/kg) may be useful in treating trematodes.

Arthropods

Ectoparasites, including blood-sucking mites (*Dermanyssus gallinae* and *Ornithonyssus sylviarum*), skin mites (e.g. *Backericheyla* spp. and *Neocheyletiella media*) and feather mites (e.g. Epidermotidae, *Dermation* spp.), are found in the calamus of the feathers. Meal-mites (*Tyroglyphus farinae*) are not parasites, but their large number on a bird can cause unrest and irritation.

The red mite (*Dermanyssus gallinae*) is a blood-sucking mite that can cause serious mortality among fledglings as well as adult birds. The common clinical sign in affected patients is anaemia. A bird with respiratory symptoms and a PCV of less than 30% should be suspected of having serious problems with blood-sucking mites. The main complaint from the owner is a general depression; the mites are often not detected or their presence is even denied. The red mite spends the day in the nest or bird-room crevices, and ventures out at night to attack the birds (Fig. 8.37). Treatment should be prompt, and consists of dusting or spraying the victims with an insecticide and vacating the cage or room during the day and thoroughly cleaning it.

The white or northern mite (*Ornithonyssus sylviarum*) is increasingly found to cause problems in aviaries. This blood-sucking mite spends its entire life on the host. Dusting with insecticides can be hazardous, especially to nestlings. A relatively safe method of treatment is to put one drop of 0.1% ivermectin in propylene glycol on the bare skin; however, the mites are killed only after sucking blood.

Other ectoparasites may cause some irritation or feather damage. They are considered a sign of inadequate hygiene and management.

Quill mites have been described in passerines, and infested birds show clinical signs of irritation, pruritus, feather-picking and feather-loss. These signs are rarely severe. The mites seem to feed on the quill tissue, and not on blood or sebaceous fluid. Many different species of quill mites are described, including *Syringophylus* spp., *Harpyrhynchus* spp., *Dermatoglyphus* spp. and *Picobia* spp. Regularly new quill mites are being described in all bird species (Bochkov et al 2004). The diagnosis is made by inspection (usually with magnification) of quill material. Treatment with ivermectin (spot-on 0.1% ivermectin in propylene glycol) is very effective (Dorrestein et al 1997).

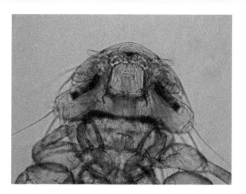

Fig 8.38 Canary feather lice, *Menacanthus spinosus*.

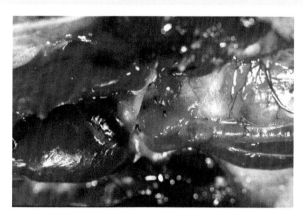

Fig 8.39 Gouldian finch with *Sternostoma tracheacolum* in the cervical air sac and trachea.

Cnemidocoptes pilae infections, or scaly mites, are occasionally seen on the beak base of finches. In general, they tend to cause hyperkeratotic lesions on the feet in Passeriformes. These mites are easily found and recognized in scrapings from the altered areas. Treatment with any oil or 0.1% ivermectin applied locally will cure the birds. This infestation should not be confused with the so-called 'tassel foot' found in the European goldfinch (*Carduelis carduelis*), which is caused by a papillomavirus (see Fig. 8.25).

Lice are fairly common in Passeriformes. Some biting lice are not specialized for life on particular feathers, and are able to move quickly. Chewing lice are often more adapted to a particular part of the body, and are more sluggish. Signs of the presence of lice include restlessness and biting, excessive preening, and damage to the plumage. Some cases of baldness in canaries are caused by lice (Fig. 8.38). Lice undergo a complete life cycle on the bird, and a weekly dusting with pyrethrins is an effective method of control (Macwhirter 1994). Some species of Estrildidae are hypersensitive to pyrethrin, and care must be taken in its use.

Endoparasites

Air sac mites (*Sternostoma tracheacolum*) are occasionally found in canaries, but they are seen mostly commonly in Australian finches (Fig. 8.39). They are not reported in softbills. This problem is also seen in wild Gouldian finches in Australia, and may have been introduced with domestic canaries. The mites' life cycle is unknown, but it is theorized that nestlings become infected by parents regurgitating nutrients with mites. Adults may be exposed via contamination of water and food, and by coughing or sneezing.

Clinical signs include a decline in physical condition, respiratory distress, wheezing, squeaking, coughing, sneezing, nasal discharge, loss of voice, head shaking and gasping. The mortality is low. Diagnosis of air sac mites can sometimes be made by transillumination of

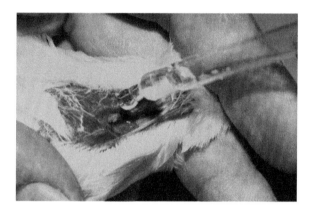

Fig 8.40 Canary spot-on application.

the trachea in live birds, with the mites visible as tiny black points in the trachea. The throat of the bird must be wetted (e.g. with alcohol) and the feathers parted. Post-mortem examination, however, is more reliable, and the condition is diagnosed by finding in the mites in the air sacs, the lungs and/or the trachea. Air sacculitis, tracheitis and focal pneumonia may be evident.

Several therapeutic regimens have been described for air sac mite infestations. Pest strips make a reasonable good air sac mite preventative, provided the bird does not come into direct contact, and only if the bird is not held within a small enclosure. Ivermectin can be used for individual treatment by a spot-on method of 0.1% ivermectin in propylene glycol, one drop on the bare skin dorsolateral to the thorax inlet or on the chest (Fig. 8.40). A small amount of alcohol is necessary to view the site of application.

Cytodites nudus is another mite that has occasionally been associated with respiratory disease in free-ranging passerines. It may be found in the abdominal cavity as well as the respiratory system.

Zoonoses

Zoonotic diseases of passerines are listed in Table 8.6.

Table 8.6 Zoonotic diseases of passerines

Allergy	Although known to be associated with finches it is very rare, more commonly associated with pigeons
Viruses	Very unlikely; Newcastle disease is always mentioned and might play a role with chickens
Bacteria	
Ornithosis or *Chlamydophila psittaci*	Infection: uncommon infection in passerines. However, if influenza-type symptoms occur in a person, with high fevers, atypical pneumonia, muscle pain and serious headache, a physician should be consulted. Transmission is aerogenic. Treatment in people is generally with doxycycline
Tuberculosis	In Passeriformes, only *Mycobacterium-avium-intracellulare* complex, which is of minor importance as a direct zoonosis. *M. genavense* is a new species that is mainly isolated from patients with AIDS and has also been identified in 20% of the culturally confirmed avian tuberculosis cases (Hoop et al 1995, 1996). Only a danger in those who are immunocompromised. Recently a case of *M. tuberculosis* in a canary has been documented (Hoop 2002)
Salmonella Typhimurium, *S. enteritidis*	Sometimes isolated from passerines. Confirmed transmissions to humans have only been incidental findings. In humans these cause gastroenteritis, headache, shivering, stomach ache and retching, followed by vomiting and diarrhoea
Other bacteria	These include *Campylobacter* spp., *Yersinia pseudotuberculosis*, *Listeria monocytogenes*, and possible many others such as *E. coli*, *Klebsiella pneumoniae*, etc. However, human involvement is very uncommon and incidental and occurs only in the most extreme situations
Fungi	*Trichophyton* spp., *Candida albicans* and *Aspergillus* spp. are all mycotic species that have been isolated from immunocompromised people, but under normal hygienic circumstances problems with these fungi are rare
Parasites	*Dermanyssus* mites can bite people when they are cleaning cages, causing itching erythromatosis, urticaria or papillomatous exanthema

References

Altman R B, Clubb S L, Dorrestein G M, Quesenberry K E (eds) 1997 Avian medicine and surgery. W B Saunders, Philadelphia, PA, p 1021

Bakonvi T, Erdelvi K, Ursu K et al 2007 Emergence of Usutu virus in Hungary. Journal of Clinical Microbiology Oct 3 Epub ahead of print

Bochkov V, Fain A, Skoracki M 2004 New quill mites of the family Syringophilidae (Acari: Cheyletoidea). Systematic Parasitology 57:135–150

Carpenter J W 2005 Exotic animal formulary, 3rd edn. Elsevier Saunders, St Louis, MO, p 272

Chvala S, Kolodziejek J, Nowotny N, Weissenbück H 2004 Pathology and viral distribution in fatal Usutu virus infections of birds from the 2001 and 2002 outbreaks in Austria. Journal of Comparative Pathology 131:176–185

Cornelissen H, Dorrestein G M 2003 A new dermatological disease in canaries (*Serinus canarius*) possibly caused by flagellates in the gastrointestinal tract. Proceedings of the 5th ECAMS Scientific Meeting Tenerife, p 17–18

Cornelissen H, Ducatelle R, Roels S 1995 Successful treatment of a channel-billed toucan (*Ramphastos vitellinus*) with iron storage disease by chelation therapy: sequential monitoring of the iron content of the liver during the treatment period by quantitative chemical and image analyses. Journal of Avian Medicine and Surgery 9:131–137

Coutteel P 1995 The importance of manipulating the daily photoperiod in canary breeding. In: Proceedings of the 3rd Conference of the European AAV, Jerusalem. European Association of Avian Veterinarians, p 166–170

Coutteel P 2003 Veterinary aspects of breeding management in captive passerines. Seminars in Avian and Exotic Pet Medicine 12:3–10

Crosta L, Sironi G, Rampin T 1997 Polyomavirus infection in Fringilidae. Proceedings of the 4th Conference of the European AAV, London. European Association of Avian Veterinarians, p 128–131

De Herdt P, Ducatelle R, Devriese L A et al 1997 Megabacterium infections of the proventriculus in passerine and psittacine birds: practice experiences in Belgium. In: Proceedings of the 4th Conference of the European AAV, London. European Association of Avian Veterinarians, p 123–127

Dhondt A A, Dhondt K Y, Hawley D M, Jenelle C S 2007 Experimental evidence for transmission of *Mycoplasma gallisepticum* in house finches by fomites. Avian Pathology 36:205–208

Dierenfield E, Sheppard C D 1989 Investigations of hepatic iron levels in zoo birds. In: Proceedings of 8th Dr Scholl Conference on the Nutrition of Captive Wild Animals. Lincoln Park Zoological Society, Chicago, p 101–114

Dodwell G T 1986 The complete book of canaries. Howell Book House, New York

Dorrestein G M 1997a Passerines. In: Altman R B, Clubb S L, Dorrestein G M, Quesenberry K E (eds) Avian medicine and surgery. W B Saunders, Philadelphia, PA, p 867–885

Dorrestein G M 1997b Diagnostic necropsy and pathology; avian cytology. In: Altman R B, Clubb S L, Dorrestein G M, Quesenberry K E (eds) Avian medicine and surgery. W B Saunders, Philadelphia, PA, p 158–169, 211–222

Dorrestein G M, Schrijver J 1982 A genetic defect in the vitamin A metabolism in recessive white canaries. Tijdschrift voor Diergeneeskunde 107:795–799

Dorrestein G M, van der Hage M H 1988 Veterinary problems in mynah birds. In: Proceedings of the AAV, Houston. Association of Avian Veterinarians, p 263–274

Dorrestein G M, Grinwis G M, Dominguez L et al 1992 An induced iron storage disease syndrome in doves and pigeons: a model for haemochromatosis in mynah birds? (a preliminary report). Proceedings of the Annual Conference of the AAV, New Orleans. Association of Avian Veterinarians, p 108–112

Dorrestein G M, van der Hage M H, Grinwis G 1993 A tumour-like pox lesion in masked bull finches (*Pyrrhula erythaca*). In: Proceedings of the 2nd Conference of the European AAV, Utrecht European Association of Avian Veterinarians, p 232–240

Dorrestein G M, van der Hage M H, van Garderen E 1996 Virus infections in passerines with special reference to a Coronavirus-like infection in canaries (*Serinus canaria*). In: Proceedings Main Conference AAV. Association of Avian Veterinarians, p 171–176

Dorrestein G M, Cremers S H J, van der Horst H J et al 1997 Quill mite (*Dermoglyphus passerinus*) infestation of canaries (*Serinus canaria*): diagnosis and treatment. Avian Pathology 26:195–199

Dorrestein G M, van der Hage M H, Fuchs A et al 1998 A Coronavirus-like infection in canaries (*Serinus canaria*): pathology and diagnosis. In: Proceedings XI Tagung über Vogelkrankheiten, München, p 110–119

Dorrestein G M, Cremers H J W M, van der Hage M et al 2001 *Dispharynx nasuta* (Rudolphi 1819): a gastric worm in birds in an exhibit with a tropical ecosystem. Proceedings of the 40th International Symposium on Diseases of Zoo Animals and Wildlife, Rotterdam, p 71–76

Dorrestein G M, Crosta L, Steinmetz H W et al 2007 Usutu virus activity is spreading in Europe. Proceedings of the 7th ECAMS Scientific meeting, Zurich 2007, p 7–8

Dublin A, Mechani S, Malkinson M et al 1995 A 4-year survey of the distribution of *Chlamydia psittaci* in 19 orders of birds in Israel with emphasis on seasonal variability. In: Proceedings of the 3rd Conference of the European AAV, Jerusalem. Association of Avian Veterinarians, p 1

Fallon S M, Ricklefs R E, Swanson B L, Bermingham E 2003 Detecting avian malaria: an improved polymerase chain reaction diagnostic. Journal of Parasitology 89:1044–1047

Fang Y, Reisen W K 2006 Previous infection with West Nile or St. Louis encephalitis viruses provides cross protection during reinfection in house finches. American Journal of Tropical Medicine and Hygiene 75:480–485

Filippich L J, Parker M G 1994 Megabacteria and proventricular/ventricular disease in psittacines and passerines. In: Proceedings AAV, Reno. Association of Avian Veterinarians, p 287–293

Fischer J R, Converse K A 1995 Overview of conjunctivitis in house finches in the eastern United States, 1994–1995. In: Proceedings of the Joint Conferences AAZV, WDA, AAWV. American Association of Zoo Veterinarians, p 508–509

Fitzgerald S D, Sullivan J M, Everson R J 1990 Suspected ethanol toxicosis in two wild cedar waxwings. Avian Diseases 34:488–490

Gelis S, Raidal S R 2006 Microsporidiosis in a flock of tricolor parrot finches (*Erythrura tricolor*). Veterinary Clinics of North America. Exotic Animal Practice 9:481–486

Gill F B 1994 Ornithology. Freeman and Company, New York

Goldsmith T 1995 Documentation of passerine circoviral infection. In: Proceedings Main Conference AAV. Association of Avian Veterinarians, p 349–350

Grifois J, Bargallo F, Perpinan D, Ramis A 2005 Circovirus infection in a canary breeding flock. Proceedings of the 8th European AAV Conference, Arles, p 148–150

Hannafusa Y, Bradley A, Tomaszewski E E, Libal M C, Phalen D N 2007 Growth and metabolic characterization of *Macrorhabdus ornithogaster*. Journal of Veterinary Diagnostic Investigation 19:256–265

Hargis A M 1989 Avocado (*Persea americana*) intoxication in caged birds. Journal of the American Veterinary Medical Association 194:64–66

Hawkins M 2003 Passerine birds. Seminars in Avian and Exotic Pet Medicine 12:1–36

Hoop R K 2002 *Mycobacterium tuberculosis* infection in a canary (*Serinus canaria* L.) and a blue-fronted Amazon parrot (*Amazona amazona aestiva*). Avian Diseases 46:502–504

Hoop R K, Ossen P, Pfyffer G 1995 *Mycobacterium genavense*: a new cause of mycobacteriosis in pet birds? In: Proceedings of the European Conference of the AAV, Jerusalem. European Association of Avian Veterinarians, p 1–3

Hoop R K, Bottger E C, Pfyffer G 1996 Etiological agents of mycobacteriosis in pet birds between 1986 and 1995. Journal of Clinical Microbiology 34:991–992

Kaleta E F, Hönicke A 2005 A retrospective description of a highly pathogenic avian influenza A virus (H7N1/Carduelis/Germany/72) in a free-living siskin (*Carduelis spinus* Linnaeus, 1758) and its accidental transmission to yellow canaries (*Serinus canaria* Linnaeus, 1758). Deutsche tierärztliche Wochenschrift 112:17–19

Klasing K C 1998 Vitamins. In: Klasing K C (ed) Comparative avian nutrition. CAB International, New York, p 277–329

Korbel R, Kösters J 1998 Beos. In: Gabrisch K, Zwart P (eds) Krankheiten der Heimtiere, 4th edn. Schlütersche, Hannover, p 397–428

Kübber-Heiss A, Juncker M 1997 Spiruridosis in birds at an Austrian Zoo. In: Proceedings of the 4th Conference of the European AAV, London, p 102–106

Labonde J 1996 Medicine and surgery of mynahs. In: Rosskopf R W Jr., Woerpel R W (eds) Diseases of cage and aviary birds, 3rd edn. Williams & Wilkins, Baltimore, MD, p 928–932

Ley D H, Shaeffer D S, Dhondt A A 2006 Further western spread of *Mycoplasma gallisepticum* infection of house finches. Journal of Wildlife Diseases 42:429–431

Macwhirter P 1994 Passeriformes. In: Ritchie B, Harrison G, Harrison L (eds) Avian medicine: principles and application. Wingers, Lake Worth, FL, p 1172–1199

Marlier D, Leroy C, Sturbois M et al 2006 Increasing incidence of megabacteriosis in canaries (*Serinus canarius domesticus*). Veterinary Journal 172:549–552

Martinez del Rio C, Bozinovic F, Dsabat P, Novoa F 1996 Digestive ability and dietary flexibility in passerine birds: a collection of 'not so stories'. In: Symposium of the Comparative Nutrition Society 1, p 87–91

Mashima T Y, Ley D H, Stoskopf M K. et al 1997 Evaluation of treatment of *Mycoplasma gallisepticum*-associated conjunctivitis in house finches (*Carpodacus mexicanus*). Journal of Avian Medicine and Surgery 11:20–24

Massey J G 1996 Clinical medicine in small passerines. In: Proceedings of the Main Conference AAV. Association of Avian Veterinarians, p 49–53

Mete A, Dorrestein G M, Marx J J et al 2001 A comparative study of iron retention in mynahs, doves and rats. Avian Pathology 30:479–486

Mete A, Hendriks H G, Klaren P H et al 2003 Iron metabolism in mynah birds (*Gracula religiosa*) resembles human hereditary haemochromatosis. Avian Pathology 32:625–632

Norton T M, Seibels R E, Greiner E C, Latimer K S 1995 Bali mynah captive medical management and reintroduction program. In: Proceedings of the Main Conference AAV. Association of Avian Veterinarians, p 125–136

Olsen G P, Russell K E, Dierenfeld E, Phalen D N 2006 A comparison of four regimens for treatment of iron storage disease using the European starling (*Sturnus vulgaris*) as a model. Journal of Avian Medicine and Surgery 20:74–79

Otten B A, Orosz S E, Auge S, Frazier D L 2001 Mineral content of food items commonly ingested by keel billed toucans (*Ramphastos sulfuratus*). Journal of Avian Medicine and Surgery 15:194–196

Patton S 1996 Diagnosis of *Toxoplasma gondii* in birds. In: Proceedings of the Main Conference AAV. Association of Avian Veterinarians, p 75–78

Perpinan D, Fernandez-Bellon H, Lopez C, Ramis A 2005 Myenteric ganglioneuritis in four non-psittacine birds. Proceedings of the 8th European AAV Conference, Arles, p 257–259

Phalen D 2005 Diagnosis and management of *Macrorhabdus ornithogaster* (formerly megabacteria). Veterinary Clinics of North America. Exotic Animal Practice 8:299–306

Phalen D N, Tomaszewski E 2003 Investigation into the identification, detection, and treatment of the organism formally known as Megabacterium. Proceedings of the 7th European AAV Conference, Tenerife, p 79–83

Phenix K V, Weston J H, Ypelaar I et al 2001 Nucleotide sequence analysis of a novel circovirus of canaries and its relationship to other members of the genus Circovirus of the family Circoviridae. Journal of General Virology 82:2805–2809

Poelma F G, Zwart P, Dorrestein G M, Iordens C M 1978 Cochlosomose, a problem in raising Estrildidae in aviaries. Tijdschrift voor Diergeneeskunde 103:589–593

Pohl U 1995 *Chlamydia psittaci* in Austrian wild birds. In: Proceedings of the 3rd Conference of the European AAV, Jerusalem. European Association of Avian Veterinarians, p 15–17

Quesada O, Rodriguez F, Herriaez P 2007 Mucor ramosissimus associated with feather loss in canaries (*Serinus canarius*). Avian Diseases 51:643–645

Račnik J, Slavec B, Trilar T et al 2007 Avian influenza surveillance in wild living migratory passerine birds in Slovenia. Proceedings of the 9th European AAV Conference, Zürich, p 130–106

Rampin T, Manarolla G, Pisoni G et al 2006 Circovirus inclusion bodies in intestinal muscle cells of a canary. Avian Pathology 35:277–279

Ravelhofer K, Rothender R, Gareis M et al 1998 Megabacteria infections of various avian species. In: Proceedings XI Tagung über Vogelkrankheiten, München. DVG, p 95–104

Reisen W K, Fang Y, Martinez V M 2005 Avian host and mosquito (Diptera: Culicidae) vector competence determine the efficiency of West Nile and St. Louis encephalitis virus transmission. Journal of Medical Entomology 42:367–375

Ritchie B W 1995 Avian viruses: function and control. Wingers, Lake Worth, FL

Rossi G, Taccini E, Tarantino C 2005 Outbreak of avian polyomavirus infection with high mortality in recently captured Crimson's seedcrackers (*Pyrenestes sanguineus*). Journal of Wildlife Diseases 41:236–240

Rottenberg H 2007 Exceptional longevity in songbirds is associated with high rates of evolution of cytochrome b, suggesting selection for reduced generation of free radicals. Journal of Experimental Biology 210:2170–2180

Sandmeier P 2003 Circovirus infections in non-psittacine avian species. In: Proceedings of the 7th Conference of the European AAV, Tenerife. European Association of Avian Veterinarians, p 23–24

Sandmeier P, Coutteel P 2006 Management of canaries, finches and mynahs. In: Harrison G, Lightfoot T (eds) Clinical avian medicine, Vol. II. Spix Publishing, Palm Beach, FL, p 879–913

Sandmeier P, Hoop R K, Bosshart G 1997 Cerebral mycobacteriosis in zebra finches (*Taeniopygia guttata*) caused by *Mycobacterium genavense*. In: Proceedings of the 4th Conference of the European AAV, London, p 119–122. European Association of Avian Veterinarians

Scanlan C M, Graham D L 1990 Characterization of a gram-positive bacterium from the proventriculus of budgerigars (*Melopsittacus undulatus*). Avian Diseases 34:779–786

Scheuerlein A, Ricklefs R E 2004 Prevalence of blood parasites in European passeriform birds. Proceedings of the Royal Society B: Biological Sciences 271:1363–1370

Schmidt R E, Reavill D R, Phalen D 2003 Pathology of pet and aviary birds. Iowa State Press, Ames, IA

Schnebel B, Dierschke V, Rautenschlein S, Ryll M 2005 No detection of avian influenza A viruses of the subtypes H5 and H7 and isolation of lentogenic avian paramyxovirus serotype 1 in passerine birds during stopover in the year 2001 on the island Heligoland (North Sea). Deutsche tierärztliche Wochenschrift 112:456–460

Scullion F T, Scullion M G 2004 Successful treatment of megabacteriosis in a canary (*Serinus canaria*) with nystatin. Veterinary Record 155:528–529

Shivaprasad D L, Hill D, Todd D, Smyth J A 2004 Circovirus infection in a Gouldian finch (*Chloebia gouldiae*). Avian Pathology 33:525–529

Sibley C G, Ahlquist J E 1990 Phylogeny and classification of birds. Yale University Press, New Haven, CT

Steward M N, Perry R, Raidal S R 2006 Identification of a novel circovirus in Australian ravens (*Corvus coronoides*) with feather disease. Avian Pathology 35:86–92

Suedmeyer W K 1997 Clinical management of endoventricular mycosis in a group of African finches. In: Proceedings of the Main Conference AAV, Reno, p 225–227

Taylor E J 1996 An evaluation of the importance of insoluble versus soluble grit in the diet of canaries. Journal of Avian Medicine and Surgery 10:248–251

Tomaszewski, E K, Logan K S, Snowden K F et al 2003 Phylogenetic analysis identifies the 'megabacterium' of birds as a novel anamorphic ascomycetous yeast, *Macrorhabdus ornithogaster* gen. nov., sp. nov. International Journal of Systematic and Evolutionary Microbiology 53:1201–1205

Tscherner W, Wittstatt U, Goltenboth R 1997 *Geopetitia aspiculata* Webster, 1971 – a pathogenic nematode in tropical birds in zoological gardens. Der Zoologische Garten 67:108–120

Tung K C, Liu J S, Cheng F P et al 2007 Study on the species-specificity of *Isospora michaelbakeri* by experimental infection. Acta Veterinaria Hungarica 55:77–85

Van der Hage M H, Dorrestein G M 1991 Flagellates in the crop of canary bird. In: Proceedings of the 1st European AAV, Vienna. European Association of Avian Veterinarians, p 303–307

Vereecken M, de Herdt P, Charlier G et al 1998 An outbreak of polyomavirus infection in Shamas (*Copsychus malabaricus*). In: Proceedings XI Tagung über Vogelkrankheiten, München, p 176–183

Vitali S D, Eden P A, Payne K L, Vaughan R J 2006 An outbreak of mycobacteriosis in Gouldian finches caused by *Mycobacterium peregrinum*. Veterinary Clinics of North America. Exotic Animal Practice 9:519–522

Walsberg G E 1983 Avian ecological energetics. Avian Biology 7:161–220

Weissenböck H, Kolodziejek J, Url A et al 2002 Emergence of Usutu virus, an African mosquito-borne flavivirus of the Japanese encephalitis virus group, central Europe. Emerging Infectious Diseases 8:652–666

White J 1997 Neotropical songbirds and veterinary medicine: are we giving them the attention they deserve? In: Proceedings of the Main Conference AAV, Reno. Association of Avian Veterinarians, p 77–81

Williams S M, Fulton R M, Render J et al 2001 Ocular and encephalic toxoplasmosis in canaries. Avian Diseases 45:262–267

Wittig W, Hoffmann K, Müller H, John E R 2007 Detection of DNA of the finch polyomavirus in diseases of various types of birds in the order Passeriformes. Berliner und Münchener Tierärztliche Wochenschrift 120:113–119

Wolf P, Kamphues J, Bartels T, Dehning S 1997 Enzyme activities along the intestinal tract of pet birds (Abstract). 1st International Symposium on Pet Bird Nutrition, Hannover, p 27–28

Wolf P, Rebehl N, Kamphues J 2003 Investigations on feathering, feather growth and potential influences of nutrient supply on feathers' regrowth in small pet birds (canaries, budgerigars and lovebirds). Journal of Animal Physiology and Animal Nutrition (Berlin) 87:134–141

Raptors

Patrick T. Redig and Luis Cruz-Martinez

9

Part I: Overview

Introduction

In Latin, the term 'raptor' means 'plunderer' (from the verb 'rapere' meaning 'to seize'). The term is also descriptive of the powerful, grasping, talon-tipped feet found in all birds of prey, and is used as a name for the group of birds whose members have this common feature. Raptors include all species in the orders Strigiformes and Falconiformes (Cooper 1996). There were five families within the order Falconiformes: the Accipitridae (hawks), the Cathartidae (vultures), the Falconidae (falcons), the Pandionidae (osprey) and the Sagittariidae (secretary bird). However, recently the family Cathartidae has been moved to the order Ciconiiformes. Within Accipitridae are three distinct groups; accipiters, buteos and eagles. The order Strigiformes has two families; the Tytonidae (barn owl) and the Strigidae (all other owls). Taxonomically unrelated relatives, but usually included with raptors because of behavioural similarities, are ravens, a member of the Corvidae (crow and jay) family within the order Passeriformes.

Raptors have a longstanding association with human beings. They have been incorporated into ancient religions and mythologies as well as modern-day culture, and have been and still are used in the sport of falconry. Falconry, hunting with trained raptors, had its origins in Eastern cultures, peaked in popularity in Western civilization during medieval times in Europe, and has seen a marked resurgence in recent times throughout North America and Europe whilst continuing to be practised in the Middle East.

In the last three decades there has been an increase in environmental awareness and conservation efforts involving raptors. These efforts include captive propagation, rehabilitation and reintroduction. Keeping birds of prey in zoos and education facilities is part of this conservation effort. As a result, more raptors are being brought to veterinarians and wildlife rehabilitation facilities for treatment. This chapter will be a basic introduction to raptor biology, husbandry and medical care. The reader is referred to cited literature for more in-depth information on these topics as well as the chapter of the same name in the first edition of this book.

There are many legal requirements that must be met by persons who choose to handle and keep birds of prey. All species of raptors in the US are federally protected, and most also have state protection. Special permits, acquired from the United States Fish and Wildlife Service at their regional offices and respective state agencies, are needed for both falconers and rehabilitators. Varying legislation exists in Europe and other countries.

Biology and anatomy

Special senses

All raptors are predatory carnivores, and they have specialized anatomical and physiological characteristics that give them great hunting capabilities. These characteristics vary, depending on the lifestyle of the birds. Diurnal raptors rely heavily on sight to locate food, and have evolved very large and sensitive eyes. As with all other avian species, they have striated muscles in their ciliary bodies, which allows them to focus quickly on their prey. Nocturnal raptors, such as the owls, have even larger eyes; however, they also rely heavily on hearing to locate their prey. The ear openings are very large and are bilaterally asymmetrical, resulting in differential sound detection, which is an aid to auditory prey location in reduced light conditions. The ear tufts found on many of the owl species do not aid in hearing, as is often thought; rather, they are part of the bird's camouflage silhouette. **Assessment of visual capacity is an important factor in determining overall fitness of a raptor; auditory function is not readily amenable to evaluation.**

Feathers and plumage

The wings and feathers of raptors are shaped in accordance with their specialization. The falcons possess long, tapered, pointed wings that enable them to achieve great speed in their flight. They are perfectly adapted to hunting other avian species on the wing in vast open spaces. The accipiters have shorter, rounded wings and very long tails, which give them great manoeuvrability with short, sudden bursts of speed. They hunt prey, both small rodents and avian species, in heavily wooded habitats. Finally, the buteos (or soaring hawks) have broad, rounded wings and tails, which facilitate soaring on the rising currents of warm air called thermals.

In owls all the flight feathers have a serrated leading edge. This condition permits almost soundless flight, which helps them catch nocturnal prey species that are also dependent on hearing for survival in the low light conditions.

Most raptors moult their feathers once per year in the early summer. The timing and pattern vary with the species, age and sex of the individual bird. Young raptors grow all their feathers in at the same time. The juvenile or first year plumages are often distinctly different from the adult plumages. Adult plumages are acquired in birds over one year of age. In subsequent annual moults the wing feathers develop in symmetrical pairs, one from the right and one from the left. This graduated symmetrical moult means there is only a slight flying handicap during the 6 months required for moulting, unlike waterfowl, which lose all their primary feathers at one time and are flightless for 4–6 weeks. Some owls, such as barred owls (*Strix varia*), moult all their tail feathers at once. Small owls, such as the saw whet owl (*Aegolius funerous*), moult into adult plumage in the late summer of their first year.

With the exception of the northern harrier (*Circus cyaneus*), American kestrel (*Falco sparverius*), merlin (*Falco columbarus*) and osprey (*Pandion haliaetus*), the plumages of North American raptors are not sexually dimorphic, which results in no distinct observational differences between genders. **In most situations it is not possible to reliably determine the sex of raptors based on plumage or other external characteristics.**

Tail feathers of hospitalized raptor patients should be protected from breakage and soiling by covering them with a sheath made from an envelope of heavy paper or polypropylene file folders that fits over the tail feathers and is affixed to the covert feathers with adhesive tape (Arent 2006). Feathers broken during medical treatment and/or the rehabilitation process should be repaired before the raptor is released back into the wild. This repair process is called 'imping' and best prepares the bird for survival after release (Heidenreich 1997, Arent 2006).

Beaks and feet

Another feature unique to raptors that complements their hunting capabilities is their stout, sharply hooked bill (Fig. 9.1). The bill is made of keratin and grows from the cere. It is a highly specialized tool that has functional morphologic variations related to specific dietary habits. For example, the snail kite has a very long, sharply hooked maxilla to allow it to extract the soft flesh of apple snails from their shells. Falcons have a notch on their maxilla which forms an almost tooth-like structure, called a tomial tooth, that is believed to enable them to easily sever the neck of vertebrate prey. **It is important to preserve the tomial tooth when performing any repairs or trimming the bill unless this structure itself is involved in a crack in the bill.** The nares of falcons, buteos and eagles have a bony baffle, or operculum (Fig. 9.1), which is thought to facilitate air flow in the nostrils during high speed flight (Heidenreich 1997).

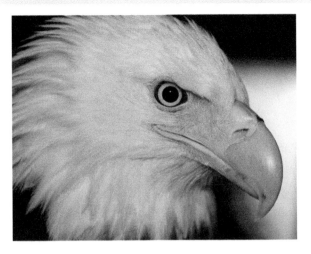

Fig 9.1 All raptors possess strongly curved bills.

Another important area of morphological specialization of raptors is their feet, which have thick scales to protect them from injury, and strong toes that terminate in curved talons.

Again, distinct differences occur among the various groups of raptors. The falcons (e.g. peregrine falcon, *Falco peregrinus*) and accipiters (e.g. sharp-shinned hawk, *Accipiter nisus*; Cooper's hawk, *Accipiter cooperi*), whose diets consist largely of light, agile prey, have long slender toes and a longer tarsometatarsus than the buteos (e.g. red-tailed hawks, *Buteo jamaicensis*; broad-winged hawks, *Buteo platypterus*), which have thick strong toes enabling them to capture difficult quarry. Ospreys have specialized pads with little spines called spicules on the ventral surface of the foot, which enable them to grab and hold slippery fish. Ospreys also have the ability to swivel their fourth digit to the rear, making them semi-zygodactylous, which gives them more dexterity in handling heavy or awkward prey items. Owls are also semi-zygodactylous, while all of the other falconiforms are syndactylous, and most owls have feathers extending to the ends of their digits. Ospreys have round talons, but the talons of all other raptors are either flat or slightly concave along the ventral surface. The medial side of the talon of the third digit has a specialized sharp edge that is used for feather grooming. This structure should be preserved during any talon trimming and reshaping procedure.

Clinically, there are four aspects of talons that require attention:

1. Captive-held birds should have the ends of the talons blunted to prevent self-inflicted injury. Conversely, birds about to be released to the wild should have their talons sharpened.
2. Talons need to be kept trimmed to a proper length. There is no exact landmark that can be

used to determine length, but a sense of this is gained by experience. Trimming them too short will cause profuse bleeding, and excessive length predisposes to self-inflicted foot injuries.

3. The groove on the ventral (or back) side of the talons needs to be kept free of debris, especially at the junction with the end of the toe. Failure to do this leads to pressure necrosis and infection of the distal toe.

4. Talons can be accidentally torn off, exposing the white, curved bone of the distal phalanx. Treatment of talon avulsion is accomplished by quickly controlling bleeding, painting the surface with a protective material (finger nail polish, New-skin®), and affixing a protective sheath such as that made from a plastic syringe case or using Soft Paws® (Softpaws.com, Three Rivers, CA, USA). Soft Paws® are vinyl nail caps manufactured for dogs and cats. **Regrowth of a talon will take up to 6 months.**

Gastrointestinal tract

There are also differences in the gastrointestinal (GI) tract anatomy of raptors (Duke 1986). Owls do not have crops, whereas most other raptors do (Fig. 9.2). The crop is used for the storage of food. The stomach of all raptors is essentially a simple glandular stomach. The pH of the stomach during digestion is approximately 1 in diurnal raptors, while owls have a pH of about 3. The former are capable of completely digesting bones, while the latter do not. The undigested bone is incorporated into the 'pellet', the mass of indigestible material that is regurgitated in the late phases of the digestive cycle prior to ingestion of another meal (Duke 1986). In falcons and hawks the caeca are vestigial, while in the owls they are large and functional. The caeca may serve to facilitate microbial fermentation and water reabsorption in owl species (Duke 1986).

Musculoskeletal anatomy

While anatomists will delineate significant differences in skeletal anatomy among raptors, the clinician will find variations among the elements of the appendicular skeleton to be minor. **The surgical anatomy of all raptor species is fundamentally the same, as it relates to orthopaedic surgery, whether a kestrel or an eagle is being evaluated.** Avian surgical anatomy is well described in *Avian Surgical Anatomy* (Orosz et al 1992) and *Avian Medicine and Surgery* (Altman et al 1997).

Management

Housing

Housing and feeding practices for raptors vary widely depending on the species and the purposes for which they are kept. In general, both indoor and outdoor

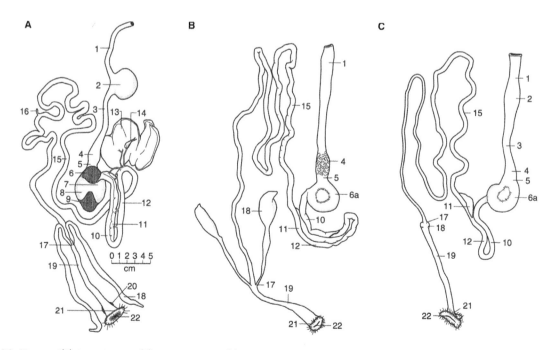

Fig 9.2 GI tracts of (**A**) domestic turkey; (**B**) great-horned owl; (**C**) red-tailed hawk. Included are: (1) pre-crop oesophagus; (2) crop; (3) post-crop oesophagus; (4) glandular stomach; (5) isthmus; (6) thin craniodorsal muscle; (6a) muscular stomach of raptors; (7) thick cranioventral muscle; (6 to 9) muscular stomach; (10) proximal duodenum; (11) pancreas; (12) distal duodenum; (13) liver; (14) gallbladder; (15) ileum; (16) Meckel's diverticulum; (17) ileocaecocolic junction; (18) caecum; (19) colon; (20) bursa of Fabricius; (21) cloaca; (22) vent; (Gc) greater curvature.

facilities should be provided. Protection from direct sunlight is mandatory, but birds may be allowed to choose their own level of exposure to inclement weather. **Many birds prefer limited exposure to rain and snow; however, protection from wind, especially in very cold weather, is essential.**

Indoor facilities for raptors are referred to as a mews. This is the term for the facility used by falconers to house their birds during the moulting season; the mews is also used as a place to protect birds from inclement weather. Some keepers move birds into the mews each night and out to the weathering yard in the day. Dimensions and shape vary tremendously depending on the species, and readers should confer with current keepers or consult other references (Beebe & Webster 1994, Heidenreich 1997, Arent 2006). Housing for display birds and birds used in education programmes may differ from that used for falconry birds. Examples of building configurations meeting the requirements for suitable housing of raptors are given in Figure 9.3 and Tables 9.1 (a) and (b). Many states in the USA have regulations affecting house design. **The mews should have at least one window obstructed by vertical dowels made of wood, plastic or metal (e.g. electrical conduit), and wall surfaces and flooring that are easily cleaned.**

Perches must be carefully considered with regard to size, shape, covering materials and placement, both for comfort and to maintain foot health. Falcons require broad, flat perches, usually covered with artificial turf (Astroturf® Monsanto Solutia Inc., St Louis, Montana USA), whereas buteos and goshawks are maintained on perches that are elliptical in cross-section, sized proportionately to their feet and wrapped with sisal rope (Arent 2006). **Care must be taken to ensure that there are no sharp edges present that may lead to puncture wounds in the bird's foot.** Perches should be positioned well off the floor, enabling the handler to approach the bird at chest level. Proximity to the barred window is desirable in most cases. Multiple perches within the mews are not required, and may be detrimental to foot health – when moving about in small areas birds hop rather than fly thus subjecting their feet to bruising from harder landing loads.

Problems related to improper perching surfaces can be assessed in part by wear patterns on the feet. Lesions occurring in the centre of the metatarsal pad arise from perches that are too small for that particular bird, resulting in excess amounts of pressure being applied to that portion of the foot. Conversely, lesions appearing on the toe pads are indicative of perches that are too large.

Outdoor pens, often referred to as weathering areas, are also required. Minimum dimensions of a weathering area for a typical raptor of approximately 1 kg housed singly are 2 m × 3 m × 2.5 m high (Heidenreich 1997). Configuration and size vary greatly, and advice should be taken from experienced individuals and appropriate references for specifics concerning the species that are being kept (Heidenreich 1997, Arent 2006). Falconry birds and those trained for handling and demonstration flights should be tethered in most instances. Where housing for multiple birds is provided, it is desirable for such birds to be separated by partitions within the facility. If separation is not practised, extreme diligence is required to maintain equipment in top condition so that a bird cannot break loose and attack one of the others. Convalescing birds undergoing rehabilitation are not tethered, and may be housed in groups of compatible individuals so long as sufficient food is available to keep all of them satiated (Table 9.2) (Arent 2006). **Certain species (e.g. accipiters) cannot be housed with other species, and the sexes of these should also be housed separately.** Similarly, with kestrels and merlins, males and females should not be housed together. Great horned owls and barred owls should be housed separately from each other and from other raptors. In all of these instances, the probability of attack and kill events is high if these separations are not observed.

Shade is important for all birds, especially gyrfalcons (*Falco rusticolus*) and snowy owls (*Nyctea scandiaca*). Conversely, some species, such as the Harris hawks (*Parabuteo unicinctus*), northern harriers, small buteos and ospreys, cannot tolerate the cold and must have supplemental heat when the ambient temperature drops below 0°C. Harris hawks, which are desert natives, require modest exposure to strong sunlight. Temperature tolerance guidelines are given in Tables 9.1 (a) and (b) (Heidenreich 1997).

Water must be available at all times for drinking and bathing, but care must be taken to prevent a tethered bird from getting tangled and drowning in a deep water pan. The water must be changed daily in the summer to prevent algae growth, and protected from freezing in the winter.

Feeding

Raptors are carnivores, and an appropriate diet is critical to their health and well-being. In nestling-stage raptors, all-meat diets with no bones cause nutritional secondary hyperparathyroidism (metabolic bone disease; Fowler 1986). This presents as a progressive, rapid demineralization of the bones, with multiple fractures and/or pathological folding of the long bones (Fig. 9.4). From within a few hours after hatching, raptors need a diet consisting of the whole bodies of typical prey species. Domestic quail, mice, and other small birds and rodents are appropriate. **A commercial diet is available (Bird of Prey Diet®, Spectrum Inc., North Platte, NE, USA), and is a good short-term source of nutrition; however, it should not be the only source of food, remembering a natural diet is always preferred.** Falcons thrive on quail and chicken, ospreys require fish, bald eagles (*Haliaeetus leucocephalus*) receive a mixture

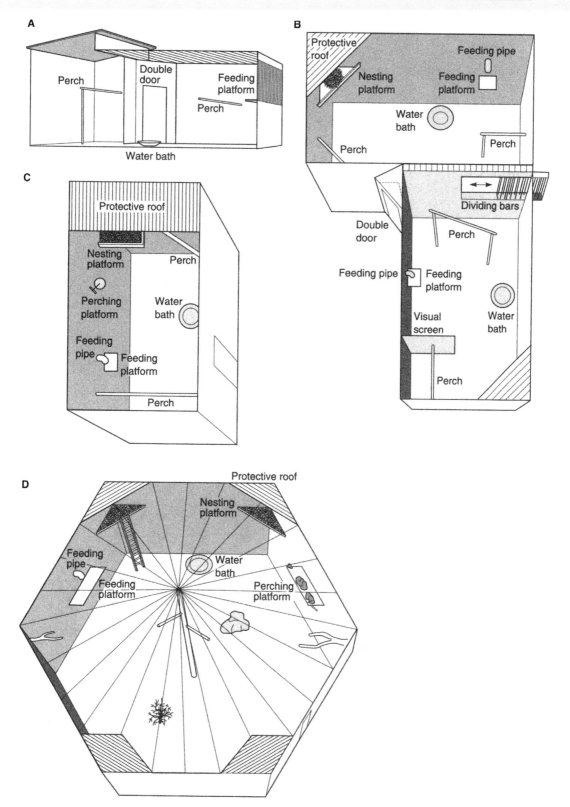

Fig 9.3 Size and configuration of mews, breeding chambers and weathering areas vary with purpose and species. A two-chamber, double-door system (**A**) provides comfort and safety. Breeding chambers (**B**, **C**, **D**) may also be used for moulting or weathering raptors.

of fish, rodents, rabbits and poultry, and most buteos and owls prefer rodents. If frozen fish is to be used for food for bald eagles and ospreys, thiamine needs to be supplemented at 1–3 mg/kg per week. For more specific information, the reader is referred to Beebe & Webster (1994) and Arent (2006). As a general rule of thumb, the smaller raptors eat approximately 20%, the medium-sized birds approximately 10–15% and the larger birds 6–8% of their body weight daily. Regular weighing of birds is an effective means of ensuring adequate dietary intake (Arent 2006).

Adequate water intake is essential for health maintenance of wild birds maintained in captivity. **Raptor patients are not guaranteed to drink water provided *ad lib* and they do not obtain adequate amounts of water from the food they ingest, particularly if it is frozen and thawed; the so-called 'metabolic water' does not make up the difference.** Therefore, to avoid dehydration, it is useful to soak food items in water for 1 to 2 minutes prior to feeding.

Clinical aspects of raptors – infectious and non-infectious diseases

There are many diseases, especially those of bacterial origin, which raptors share in common with other avian species. These are covered in other sections of this book. This chapter will focus on diseases and conditions that are unique to or commonly found in raptors.

Endoparasitic diseases of raptors

There are numerous endoparasites in birds of prey (Table 9.3; Cooper 1985, Greiner 1997). The most commonly encountered endoparasitic diseases among raptors are protozoan infections caused either by coccidia or by trichomonads, fluke and roundworm infestation of the GI tract, and two types of nematodes found in the respiratory tract. **Many endoparasites are capable of causing or contributing to a debilitated state; hence detection and treatment is recommended.**

Syngamus trachea and *Cyathstoma* spp. are occasional upper respiratory parasites, although the latter can also be found in air sacs. The life cycle of these respiratory parasites is either direct, or via paratenic hosts such as earthworms, snails and other invertebrates. Raptors that eat the paratenic hosts, such as the snail kite, kestrels and small owls, are more likely to be infected than other species of raptors (Hunter et al 1993). After ingestion, the larvae pass from the GI tract to the respiratory system via the bloodstream. The eggs move into the trachea and oropharynx, where they are swallowed, and pass through the GI tract to be shed with the faeces.

Serratospiculum spp. and *Serratospiculoides* spp. (e.g. *S. amaculata*) are filarid worms found in the air sacs of some falcon species. *S. amaculata* may be

Table 9.1a Categories of minimum size requirements for raptor enclosures (given per animal; young birds are not included until they gain independence) (Heidenreich 1997)

A	Aviary: outdoor area 2 m², width 1 m, height 2 m. Each additional animal: 1 m² added to outdoor area, and 1 m² shelter area. If kept exclusively in heated indoor chamber: area 2 m², height 1 m, each additional animal 1 m² more.
B	Aviary: outdoor area 5 m², width 2 m, height 2 m. Each additional animal 1 m² added to outdoor area, and shelter, if necessary: 1.5 m², height 2 m, width 1 m.
C	Aviary: outdoor area 7.5 m², width 2 m, height 2.5 m. Each additional animal: 3 m² added to outdoor area, and shelter, if necessary: 2 m², height 2 m, width 1 m.
D	Aviary: outdoor area 12 m², width 2 m, height 2.5 m. Each additional animal: 6 m² added to outdoor area, and shelter, if necessary: 4 m², height 2 m, width 2 m.
E	Aviary: outdoor area 18 m², width 3 m, height 2.5 m. Each additional animal: 6 m² added to outdoor area, and shelter, if necessary: 4 m², height 2 m, width 2 m.
F	Aviary: outdoor area 24 m², width 3 m, height 3 m. Each additional animal: 10 m² added to outdoor area, and shelter, if necessary: 4 m², height 2 m, width 2 m.
G	Outdoor aviary for a pair of birds at least 100 m².

Categories of temperature requirements

I	Hardy in winter, requires only protection from rain and wind.
II	Sensitive to very cold temperatures, requires an unheated enclosure or chamber.
III	Sensitive to moderately cold temperatures, requires indoor room protected from frost and draughts.

endemic in North American prairie falcons and Asian saker falcons (*Falco cherrug*). The host range for this species is described by Smith (1993) and Cooper (1985), and other species affected include peregrine falcons, Cooper's hawks and goshawks (*Accipiter gentilis*). Diagnosis is typically made following an incidental finding of lemon-shaped embryonated eggs on routine faecal flotation (Smith 1993), rather than as a result of a search for aetiology of medical problems with vague signs. Poor performance or unthriftiness in a falcon could indicate an air-sac worm infestation as part of a differential diagnosis. The mode of transmission, the intermediate hosts and other aspects of the biology of these parasites are largely unknown. They are easily eliminated with ivermectin (Ivomec® ivermectin, MSD AGVET Division of Merck and Co., Inc., Rahway, NJ, USA) or fenbendazole (Panacur® fenbendazole, Hoechst-Roussel Pharmaceuticals, Inc., Somerville, NJ, USA); however, advisability of treatment is controversial.

Table 9.1b Categories of minimum size requirements for many species of raptors along with temperature tolerances (Heidenreich 1997)

Family	Species	Category of aviary size requirement	Category of temperature requirement
New World vultures			
Cathartidae			
Genus *Cathartes*	Black vulture *Cathartes atratus*	D	III
	Turkey vulture *Cathartes aura*	D	IV
Genus *Sarcoramphus*	King vulture *Sarcoramphus papa*	D	IV (very sensitive to frost)
Genus *Vultur*	Andean condor *Vultur gyphus*	F	I
Osprey			
Pandionidae			
Genus *Pandion*	Osprey *Pandion haliaetus*	D	II
Secretary birds			
Sagittariidae			
Genus *Sagittarius*	Secretary bird *Sagittarius serpentarius*	G because they are ground birds, can also be maintained with unilaterally trimmed flight feathers	
Hawks			
Accipitridae			
Genus *Elanus*	Black-shouldered kite *Elanus caeruleus*	C	IV
Genus *Milvus*	Black kite *Milvus migrans*	D	I–II
			Consider origin[a]
	Red kite *Milvus milvus*	D	I
Genus *Haliastus*	Brahminy kite *Haliastus indus*	D	IV
Genus *Ichthyophaga*	Grey-headed fishing eagle *Ichthyophaga ichthyaetus*	D	IV
Genus *Haliaeetus*	White-tailed sea eagle *Haliaeetus albicilla*	F	I
	Bald eagle *Haliaeetus leucocephalus*	F	I
	White-bellied sea eagle *Haliaeetus leucogaster*		
	Pallas' sea eagle *Haliaeetus leucoryphus*	D	I
	Steller's sea eagle *Haliaeetus pelagicus*	F	I
	African fish eagle *Haliaeetus vocifer*	D	IV
Genus *Gypaetus*	Bearded vulture *Gypaetus barbatus*	F	I
Genus *Aegypius*	European black vulture *Aegypius monachus*	F	I
Genus *Gypohierax*	Palm nut vulture *Gypohierax angolensis*	D	IV
Genus *Neophron*	Egyptian vulture *Neophron percnopterus*	D	II–III
			Consider origin[a]
Genus *Necrosyrtes*	Hooded vulture *Necrosyrtes monachus*	D	IV
Genus *Sarcogyps*	Indian black (King) vulture *Sarcogyps calvus*	F	IV
Genus *Torgos*	Lappet-faced vulture *Torgos tracheliotus*	F	IV
Genus *Trigonoceps*	White-headed vulture *Trigonoceps occipitalis*	F	III
Genus *Gyps*	Griffon vulture *Gyps fulvus*	F	I
	Himalayan griffon *Gyps himalayensis*	F	I
	Rüppell's griffon *Gyps rueppellii*	F	III

(*continued*)

Table 9.1b *(continued)*

Family	Species	Category of aviary size requirement	Category of temperature requirement
Genus *Pseudogyps*	Indian white-backed vulture *Pseudogyps bengalensis*	D	III
	African white-backed vulture *Pseugogyps africanus*	D	III
Genus *Circaetus*	Brown harrier (snake) eagle *Circaetus cinereus*	D	IV
	Short-toed (serpent) eagle *Circaetus gallicus*	D	IV
Genus *Terathopius*	Bateleur eagle *Terathopius ecaudatus*	D	IV
Genus *Spilornis*	Crested serpent eagle *Spilornis cheela*	D	IV
Genus *Circus*	Marsh harrier *Circus aeruginosus*	D	II
	Hen harrier *Circus cyaneus*	D	I
Genus *Melierax*	Pale chanting goshawk *Melierax canorus*	D	IV
Genus *Polyboroides*	African harrier hawk *Polyboroides typus*	D	IV
Genus *Accipiter*	Northern goshawk *Accipiter gentilis*	D	I
	European sparrow hawk *Accipiter nisus*	C	I
Genus *Kaupifalco*	Lizard buzzard *Kaupifalco monogrammicus*	C	IV
Genus *Geranoaetus*	Grey eagle-buzzard *Geranoaetus melanoleucus*	D	II
Genus *Buteo*	Common buzzard *Buteo buteo*	C[b]	I
	Red-tailed hawk *Buteo jamaicensis*	C[b]	I–II
			Consider origin[a]
	Rough-legged buzzard *Buteo lagopus*	D	I
	Red-backed buzzard *Buteo polyosoma*	D	II
	Ferruginous hawk *Buteo regalis*	D	I
	Jackal (Augur) buzzard *Buteo rutofunus*	D	III
	Long-legged buzzard *Buteo rufofuscus*	D	I
Genus *Pernis*	Honey buzzard *Pernis apivorus*	C[b]	III
Genus *Harpia*	Harpy eagle *Harpia harpyja*	F	III
Genus *Morphnus*	Guiana crested eagle *Morphnus guianensis*	F	III
Genus *Pithecophaga*	Philippine monkey-eating eagle *Pithecophaga jefferyi*	F	IV
Genus *Polemaetus*	Martial eagle *Polemaetus bellicosus*	F	III
Genus *Stephanoaetus*	Crowned eagle *Stephanoaetus coronatus*	F	IV
Genus *Lophaetus*	Long-crested eagle *Lophaetus occipitalis*	D	IV
Genus *Hieraaetus*	Bonelli's eagle *Hieraaetus fasciatus*	D	I–II
			Consider origin[a]
Genus *Spizaetus*	Ornate hawk eagle *Spizaetus ornatus*	D	IV
Genus *Aquila*	Wedge-tailed eagle *Aquila audax*	F	I
	Greater spotted eagle *Aquila clanga*	D	II
	Golden eagle *Aquila chrysaetos*	F	I
	Imperial eagle *Aquila heliacea*	F	I
	Lesser spotted eagle *Aquila pomarina*	D	II

(continued)

Table 9.1b *(continued)*

Family	Species	Category of aviary size requirement	Category of temperature requirement
	Tawny (Steppe) eagle *Aquila rapax*	E	I–II
			Consider origin[a]
	Verreaux's (Black) eagle *Aquila verreauxii*	F	III
Falcons			
Falconidae			
Genus *Milvago*	Chimango *Milvago chiachima*	C	III
	Yellow-headed caracara *Milvago chiachima*	C	III
Genus *Phalcoboenus*	Forster's caracara *Phalcoboenus australis*	D	I
	Mountain caracara *Phalcoboenus megalopterus*	D	II
Genus *Polyborus*	Common caracara *Polyborus plancus*	D	II
Genus *Polihierax*	African pygmy falcon *Polihierax semitorquatus*	B	IV
Genus *Microhierax*	Red-legged falconet *Microhierax caerulescens*	A	IV
Genus *Falco*	Lanner falcon *Falco biarmicus*	D	I–II
			Consider origin[a]
	Saker falcon *Falco cherrug*	D	I–III
			Consider origin[a]
	Merlin *Falco columbarius*	C	I
	Eleonora's falcon *Falco eleonorae*	D	III
	Laggar falcon *Falco jugger*	D	II
	Prairie falcon *Falco mexicanus*	D	I
	Peregrine falcon *Falco peregrinus*	D	I
	Gyrfalcon *Falco rusticolus*	D	I
	American kestrel *Falco sparverius*	B	II–III
			Consider origin[a]
	European hobby *Falco subbuteo*	C[b]	III
	Common kestrel *Falco tinnunculus*	B	I
	Red-footed falcon *Falco vespertinus*	B	III

[a]*Consider origin: Temperature requirements will vary with regional geographic origin. Other categories may be more appropriate.*
[b]*Individually housed birds require the same space as pairs do, 10.5 m².*

Some experts fear that a mass of dead worms in the air sacs may lead to a necrotizing nidus of infection there (Cooper 1985); however, based on the numbers of worms typically found, this concern may be unfounded (Redig, unpublished). Some clinicians prefer to 'partially paralyse' the worms with ivermectin, then remove them endoscopically (Samour & Naldo 2001).

The most common parasite of clinical significance is *Trichomonas gallinae*, the causative organism of 'frounce' (Samour & Naldo 2003). The organism is found in nearly all wild pigeons but seldom causes disease in them. The disease is readily transmitted to captive raptors that have fed upon a warm, freshly killed pigeon. It is also seen in wild birds that feed on pigeons, most frequently in goshawks, barred owls, and great horned owls (*Bubo virginianus*), especially in late spring when the low availability of normal prey has them resorting to alternative sources such as pigeons. It is also common in juvenile Cooper's hawks (Boal et al 1998) and affected kestrels and screech owls are encountered in summer during times of drought (Ueblacker 2000). **Interestingly, wild peregrine falcons appear to develop or have an innate resistance, as the disease seldom occurs in this species despite regular consumption of feral pigeons.**

Table 9.2 Raptor species that can be safely housed together (Arent 2006)

Species	American kestrel	Bald eagle	Barn owl	Barred owl	Broad-winged hawk	Burrowing owl	Cooper's hawk	Golden eagle	Great horned owl	Northern goshawk	Peregrine falcon	Prairie falcon	Long-eared owl	Red-tailed hawk	Rough-legged hawk	Saw-whet owl	Screech owl	Sharp-skinned hawk	Short-eared owl	Swainson's hawk	Turkey vulture
American kestrel	S					X															
Bald eagle		X						X													X
Barn owl			X																		
Barred owl				X																	
Broad-winged hawk					X								X						X		
Burrowing owl	X					X															
Cooper's hawk							S														
Golden eagle		X						X													X
Great horned owl									X					X	X						X
Northern goshawk										S											
Peregrine falcon											X	X									
Prairie falcon											X	X									
Long-eared owl					X								X						X		
Red-tailed hawk									X					X	X					X	X
Rough-legged hawk									X					X	X					X	X
Saw-whet owl																X					
Screech owl																	X				
Sharp-skinned hawk																		S			
Short-eared owl					X								X						X		
Swainson's hawk														X	X					X	X
Turkey vulture		X						X	X					X	X					X	X

S = *Same sex only.*

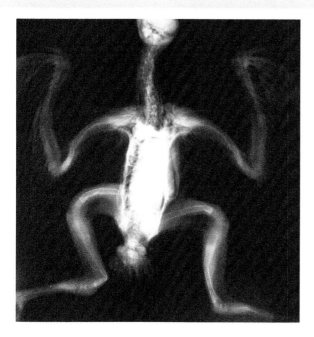

Fig 9.4 Hatch year red-tailed hawk showing pathological fractures due to severe metabolic bone disease. (Radiograph by L. Cruz-Martinez.)

Clinical signs of frounce are yellow caseous plaques on and under the tongue, pharyngeal surfaces, and crop (Fig. 9.5). It may also invade the sinuses and trachea. Affected birds have difficulty swallowing, often flicking away bites of meat. Ultimately they are unable to swallow, and starvation ensues. Diagnosis is confirmed by recovering the protozoan organisms with a swab or scraping (wet mount, examine at 40×). The organism is very sensitive to treatment with metronidazole (Flagyl, Watson Laboratories, Inc., Grona, CA, USA) at 30–50 mg/kg daily for 3–5 days (depending on severity). Samour & Naldo (2003) recommend oral metronidazole at a dose of 100 mg/kg every 24 hours for 3 days.

Carnidazole (Spartrix®, Foy's Pigeon Supplies, Beavertown, PA, USA) at 30 mg/kg given once daily for 2–3 days is an effective alternative (Forbes 1996). Where invasion of the palate and development of large caseous lesions has occurred, treatment is ineffective. Samour (2000) has reported infection with *Pseudomonas* spp. as a sequela to severe trichomoniasis infections.

Among nematodes, *Capillaria* spp. (e.g. *C. contorta*) are the most frequently encountered and are likely to be a source of pathology, occurring at any location within the GI tract. Morbidity and mortality have been associated with capillaria in the oral cavity, where they cause a lesion resembling that of trichomoniasis (Boydell & Forbes 1996). The bipolar ova of *Capillaria* spp. are readily recognized in a faecal flotation (Smith 1993). Stomach worms of the genera *Porrocaecum* spp. and *Contracaecum* spp. are frequently encountered by faecal examination. Pathology and clinical signs are rare;

however, verminous granulomatous inflammation of the ventriculus of undetermined aetiology, possibly due to such nematodes, has been encountered (Redig, unpublished). The affected owls (two cases in great horned owls) exhibited anorexia, vomiting and severe weight loss.

Other roundworms (e.g. *Acanthocephalan* spp.) and tapeworms rarely cause clinical problems. Finding their eggs or motile segments in faeces will prompt treatment. The former are easily eliminated by periodic treatments with either fenbendazole, mebendazole or ivermectin, while praziquantel (Droncit®, Bayer Corporation, Animal Health, Shawnee Mission, Kansas, USA) dosed at 2.5 mg/kg once effectively eliminates the latter (Cooper 1985, Smith 1993).

Trematodes are the second most prevalent parasite detected by faecal examinations. There are many species, indistinguishable by their large, operculated eggs, but known to inhabit the intestine, and bile and pancreatic ducts (Cooper 1985). While pathology is not a constant feature of their presence, fatal syndromes and poor condition have been reported in several raptor species. One case of intestinal intussusception and prolapse was encountered in an American kestrel with a heavy fluke (dicrocoelid type) infestation. Trematodes are eliminated by dosing with praziquantel at 5–10 mg/kg p.o. (repeating dose after 2–4 weeks) (Carpenter 2005).

Coccidians are a frequent cause of lethargy accompanied by weight loss, anorexia and passage of abnormal stools, varying from green, stringy masses to bloody pools of faeces (Heidenreich 1997). Eimeriad types and *Caryospara* spp. (e.g. *C. neofalconis*, Forbes & Simpson 1997) are most common. The latter are frequently found in juvenile and sub-adult falconiforms in captivity (Zucca 2000). Other coccidian genera found in raptors include *Sarcocystis* spp. and *Frankelia* spp. (Cawthorne 1993). An aberrant occurrence of the former was reported to be associated with a neurological syndrome in a goshawk (Aguilar et al 1991), and Dubey et al (1991) reported on a similar case in a golden eagle (*Aquila chrysaetos*). While the latter types of coccidial infections are clearly untreatable, most others occurring in the GI tract are amenable to treatment with sulfa drugs or, preferably, two treatments at a 24-hour interval of toltrazuril (Baycox®, Bayer Austria, Vienna) (Carpenter 2005, Forbes 1996) at 10 mg/kg p.o. This is repeated in 2 weeks. In our experience, direct administration of this drug results in regurgitation but this treatment side effect may be avoided by loading the drug in a gelatin capsule and administering it in a small piece of meat.

Ectoparasitic diseases

A wide variety of ectoparasites, such as lice, black flies, mosquitoes, ticks, and hippoboscid and acarid flies, are found on raptors (Heidenreich 1997). Ectoparasites can be seen and identified on physical examination of the bird. Most ectoparasites are commensal on raptors.

With debilitation and concomitant decreased grooming by the host, their numbers can increase resulting in immunosuppression and clinical disease. **Ectoparasites cause anaemia, both directly from their obtaining blood meals and indirectly by the transmission of the blood parasites.** Pyrethrin sprays (Adams® Tick and Flea Mist, Pet Chemicals. Memphis, TN, USA) and fipronil spray (Frontline®, Merial Inc., Duluth, GA, USA) effectively kill these ectoparasites.

Blow-fl y larvae of the genus *Protocalliphora* are found with regularity in the external auditory canals of nestling raptors (Smith 1993), especially the buteoine hawks (e.g. red-tailed hawks, broad-winged hawks, red-shouldered hawks (*Buteo linneatus*)). Though the ear canal becomes soiled with dried blood and excreta from the worms, permanent damage is not done to the host. Ordinarily, these larvae leave the ear canal to pupate in the nest. When encountered among orphaned birds submitted for rehabilitation, they can and should be mechanically removed. This is easily accomplished by placing a drop of mineral oil or saline in the ear, thereby forcing the worms to stretch to get their spiracles in open air for breathing. They can then be removed with a pair of forceps.

Table 9.3 Endoparasitic diseases (after Cooper 1985)

Parasite	Location	Detection	Treatment (after Carpenter et al 2005)
Nematodes			
Capillaria	Oral, GI, caeca	Faecal exam, oral scraping	Ivermectin (0.2 mg/kg one dose)
Ascarids	Intestines	Faecal exam	Ivermectin (see above)
Spirurids	Intestines	Faecal exam	Ivermectin (see above)
Porrocaecum	Stomach	Faecal exam	Ivermectin (see above)
Contracaecum	Stomach	Faecal exam	Ivermectin (see above)
Syngamus spp.	Trachea, bronchi	Faecal exam, tracheal wash	Ivermectin (see above)
Cyathostoma spp.	Air sacs	Faecal exam	Ivermectin (see above)
Serratospiculum spp.	Air sacs	Faecal exam	Ivermectin (see above) Endoscopic removal of the parasites
Cestodes	Intestines	Motile segments in faeces	Praziquantel (30 mg/kg) repeat in 10 days
Trematodes	Intestines, bile ducts, pancreatic ducts	Faecal exam	Praziquantel (see above)
Protozoans			
Trichomonads	Oral, intestines	Oral scrapings	Metronidazole 50 mg/kg b.i.d. for 5–7 days Carnidazole 20 mg/kg – one dose
Coccidia	Intestines	Faecal exam	Albon (55 mg/kg day 1, then 25 mg s.i.d. for 10 days) Clazuril 10 mg/kg s.i.d. for 3 days, repeat 1 − 2 × with 2 days off (Tully 1997) Toltrazuril 0.25 mL/kg p.o., two doses 24 hours apart
Sarcocystis	Skeletal muscle		None
Frankelia	Intestines		
Toxoplasma			
Haematozoa			
Leucocytozoon	Peripheral blood	Blood smear	None
Haemoproteus	Erythrocytes	Blood smear	Chloroquine (10 mg/kg) plus primaquine (0.75 mg/kg). Questionable efficacy
Plasmodium	Erythrocytes	Blood smear	Chloroquine/primaquine (see above for dosage), dose at $t_{0,12,24,48}$ hours, primaquine first dose only. Combination also used as a once-weekly prophylactic during mosquito season for gyrfalcons and their hybrids Mefloquine (alternative treatment/prophylactic – better acceptance than C/P, but utilized sufficiently to know efficacy

Haematozoa

Blood parasites can also be found in raptors and their pathogenicity depends upon the type of parasite, age of the bird and the level of parasitaemia. *Leucocytozoon* spp. are considered non-pathogenic in adult raptors, although they have been associated with mortality in nestlings. *Haemoproteus* spp. are also considered non-pathogenic; however, there are recent reports of fatalities in owls (Remple 2004). *Plasmodium*, of which there are 11 species known to affect raptors, is the true malarial parasite (Remple 2004); among North American raptors, gyrfalcons and snowy owls are known to be particularly susceptible. The treatment protocol for avian malaria used at The Raptor Center at the University of Minnesota consists of 30 mg/kg oral

mefloquine (Lariam® Hoffmann-La Roche Inc., NJ, USA) at 0, 12, 24 and 48 hours (Tavernier et al 2005). **Routine prophylaxis in susceptible species (gyrfalcons (*Falco rusticolus*), gyr-hybrids, and snowy owls) with mefloquine (30 mg/kg) given per os once weekly during the insect season is recommended.** *Babesia* spp. have also been reported in raptors and may cause anaemia and blindness in young falcons. *Babesia* has been diagnosed recently in a great horned owl (Redig, unpublished) and reported in other raptor species. Imidocarb dipropionate (Imizol® Schering-Plough Animal Health Corp. Union, NJ, USA) 5 mg/kg i.m. given once and repeated 1 week later, constitutes the treatment of choice (Samour et al 2005).

Bumblefoot

Bumblefoot is a degenerative, inflammatory condition affecting the feet of raptors and occasionally in other birds, most notably waterfowl (Redig 1996a). **Though common in captive raptors, bumblefoot is a by-product of captive management and is not an infectious disease.** This condition is rare among wild birds and, in them, it is typically associated with pre-existing injury to one or both feet (Ellis 1986, Gentz 1996). It is initiated by abnormal pressures placed on the feet by improperly shaped perches and inappropriate perching substrate, and by housing arrangements in which raptors traumatize the metatarsal pad by jumping from perch to perch. In some instances, the condition may result from self-inflicted puncture wounds (Cooper 1985), foreign body penetration, or bite wounds from prey or other trauma. In all cases, trauma to the bottom of the foot or toe is the inciting factor. Infection, usually with *E. coli* or *Staphylococcus* spp., is secondary. We agree with Harcourt-Brown's (1996) analogy of the pathogenesis to that of a bedsore. This disorder is graded in five categories (Oaks 1996), depending on the severity and prognosis (Fig. 9.6 A–D); type I is a non-disrupting hyperaemic or hyperkeratotic devitalization of the plantar epithelium

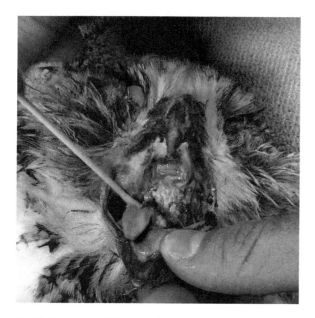

Fig 9.5 Extensive oral *Trichomonas* lesion in a great horned owl. (Photo by L. Cruz-Martinez.)

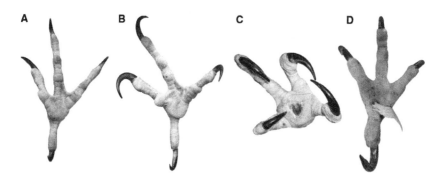

Fig 9.6 Plantar aspect of a raptor foot showing (**A**) normal, healthy epithelium layer; (**B**) bumblefoot type I, note the pink coloration and the flat appearance of the epithelium as well as overgrown talons; (**C**) bumblefoot type III, note the large scab/plug and swelling of the plantar surface of the foot; (**D**) gauze seton insertion to the wound in order to establish drainage and provide contact to a wet-to dry-bandage. (Photos by L. Cruz-Martinez.)

and carries a good prognosis (Fig. 9.6B), while type V is characterized by deep infection of the soft tissue and osteomyelitis; it is most often treated by euthanasia.

The treatment of bumblefoot is complex and prolonged. It involves removal of the underlying cause(s) and management of the wound. In early type I cases, where the papillae of the plantar epithelium are flattened and there is slight reddening of the skin, application of skin tougheners and protectants (Camphor Spirit and Benzoin Tincture, Humco™ Texarkana, TX, USA, NewSkin® Liquid Bandage, Medtech Laboratories Inc., Jackson, Wyoming, USA) along with alteration of perch size and/or covering material will suffice. In types II (Fig. 9.6C) and III, where there is ulceration, swelling and inflammation, management consists of surgical debridement, establishing and maintaining drainage, and protective bandaging. Culture and determination of antibiotic sensitivity for systemic antibiotics is essential. The course of treatment typically involves surgically removing the scab, gently removing loose tags of exudate and inflammatory tissue, and irrigating the wound with warmed, sterile saline or 0.5% chlorhexidine (not iodine-containing solutions). A sterile strip of saline-soaked gauze or umbilical tape is inserted into the wound as a seton (Fig. 9.6D) and the foot is bandaged into a 'ball bandage' (Fig. 9.7), using a 'ball' of sterile gauze in contact with the bottom of the foot, thereby forming a wet-to-dry bandage. This bandage is changed daily, with continued copious, irrigation, replacement of the seton and application of a ball bandage for a period of 10–20 days, pending the cessation of drainage and the appearance of granulation tissue in the wound. Appropriate systemic antibiotic therapy should be given for 5–7 days (cephalosporins and fluoroquinolones typically yield the best results). From this point, the wound should be packed with a granulation-stimulating product (Intra-site Gel®, Smith and Nephew SAS Espace Novaxis, Le Mans Cedex 2, France or equivalent) and covered with a non-adherent absorbent dressing (Release® non-adhering dressing, Johnson and Johnson Medical Inc., Arlington, Texas, USA) held in place with adhesive tape or semipermeable membrane wound dressing material (Tegaderm®, 3M Medical-Surgical Division, St Paul, MN, USA). All of this is overwrapped with conforming bandaging material (Vetrap® bandaging tape, 3M Animal Care Products, St Paul, Minnesota) to form a ball (Rupley 1997). The ball bandage is maintained until the wound has closed by secondary intention healing. Alternatively, healing may be expedited at the point where abundant granulation tissue is present by suturing the wound. **It will take 1 to 2 months from the point of closure to the point where the epithelium is strong enough to withstand normal use.** During this time, the foot should be protected in a polypropylene shoe (Fig. 9.7). In the final stages, it is useful to switch from a shoe to a padded interdigitating bandage for

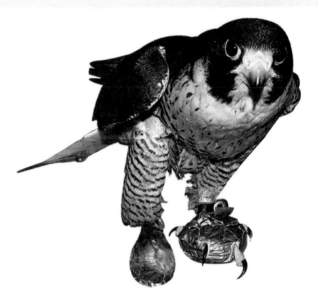

Fig 9.7 Peregrine falcon wearing a polypropylene shoe on the right foot and a ball bandage on the left foot. With either bandage the bird is able to stand and/or perch. Note the layer of duct tape used in order to prevent bandage destruction by the bird.

several weeks until the integrity of the tissue allows normal use. At this stage it is useful to apply skin tougheners to the healing tissues on a twice-weekly basis.

Adjuncts to therapy of bumblefoot

Where significant swelling is present, it can be reduced in 1 to 2 days prior to conducting any surgical debridement by the application of a dimethylsulfoxide-antibiotic-steroid cocktail (0.5 mL DMSO, 0.2 mL dexamethasone, 0.3 mL of concentrated enrofloxacin (100 mg/mL). This is painted over the surface of the affected area once, after which the foot is placed overnight in a ball bandage. In cases with extensive infection, control may be enhanced by the insertion of antibiotic-impregnated methylmethacrylate beads (Remple 2005). These may be left in place for several days with the foot bandaged and in some cases, even after the wound has healed.

Preventionof b umblefoot

Since the causes of bumblefoot are management-related and the course of treatment is complicated and protracted, prevention is extremely important. Five important elements include:

1. Provision of a nutritious, balanced diet suitable for the species of raptor in question and avoidance of obesity.
2. Provision of perches that are sized, shaped and covered appropriately for the species and sex.
3. Provision of adequate manoeuvring space for free-lofted birds so they can land normally.

4. Keeping talons at appropriate lengths and blunting the tips unless the bird is used for hunting.
5. Provision of adequate exercise and observing the condition of the feet on a regular basis.

A special form of bumblefoot, seen in large, highly athletic hunting falcons, is described by Heidenreich (1997). Because it occurs when hunting hawks are idled at the end of the hunting season, it is likened to similar conditions seen in horses and human athletes. The high level of cardiovascular condition and blood volume present in such animals is not compatible with abrupt onset of inactivity, and this leads to oedema and swelling of dependent limbs. In falcons, these events can lead to bumblefoot. Prevention of this form can be accomplished by placing the birds on a schedule of progressively decreasing exercise as the field season draws to a close.

Feather abnormalities

Issues relating to the protection of feathers, repairing broken feathers by imping, and moulting have been discussed above. **Pathological conditions involving feathers of raptors include the occurrence of 'stress marks', and a peculiar 'pinching-off' syndrome which may be related to transient, clinically inapparent viral infections of unknown aetiology.**

Stress marks appear as lines across one or more feathers, which occur due to an interruption in the normal flow of nutrients to the feather or exposure to stress during its growth. In young raptors taken into captivity as mid-growth nestlings, a continuous line of stress marks across the tail feathers will often be seen; these reflect the stress of adjustment to a new environment and possibly a day or two of below-normal food intake. Injury, administration of corticosteroids, or illness during feather growth are other purported causes (Malley & Whitbread 1996).

Pinching off of individual feathers (Fig. 9.8) is an occasional cause for presentation of wild and captive raptors (Mueller et al 2007). The pattern is for normal growth of

a retrix or remige for one-half to two-thirds of its normal growth, after which the blood supply withdraws and the feather pinches off in a characteristic hourglass presentation. A new feather usually grows after removal of the remaining stump (by the bird or by human intervention), and this may or may not pinch off. In time the problem self-corrects, but it may require more than a couple of moult sequences to do so. Heidenreich (1997) attributes the cause to quill mites (*Harpyrhyncthus* spp.), and suggests treatment with ivermectin during feather growth stages as a possible means of management. Recently, this phenomenon has been seen regularly in birds recovering from West Nile virus infections, begging the question whether some of the other cases of pinched off feathers may have a viral aetiology.

Manipulating the moult

The information about the induction of moulting for the purpose of extra-seasonal feather replacement is scant and anecdotal, but varying degrees of success have been had by manipulating the photoperiod adjustment or by oral administration of exogenous thyroid hormone (Van Wettere, unpublished). The former is a preferred method as it results in a more natural moult with better feather quality. It is accomplished by advancing the photoperiod to 18–20 hours of light/day after a period of a month to 6 weeks of less than 10 hours of light per day. Lighting sources have ranged from fluorescent to incandescent bulbs to full spectrum lighting with little indication that any one is better than the other. Results vary with species. Moulting will start within a few weeks and may be completed over a period of 4 to 5 months. Synthetic thyroid hormone is used with dosages ranging between 100μg/kg to 800μg/kg daily for several days to weeks. If the bird is responsive, the onset and rate of moult tends to be very rapid, some birds losing most of their flight feathers nearly simultaneously. **Quality of regrown feathers from a forced moult often is less than that of the natural moults.**

Viruses

Herpesviruses

While herpesviruses are known to occur in a wide range of vertebrate animals, three distinct serotypes have been encountered in various raptor species; the one responsible for fatal hepatosplenitis or inclusion body disease seen in falcons is the most commonly encountered. There are three subfamilies of the herpesvirus, alpha, beta and gamma, which determine the biological properties, host range, cytopathology and other characteristics of that subfamily (Wheler 1993). Other avian diseases known to be caused by herpesviruses are Marek's disease, duck viral enteritis, and Pacheco's disease in psittacines (Ritchie et al 1994). The pathogenic herpesvirus for falcons causes a fatal disease process that is characterized by multifocal necrosis of the liver, spleen

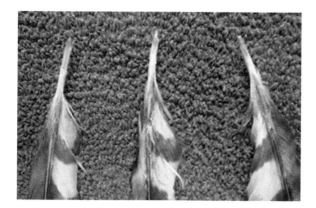

Fig 9.8 Pinched feathers. (Photo by L. Cruz-Martinez.)

and other organs, with the formation of intranuclear inclusion bodies. In two owl cases, the gross pathological findings resembled trichomoniasis or avian tuberculosis (Gough et al 2000). The clinical course lasts from several hours to several days, with weakness, depression, anorexia, regurgitation and diarrhoea following a pre-patent period of 7–10 days. A profound leucopenia is exhibited in the 24–48 hours preceding death. Presumptive diagnosis is based on gross lesions (Heidenreich 1997) and demonstration of intranuclear inclusion bodies. The diagnosis is confirmed by virus isolation. Natural transmission of this disease occurs via ingestion of the viral particle, usually from the consumption of infected prey – most commonly pigeons.

Paramyxovirus

The most important member of the Paramyxoviridae family is Newcastle disease virus (NDV) (paramyxovirus-1:PMV-1). It occurs worldwide and has the broadest host range infecting most species of free-ranging and captive birds (Clubb et al 1980) and many species of mammals, including humans. Okoh (1979) has described this disease in falcons.

The incubation period can vary from 3 to 28 days and the clinical progression of disease varies widely depending on the species of bird and the strain of the virus. Almost any combination of mild to severe disease signs involving the respiratory, gastrointestinal or nervous system (e.g. torticollis, ataxia, convulsions, head twitching) can be observed in birds infected with PMV-1. Experiences at The Raptor Center at the University of Minnesota have not revealed any cases of Newcastle disease among raptors. However, since an American kestrel yielded an isolate serologically identical to pigeon paramyxovirus-1 (Ritchie et al 1994), it is suggested that raptors are susceptible to pigeon PMV-1.

In the eastern hemisphere, several strains of Newcastle disease virus have been identified and characterized. This disease was an important infectious disease in the United Arab Emirates (UAE). Birds of prey can become infected by eating a virus-contaminated food source. It is known that lentogenic strains from poultry can be velogenic in raptors. A velogenic viscerotropic strain of NDV was the suspected cause of death of a bearded vulture without any previous signs of illness (Lublin et al 2001). Vaccines containing Hitchner B-1/LaSota strains (Lohmann Animal Health International, Gainesville, GA, USA) used for poultry have been administered in isolated circumstances among captive birds (Heidenreich 1997, Manvell et al 2000), but should never be given to birds intended for release to the wild. Despite being enveloped, these viruses are relatively stable in the environment and are resistant to many commonly used disinfectants. Insects, rodents and humans should be considered potential mechanical vectors.

Adenovirus

Adenovirus is a fatal disease, especially of young birds, and has been reported recently in a number of species (Forbes 1997, Oaks et al 2005). The causative agent has been clearly identified as an adenovirus. Adenoviruses are currently classified into four genera (*Mastadenovirus*, *Aviadenovirus*, *Siadenovirus* and *Atadenovirus*), with the falconid adenovirus the best characterized of raptor viruses (Zsivanovits et al 2006). The virus can be transmitted by the faecal/oral route and by aerosols. It was thought that the source of infection was food items. However, epidemiological and serological data from recent outbreaks implicates peregrine falcons as the possible reservoir species and the source of contamination to other falcon species (Oaks et al 2005, Van Wettere et al 2005). Non-native falcons appear extremely susceptible when exposed to this particular adenoviral disease.

The disease has been encountered in both free-ranging and captive-held birds. Taita falcons (*Falco fasciinucha*), northern aplomado falcons (*Falco femoralis*), merlins (*Falco columbarus*), American and Mauritius kestrels (*Falco sparverius*, *Falco punctatus*), northern goshawks, Harris hawks (*Parabuteo unicinctus*), Bengal eagle owl (*Bubo bengalensis*), a Verreaux's eagle owl (*Buteo lacteus*), white-tailed sea eagle (*Haliaeetus albicilla*) and common buzzards (*Buteo buteo*) have been reported to be susceptible to this disease (Dean et al 2006, Zsivanovits et al 2006).

Clinical characteristics of the adenoviral infection are sudden death or an acute illness (2–4 days) with clinical signs of anorexia and lethargy. The morbidity reaches 100% while the mortality is 50% within an infected population. There is no definitive ante-mortem diagnosis nor is treatment, aside from supportive care, feasible. At post-mortem, a tentative diagnosis can be achieved by histopathology. Basophilic, intranuclear inclusions are identified from spleen, liver, intestine and pancreas tissue sections obtained from dead birds. Adenoviral nucleic acid may be detected by testing using PCR technology, thus confirming the diagnosis.

Management recommendations to reduce a bird's exposure to adenovirus during nestling age include avoiding co-housing of falcon species originating from isolated populations with other falcon species, especially peregrine falcons and gyrfalcons; quarantine protocols for newly acquired birds; and application of strict hygiene standards in all aspects of management. Recommended disinfection for aviadenoviruses in poultry consists of chlorine-releasing agents, iodophors and quaternary ammonium compounds. Chlorhexidine may be a fairly ineffective disinfecting agent when used for this viral organism. Removal of any organic matter, rinsing of the soap before the application of the disinfectant, and a sufficiently long incubation time with the disinfectant at room temperature are known to be important factors for successful disinfection.

Poxvirus

Pox is another viral disease diagnosed in raptor species (Ritchie et al 1994, Heidenreich 1997). Usually only the dry form is noted in birds of prey, and it is spread by mosquitoes. As a group, avipoxes are species specific, although they may cross species barriers to cause a less severe form of the disease in the new host (Heidenreich 1997). **Clinical signs of poxvirus infection include nodular encrustations on the cere, eyelids and feet that progress through the papule state to vesicles, pustules and then scabs.** Pox-injected birds are prone to secondary bacterial infections. Diagnosis is made typically by histological examination of biopsies of affected epithelial tissue, which show intracytoplasmic inclusions (Bollinger bodies). Affected birds typically do not exhibit outward signs of illness unless the lesion is obstructing part of the mouth or an eye, which may debilitate the patient. Early lesions may be managed by topical application of antiseptic-astringent compounds (merthiolate, mercurichrome or povidone iodine). Treatment of larger lesions may be accomplished by surgical removal (cautery), topical and systemic antibiotics, and wound treatment for control of secondary bacterial infection. The disease is self-limiting.

WestN ilev irus

West Nile virus (WNV) was introduced into the USA in 1999 and became a significant cause of morbidity and mortality among wild birds. The principal vector appears to be *Culex* spp. mosquitoes. Incubation is reported to be 7–10 days and viraemias are of short duration, lasting 3–4 days. The viraemia subsides before the onset of severe clinical signs (Nemeth et al 2006). West Nile virus has been reported in virtually all species of raptors (USGS 2006); however, the overall incidence is highest in red-tailed hawks, Cooper's hawks, goshawks, great horned owls and golden eagles, occasional in bald eagles, screech owls (*Macroscops asio*), barred owls (*Strix varia*), kestrels and merlins, rare in peregrine falcons and gyrfalcons, and incidental in other species of raptors. Great grey owls (*Strix nebulosa*) and snowy owls were also found to be very susceptible (Gancz et al 2004). Hull et al (2006) describe a variation in antibody prevalence in migrating and wintering hawks.

At The Raptor Center at the University of Minnesota the first case of WNV was encountered in great horned owls in mid-August 2002. By mid-October 2002, approximately 80 cases had been seen, affecting a wide range of falconiforms and strigiforms. However, the highest incidence was seen among great horned owls and red-tailed hawks. In the summer of 2003, a different pattern emerged. Juvenile Cooper's hawks and juvenile red-tailed hawks were the primary species admitted to The Raptor Center with clinical signs and serology consistent with WNV.

Clinically affected diurnal raptors most often exhibited lethargy, ataxia and reduced mental state, and mild tremors. Some had overt visual impairment due to retinal inflammation. Accipiter hawks (goshawks and Cooper's hawks) and red-tailed hawks exhibited seizures. Nocturnal raptors, especially great horned owls, characteristically exhibited altered mental state, star-gazing, and dyskinetic movements of the head, a condition described as a 'bobble-head bird'. Some owls exhibited an apparent brachial plexus neuritis manifested by unilateral paralysis of the wing, often accompanied by central blindness. Affected birds of both types presented with elevated white cells counts characterized by heterophilia, and, radiographically, a swollen spleen was often detected. WNV appeared to cause chronic disease and death that was frequently characterized by a complex of inflammatory lesions including myocarditis (especially in goshawks), lymphoplasmacytic and histiocytic encephalitis, endophthalmitis and pancreatitis (Wunschmann et al 2005). Cachexia was a common physical abnormality noted during an examination of a clinically affected bird.

The biology of the disease caused by WNV made real-time diagnosis difficult. Viraemia was of short duration (Komar et al 2003) and typically waned before the onset of overt clinical signs, making diagnosis by virus isolation or PCR technology a low yield process. Antibody production takes 10–14 days. Therefore, there was a window of time when neither viral detection methods nor serological methods yielded definitive diagnostic information. Further, antibodies persisted after infection, so effective use of serology required evidence of a rising antibody titre in order to be meaningful for diagnostic evaluation. Cross-reactivity with other flaviviruses required simultaneous testing of all samples for St Louis encephalitis virus to ensure antibodies were due to WNV. Though ELISA tests are available for antibody screening, titering requires the use of a plaque reduction neutralization test (PRNT) and this can be done only in a laboratory certified for handling organisms requiring a Biosafety Level III facility.

Treatment recommended for raptors infected with WNV was entirely supportive in nature, consisting of fluid therapy, assisted feeding, and administration of NSAIDs (Metacam® Boehringer Ingelheim, Vetmedica, Inc., St Joseph, MO, USA) dosed at 0.2–0.5 mg/kg b.i.d. to reduce the inflammatory response. NSAIDs were most effective if administered early in the progression of the disease. Birds presenting with neurological signs were recovered, but often were not completely sound. Diurnal raptors often had visual impairment in one or both eyes owing to retinal inflammation and degeneration. The extent of ocular impairment was assessed by fundoscopic examination.

West Nile virus vaccination for raptors in the high prevalence group is recommended. The product used to date has been the Fort Dodge Animal Health equine vaccine (West Nile-Innovator™). Initially, two doses spaced 4 weeks apart are recommended in the early spring, followed by a booster shot in mid to late summer, when WNV tends to peak. In subsequent years, a single late spring booster shot is recommended. A full 1 mL dose is recommended for birds weighing 800 grams or more. Proportionally scaled down doses may be given to smaller raptors, but the effect of this on vaccine efficacy is unknown. Raptors in other categories may be vaccinated as added insurance. No raptor that has been vaccinated, as discussed, has been subjected to an experimentally controlled challenge and the actual vaccine efficacy is not known. However, since 2003, many hundreds of vaccinated captive raptors in areas of intense WNV activity have been apparently protected while unvaccinated wild birds experienced disease (Redig, unpublished). As WNV has become endemic, the incidence among wild birds has waned considerably. However, it remains a threat to unprotected captive birds, especially when weather conditions favour a rise in mosquito populations. Therefore, preventive measures including protective screening and vaccination should be continued for the indefinite future.

Influenza virus

The influenza viruses are contained in the Orthomyxoviridae family and birds are natural reservoirs. Serotypes are differentiated by the different combinations of haemagglutinin (H) and neuraminidase (N) proteins found on the surface of the virus. They are further distinguished as high pathogenicity (HP) or low pathogenicity (LP) viruses. Prior to 2006, influenza viruses were not a significant pathogen for raptors. **Recently (spring 2006), occurrences of fatal infections in raptors in the eastern hemisphere related to the highly pathogenic influenza A (HP H5N1) have occurred (ProMED 2006, FAO 2005).** These have been associated presumably with direct ingestion of dead infected prey or close physical contact with viral-shedding birds. HP H5N1 in a captive hunting falcon in Saudi Arabia has been reported (Samour et al 2007). At the time of this writing, the HPAI H5N1 virus has not been reported in the western hemisphere in raptors or any other avian species.

There are reports of raptors harbouring other type A influenza viruses. Magnino et al (2000) reported an H7 serotype in a saker falcon (*Falco cherrug*) in Italy. A survey of raptors in a rehabilitation facility in Italy showed two seropositive birds, a common buzzard (*Buteo buteo*) and a peregrine falcon, out of a sample of 192 hawks and owls (DeMarco et al 2003). It is likely that falcons used for duck hunting carry antibodies to various influenza viruses. Should HPAI H5N1 ever arrive in the western hemisphere and presently for falconers in the eastern hemisphere, exposure to HP H5N1 influenza may be a concern. For the reasons stated above strict hygiene and use of basic protective equipment (mask, gloves) when handling wild waterfowl taken by a raptor should be followed. **Surveillance protocols and monitoring of movements of birds (poultry, smuggling of birds) are important methods for both prevention and control of this zoonotic disease.**

Bacteria

Mycobacterium

Avian tuberculosis is uncommon in raptors in North America; however, in other parts of the world it is endemic (Cooper 1985). It is usually fatal for the affected bird, and is considered a low risk zoonotic disease. *Mycobacterium avium/intracellulare complex* or *M. genavense* are the causative organisms most frequently encountered, and they cause a chronic wasting disease syndrome accompanied by weakness, anorexia and diarrhoea (Boydell & Forbes 1996). Tuberculosis may affect the liver, intestine, lungs and bone marrow and occasionally subcutis. Ante-mortem diagnosis by acid-fast staining of the faeces and/or bone marrow aspirate (if the bones display the pathognomonic punched out lesions; Fig. 9.9) or other tubercles that can be sampled directly or via endoscopy (Heatley et al 2007). In general, due to the disease's zoonotic potential and poor treatment success, most authors recommend euthanasia for all tuberculosis patients.

Pasteurella

Pasteurella multocida, the aetiological agent for fowl cholera, is known to cause an acute, septicaemic disease in raptors. The disease is endemic in waterfowl in the western USA (especially Nebraska, California and Oregon), particularly where birds congregate in large numbers during spring migrations. While little is known about the actual occurrence of pasteurellosis among wild birds, it is problematic for falconers that hunt waterfowl. Following an encounter with an infected duck, an infected raptor may begin to show lethargy and deteriorate rapidly, dying in 24–36 hours unless treatment is provided. Rapid clinical improvement is often noted with aggressive antibiotic therapy consisting of penicillin G and trimethoprim-sulfa (Morishita et al 1996) or cefazolin (Cefazolin for injection, USP, G.C. Handford Mfg. Co., Syracruse, NY, USA) and amikacin (William Ferrier, personal communication), along with supportive care (fluids and short-acting steroids to protect against endotoxin shock). Recovered birds are likely to be carriers of the organism. Vaccination with killed vaccine products used for poultry may be advisable for high risk birds.

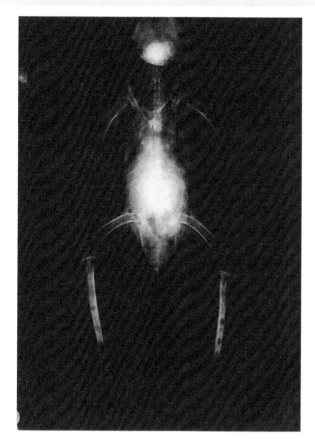

Fig 9.9 In this radiograph, the 'punched out' lesions characteristic of tuberculosis are seen in the long bones. (Photo by P. T. Redig.)

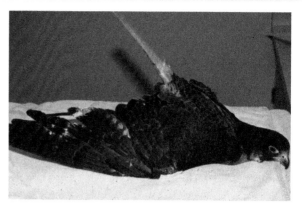

Fig 9.10 Tetanus in a female peregrine falcon. (Photo by P. T. Redig.)

Clostridia

Clostridial enterotoxaemia is caused by either a bloom of endogenous *C. perfringens*, part of the normal GI tract flora, or by exogenously provided toxin in food-stuffs that have been improperly managed (Heidenreich 1997). The former situation is likely to occur when a bird has been stressed through over-exercise, excessive food deprivation and attendant dehydration, or some other process that slows or stops GI motility. Clostridial organisms will proliferate, causing low-grade depression and little else in the way of clinical signs. A Gram stain performed on a direct faecal smear will reveal moderate to heavy occurrence of Gram-positive rods with an intracellular spore. Treatment with metronidazole (30 mg/kg b.i.d. for 5 days) will effect a cure. **The second instance where C. perfringens is problematic occurs when food has not been properly frozen.** This is most likely to occur when a mass of food items (e.g. quail, rats, mice) is bagged together in a freezer. This is especially problematic if they have not been allowed to cool down prior to being bunched. The items near the centre of the mass may take several days to freeze, allowing for an abundant growth of clostridial organisms and the production of endotoxin. When fed to raptors, there is an almost immediate adverse response, with affected birds becoming moribund and most dying. Treatment options extend no further than immediate emptying of the stomach, administration of activated charcoal and supportive care.

Infections with *Clostridium tetani* are rare in birds and the few known cases have been diagnosed on circumstantial evidence vis-à-vis history of puncture wound and clinical signs. A single case has been noted by Heidenreich (1997) and these authors have encountered two cases in 30 years of practice, one a falcon that punctured its foot on a barbed wire fence and developed an ascending paralysis that culminated in widespread tetany and death over a course of 4 days. The other was a female peregrine in a breeding chamber that was footed in the middle of the back by her mate (wounds found on necropsy). She presented initially with ataxia, after an unknown passage of time from the wounding, that progressed to full body tetany (Fig. 9.10). There was no response to equine toxoid and antitoxin products, resulting in a decision to terminate the case with euthanasia.

Fungi and yeast
Candida

A common yeast infection of raptors and other species of birds is *Candida albicans*. It primarily targets the anterior gastrointestinal tract, with particular affinity for the crop. Clinical signs range from inappetence to flinging food, and regurgitation to complete anorexia. When the lower GI tract is involved, the bird may present with diarrhoea. Usually no lesions are observed, but the mucous membranes have a somewhat milky and occasionally doughy appearance. There is often a layer of mucus, which adheres to the membranes and causes an audible clicking sound when the bird opens its mouth.

Diagnosis of *Candida albicans* is made by cytology and culture; the former is performed using Diff-Quik® or a Gram's stain on a glass slide preparation, the latter on Sabouraud's agar, where culture takes 2–3 days at 37°C. Treatment is a course of nystatin (20 000 IU/kg b.i.d. for 10 days painted on the surface of the oral mucous membranes). Alternatively, fluconazole (Diflucan®, Janssen Pharmaceutical, Titusville, New Jersey, USA) at 5–10 mg/kg p.o. once daily is an effective treatment (Plumb 2005), and Samour & Naldo (2002) have reported on the effective use of miconazole gel.

Aspergillosis

One of the most devastating diseases of raptors is the fungal infection of the respiratory system caused by *Aspergillus fumigatus* (Redig 2008, Aguilar & Redig 1995). Infection occurs by inhalation of the spores, which are ubiquitous within the environment. The incubation period is extremely variable, depending on the immunocompetency of the host and exposure dose. Acute aspergillosis is the product of inhalation of overwhelming numbers of spores from the environment, while the chronic forms, in most instances, develop clinically over a period of 1 to 3 weeks.

A diagnosis is made by evaluation of a combination of clinical signs, complete blood count (elevated total white cell count and dystrophic heterophilia), radiography, and deep tracheal cultures. A specific ELISA test is available that detects antibodies to *A. fumigatus* (The Raptor Center, University of Minnesota, USA). Antigen detection tests and plasma protein electrophoresis (University of Miami, School of Medicine, Miami, FL, USA) are showing promise as useful tools in diagnosing this disease. Endoscopic examination of the trachea (to the level of the syrinx) and air sacs is invaluable in confirming the diagnosis and establishing a prognosis.

The currently recommended treatment consists of oral itraconazole (Sporonox®, Janssen Pharmaceutica, Titusville, NJ, USA) given with food at 7–10 mg/kg b.i.d. for 5 days, then once daily for 1–3 months as necessary; nebulization with clotrimazole (clotrimazole 5–10% solution in polyethylene glycol (PEG) with 5% dimethylsulfoxide from a compounding pharmacy); and amphotericin B (Fungizone® Bristol-Meyers Squibb Co., Princeton, NJ, USA) given intratracheally or injected transcostally into left and right posterior thoracic air sacs (percutaneous puncture – approximately 1 mg/kg diluted to 1–3 mL in water (not saline) – and injected in selected target sites at each treatment) or otherwise applied directly to air sac lesions in other locations via endoscope. Itraconazole alone is effective in controlling clinically inapparent cases detected by ELISA and accompanied by an elevated white cell count. **Itraconazole, when administered at higher dosages, often causes patients to become transiently anorexic.** Nebulization

with clotrimazole (two 1-hour sessions/day for 4–8 weeks) is indicated where clinical signs of inappetence, reduced endurance or mild respiratory signs are observed or disease is confirmed by endoscopic or radiological evaluation. Birds with severe respiratory signs have a poor prognosis. Surgical removal of lesions that are blocking the trachea or syrinx is an effective therapeutic adjunct. Prophylaxis using itraconazole at 8 mg/kg, as above, is recommended for captive-held raptors undergoing a change in management, and for certain species with a known high risk (Redig 1996b). The drug should be administered for 3–4 weeks in as close a proximity to the event as possible.

Voriconazole (Vfend, Pfizer), introduced to the avian veterinary community in 2005 (Di'Somma et al 2007, Silvanose et al 2006), may provide another effective pharmacological tool for treating aspergillosis. Working doses are stated to be at 12.5 mg/kg. Frequency of administration and subsequent bioavailability appears to vary among species of birds (Scope et al 2005, Flammer 2006). **Food in the gastrointestinal tract has been shown to reduce absorption of voriconazole; therefore it is recommended there be at least a 1-hour delay between drug administration and feeding.**

Toxins

Presently, the most commonly occurring toxicities are due either to cholinesterase-inhibiting compounds (Porter 1993) or lead (Kramer & Redig 1997). Laboratory tests for toxins are run on suspicion of which toxin is involved from the clinical signs and history, if any is available. When a toxin is suspected, but the exact one is undetermined, it is advisable to treat with supportive care. This includes activated charcoal orally to stop any further gastrointestinal absorption of the toxin, intravenous and subcutaneous fluids, and diazepam if seizures are occurring.

Organochlorines

Organochlorine pesticides remain a source of potential toxicity for raptors in parts of the world where these compounds are still used. The likelihood of encountering a raptor intoxicated from these compounds is small, and treatment recommendations are unknown.

Leadp oisoning

Lead poisoning remains one of the most significant causes of nervous and multisystemic diseases in raptors that have consumed hunter-killed or injured prey. Bald and other sea eagles and golden eagles are the most frequent victims where big game or varmint remains containing spent ammunition fragments left in the field appear to be a major source of toxin. California condors *(Gymnogyps californianus)* are severely affected also. However, any raptor that ingests lead can become intoxicated. Clinical toxicosis occurs when the ingested lead is dissolved in the acid environment of the stomach and absorbed in sufficient quantity to cause disruption of various organ systems. Clinical signs associated with lead toxicity include anaemia, lethargy, anorexia, paralysis of the anterior gastrointestinal tract, vomiting, ataxia, diarrhoea, and paralysis of the neck, wings or legs. Seizures and blindness may occur in some severe cases. The diagnosis of lead toxicity is made from the clinical signs and from assays of the blood lead levels using atomic absorption spectrophotometry. Toxicity is typically apparent at blood lead levels greater than 0.4 ppm, although treatment should be instituted at blood lead levels of 0.2 ppm and above. If lead particles are seen in the ventriculus on radiographic evaluation, they must be removed by one of several means: (a) force-feeding of casting material (rat skin), (b) gastric lavage, or (c) passage through the GI tract if the patient has a functional tract and is eating. Chelation treatment with calcium-EDTA (CaEDTA, Sigma Chemical Co., St Louis, Montana, USA), 50–100 mg/kg diluted in 50 mL of saline subcutaneously b.i.d. (Samour & Naldo 2005), is initiated on the basis of clinical signs and blood lead levels and maintained for 5 days. After a 2–3 day hiatus, the regimen is repeated again and continued in this fashion until blood lead levels are below 0.2 ppm. The chelation process may be augmented by the simultaneous utilization of dimercaptosuccinic acid (DMSA) at 30 mg/kg b.i.d. (Redig & Arent 2008). Treatment should continue until blood lead levels are below 0.2 ppm. Treatment has not been effective in most raptors if initial blood lead levels are greater than 1.2 ppm (Kramer & Redig 1997).

Cholinesterase inhibitors

Toxicity due to cholinesterase-inhibiting compounds (e.g. organophosphates, carbamates) is another form of poisoning in raptors (Porter 1993). The onset of clinical signs is peracute, although there may be a delayed onset of 1–3 weeks, depending on the dosage received. These signs include ataxia and weakness, salivation, bradycardia and mild head tremors. Paralysis may be noted as a clinical sign associated with cholinesterase-inhibiting compound toxicity. The mechanism of action is similar to that in mammals, where acetylcholinesterase is inhibited at the neuromuscular junctions. The treatment consists of atropine (Atropine sulfate 1/120 g, Vedco Inc., St Joseph, Montana, USA) and diazepam (Valium®, Steris Laboratories Inc., Phoenix, Arizona, USA) to control seizures.

Barbiturate toxicity

Pentobarbital intoxication has been previously described by Hayes (1988) and Langelier (1993). The source appears to be pentobarbital-euthanized animals, improperly disposed of and scavenged by eagles.

Other conditions
Low condition and sour crop

'Low condition' is a term taken from the literature of falconry describing a metabolic condition where the raptor, trained and used in falconry, has been reduced in body weight, inadvertently, to a critical point. This problem may come as a result of having been maintained at flying weight for too long (e.g. several weeks during the peak of hunting season), an unforeseen event that prevents adequate daily provision of food, or a judgement error. **Sudden increased metabolic demand from an abrupt decrease in temperature often serves as a trigger for 'low condition'.** The affected bird will deteriorate rapidly, becoming depressed, weak, profoundly anaemic (PCV often around 20% or less), hypoproteinaemic (total solids often not registering on the refractometer scale), cachectic, dehydrated and hypotensive. The bird will have a weak wing beat and the eyes will have a dull or glazed appearance and exhibit an oval shape owing to partial closure of the lids (i.e. so-called 'almond-eyed'). The falconer may have realized the problem and fed the bird, either by voluntary intake or by force-feeding. In most cases, there is gastrointestinal stasis and the food in the crop begins to putrefy, leading to a condition known as 'sour crop'. Collectively, these circumstances represent a critical medical emergency that must be carefully managed over several days.

Treatment consists of re-establishing circulating blood volume through aggressive fluid therapy (crystalloid and colloidal agents) and should include a blood transfusion if the PCV is below 20%, keeping the bird in a warm environment, and providing antimicrobial therapy to ward off bacterial and fungal infections. **Feeding the bird is not the first priority and should not be attempted until after the first 6–12 hours.** If the crop has soured, the contents should be removed by retrograde massage and irrigation of the crop with warmed saline, although this may be deferred for a couple of hours until the bird has responded to the initial administration of fluids. In the authors' experience the use of injectable ranitidine at 0.2–0.5 mg/kg i.m. every 12 hours (Ranitidine injection USP, Bedford Laboratories™ Bedford, OH, USA), will stimulate crop motility. A treatment outline is detailed in Table 9.7. This protocol should be repeated on a 6-hour basis for the first 48 hours. For the first two or three applications, fluids should be given intravenously or intraosseously as the absorption of subcutaneous fluids is inadequate to meet the needs of the critical patient. Indirect blood pressure monitoring as described by Lichtenberger (2004, 2005) during this stage is both an effective and useful tool for assessing the patient's response to fluid therapy.

Food, in the form of a hyperalimentation preparation, given by crop or stomach tube is introduced after a minimum of 12 hours of fluid therapy. A useful indicator of ability of the patient to process food is the production of urine and the passage of small amounts of faecal material. **Solid food should be reintroduced only slowly and not before the second or third day.** It is given as 'clean meat' (i.e. devoid of feathers, fur or bone), well moistened in saline, and fed by direct placement in the mouth or crop with a forceps. A target for daily caloric intake is 250 kcal/kg/day. As the bird responds, fluids may be given on a twice daily basis by the subcutaneous route. Progress is monitored by the bird's overall appearance and twice daily weighing to ensure adequacy of calorie intake. **Regardless of how 'well' the bird appears to be responding to the overall treatment, fluid supplementation should not be discontinued in less than 5 days of treatment.**

Once recovered, the bird should be fed to a level well above its flying weight before being released to train. Antibiotics may be discontinued once the bird is eating well, but antifungal therapy should be continued for a full 3 weeks.

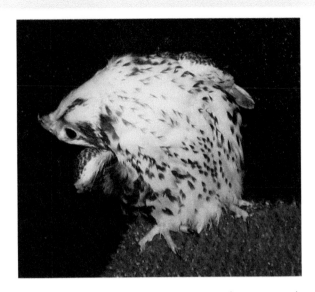

Fig 9.11 The star-gazing posture of this prairie falcon (*Falco mexicanus*) is attributed to a deficiency of B vitamins, possibly as a result of malabsorption arising from an enteritis. (Photo by L. Cruz-Martinez.)

Miscellaneousn eurologicalc onditions

Aberrant parasitism due to *Sarcocystis* spp. (Cawthorne 1993) infections present as vague neurological signs. Typically, a coccidian parasite that encysts in muscle tissue, *Sarcocystis* spp. are known to invade neurological tissue also, including both peripheral and central nerves. Clinical signs vary with the location of the parasite and have ranged from flaccid bilateral paralysis of the wings to seizuring (Aguilar et al 1991, Dubey et al 1991). Diagnosis of sarcocystosis is typically made at post-mortem examination.

Presumed vitamin B deficiency is principally seen in large falcons, where it causes a star-gazing syndrome (Fig. 9.11) (Ward 1971). In other raptors, it presents as muscle weakness and tremors. The aetiology is obscure; however, Heidenreich (1997) proposed that it is caused by an enteritis that interferes with the absorption of B vitamins and leads to the neurological disorder. In other cases, the occurrence appears to have been associated with a poor quality diet such as chicken necks. Aggressive parenteral therapy with a B complex in the acute stages is said to reverse the disease, and indeed, mild cases are responsive. However, the derangement can become permanent and unresponsive to therapy if not dealt with immediately.

Spinaltr auma

The clinical signs typically associated with spinal trauma in a raptor include partial or complete flaccid paralysis of the pelvic limb, inability to manipulate tail feathers, and loss of cloacal tone. This condition is the result of blunt trauma from a window collision or moving vehicle impact, occasionally other immovable objects. **Radiology is generally not useful as a diagnostic tool to detect acute cases of spinal trauma;** however, increased areas of density may be seen 2 to 3 weeks after injury in the area of the spinal column where the synsacrum attaches to the notarium as the healing fracture begins to calcify. Recently, MRI has been demonstrated to more effectively define spinal damage in raptors (Stauber et al 2007). Differential diagnoses to consider in a bird presenting with these signs include lead poisoning, organophosphate or carbamate poisoning, and osteomyelitis involving the vertebral bodies at the notarial–synsacral junction. The latter usually presents as a slow development of ataxia leading to paralysis when the vertebral column finally fractures. Treatment of acute, blunt-trauma-induced spinal trauma consists of supportive care including manual voiding of the cloaca at least once a day, and short-acting steroids (prednisolone 10 mg/kg), which are thought to be controversial and effective only if given within 12–24 hours of the traumatic event. A withdrawal response within the first 3–5 days of treatment is an indicator of a favourable outcome. Conversely, experience has shown that failure to mount a response within that time frame is indicative of a grave prognosis and euthanasia is recommended.

Zoonoses

Diseases among raptors with zoonotic potential include avian chlamydiosis, tuberculosis, salmonellosis, and West Nile virus, although actual occurrence of disease transmission to humans is extremely rare. Avian chlamydiosis, itself very rare among raptors (Schlosberg 1976), is clearly a concern should the disease ever be encountered in raptors. There is no indication that they are subclinical carriers of this disease. Tuberculosis produces a debilitating disease in raptors with varying clinical signs, depending on which organ systems are involved. This disease, caused by *M. avium/intracellulare complex* in birds, is encountered with low frequency in raptors, and presently there is limited concern of zoonosis (Lennox 2007).

While salmonellosis has zoonotic potential, it is occasionally encountered in either captive or wild raptors (Smith 1993, Palmgren et al 2004), human handlers are more likely to encounter *Salmonella* spp. in the food items prepared for the birds. Proper sanitation and hygiene precautions are generally sufficient to prevent these and other infections with zoonotic potential.

Birds infected with West Nile virus may shed the virus in faeces and secretions for a short period of time. Appropriate hygiene and sanitation should be employed by hospital staff in the handling of West Nile virus suspects.

Part II: Clinical approach to management of medical problems in raptors

Introduction

Part I of this chapter gave an overview of what raptors are and the significant medical problems encountered with these species, along with general treatment modalities that may be applied. In this section, approaches to patient assessment, establishment of a minimum database, and generalized and specific treatment modes for the most frequently encountered disease complexes will be presented.

While there is increased likelihood that captive-held raptors (such as are used in falconry or bird shows) may present with a defined problem or complaint, they (like the many wild casualty birds) often have multiple problems or complexes for which the presenting sign is only the most obvious indicator. In order to expedite diagnosis and application of appropriate treatment, a basic core of assessment and diagnostic procedures should be applied to all birds at admission, thereby avoiding the need for return visits for further diagnostics and a potential delay in the administration of what may be life-saving treatment.

Overall approach

The general approach to treatment of raptors is presented in Figure 9.12. Phase I (assessment) includes anamnesis accompanied by a four-element minimum database, consisting of complete blood count (CBC), microbiological evaluation (bacteria and pathogenic fungi), radiological examination and, optionally, a parasite examination. **Raptors, due to their strength, inherent ability to inflict**

damage on handlers and stressful response to restraint, are best handled under gas anaesthesia (Isoflo® isoflurane, USP Abbot Laboratories, North Chicago, Illinois, USA) (Redig 1998) for all of these procedures except, history taking, observation and parasitological collections.

Phase II events flow directly from phase I so that the initial stabilization and treatment modalities are instituted essentially at the time of admission. It is useful to have radiology facilities available in the admission arena, and to conduct the haematology and microbiological procedures on an in-house basis to facilitate rapid return of results. Facilities and operational procedures should be designed with this arrangement in mind. Phases III and IV are separated in time and space from the first two phases, depending on the patient's needs and response to admission treatment. Surgical management of fractures, especially fractures of the extremities, may be delayed for 3–5 days to allow for soft tissue management and overall patient recovery.

Phase V addresses the outcomes and preparation for return to normal function. For birds being returned to the wild, recovery means not only restoration to function from disease or injury, but also returning the animal to the full athletic capability required for survival in the wild. It will severely diminish the likelihood of post-release survival if adequate exercise evaluation regimens and ophthalmological considerations are not included in the management scheme prior to release.

History and background information

For wild birds, the following information should be acquired:

1. Name and address of person recovering the bird if different from presenter
2. Date of recovery
3. Location of recovery
4. Circumstances of recovery
5. Proximity to fences or power lines
6. Proximity to roads and vehicular traffic
7. Proximity to windows or glass buildings
8. Proximity to water
9. Proximity to areas of recent pesticide application
10. Presence of any other affected birds or mammals in the vicinity
11. Any food, water, or medical treatments administered prior to presentation
12. Any identifying markers, rings or bands carried by the bird.

Captive-held birds used for falconry or bird shows will most often be presented perched on the fist, with or without a hood, or inside a carrying box with which they are very comfortable and familiar. Before the bird

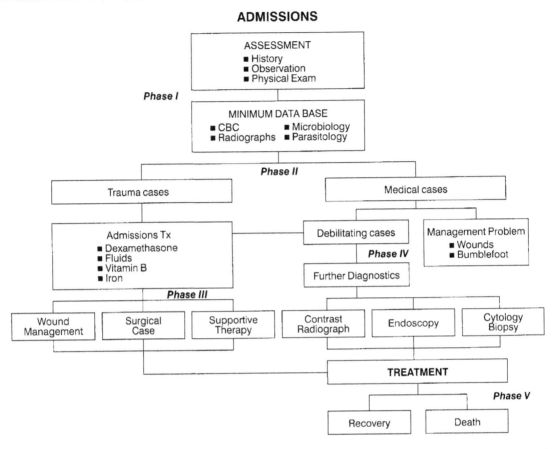

ADMISSIONS

ASSESSMENT
- History
- Observation
- Physical Exam

Phase I

MINIMUM DATA BASE
- CBC
- Radiographs
- Microbiology
- Parasitology

Phase II

Trauma cases

Medical cases

Admissions Tx
- Dexamethasone
- Fluids
- Vitamin B
- Iron

Debilitating cases

Phase IV

Management Problem
- Wounds
- Bumblefoot

Further Diagnostics

Phase III

Wound Management

Surgical Case

Supportive Therapy

Contrast Radiograph

Endoscopy

Cytology Biopsy

TREATMENT

Phase V

Recovery

Death

Fig 9.12 The treatment programme for injured and ill raptors follows a five-phase process. Phase I is admission, examination and history taking. Phase II is stabilization treatments. Phase III is specific treatment for trauma cases, while phase IV entails the application of specific diagnostic tests to further elucidate problems in medical cases. Phase V is the outcome phase.

is restrained for any further work, a few minutes should be spent observing the bird as it is perched. The key observations are listed in Table 9.4.

Wild birds are more difficult to observe. However, the task can be accomplished by releasing the bird into an unoccupied room or large cage and observing it clandestinely for the above parameters. Often such observations are made following admission and physical examination in wild birds.

Faecal and urine examination

In raptors, intestinal and urinary tract outputs are collectively referred to as a 'mute'. Birds in boxes for any amount of time will have muted in the box, and this material should be examined. Hooded falcons will usually mute when the hood is removed. As indicated in Table 9.4, the normal mute of a raptor consists of a dark black centre surrounded by a pure chalky white urate mass, sometimes accompanied by a larger ring

of clear urine. Any presentation other than this should raise a question. **A fatty diet (such as day-old cockerels) will cause the faecal portion to turn tan, and the small feathers of such cockerels may be passed through the GI tract and appear in the mute.** A fasted bird (one normally fed at the same time every day and approaching feeding time when examined) will pass unutilized bile in the faecal portion, which has a bright green appearance. Any other shades of green or other colours in either the stool or the urine are indicative of serious liver, kidney or urinary tract problems. A very thorough review of the various mute presentations, enhanced by vivid colour pictures, is available in Heidenreich (1997). Comprehensive urinalysis data from healthy falcons has been reported by Tschopp et al (2007).

Physical examination

It is difficult – if not impossible – to conduct an adequate physical examination on a strong, frightened and

Table 9.4   Key observations to be made in assessing a raptor patient

Parameter	Normal appearance	Common abnormalities
Posture	Erect, near vertical	Hunched over, wings drooped, leaning to one side, hocks straight
Respiratory rate and character	10–15/minute, little to no evidence of movement of body parts, especially in areas over the shoulders, tailhead or in the abdominal area	Tail bobbing with each breath Exaggerated movements of abdominal panel between legs Movement of wings in shoulder area with each breath
Eyes	Round, bright, adnexa clean and dry	Dull appearance to cornea Squinted or almond shaped Lids closed Moisture on feathers below eye
Feathers	Clean, straight, rounded edges	Soiling with mutes or dirt on tips of tail and wing feathers Broken, frayed Damage to top of head Fluid or blood on body feathers
Mutes (stool)	Dark black centres with chalk white urates, occasionally tan centres if fed day-old chicks Urates occasionally have a reddish pigment in them (cause unknown) Bright green centres in a fasted bird	Lime-green staining to faecal or urine component Yellow urates Dark blood flecks
Condition of scales on legs and feet	Bright yellow, clean, undamaged	Brown lumps Missing or worn scales Swellings
Talon condition	Even curvature, sharp points	Thick, dull Twisted Missing Too long and curved
Beak and cere	Beak black, cere a bright shiny yellow Beak of normal length, coming to a sharp point	Cere traumatically damaged Beak cracked and delaminating, especially around tooth in falcons Mandible or maxilla overgrown

struggling raptor. Not only is it difficult, it is also dangerous for both restrainer and examiner, and stressful for the patient. The safety and efficacy of isoflurane anaesthesia alleviates all of these concerns, and its use is highly recommended. Exercise caution if there is food in the crop. Anaesthesia can be administered safely by mask immediately upon restraining the bird. Birds wearing hoods can be anaesthetized while perching on their owner's fist, by placing a cone with a large opening over the bird's head and shoulders. Mild restraint may be necessary with the onset of anaesthesia-induced ataxia.

A checklist of parameters is presented in Table 9.5.

Laboratory assessment

The haematological assessment can be quickly accomplished by drawing 0.1–0.2 mL blood from the basilic, metatarsal, cutaneous ulnar or jugular veins, then preparing two or three good blood smear slides and two haematocrit tubes. The tubes are spun immediately for determination of packed cell volume and total plasma solids (refractometer), while the slides can be stained with a rapid staining method (e.g. Diff-Quik®, American Scientific Products, Harleco, Gibbstown, NJ, USA), dried

Table 9.5 Checklist of parameters for physical examination in a raptor

	Important items to note
Head region:	
Beak (maxilla)	Length
	Normal notch or tomial tooth in falcons
	Absence of cracking or delaminating
	Proper approximation to mandible when closed
Beak (mandible)	Length normal – not forcing maxilla outward
	Mandibular rami intact
Cere	Note colour, evidence of trauma, nodular lesions
Nostril and operculum	Rhinoliths
Mouth	Membranes pink in most species, blue in accipiters and merlins
	Membranes doughy consistency, clinging mucus (associated with *Candida* spp. infections)
	Proliferative lesions, diphtheritic membranes (associated with pox)
Tongue	Ingested tendon or other fibrous material entangled around base
	Caseous lesions sublingually
Palate	Caseous lesions
	Penetrating wounds
Choanal slit	Mucus
	Palatine fringes with caseous lesions
Eyes:	
Adnexa	Normally feathered, not damp, not reddened, no crepitus when palpated
Conjunctiva	White, not inflamed or infiltrated with blood vessels
Lacrimal duct	Normal, bilaterally symmetrical distension, not oedematous, fluorescein dye test – no retention
Cornea	Normal, bilaterally symmetrical distension, not oedematous, fluorescein dye test – no retention
Iris	Normally pigmented, round, responsive to light
Anterior chamber	Filled with clear fluid, no blood or fibrin strands, no turbidity, no synechia
Lens	In normal position, translucent, not containing a cataract
Posterior chamber	
Posterior segment and retina	Uninterrupted retinal pattern, pecten in normal position, absence of focal areas of depigmentation
Ears	Free of blowfly larvae and blood
Pharynx	Colour of mucous membranes (pigmented blue in accipiters), devoid of lesions, foreign bodies
Neck region	Free of obstructing foreign bodies, fistulas, no crepitus
Crop	Empty or solid distension from food, not soft and fluctuant as with fluid content, not fistulated
Thoracic inlet	Free of obstructing foreign bodies
Shoulder girdle	Symmetrical range of motion of humeral head, no crepitus or joint laxity
Joint palpation	Elbows, metacarpi, stifles, hocks – not swollen, full range of motion
Forelimb	Functional mechanical extension, integrity of patagium
Alula	Not turned over leading edge of wing
Secondary feathers	Not broken, frayed, or abnormally sheathed
Primary feathers	Not broken, frayed, or abnormally sheathed while still growing, look for evidence of fault bars
Pelvic limb	
Femur and hip	Absence of fractures, crepitus, weight-bearing symmetry

(continued)

Table 9.5 *(continued)*

	Important items to note
Tibiotarsus	Asymmetrical muscle mass between legs
	Lack of tension when stretched, weight-bearing
Tarsometatarsus	Nodular lesions, cuts, bite wounds, trap injuries, weight-bearing
Hallux	Held in flexed position from extensor tendon rupture, erosive lesions on joint pads
Forward digits	Erosive lesions on digital pads
	Accumulation of debris under talons at end of P1
	Held in flexed position from extensor tendon rupture
Metatarsal pad	Erosive lesions
	Puncture wounds
	Swelling ulceration
Abdominal region	Brood patch in laying females – normal
	Swollen liver
	Distended ventriculus

Table 9.6a–c Basic haematology (Redig in Altman et al 1997). Haematological, biochemical and morphometric reference ranges of selected raptor species
Table 9.6a Haematological reference ranges of selected healthy adult captive raptors[a]

Value	Red-tailed hawk (n = 10)	Great-horned owl (n = 10)	Bald eagle (n = 8)	Peregrine falcon (n = 14)	Gyrfalcon (n = 12)
PCV (%)	44.6 (2.6)[b]	43.3 (2.9)	44 (4)	44 (4)	49 (2)
Total protein (g/dL)	4.3 (0.5)	5.1 (0.6)	4.0 (1)	2.65 (1.18)	2.94 (0.38)
White blood cells ($\times 10^3/\mu L$)	6.0–8.0	10.0–20.0	12.8 (4.8)	8.7 (2.2)	4.6 (1.7)
Heterophils (%)	35 (11.1)	47 (10.7)	75 (13)	65 (12)	51 (5)
Lymphocytes (%)	44 (8.9)	27 (7.0)	18 (10)	35 (13)	47 (5)
Monocytes (%)	6 (3.2)	9 (3.6)	3 (3)	0 (0)	1 (1)
Basophils (%)	2 (1.3)	Rare	Rare	0 (0)	Rare
Eosinophils (%)	13 (3.8)	1 (1.2)	4 (3)	0 (1)	1 (1)

[a]*From Dr P. Redig, The Raptor Center, University of Minnesota, St. Paul, MN 55108.*
[b]*Standard deviation in parentheses.*

with a blow-drier or exposure to room air, and examined by microscope within a few minutes of drawing. An estimated white cell count and differential will yield the necessary data for interpretation. Presently, the parameters assessed are total white cell count, differential white cell count (percentages), and examination for blood parasites. The use of absolute counts for different white cells has not typically been pursued, hence no reference values for this parameter or indications of its clinical use are available. Table 9.6a–c contains reference values for haematological parameters in raptors (Redig 1996b).

Microbiological examination may consist of cultures taken from the oral pharynx and trachea, and from freshly voided faeces. In cases where aspergillosis may be a concern, the trachea should be cultured as a routine matter, using a nasopharyngeal swab thrust deeply into the trachea and cultured on half of a Sabouraud's dextrose plate for *Aspergillus* spp. organisms. The other half of this same plate can be used to culture the pharynx for *Candida* spp. Growth will be evident in 48–72 hours if plates are incubated at 37°C.

Intestinal parasites are screened by faecal examination – both direct smear as well as flotation. Patients are treated as appropriate (Table 9.3). If external parasites are present, the raptors are sprayed lightly with a pyrethrin or fipronil spray. Signs specifically referable to coccidia or

Table 9.6b   Haematological and morphometric measurement of wild red-tailed nestlings[a]

Stage of development	Primary feather length (cm)	Central tail feather length (cm)	PCV (%)	Total protein (g/dL)	RBC (×10³/μL)	Haemoglobin (g/dL)
Early (n = 5)	0–10	0–8	28 (1)[b]	3.4 (0.1)	1.74 (0.09)	9.79 (0.40)
Late (n = 5)	11–18	9–16	33 (1)[b]	4.0 (0.1)	2.35 (0.03)	10.98 (0.14)

[a]From Dr. P Reding, The Raptor Center, University of Minnesota, St. Paul, MN 55108.

[b]Means ± standard deviations in parentheses.

Table 9.6c   Serum biochemical reference values of selected raptor species[a]

Value	Bald eagle (n = 8)	Peregrine falcon (n = 14)	Gyrfalcon (n = 12)	Red-tailed hawk (n = 10)	Great-horned owl (n = 10)
Acetylcholinesterase (delta pH units/h)	0.16 (0.06)	–	–	–	–
Alanine aminotransferase (ALT) (U/L)	25 (13)	62 (56)	–	31(5)	39 (14)
Albumin (g/dL)	1.09 (0.18)	0.96 (0.13)	0.73 (0.09)	1.34 (0.41)	1.27 (0.35)
Alkaline phosphatase (U/L)	57 (12)	99 (44)	257 (61)	53 (18)	31 (7)
Amylase (U/L)	1158 (376)	–	–	–	–
Aspartate aminotransferase (AST) (U/L)	218 (63)	78 (31)	97 (33)	303 (22)	287 (65)
Bilirubin, total (mg/dL)	0.31 (0.08)	4.57 (2.04)	–	0.16 (0.08)	0.07 (0.06)
Blood urea nitrogen (BUN) (mg/dL)	3.10 (2.47)	3.25 (1.39)	4.67 (0.82)	4.67 (0.47)	5 (2.94)
Calcium (mg/dL)	9.94 (0.45)	8.93 (0.46)	9.61 (0.24)	–	10.19
Chloride (mmol/L)	120 (3)	114.38 (43.36)	125 (2)	125 (3)	122
Creatine kinase (U/L)	383 (300)	783 (503)	402 (163)	1124 (251)	977 (407)
Creatinine (mg/dL)	0.70 (0.26)	0.51 (0.22)	–	–	–
Glucose (mg/dL)	302 (25)	366 (29)	318 (39)	356 (16)	356
Osmolality (mmol/kg)	319 (6)	–	–	–	–
Phosphorus (mg/dL)	3.03 (0.51)	3.35 (0.70)	3.57 (1.13)	3.14 (0.5)	4.34
Potassium (mmol/L)	3.0 (0)	2.04 (0.81)	1.99 (0.56)	2.42 (0.73)	2.8
Protein, total (g/dL) (biuret)	3.51 (0.75)	2.63 (0.48)	2.89 (0.31)	4.17 (0.69)	4.33
Sodium (mmol/L)	156 (4)	143 (54)	160 (3)	157 (1)	156
Uric acid (mg/dL)	5.07 (3.33)	4.50 (4.24)	13.93 (5.64)[b]	10.84 (5.1)[b]	13.7 (10.8)[b]

[a]From Dr P. Redig, The Raptor Center, University of Minnesota, St. Paul, MN 55108. All samples were collected from healthy adult birds – either display/education or breeders or birds flown in falconry. All samples were collected after the birds had been anaesthetized for a minimum of 10 minutes with isoflurane.

[b]Postprandial samples.

trichomoniasis trigger further verifying diagnostics and treatment, as described in the previous section.

Other essential procedures

Radiologicale xamination

Radiology is mandatory for proper evaluation of any trauma case, and very useful in medical cases where the source of the problem is not immediately obvious. It is recommended that ventrodorsal and lateral (right side down, head to the left) views be taken (Fig. 9.13). The following diagnoses can be made radiographically, and are relatively inapparent without radiographs: fractures of the coracoid and furcula; luxations of joints in the limbs; foreign bodies in the GI tract; swelling of

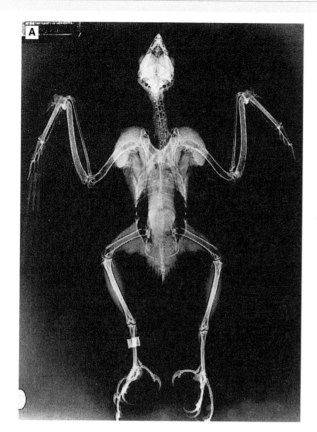

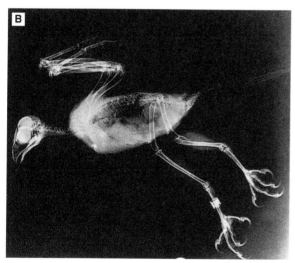

Fig 9.13A, B These figures show the proper radiographic positioning for the radiographic anatomy of a raptor (red-tailed hawk) in lateral and ventrodorsal views. Note healed radial fracture. (Radiograph by T. Guarnera.)

the liver, kidneys and spleen; lung contusions; air sac ruptures with internal organ displacement, and hyperinflated air sacs. A comprehensive overview of avian radiology is available (Samour & Naldo 2007).

Ophthalmologicale xamination

The last of the general procedures conducted at admission is ophthalmoscopy (Davidson 1997). Vision assessment is challenging in raptors, requiring the combination of a complete ophthalmic examination and functional vision assessment tests. Given the importance of vision for these animals, it should not be overlooked.

The eyes and orbit should first be evaluated for the presence of any asymmetries between the two eyes or facial structures. The adnexa then must be assessed. The lower lid should be pulled away from the eye and examined for foreign bodies or inflammation of the palpebral conjunctiva. Examination of the clarity of the cornea and ocular media is performed using a slit-lamp biomicroscope or a bright focal light source, such as a Finoff transilluminator, and the cornea is examined for evidence of scratches, ulceration or iris prolapse. Fluorescein stain application can confirm presence of corneal ulceration. Steroid-containing preparations should be avoided if there is ulceration of the cornea. Cautious application of topical non-steroidal anti-inflammatories can be considered in cases of concurrent corneal ulceration and anterior uveitis. The anterior chamber should be examined for aqueous flare (sign of intraocular inflammation), hyphaema, anterior synechia or posterior synechia.

The iris sphincter is composed of skeletal muscle, thus mydriasis for detailed lenticular and fundic examination cannot be achieved with topical parasympatholytics, such as tropicamide or atropine. Intracameral injection and topical application of non-depolarizing neuromuscular blocking agents have been described for this purpose (turbocurare), although the risk of respiratory paralysis and death is present with their use (Ramer et al 1996). However, if an ophthalmic examination is conducted as part of the general examination under anaesthesia, no additional mydriatic agents are needed. Alternatively, conducting an eye examination in a darkened room often affords adequate pupillary dilatation. The lens can be examined for evidence of cataracts or luxation. A luxated lens may present with a ring of pigment (from the avulsed tips of the ciliary body) outlining the equatorial region of the lens.

Funduscopy can be performed using both indirect and direct ophthalmoscopes (Murphy & Howland 1987). Indirect ophthalmoscopy provides the operator with a wide field of view with less magnification; thus it is a good screening tool, allowing visualization of a greater area of the fundus in a single view. It also facilitates examination of peripheral fundus and permits a safe distance from patients. Direct ophthalmoscopy offers greater magnification with a narrow field of view and is best for detailed examination of specific lesions. The fundic examination should entail a systematic assessment of the retina, optic nerve, pecten and choroid. There are two foveas in diurnal raptors and one fovea in owls. The retina is avascular, and the retinal epithelium is heavily pigmented in diurnal raptors (Fig. 9.14A) and poorly pigmented in nocturnal raptors (Fig. 9.14B). This feature of owls allows the visualization of choroidal vasculature. **The optic nerve head is largely obscured by the pecten, a uveal appendage which projects from the optic nerve into the vitreous.** Common abnormalities of the fundus include retinal detachment and/or tears (Fig. 9.15A), inflammatory and haemorrhagic processes of the retina (Fig. 9.15B), choroid and vitreous, luxation and/or haemorrhage of the pecten, and chorioretinal scarring (Murphy 1993, Korbel 2000). Retinal detachments can be identified by grey, raised regions, and retinal tears are identified by their well-delineated edges which are occasionally curled. Such tears and detachments may also be detected using ultrasonographic diagnostic techniques. Active chorioretinal lesions appear white and raised with fuzzy, irregular margins while inactive scarring appears as flat, well-delineated, mottled variation in pigmentation, and will not progress over time. Traumatic and infectious aetiologies should be considered, especially West Nile virus, which causes damage to the retina producing an exudative, white lesion (Fig. 9.15C) (Wunschmann et al 2004, 2005).

It is important to notice that the pupillary light reflex is very brisk due to voluntary striated muscle control; the absence of this reflex suggests a severely impaired retina. Raptors, as all birds, lack consensual pupillary reflexes.

Further assessment of visual function can be made in the awake patient by:

- testing the ability of the bird to track a finger or hand moved in front of it across the field of vision
- assessing the response to a menace by quickly thrusting a hand or object toward the bird
- test flying the bird in a corridor with a perch at each end.

Admission treatments

The majority of wild birds are submitted for traumatic injuries and related debilitating conditions. Accordingly, they can be assumed to have undergone food deprivation, weight loss, dehydration and blood loss. They are mildly to severely azotaemic, and in a state of metabolic acidosis. The standardized regimens described in Table 9.7 are recommended for all incoming raptors at the time of admission. Parts (or all) of these regimens are also recommended for captive-held birds that have been severely injured or are afflicted by debilitation.

Triage

Once the initial assessment and stabilization is complete, the patient should be further assessed for the prospects of recovery and meeting programmatic goals. Where return to the wild or full flight status is the desired outcome, birds that are clearly blind in one or both eyes or have irreparable damage to a wing or leg or such debilitating disease that full recovery is an obvious impossibility should be candidates for euthanasia. **Where wild casualty birds are being received, about 25–30% will be euthanized after the initial assessment.**

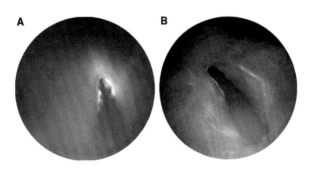

Fig 9.14 Normal fundus of (**A**) a diurnal raptor and (**B**) a nocturnal raptor. (Photo by A. Pauli and G. Klauss.)

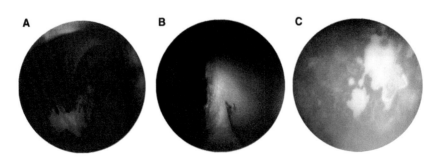

Fig 9.15 Fundic photographs showing (**A**) a retinal tear and detachment in great horned owl (photo by E.A. Giuliano), (**B**) vitreal haemorrhage in a red-tailed hawk (photo by G. Klauss) and (**C**) West Nile virus lesions (photo by A. Pauli).

Table 9.7 Therapeutics used in treatment of low condition – see text for detail

Therapeutic agents	Dose	Purpose	Comment
Lactated Ringer's	Calculate based on an expected 10% rate of dehydration	Rehydration	For working purposes, an estimate of 10% dehydration is a reasonable approximation. A 1 kg red-tail would have a total fluid deficit of 100 mL with a daily maintenance requirement of 50 mL. On day 1, the goal is to replace one half of deficit (50 mL) plus provide maintenance, yielding a total volume of 100 mL in four divided doses. Replace one half of the remaining deficit per day over the next 4–5 days
Hetastarch	10 mL/kg i.o. or i.v. until blood pressure is higher than 90 mmHg	Re-establishment of osmotic pressure	Give for first 2–3 days, reducing the amount of lactated Ringer's solution given by the amount of hetastarch
Oxyglobin®	5 mL/kg	Oxygen carrier to tissues	Useful in treatment of acute blood loss if transfusion is not feasible
5% Dextrose	In place of lactated Ringer's solution	Energy and fluid source	Use in place of lactated Ringer's solution for first 24 hours of treatment
Whole blood	10 mL/kg	Re-establish oxygen carrying capacity, plasma proteins	Best results obtained with homologous transfusion
Metronidazole	30 mg/kg b.i.d.	Intestinal antibiosis	
Itraconazole	7 mg/kg b.i.d.	Antifungal	Give for a full 3 weeks
Ranitidine/Metoclopramide[a]	0.2–0.5/0.5–2 mg/kg	Stimulate GI motility	Scattered clinical reports, mostly from anecdotal experiences
B-complex vitamins	5 mg/kg thiamine	Nutritional support	
Hyperalimentation diet[b]	Variable	Provision of easily absorbed dietary materials	Sufficient density to provide 250 kcal in 4–6 divided doses per day, volume of each dose not exceeding 20% body weight w/v
Iron dextran	10 mg/kg	Erythropoiesis	
Broad-spectrum antibiotics		Control of secondary bacterial infections	Depending on each individual case

[a]Metoclopramide 0.5–2 mg/kg s.c., i.m., i.v. every 12 hours (Reglan injection, Metoclopramide injection USP Deerfield, IL 60015 USA).

[b]Oxbow Carnivore Care Diet. Oxbow 29012 Mill Road Murdock, NE 68407 800 249 0366 Fax: (402) 867 3222 USA.

As the treatment programme progresses, further triage should be frequently conducted.

Further clinical management

Wound management

For patients going forward, wound management is the next procedure undertaken, taking advantage of the anaesthesia already in use for the examination and stabilization phase. Dead tissue and blood-matted feathers are carefully plucked and removed, avoiding skin tears. If the affected area is too friable and swollen, the feathers are cut next to the skin using an iris scissors. The removal of flight feathers (retrices and remiges) in order to clean a wound should be avoided. The area around the wound is then cleaned with 2.5% chlorhexidine solution, also flushed several times with volumes (50–100 mL) of warmed fluid – some clinicians recommend saline, others recommend lactated Ringer's solution. The cleaned and debrided wound is then daubed dry with sterile sponges and drawn partially closed; temporary closure can be rapidly obtained using skin staples. If the wound is more than 8 hours old, a gauze seton should be left in place for drainage. The wound should then be covered temporarily with a transparent semipermeable membrane dressing to prevent desiccation, and the surrounding area dried with a hairdryer. After removing the temporary wound dressing, sterile absorbent wound dressing material is applied over the wound and held in place with another piece of membrane dressing before applying further support bandaging using gauze and materials such as Vetrap®. It is recommended to change bandages daily for as long as drainage is evident.

Other treatments

Management beyond the stages of admission, stabilization and wound management consist of various medical procedures ranging from infectious diseases to internal medicine to orthopaedic management. Many aspects of the first two are detailed in the first part of this chapter; for detailed information on orthopaedics, readers are referred to other published material (Redig 2008).

Conclusion

While raptors have many clinical aspects in common with other species of birds, their presentation either as casualty patients or as athletic working birds used in the sport of falconry or flown in bird shows sets them apart and generates unique circumstances. Shock, dehydration and massive soft tissue and orthopaedic injuries challenge the clinician, and metabolic problems due to food restriction and heavy exercise create challenges on the medical side. The recent introduction of West Nile virus has added a novel aspect to raptor management, requiring previously unneeded levels of biosecurity and consideration of vaccination. Overall, however, they are sturdy birds that are easily maintained on a properly balanced carnivore diet. They are easy to anaesthetize, and are very tolerant of surgical and medical treatments. Those who wish to develop expertise in their management should become thoroughly familiar with their natural history and the sport of falconry. Combining knowledge of these elements with a specific background in avian medicine will give specialists the tools needed to engage competently in the care and treatment of raptors.

Acknowledgements

The authors gratefully acknowledge Dr Julia Ponder for critical review of this manuscript and Giovanni Rogas for rendering the digital images used in the figures. We also thank the many students, interns, residents and raptors who have supplied raw materials and applied and refined knowledge gained in over 30 years of practice of raptor medicine at The Raptor Center, University of Minnesota.

References

Aguilar R F, Redig P T 1995 Diagnosis and treatment of avian aspergillosis. In: Bonagura J D, Kirk R W (eds) Kirk's Current veterinary therapy XII. W B Saunders, Philadelphia, PA, p 1294–1298

Aguilar R F, Shaw D P, Dubey J P et al 1991 Sarcocystis-associated encephalitis in an immature northern goshawk (*Accipiter gentilis actricapillus*). Journal of Zoo and Wildlife Medicine 22(4):466–469

Altman R B, Clubb S L, Dorrestein G M, Quesenberry K (eds) 1997 Avian medicine and surgery. W B Saunders, Philadelphia, PA

Arent L 2006 Raptors in captivity, guidelines for care and management. Hancock House, Blaine, WA

Beebe F L, Webster H M 1994 North American falconry and hunting hawks. North American Falconry and Hunting Hawks, Denver

Boal C W, Mannan R W, Hudelson K S 1998 Trichomoniasis in Cooper's hawks from Arizona. Journal of Wildlife Diseases 34(3):590–593

Boydell I P, Forbes N A 1996 Diseases of the head (including the eyes). In: Beynon P H, Forbes N A, Harcourt-Brown N (eds) Manual of raptors, pigeons and waterfowl. British Small Animal Veterinary Association, Cheltenham, p 40–46

Carpenter J W 2005 Exotic animal formulary, 3rd edn. Elsevier Saunders, St Louis, MO, p 190, 196–197, 238–239

Cawthorne R A 1993 Cyst-forming coccidia of raptors: significant pathogens or not? In: Redig P T, Cooper J E, Remple J D, Hunter D B (eds) Raptor biomedicine. University of Minnesota Press, Minneapolis, p 14–20

Clubb S L, Levine B M, Graham D L 1980 An outbreak of viscerotropic velogenic Newcastle disease in pet birds. Proceedings American Association of Zoo Veterinarians. American Association of Zoo Veterinarians, p 105–109

Cooper J E 1985 Veterinary aspects of birds of prey. Standfast Press, Saul, Gloucestershire

Cooper J E 1996 Introduction. In: Beynon P H, Forbes N A, Harcourt-Brown N (eds) Manual of raptors, pigeons and waterfowl. British Small Animal Veterinary Association, Cheltenham, p 9–16

Davidson M 1997 Ocular consequences of trauma in raptors. Seminars in Avian and Exotic Pet Medicine 6(3):121–130

Dean J, Latimer K, Oaks J et al 2006 Falcon adenovirus infection in breeding Taita falcons (*Falco fasciinucha*). Journal of Veterinary Diagnostic Investigation 18(3):282–286

DeMarco M A, Foni E, Campitelli L et al 2003 Long-term monitoring for avian influenza viruses in wild bird species in Italy. Veterinary Research 27(1):107–114

Di Somma A, Bailey T A, Silvanose C et al 2007 The use of voriconazole for the treatment of aspergillosis in falcons. Journal of Avian Medicine and Surgery 21(4):307–316

Dubey J P, Porter S L, Hattel T et al 1991 *Sarcocystosis*-associated clinical encephalitis in a golden eagle (*Aquila chrysaetos*). Journal of Zoo and Wildlife Medicine 22(4):233–236

Duke G E 1986 Alimentary canal: anatomy, regulation of feeding and motility. In: Sturkie P D (ed) Avian physiology, 4th edn. Springer-Verlag, New York, p 269–288

Ellis K L 1986 Bilateral bumblefoot in a wild red-tailed hawk. Journal of Raptor Research 20(3):132

FAO 2005 Reported cases of HPAI in wild birds in 2004/2005. FAO AIDE News, Update on the Avian Influenza situation as of 10 Oct 2005, Issue no. 34. Online. Available: http://www.fao.org/ag/againfo/subjects/documents/ai/AVIbull034.pdf

Flammer K 2006 Antifungal drug update. In: Proceedings of Association of Avian Veterinarians. Association of Avian Veterinarians, San Antonio, Texas, p 3–6

Forbes N A 1996 Chronic weight loss, vomiting and dysphagia. In: Beynon P H, Forbes N A, Harcourt-Brown N (eds) Manual of raptors, pigeons and waterfowl. British Small Animal Veterinary Association, Cheltenham, p 189–196

Forbes N A 1997 Adenovirus infection in Mauritius kestrels (*Falco punctatus*). Journal of Avian Medicine and Surgery 11(1):31–33

Forbes N A, Simpson G N 1997 *Caryospora neofalconis:* an emerging threat to captive-bred raptors in the United Kingdom. Journal of Avian Medicine and Surgery 11(2):110–114

Fowler M E 1986 Metabolic bone disease. In: Fowler M (ed) Zoo and wild animal medicine, 2nd edn. W B Saunders, Philadelphia, PA, p 69–90

Gancz A Y, Barker I K, Lindsay R et al 2004 West Nile virus outbreak in North American owls, Ontario, 2002. Emerging Infectious Diseases 10(12):2135–2142

Gentz E J 1996 *Fusobacterium necrophorum* associated with bumblefoot in a wild great horned owl. Journal of Avian Medicine and Surgery 10(4):258–261

Gough R E, Capua I, Wernery U 2000 Herpesvirus infections in raptors. In: Lumeij J T, Remple J D, Redig P T et al (eds) Raptor biomedicine III. Zoological Education Network, Lake Worth, FL, p 9–11

Greiner E 1997 Parasitology. In: Altman R B, Clubb S L, Dorrestein G M, Quesenberry K (eds) Avian medicine and surgery. W B Saunders, Philadelphia, PA, p 332–349

Harcourt-Brown N 1996 Foot and leg problems. In: Beynon P H, Forbes N A, Harcourt-Brown N (eds) Manual of raptors, pigeons and waterfowl. British Small Animal Veterinary Association, Cheltenham, p 147–168

Hayes B 1988 Deaths caused by barbiturate poisoning in bald eagles and other wildlife. Canadian Veterinary Journal 29(2):173–174

Heatley J L, Mitchell M M, Roy A, Williams D L, Tully T N 2007 Disseminated mycobacteriosis in a bald eagle (*Haliaeetus leucocephalus*). Journal of Avian Medicine and Surgery 21(3), p 201–209.

Heidenreich M 1997 Birds of prey: medicine and management. Blackwell Wissenschafts – Verlag, Oxford, p 12–14, 52, 103–105

Hull J, Hull A, Reisen W et al 2006 Variation of West Nile virus antibody prevalence in migrating and wintering hawks in Central California. The Condor 108:435–439

Hunter D B, McKeever K, Barlett C 1993 Cyathostoma infections in screech owls, saw whet owls, and burrowing owls in southern Ontario. In: Redig P T, Cooper J E, Remple J D, Hunter D B (eds) Raptor biomedicine. University of Minnesota Press, Minneapolis, p 54–56

Komar N, Langevin S, Nemeth N et al 2003 Experimental infection of North American birds with the New York 1999 strain of West Nile virus. Emerging Infectious Diseases 9:311–322

Korbel R T 2000 Disorders of the posterior eye segment in raptors – examination procedures and findings. In: Lumeij J T, Remple J D, Redig P T et al (eds) Raptor biomedicine III. Zoological Education Network, Lake Worth, FL, p 179–193

Kramer J, Redig P T 1997 Sixteen years of lead poisoning in eagles. Journal of Raptor Research 31(4):327–332

Langelier K M 1993 Barbiturate poisoning in twenty-nine bald eagles. In: Redig P T, Cooper J E, Remple J D, Hunter D B (eds) Raptor biomedicine. University of Minnesota Press, Minneapolis, p 231–232

Lennox A G 2007 Mycobacteriosis in companion psittacine birds: a review. Journal of Avian Medicine and Surgery 21(3):181–187

Lichtenberger M 2004 Principles of shock and fluid therapy in special species. Seminars in Avian and Exotic Pet Medicine 13(3):142–153

Lichtenberger M 2005 Determination of indirect blood pressure in the companion bird. Seminars in Avian and Exotic Pet Medicine 14(2):149–152

Lublin A, Mechani S, Simantov Y et al 2001 Sudden death of a bearded vulture (*Gypaetus barbatus*) possibly caused by Newcastle disease virus. Avian Diseases 45(3):741–744

Magnino S, Fabbi M, Moreno A et al 2000 Avian influenza virus (H7 serotype) in a saker falcon in Italy. Veterinary Record 146(25):740

Malley A D, Whitbread T J 1996 The integument. In: Beynon P H, Forbes N A, Harcourt-Brown N (eds) Manual of raptors, pigeons and waterfowl. British Small Animal Veterinary Association, Cheltenham, p 129–139

Manvell R J, Wernery U, Alexander D J et al 2000 In: Lumeij J T, Remple J D, Redig. P T et al (eds) Raptor biomedicine III. Zoological Education Network, Lake Worth, FL, p 9–11

Morishita T Y, Lowensteine L J, Hirsch D C et al 1996 *Pasteurella multocida* in raptors: prevalence and characterization. Avian Diseases 40(4):908–918

Mueller K, Altenkamp R, Brunnberg R et al 2007 Pinching off syndrome in free-ranging white-tailed sea eagles (*Haliaeetus albicilla*) in Europe: frequency and geographic distribution of a generalized feather abnormality. Journal of Avian Medicine and Surgery 21(2):103–109

Murphy C J 1993 Ocular lesions in birds of prey. In: Fowler M E (ed) Zoo and wild animal medicine, 3rd edn. W B Saunders, Philadelphia, PA, p 211–221

Murphy C J, Howland H C 1987 The optics of comparative ophthalmology. Vision Research 27:599–607

Nemeth N, Gould D, Bowen R et al 2006 Natural and experimental West Nile virus infection in five raptor species. Journal of Wildlife Diseases 42(1):1–13

Oaks J L 1996 Immune and inflammatory responses in falcon staphylococcal pododermatitis. In: Redig P T, Cooper J E, Remple J D, Hunter D B (eds) Raptor biomedicine. University of Minnesota Press, Minneapolis, p 72–87

Oaks L, Schrenzel M, Rideout B et al 2005 Isolation and epidemiology of falcon adenovirus. Journal of Clinical Microbiology 43:3414–3420

Okoh A E 1979 Newcastle disease in falcons. Journal of Wildlife Diseases 15:479–480

Orosz S E, Ensley P K, Haynes C J 1992 Avian surgical anatomy: thoracic and pelvic limbs. W B Saunders, Philadelphia, PA

Palmgren H, Broman T, Waldenstroem J et al 2004 *Salmonella* Amagar, *Campylobacter jejuni*, and urease-positive thermophilic *Campylobacter* found in free-flying peregrine falcons (*Falco peregrinus*) in Sweden. Journal of Wildlife Diseases 40(93):583–587

Plumb C D 2005 Plumb's Veterinary drug handbook, 5th edn. Blackwell Publishing, Oxford, p 336–337

Porter S A 1993 Pesticide poisoning in birds of prey. In: Redig P T, Cooper J E, Remple J D, Hunter D B (eds) Raptor biomedicine. University of Minnesota Press, Minneapolis, p 239–425

ProMED 2006 PRO/AH/EDR> Avian influenza – worldwide (86): Germany, Denmark, Indonesia X-ProMED-Id: 20060412.1085

Ramer J C, Paul-Murphy J, Brunson D et al 1996 Effects of mydriatic agents in cockatoos, African grey parrots and blue-fronted Amazon parrots. Journal of American Veterinary Medical Association 208(2):227–230

Redig P T 1996a Nursing avian patients. In: Beynon P H, Forbes N A, Harcourt-Brown N (eds) Manual of raptors, pigeons and waterfowl. British Small Animal Veterinary Association, Cheltenham, p 42–46

Redig P T 1996b Raptors. In: Altman R B, Clubb S L, Dorrestein G M, Quesenberry K (eds) Avian medicine and surgery. W B Saunders, Philadelphia, PA, p 918–928

Redig P T 1998 Recommendations for anaesthesia in raptors with comments on trumpeter swans. Seminars in Avian and Exotic Pet Medicine 7(1):22–30

Redig P T 2008 Fungal diseases – aspergillosis. In: Samour J H (ed) Avian medicine, 2nd edn. Mosby Elsevier, Edinburgh. p 373–387

Redig P T, Arent L A 2008 Raptor toxicology. Veterinary Clinics of North America: Exotic Animal Practice 11(2)

Redig P T, Cruz L 2008 Fractures. In: Samour J H (ed) Avian medicine, 2nd edn. Mosby Elsevier, Edinburgh, p 215–248

Remple J D 2004 Intracellular hematozoa of raptors: a review and update. Journal of Avian Medicine and Surgery 18(2):75–88

Remple J D 2005 Antibiotic-impregnated polymethylmethacrylate beads: advantages, antibiotic choices, and production. In: Proceedings of Association of Avian Veterinarians. Association of Avian Veterinarians, California, p 287–292

Ritchie B W, Harrison G J, Harrison L R 1994 Avian medicine: principles and application. Wingers, Lake Worth, FL

Rupley A E 1997 Manual of avian practice. W B Saunders, Philadelphia, PA, p 223

Samour J 2000 *Pseudomonas aeruginosa* stomatitis as a sequel to trichomoniasis in captive saker falcons (*Falco cherrug*). Journal of Avian Medicine and Surgery 14(2):113–117

Samour J, Naldo J L 2001 Serratospiculiasis in captive falcons in the Middle East: a review. Journal of Avian Medicine and Surgery 15(1):2–9

Samour J J, Naldo J L 2002 Diagnosis and therapeutic management of candidiasis in falcons in Saudi Arabia. Journal of Avian Medicine and Surgery 16(2):129–132

Samour J, Naldo J L 2003 Diagnosis and therapeutic management of trichomoniasis in falcons in Saudi Arabia. Journal of Avian Medicine and Surgery 17(3):136–143

Samour J, Naldo J L 2005 Lead toxicosis in falcons: a method for lead retrieval. Seminars in Avian and Exotic Pet Medicine 14(2):143–148

Samour J H, Naldo J L 2007 Anatomical and clinical radiology of birds of prey including interactive advanced anatomical imaging. Saunders, Elsevier

Samour J, Naldo J L, John S K 2005 Therapeutic management of *Babesia shortii* infection in a peregrine falcon (*Falco peregrinus*). Journal of Avian Medicine and Surgery 19:294–296

Samour J, Naldo J L, Wernery U, Beer M 2007 Highly pathogenic avian influenza H5N1 phenotype infection in a saker falcon (*Falco cherrug*). Falco (Newsletter of the Middle East Falcon Research Group) #30: 14–16

Schlosberg A 1976 Treatment of monocrotophous-poisoned birds of prey with pralidoxine iodide. Journal of American Veterinary Medical Association 169(11):989–990

Scope A, Burhenne J, Haefeli W et al 2005 Pharmacokinetics and pharmacodynamics of the new antifungal agent voriconazole in birds. In: Proceedings of the 8th European Association of Avian Veterinary. Arles, France, p 217–221

Silvanose C, Bailey T A, Di'Somma A 2006 Susceptibility of fungi isolated from the respiratory tract of falcons to amphotericin B, itraconazole and voriconazole. Veterinary Record 159:282–284

Smith S A 1993 Diagnosis and treatment of helminths in birds of prey. In: Redig P T, Cooper J E, Remple J D, Hunter D B (eds) Raptor biomedicine. University of Minnesota Press, Minneapolis, p 21–27

Stauber E, Holmes S, DeGhetto D L, Finch N 2007 Magnetic resonance imaging is superior to radiograpy in evaluating spinal cord trauma in three bald eagles (*Haliaeetus leucocephalus*). Journal of Avian Medicine and Surgery 21(3):196–200

Tavernier P, Saggese M, Van Wettere A et al 2005 Malaria in an Eastern Screech Owl (*Otus asio*). Avian Diseases 49:433–435

Tschopp R, Bailey T, Di Somma A, Silvanose C 2007 Urinalysis as a noninvasive health screening procedure in Falconidae. Journal of Avian Medicine and Surgery 21(1):8–12

Ueblacker S 2000 Trichomoniasis in American kestrels (*Falcon sparverius*) and Eastern Screech Owls (*Otus asio*). In: Lumeij J T, Remple J D, Redig P T et al (eds) Raptor biomedicine III. Zoological Education Network, Lake Worth, FL, p 59–63

USGS 2006 West Nile virus. Online. Available: http://www.nwhc.usgs. gov/disease_information/west_nile_virus/affected_species.jsp. 26 Sept 2006

Van Wettere A J, Wunschmann A, Latimer K S et al 2005 Adenovirus infection in Taita falcons (*Falco fasciinucha*) and Hybrid falcons (*Falco rusticolus x Falco peregrinus*). Journal of Avian Medicine and Surgery 19:280–285

Ward F P 1971 Thiamine deficiency in a peregrine falcon. Journal of the American Veterinary Medical Association 159(5):599–601

Wheler C L 1993 Herpesvirus disease in raptors: a review of the literature. In: Redig P T, Cooper J E, Remple J D, Hunter D B (eds) Raptor biomedicine. University of Minnesota Press, Minneapolis, p 103–107

Wunschmann A, Shivers J, Bender J et al 2004 Pathologic findings in red-tailed hawks (*Buteo jamaicensis*) and Cooper's hawks (*Accipiter cooperi*) naturally infected with West Nile virus. Avian Diseases 48(3):570–580

Wunschmann A, Shivers J, Bender J et al 2005 Pathologic and immunohistochemical findings in goshawks (*Accipiter gentilis*) and great horned owls (*Bubo virginianus*) naturally infected with West Nile virus. Avian Diseases 49(2):252–259

Zsivanovits P, Monks D J, Forbes N A et al 2006 Presumptive identification of a novel adenovirus in a Harris Hawk (*Parabuteo unicinctus*), a Bengal Eagle Owl (*Bubo bengalensis*), and a Verreaux's Eagle Owl (*Buteo lacteus*). Journal of Avian Medicine and Surgery 20:105–112

Zucca P 2000 Infectious diseases. In: Samour J (ed) Avian medicine. Mosby, London, p 230–231

Cranes

Glenn H. Olsen

10

Introduction

All cranes are found in the family Gruidae, and in two subfamilies, Balearicinae and Gruinae. In the subfamily Balearicinae there are only two species, the black crowned crane (*Balearica pavonina*) native to northern Africa and also called the West African crowned crane or Sudan crowned crane, and the grey crowned crane (*Balearica regulorum*) also called the East African crowned crane or the South African crowned crane. This subfamily is distinct in having a decorative spray of feathers emanating from the back of the head.

All other crane species are found in the subfamily Gruinae. This includes the two species of cranes native to North America; the highly endangered whooping crane (*Grus americana*), numbering less than 600 birds, and the sandhill crane (*G. canadensis*). Sandhill cranes are divided into six subspecies in North America: the migratory greater (*G. c. tabida*), lesser (*G. c. canadensis*) and Canadian (*G. c. rowani*) sandhill cranes and the non-migratory Florida (*G. c. pratensis*), Mississippi (*G. c. pulla*) and Cuban (*G. c. nesiotes*) sandhill cranes. The latter two subspecies are both listed as endangered. However, recent work (Jones et al 2005) calls for taxonomically dividing sandhill cranes into two subpopulations, lesser sandhill cranes as one subpopulation and the other five subspecies as the other. This division into two groups is thought to have resulted from Pleistocene glaciation causing a separation of the original sandhill crane species into two distinct subpopulations or subspecies. The current subspecies designations were based on geographic/breeding isolation, especially for the Mississippi, Florida and Cuban subspecies, and migratory pathways and breeding grounds for the other three subspecies.

In Africa, in addition to the two species in the subfamily Balearicinae, there are three species in the subfamily Gruinae, the wattled crane (*Bugeranus carunculatus*), the blue crane (*Anthropoides pardisea*) of southern Africa, and the demoiselle crane (*Anthropoides virgo*) found in both Africa and Asia. Other cranes of Asia include the white-naped crane (*Grus vipio*) found in East Asia, the hooded crane (*Grus monacha*) also from East Asia, the black-necked crane (*Grus nigricollis*) from the Tibetan Plateau, and the red-crowned crane (*Grus japonensis*) of the East Asian mainland and Japan. The Siberian crane (*Grus leucogeranus*) is found across Asia, though the western population is almost extinct. Found across Europe and Asia in the hundreds of thousands

is the Eurasian or common crane (*Grus grus*). The sarus crane (*Grus antigone*) is divided into three subspecies geographically, the Indian, Eastern (Southeast Asia) and Australian. Also found in Australia is the brolga crane (*Grus rubicunda*). The only continents without crane species are South America and Antarctica.

Biology and husbandry

Cranes are tall (over 1 m for sandhill cranes, and 1.25 m for whooping cranes), heavy-bodied birds (up to 6 kg for sandhill cranes and 7 kg for whooping cranes) with large wing spans (2 m for sandhill cranes and 2.5 m for whooping cranes). **One characteristic that sets cranes apart from herons and egrets is that many crane species have bright-red thick skin with an irregular surface covering parts of their head and neck.** With whooping cranes and sandhill cranes, the red skin covers the top of the head (Fig. 10.1), and the size of the patch can be varied to reflect behavioural aspects of dominance or submissiveness. Using bright antibiotic sprays (such as furazolidone) on the head or neck can adversely affect a crane's acceptance by others of its species. Another distinguishing characteristic between cranes and herons or egrets is that cranes fly with the neck extended straight

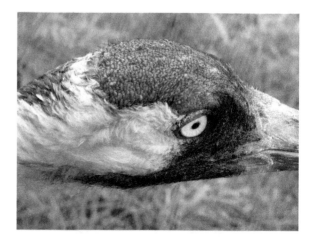

Fig 10.1 Close-up view of an adult male whooping crane (*Grus americana*) showing the red skin covering the top of the head. The size and intensity of the red coloured area can be changed to reflect the mood or attitude of the crane such as aggression, submission or even illness, when the crown may be pale, slightly grey or even cyanotic in appearance.

ahead, while herons and egrets fly with the neck held in a half circle and the head held back towards the body.

Crane feather coloration is generally grey or white for most species, with some cranes having areas of black or even brown coloration. Newly hatched chicks are covered with tan to brown down. Later they will have primarily tan to brown coloured feathers before moulting into adult plumage during the first year. A few crane species maintain some tan juvenile feathers into their second year. Cranes carry their tertiary wing feathers fluffed up over their rump.

Cranes have a long convoluted trachea that makes a loop within the sternum (Fig. 10.2). This tracheal shape, similar to some brass musical instruments such as the trombone, makes it possible for cranes to produce a loud bugling call. Cranes share this tracheal characteristic only with swans (*Cygninae*). The looping trachea can lead to the build-up of mucus or fluids at certain points, resulting in severe dyspnoea. Some cranes, such as whooping cranes, also have a tracheal stenosis that may have a genetic basis. Because of the looping anatomy of the trachea in cranes, any tracheal flushes should be used with extreme caution.

Handling/restraint

Cranes can be large, aggressive birds. In addition to a long, pointed beak, they have extremely sharp toenails, capable of slicing through the clothing or skin of the unwary handler. However, with the use of proper techniques even the larger species can be restrained safely. The best method of capturing a crane in an enclosure is to herd the bird into a corner of the pen. When the crane's head is orientated toward the fence, move forward, grasping the secondary and tertiary flight feathers of both wings with one hand to control the bird's ability to extend its wings. Move the other arm over the crane's body, keeping the crane's head pointed toward the rear of the handler (Fig. 10.3A, B). Grasp the legs at or just above the hocks and prevent the hocks from rubbing together by placing one or two fingers between the hocks (Fig. 10.4). Now the bird is lifted and tucked under the arm of the handler.

Once the crane's wings are restrained by the upper arm of the handler, the hand holding the tertiary feathers is free and can be moved around the handler's back to grasp the head of an aggressive crane (Fig. 10.5). An alternative holding method moves the hand on the tertiaries down to the hock position, and the hand on the hocks moves up under the sternum to give additional support to the crane. Safety glasses or goggles should be worn by handlers.

Anaesthesia

Cranes have been successfully anaesthetized with ketamine/xylazine (10–15 mg/kg ketamine, 1 mg/kg xylazine) or ketamine/diazepam (10–15 mg ketamine, 0.2–0.5 mg/kg diazepam) combinations. Once the injection is given, the crane should be held until anaesthetized to prevent injury when the bird begins to lose its balance. Likewise, the crane needs to be held during recovery until it can stand and move without falling. Because of these requirements and the time involved, injectable agents are now used primarily in field situations whereas gaseous anaesthetic agents are used for most captive procedures.

Isoflurane is currently the gas anaesthetic of choice for most procedures requiring general anaesthesia.

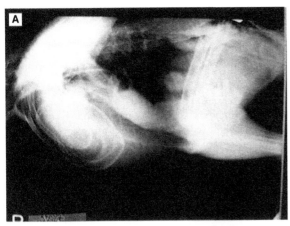

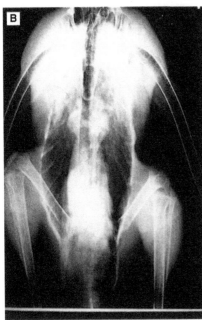

Fig 10.2 Lateral (**A**) and dorsoventral (**B**) radiographs of a crane. The lateral view shows the convoluted loops of the trachea found within the sternum.

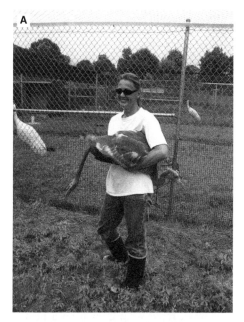

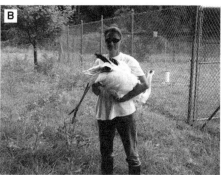

Fig 10.3A, B Technique used to hold a crane; one hand supports the body and the other grasps the legs at the hocks, juvenile whooping crane (*Grus americana*).

An appropriate facemask to accommodate the long beak of the crane can be made using a 60 mL plastic syringe case. After induction (at 4–5%), the crane can be intubated and maintained at 1–3% isoflurane and an oxygen flow of 1–2 L/min.

Proprofol (PropoFlo Injectable, Abbott Laboratories, North Chicago, IL, USA) can be used to anaesthetize cranes when gas anaesthesia is not practical. When using an injectable general anaesthetic agent such as propofol, intubation should still be done. Regurgitation of gastrointestinal fluids or food is possible with aspiration into the elongated trachea leading to disastrous results if one fails to intubate the crane. Another intravenous anaesthetic agent useful for short procedures is the mixture alphaxolone-alphadolone (Bailey et al 1999). The recommended dose for cranes is 6.5–7.0 mg/kg given intravenously. Induction is smooth and rapid (13 to 26 seconds) and the maximum anaesthetic effect lasts 5–6 minutes. Time to standing with no residual ataxia varied by species but was generally 20 to 33 minutes (Bailey et al 1999).

Alpha-chloralose ($C_6H_{11}Cl_3O_6$) is used to capture wild cranes and cranes that have escaped from zoos or private collections. Alpha-chloralose works by depressing the cortical centres of the brain (Balis & Monroe 1964). The target cranes are first fed whole corn at a bait station. On the day proposed for capture, alpha-chloralose is mixed with the corn at the rate of 0.39–0.48 g/cup (280 mL) of corn (Hayes et al 2003). Generally, a single crane needs to ingest 0.5–1.0 cup of the treated corn to receive a sufficient dose. After the crane eats the alpha-chloralose-treated corn, the first effects of sedation can start 20–30 minutes later. Usually the crane will become ataxic, spending more time resting,

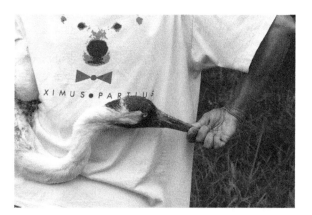

Fig 10.4 Technique used to hold a crane's legs, using a finger to separate the hocks and prevent rubbing injuries.

Fig 10.5 A normal handling position for an aggressive crane. The handler's one arm restrains the wings, while the hand grasps the legs at the hocks. The other hand is placed behind the handler's back and controls the crane's head.

having difficulty flying or not flying, and eventually going to sternal recumbency. The crane may or may not become totally unresponsive to stimuli. Effects may last from 12 to 24 hours, so provision needs to be made for a quiet dark pen space to house the crane until it recovers fully. Complications that may occur include hyperthermia, hypothermia, exertional myopathy, and if the crane is released prior to full recovery, drowning or predation (Carpenter 2003). **Exertional myopathy can be a major morbidity/mortality factor when capturing wild cranes using alpha-choralose-laced corn,** with 3.7% morbidity and 1.6% mortality in one study in Wisconsin (Hayes et al 2003). Lower levels of sedation in this study were actually correlated with a higher incidence of developing exertional myopathy. In another report (Businga et al 2007), the successful treatment of three sandhill cranes for exertional myopathy is described. Treatment consisted of dexamethasone 1–2 mg/kg q12h subcutaneously for the first 1–2 days, selenium/vitamin E 0.06 mg/kg intramuscular as a single dose on day 1 and repeated on day 7, lactated Ringer's solution 60–180 mL q12h subcutaneously for the first 2–5 days and nutritional support by gavage feeding 30–120 mL q12h (Businga et al 2007).

For tranquillization, diazepam at 0.5–1.0 mg/kg is appropriate and lasts 4–6 hours. The desirable dose for procedures such as shipping agitated cranes should be low enough to prevent loss of balance, but high enough to calm the bird. Local anaesthetics (lidocaine 0.5 mL, xylocaine 0.5 mL, or bupivacaine up to 2 mg/kg) can be infiltrated into areas for minor procedures such as wound suturing or implanting subcutaneous radio transmitters. Local anaesthetic agents may also be applied to surgery sites to reduce pain after recovery from general anaesthesia.

Blood collection

The three most common sites for blood collection in cranes are the right jugular, the medial metatarsal or brachial veins. The feathers overlying the jugular and brachial veins can be wetted with isopropyl alcohol and the vein held off proximal to the desired withdrawal site. A large volume (up to 50 mL for transfusions) can be quickly obtained from the jugular vein. However, if the crane struggles extensively – or the person assisting in holding the head fails to hold it firmly – the needle may lacerate the jugular vein, potentially leading to death of the crane. However, laceration of the jugular vein is a very rare complication of blood collection. Using the medial tarsal or brachial/ulnar veins requires further restraint of the wing or leg, and there is an increased risk of a limb injury. Due to frequently observed complications, a severe long bone fracture can result in the death of a crane (Olsen 1994). Normal blood values for North American cranes are listed in Table 10.1.

Injection sites are similar to those for most birds. **The pectoral muscles are the recommended sites for intramuscular injections.** Subcutaneous injections can be given in a number of sites, but are often administered over the lateral thigh.

Metabolic and nutritional disorders

High protein diets (32% protein) fed to Florida sandhill and greater sandhill crane chicks resulted in increased rate of growth as compared to a lower protein diet (24% protein) (Serafin 1982). However, in the larger and faster-growing greater sandhill cranes there was a 17% rate of leg deformities and 25% rate of wing deformities when the 32% protein diet was used during the period of rapid growth between days 7 and 28 post-hatch. The abnormalities observed in rapidly growing crane chicks included deformities in the proximal ends of the tibiotarsus and tarsometatarsus, the distal end of the tibiotarsus, and the intertarsal and tibiofemoral joints, due to weak legs being unable to support the rapid weight gain possible in this species. Likewise, rapid wing growth on a high protein diet leads to twisting deformities at the carpal joint, sometimes called 'angel wing'. This condition will respond to restraining the wings against the body in a normal folded position to prevent a permanent anatomical malformation. Usually restraint is needed only for a short period (48 h). Young whooping cranes are also subject to similar limb deformities (Kepler 1978), and it is thought that any of the larger crane species that breed in temperate climates are susceptible to similar problems (Serafin 1982).

Diets that promote slower growth of crane chicks are recommended. **Using a 24% protein diet with a low (0.73%) sulphur amino-acid level slows crane growth sufficiently to reduce limb deformities.** If the daily weight gain continuously exceeds 10% in crane chicks during the critical 7–28-day age period, further management techniques such as food withholding for several hours are used to help slow growth (Wellinton et al 1996). However, crane chicks raised by parent birds in a large enclosure or by human handlers, but receiving constant supervision and exercise, can be fed *ad libitum* during this period without experiencing any leg or joint problems.

Infectious diseases

Viral diseases

Viral diseases such as avian pox and Newcastle disease, which occur in most species of birds, also occur in cranes. Two viral diseases have been identified as potential problems in captive cranes maintained in North America: eastern equine encephalitis and inclusion body disease of cranes. Two other new diseases have the potential to cause morbidity and mortality in cranes: West Nile virus and infectious bursal disease.

Table 10.1 Normal reported mean blood values for cranes (Olsen et al 1996a, Olsen & Carpenter 1997)

	Whooping crane	Sandhill crane	Siberian crane	Red-crowned crane	Wattled crane
Haematocrit (%)	42	43	45	39	45
Haemoglobin (g/dL)	14.4	13.5	–	–	–
Red blood cells (10^6/mm^3)	2.2	2.5	–	–	–
White blood cells (10^3/mm^3)	13.4	17.0	10.8	14.9	12.7
Heterophils (%)	53	56	53	41	48
Lymphocytes (%)	40	41	39	48	39
Monocytes (%)	6	2	3	6	5
Eosinophils (%)	2	1	5	5	8
Total protein (g/dL)	3.8	3.9	3.6	3.3	3.1
Albumin (g/dL)	1.5	1.5	1.4	1.2	1.1
Globulin (g/dL)	2.3	2.3	2.3	2.1	2.0
Albumin/Globulin ratio	0.7	0.7	0.6	0.6	0.6
Glucose (mg/dL)	232	247	266	267	266
Uric acid (mg/dL)	8.1	9.7	9.0	7.8	7.7
Creatinine (mg/dL)	0.6	0.7	0.3	0.3	0.4
Cholesterol (mg/dL)	148	128	212	170	147
Aspartate aminotransferase (IU/L)	261	181	182	208	189
Lactic dehydrogenase (IU/L)	440	278	202	288	137
Alkaline phosphatase (IU/L)	46	164	45	226	37
Calcium (mg/dL)	9.1	9.7	10.5	10.8	10.8
Phosphorus (mg/dL)	2.8	3.6	3.8	3.5	2.7
Sodium (mmol/L)	147	148	149	148	146
Chloride (mmol/L)	107	108	109	107	108
Potassium (mmol/L)	3.4	3.4	2.9	2.8	3.2

Eastern equine encephalitis

Eastern equine encephalitis (EEE) virus is found in the eastern USA and south-eastern Canada, the Caribbean and Central and South America. Most native birds do not show signs of clinical disease, but rather act as reservoirs of the virus, promoting exposure to horses, other avian species, and/or humans through mosquito bites. The virus is transmitted by the ornithophilic mosquito *Culiseta melanura*, which breeds in wooded swamps. Whooping cranes (Dein et al 1986) and Mississippi sandhill cranes (Young et al 1996) are both susceptible to this virus.

Vaccination programmes for EEE, using commercially available equine vaccine or a formalin-inactivated human EEE vaccine, have been developed (Clark et al 1987) and used successfully in whooping cranes (Pagac et al 1992, Olsen et al 1997). Cranes are initially vaccinated with 0.5 mL of formalin-inactivated human EEE vaccine in late July of their hatch year, then have a second injection of

1.0 mL 3–4 weeks later. Human EEE vaccine has become difficult to obtain in recent years; therefore equine vaccine products are commonly used, with preference given to killed vaccines. A 0.25 mL dose of ENCEVAC (Intervet, Inc., Millsboro, Delaware, USA) given intramuscularly and repeated 3–4 weeks later appears to be effective in immunizing whooping crane chicks. A single injection of 0.25 mL, given intramuscularly, is used as an annual booster to maintain titre levels. The booster vaccinations are given in July or early August, as the mosquito activity and potential spread of EEE is greatest in late summer and autumn (Pagac et al 1992). The vaccination programme has proven effective in preventing further losses of whooping cranes due to EEE when known virus-carrying mosquitoes are trapped in the area (Olsen et al 1997).

Inclusion body disease of cranes (IBDC)

This is a viral disease that causes lethargy and loss of appetite for 48 hours followed by diarrhoea (sometimes haemorrhagic diarrhoea) and death, and was first identified in 1978 (Doeherty 1987). A previously unknown herpesvirus was isolated as the causative agent for IBDC. Mortality has occurred in blue cranes, sandhill cranes, red-crowned cranes, and hooded cranes. Antibodies have been detected in sandhill cranes, blue cranes, hooded cranes, sarus cranes, Eurasian cranes, red-crowned cranes, demoiselle cranes and East African crowned cranes. All these cranes were captive, and all but the sandhill cranes were Old World species. In sampling 95 wild greater sandhill cranes in Wisconsin and Indiana, none of the birds had antibodies to the virus (Doeherty 1987).

Gross pathological lesions include an enlarged liver and spleen with small (pinpoint to pinhead) yellowish-white lesions, and haemorrhage is seen in the thymus and intestines. Fat stores in the subcutaneous tissues were still abundant when dead birds were examined, indicating a rapid disease process (Doeherty 1987). Viral isolation from affected organs (e.g. liver, spleen) is the recommended diagnostic method of confirming IBDC. Additional confirmation of IBDC may be determined through observation of characteristic intranuclear inclusion bodies in hepatic and splenic tissue collected from suspect birds (Doeherty 1987).

At the present time there is no treatment or vaccine for IBDC. **The presence of antibodies in some captive cranes indicates that a few birds survive exposure to the virus and may develop a level of immune protection.** A complicating factor involving birds that survive the initial infection is that they may become subclinical carriers of this potentially fatal herpesvirus. However, the exact mechanism for transmission is unknown, although there does not appear to be vertical transmission of the organism (Doeherty 1987). The antibody response noted in some cranes lasts for several years, and these birds should be considered carrier animals of IBDC. A control programme is in place at many institutions that maintain crane populations. The control programme includes testing all cranes periodically for IBDC antibody titres and removing or isolating any positive birds. Since the disease has not been isolated from wild North American cranes, it is critical to isolate any potential carriers from wild birds and to test all cranes scheduled for release.

West Nile virus

West Nile virus (WNV) first occurred in the United States in 1999. Prior to that time the disease had been identified in Africa, the Middle East and Europe with no reports in the literature of crane fatalities. However, the North American cranes comprised a naive population to the virus. Since WNV has been identified in the USA there have been documented cases of sandhill cranes dying from WNV, with one adult greater sandhill crane and two 3-month-old Florida sandhill cranes dying from confimed WNV infections at Patuxent Wildlife

Research Center. In an experimental challenge of vaccinated and unvaccinated Florida sandhill crane adults, there were no deaths recorded, but some birds lost weight, up to 6%, and had elevated white blood cell counts (Olsen et al 2003). **The WNV-vaccinated sandhill cranes developed a less severe infectious response and had a quicker recovery from the disease than their non-vaccinated counterparts.** A killed equine WNV vaccine is commercially available (West Nile – Innovator®, Wyeth/Fort Dodge Laboratories, Madison, NJ, USA) and is currently being used to immunize young sandhill and whooping cranes at an intramuscular dose of 1 mL given as a three dose series, the second and third doses coming 21 and 28 days after the first dose (Olsen et al 2003). The first dose has been given as early as 7 days of age. No whooping cranes have died from West Nile virus to date that have been vaccinated intramuscularly with the equine product using a 1 mL dose schedule as outlined above for sandhill cranes.

Infectious bursal disease

Infectious bursal disease (IBD) is a viral disease with an acute onset that results in immunosuppression. Immunosuppression occurs because lymphoid tissue of the bursa is the primary target of the virus. Among young chickens IBD is highly contagious (Lukert & Saif 2003). Infectious bursal disease has been implicated in the deaths of released whooping cranes in Florida. Captive cranes have varying titres to this disease indicating some level of exposure is occurring even though the birds are in fenced enclosures. At this time the course of IBD in cranes is not well documented, but it is thought to have been associated with fatal cases. One should avoid housing cranes in an exhibit with or near chickens or turkeys to reduce exposure to IBD.

Bacterial diseases

Many of the common avian bacterial pathogens have been isolated from cranes, including *Pasteurella multocida*, *Mycobacterium avium*, *M. tuberculosis*, *Salmonella* spp., *Clostridium* spp., *Erysipelothrix* spp., *Escherichia coli*, *Streptococcus* spp. and *Staphylococcus* spp. Though pathogenesis varies between isolates, *E. coli* can be part of the normal gastrointestinal flora or responsible for gastroenteritis that presents as severe diarrhoea, dehydration and death in young birds. Various *Salmonella* spp. have been isolated from cranes during routine health maintenance examinations. In Japan from 420 samples of crane faeces, 29 strains of *Salmonella* were isolated (Maeda et al 2001). Salmonellosis was also diagnosed as the cause of gastrointestinal disease in at least one crane chick at Patuxent Wildlife Research Center. The chick developed diarrhoea, lost weight, became dehydrated and lethargic.

Supportive care and appropriate antibiotic therapy resulted in complete recovery. Eye infections involving the cornea in crane chicks caused by *Pseudomonas aeruginosa* can be severe and lead to the loss of vision in the affected eye (Fig. 10.6). Treatment with gentamicin or other antibiotics as indicated by sensitivity testing should be initiated whenever a crane chick is diagnosed with corneal trauma.

Enrofloxacin and ciprofloxacin are antibiotics commonly used in cranes to treat bacterial infections. The accepted methods of delivery include injections and a tablet for oral administration. One study (Bowman et al 2004) demonstrated that giving enrofloxacin in drinking water at 50 ppm to sandhill cranes resulted in plasma concentrations below accepted therapeutic levels, so delivery in drinking water is not recommended.

Avian tuberculosis

Wild whooping cranes have been diagnosed with *Mycobacterium avium*. One 5-year-old wild whooping crane found debilitated, had a large, palpable, splenomegaly, mid-coelomic mass, and a chronic cloacal prolapse with a mass 2 cm in diameter within the prolapsed cloacal tissues (Snyder 1996). Removal and biopsy of the cloacal mass revealed a coalescing granuloma with necrotic centres and macrophage zones, with the necrotic centres containing rod-shaped acid-fast staining bacteria. *Mycobacterium avium* was isolated from the mass, and confirmed with a DNA-specific probe. The crane was treated for 1 year with rifampin (45 mg/kg, once daily; Rifadin, Marion Merrill Dow, Inc., Kansas City, MO, USA) and ethambutol (30 mg/kg, once daily; Myambutol, Wyeth–Lederle, Pearl River, NY, USA), both given for 1 year. Isoniazid (Isoniazid USP, Rugby Laboratories, Rockville Center, NY, USA) was added at a dose of 30 mg/kg, once daily to the treatment regimen on two occasions, but discontinued because on both occasions the crane became anorectic. In an attempt to elicit an immune response two doses of *M. vaccae* antigen (0.05 mL) were given intradermally 8 weeks apart (Snyder 1996).

Approximately 10 months after discontinuing the antitubercular therapy, recrudescence was suspected, based on radiographic findings, weight loss and elevated WBC (Snyder 1996). Although *M. avium* was not isolated on faecal culture, the crane was treated with azithromycin (Pfizer Laboratories, Inc.) 20 mg/kg once daily in food, later increased to 40 mg/kg.

The clinical improvement of the bird during the 16-week course of treatment was described as dramatic (Snyder 1996). However, later treatment with a combination of azithromycin and ethambutol produced a fatal adverse reaction. At the time of necropsy, no *M. avium* was isolated from the treated crane (Snyder 1996), so one would conclude that the treatment was apparently effective.

Fungal diseases

Candida spp.

Candida spp. have been isolated on occasion from the beak or mouth of a crane, often diagnosed in immunosuppressed birds. Treatment with a topical nystatin cream has been a successful option for cranes infected with this organism.

Aspergillosis

Aspergillosis is a serious respiratory disease, especially in chicks and debilitated adult birds suffering from other disease or injuries. *Aspergillus* spp. (usually *A. fumagatus*) have caused the death of many cranes, some as young as 9 days old (Figs 10.7 and 10.8).

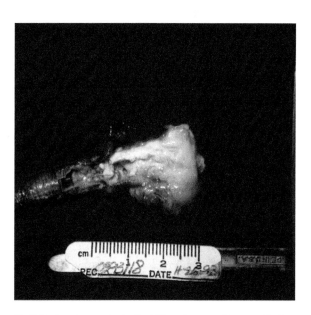

Fig 10.7 Granuloma at the tracheal bifurcation caused by aspergillosis.

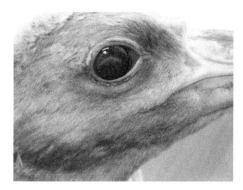

Fig 10.6 Whooping crane chick suffering from a small penetrating wound of the cornea followed by a *Pseudomonas aeruginosa* infection. Cornea is darkly pigmented and vascularized.

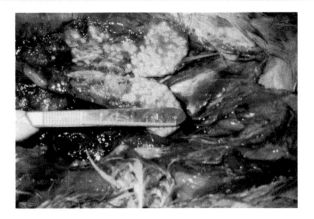

Fig 10.8 Aspergillosis in the air sac of a sandhill crane.

A treatment regimen recently developed at the Patuxent Wildlife Research Center and based on earlier work with raptors (Joseph et al 1994) has shown a high success rate and return to normal function for the cranes treated. The treatment regimen consists of oral itraconazole given at the dose rate of 10 mg/kg p.o. q12h. Itraconazole comes as a capsule containing small granules, and there are approximately 285–290 granules in each 100 mg capsule; hence each granule averages 0.35 mg. The appropriate number of granules is therefore counted out and mixed with food to be given to the crane. A cleaned smelt works well for this, as the granules can be sprinkled inside the fish, and most cranes will eat small fish readily if trained to do so. In addition to oral itraconazole, enrofloxacin is given either by intramuscular injection or, more frequently, per os, at a dose of 15 mg/kg q12h, as a prophylaxis against secondary bacterial infections.

Each crane is also nebulized with clotrimazole 10 mg/mL in polyethylene glycol (Island Pharmacy Services, Woodruff, WI, USA). The patient is placed in a small cage (tall enough to allow the crane to stand and wide enough to turn around). The clotrimazole (3–5 mL) is added to an 'up-mist' medication nebulizer (cat. no. HK8955, Metropolitan Medical, Inc., Sterling, VA, USA), and the nebulizer is connected to an oxygen source. A flow rate of 5–8 L/min is required to achieve proper nebulization. Each bird is nebulized for 20 minutes, q8h (1 h/total/day).

The combination of itraconazole/enrofloxacin orally plus clotrimazole nebulization has been used successfully to treat aspergillosis infections diagnosed in crane species for 6 years. The minimum period of treatment is usually 2 weeks, but if clinical signs are still present, nebulization is continued for an additional week and oral itraconazole for an additional 2 weeks. Itraconazole has been reported as possibly being toxic if used concurrently with clotrimazole (Carpenter et al 1996), but no toxicity problems have been observed in

cranes given this treatment. Voriconazole (Vfend, Pfizer, Amboise Cedex, France) has recently been described as very effective in treating raptors for aspergillosis (Di Somma et al 2007). The recommended dose for raptors was made by crushing a 50 mg tablet and mixing with 5 mL water. Treatment was given at 12.5 mg/kg q12h for 3 days then q24h until resolved (Di Somma et al 2007). This treatment regimen has not been tested in cranes but holds some promise.

Mycotoxins

Mycotoxins produced as secondary metabolites of fungal moulds (primarily *Fusarium graminearum*) on corn and other crops have proved to be a disease source for cranes. At least two cases of large-scale natural mortality in wild cranes have been attributed to mycotoxins (Roffe et al 1989, Windingstad et al 1989). In 1987, an epizootic in captive cranes in Maryland caused illness in 240 of 300 cranes and the death of 15 of these cranes (including two whooping cranes and two endangered Mississippi sandhill cranes) (Olsen et al 1995). Clinical signs were non-specific, and included weakness, necrosis of mucous membranes of the mouth or tongue, depression and dehydration, followed by ataxia, recumbency and death. Gross pathological findings were inconclusive, consisting of dehydration, atrophy of fat, renal insufficiency and small spleens. Further research isolated *Fusarium* spp. mould from the pelleted diet and low levels of two mycotoxins, T_2 (1–2 ppm) and deoxynivalenol (0.4 ppm). Testing of all grain-based feeds prior to feeding to cranes is recommended to prevent mycotoxin exposure.

Parasitic diseases

Parasites are often opportunistic and clinically significant where cranes are stressed or crowded, especially when kept in captivity. Clinical signs of parasitism are often non-specific, and may include lethargy, weight loss, enteritis or dyspnoea. In the captive situation, a parasite monitoring and treatment programme is important for raising and maintaining healthy cranes. Reducing crowding and other stress factors, plus annual pen rotation and treatment of new birds during quarantine, can result in a relatively parasite-free flock.

Gapeworms (*Syngamus* spp. and *Cyanthostoma* spp.) can cause severe tracheitis, bronchitis, dyspnoea and even death associated with mucus plugs forming in the trachea. A diagnosis of gapeworm infestation may be made by observing the parasites in the upper trachea, or by tracheal washes. Fenbendazole given at 100 mg/kg p.o. once daily for 5 days has been effective in eliminating the parasite in infected cranes (Olsen et al 1996a). Care must be taken to shake the fenbendazole suspension well before administration to reduce the possibility of fenbendazole toxicity in the crane patient.

Capillaria spp., *Eucoleus* spp. and *Ascaridia* spp. all infect cranes, leading to weakness, lethargy, weight loss and, occasionally, enteritis. Diagnosis of the nematodes listed above is easily made by faecal flotation (Fig. 10.9). Treatment with a combination of fenbendazole 100 mg/kg p.o. and 0.2 mg/kg ivermectin subcutaneously or per os, both given once and then repeated in 1–2 weeks, has been effective in eliminating these common parasites but management measures should be implemented to prevent the bird's re-exposure to the parasites (Olsen et al 1996a).

Acanthocephalans (spiny-headed worms, Fig. 10.10) infest cranes and can produce a perforation of the intestines, which often results in a fatal coelomitis. As with many parasite infestations this condition is more commonly seen in crane chicks than in adults. Arthropods are the most common intermediate host of spiny-headed worms. No effective treatment is known; controlling exposure is therefore of primary importance.

Cranes are especially susceptible to coccidial infections caused by *Eimeria gruis* (Fig. 10.11) and *E. reichenowi*. With sandhill and whooping cranes, coccidia are found in the intestines and in other vital organs (Carpenter et al 1980, 1984, Novilla et al 1989). Because of this extra-intestinal pathological development affecting crane species the disease is called disseminated visceral coccidiosis (DVC). In DVC, granulomatous nodules form in various tissues, and symptoms consistent with such conditions as hepatitis, pneumonia, tracheitis, myocarditis or enteritis may be identified. The disease is most severe in chicks under 60 days of age, and is often fatal. Characteristic white nodules are observed in the various affected tissues during the necropsy examination.

Even though coccidia are commonly found in wild cranes, the disease is much more of a problem in the captive situation due to husbandry practices that promote the concentration of coccidia in the soil of an enclosure. **Yearly or even every third year (three pens per group of cranes) pen rotation helps to reduce coccidia concentrations within the soil.** In addition, various food and water additives have proved useful in controlling DVC. These include amprolium (0.006% in drinking water or 0.0125–0.025 mg/kg in feed) or monensin (99 ppm in feed) (Carpenter et al 1992, 2005). Clazuril at 1.1 and 5.5 ppm in feed was not effective in preventing DVC in challenged cranes (Carpenter et al 2005).

Avian blood parasites have been identified in sandhill cranes in Florida (Dusek et al 2004) and grey crowned cranes and wattled cranes from southern Africa (Peirce & Anderson 2002). In the Florida study, *Haemoproteus antigonis* was found in 7% of sandhill crane chicks, and *H. balearicae* in 3% of chicks including one that was severely anaemic (packed cell volume (PCV) 13%). This chick was later found moribund and died. Death was attributed to severe

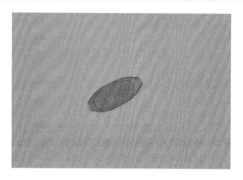

Fig 10.9 *Capillaria* spp. diagnosed on a faecal flotation examination of crane faeces.

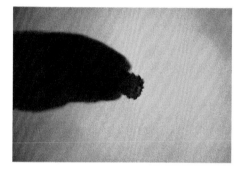

Fig 10.10 Acanthocephalan or thorny-headed worm that penetrated the jejunum causing peritonitis and death of the young whooping crane.

Fig 10.11 *Eimeria gruis* found by faecal flotation. This coccidial organism along with *Eimeria reichenowi* can cause a fatal disseminated visceral coccidiosis in crane chicks.

anaemia and early cardiomyodegeneration (Dusek et al 2004). Parasites identified in the crane study encompassing southern Africa included *H. antigonis*, *H. balearica* and *Leucocytozoon grusi* (Peirce & Anderson 2002).

Ectoparasites infest both captive and wild cranes. Five species of mites (order Acarina) and four species of biting lice (order Mallophaga) have been documented affecting crane species (Forrester et al 1976, Atyeo &

Windingstad 1979). Severe cases of ectoparasites, especially in chicks, can be debilitating. Control is achieved by dusting cranes with 5% carbaryl or 0.10% pyrethrin powders. Biting and stinging insects, including bees (*Apis* spp.), wasps (*Vepis* spp.), black flies (*Simulium* spp.) and deer flies (*Chrysops* spp.), will attack cranes, causing localized inflammation of the skin, excessive preening, discomfort and stress. Occasionally the mucous membranes in the mouth will swell due to an inflammatory response resulting from the crane trying to catch the insect and being stung in the attempt. This is a common occurrence in chicks around fledging age.

Orthopaedic problems

Cranes being large, long-legged birds that initially grow very fast, are predisposed to a number of different orthopaedic problems at various stages in their lives. Orthopaedic problems can be serious and even fatal, due to complications associated with fractures. At the International Crane Foundation in Baraboo, Wisconsin, fractures and subsequent complications were listed as the cause of death of 10% (*n* = 11) of all mortalities (Hartman 1983). At the Patuxent Wildlife Research Center in Laurel, Maryland, fractures and complications contributed to 4% (*n* = 5) of the deaths of captive Mississippi sandhill cranes (*Grus canadensis pulla*) (Olsen & Gee 1996) and 5% (*n* = 5) of mortalities in captive whooping cranes (*Grus americana*) in a 14-year period (Olsen et al 1996b). Other common orthopaedic injuries include fractures and soft tissue injuries to ligaments, tendons and/or joints. Soft tissue injuries to the intertarsal joint (hock) occur in 4% of the 120 cranes at the International Crane Foundation annually (Linn et al 2003). Fractures and soft tissue injuries in older birds are often associated with capture, handling and transport; therefore handlers should hold cranes in such a manner as to prevent or reduce orthopaedic injuries as described earlier.

Paediatric orthopaedics

Injuries and deformities in chicks are different from those seen in adult cranes. Fractures in birds <1 year of age commonly occur during the first 4 months of life, with 32% of all fractures in young birds noted in the age range of 9–12 weeks, and 64% occurring during the period of 5–16 weeks of age (Olsen 1994). The high incidence of fractures during this period coincides with the period of open epiphyseal plates – closure of the epiphyseal plates takes place at 10–14 weeks. Crane chicks reared by artificial (hand-rearing) means have more orthopaedic problems than crane chicks raised by parent birds, and one possible reason for this may be the reduced levels of exercise seen in the hand-reared

chicks. Parent-raised birds spend most of their day walking behind or near parent birds.

Nutrition definitely plays an important role in raising healthy crane chicks. Although the specific nutrient requirements of cranes are not completely known, three diets for cranes of different age/breeding status have been formulated at the Patuxent Wildlife Research Center (Table 10.2) and are commercially produced (Ziegler Bros. Inc., PO Box 95, Garners, PA, USA). Chicks are normally fed the starter diet until after fledging, at which time a maintainer diet is provided. The starter diet is higher in calcium and protein than the maintainer ration while the breeder diet is higher in calcium and only slightly lower in protein than the starter diet.

Experimentally, diets containing higher levels of protein (32%) and 1.13% sulphur-containing amino acids had a 25% incidence of wing disorders and 17%

Table 10.2 Composition of the diets for crane chicks (Starter), non-breeding adults (Maintainer) and breeding adults (Breeder) (Swengel & Carpenter 1996, Olsen & Carpenter 1997)

Ingredient/nutrient	Starter	Maintainer	Breeder
Protein (%)	23.8	19.4	20.5
Metabolizable energy (kcal/kg)	2689	2530	2533
Calcium (%)	1.4	1.0	2.45
Phosphorus (%)	0.90	0.86	0.89
Methionine and cystine (%)	0.70	–	–
Lysine (%)	1.30	–	–
Ground yellow corn (%)	24.4	38.8	41.2
Soybean meal (44% protein) (%)	–	13.1	15.0
Soybean meal (49% protein) (%)	31.5	–	–
Wheat middlings (%)	12.0	12.6	10.0
Fish meal (60% protein) (%)	–	4.0	5.0
Ground oats (%)	11.5	15.7	7.5
Meal and bone meal (%)	–	5.2	4.0
Alfalfa meal (17% protein) (%)	5.0	5.2	5.0
Corn distiller's solubles (%)	3.0	–	1.5
Brewer's dried yeast (%)	2.5	–	2.0
Corn oil (%)	3.3	–	–
Dried whey (%)	1.2	3.2	3.5
Limestone (%)	1.5	0.5	3.5
Dicalcium phosphate (%)	3.0	0.5	1.0
Iodized salt (%)	0.25	0.5	0.5
Vitamin/mineral premix (%)	0.5	0.5	0.5

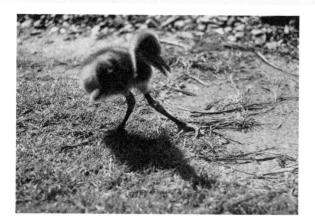

Fig 10.12 Whooping crane (*Grus americana*) chick with splay leg syndrome.

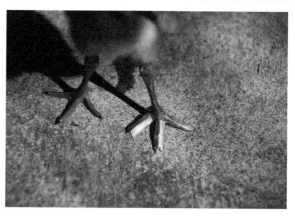

Fig 10.13 Small whooping crane chick with very crooked toes. Correction can be done with a wooden dowel and low-tack adhesive tape applied for 48 hours.

incidence of leg disorders in one study (Serafin 1982). The disorders were primarily weak and deformed proximal tibiotarsus, tarsometatarsus and distal tibiotarsus (i.e. all the typical sites for fractures in young birds). Greater sandhill crane chicks fed a diet of 24% protein and 0.73% sulphur-containing amino acids had only a 2.5% incidence of leg disorders (Serafin 1980). Similarly, wing development is also affected by diet. Greater sandhill crane chicks raised on a diet containing 24% protein and 0.87% sulphur-containing amino acids had a 16% rate of wing deformities (primarily rotation of metacarpals seen at the stage when feathers are developing). Crane chicks on a diet of 24% protein and 0.73–0.78% sulphur-containing amino acids had only a 5% rate of such wing deformities, and those deformities were correctable with bandaging.

There are several orthopaedic problems seen post-hatching that appear unrelated to diet. Improper incubation techniques or exposure to slippery surfaces early in life may contribute to a condition resulting in splay-leg (a lateral deviation of one or both legs.) Normal chicks walk with the legs parallel to each other and the central toe of each foot pointed forward. Lateral deviations that occur can often be corrected by placing temporary hobbles on the legs (Fig. 10.12). Hobbles are used intermittently over a period of 24–48 hours, and chicks must be monitored closely to ensure accommodation of the hobbles.

Curled toes are another frequently diagnosed orthopaedic condition. This abnormal anatomical problem appears to occur more often in crane chicks raised indoors by humans when compared to crane chicks reared by parent birds in natural grass-covered enclosures. The problem may be related to decreased exercise or to improper substrate. The problem is usually correctable by using a small coaptation splint for 48

hours (Fig. 10.13). **The corrective splint for curled toes can be constructed using items commonly stocked in a veterinary hospital, such as a round wooden applicator stick cut to length and taped to the outside curve of the deviated toe.** A low-tack adhesive tape (e.g. filament, packing) works well, whereas ordinary adhesive tape is difficult to remove and may cause further injury. The rapid growth noted in young crane chicks requires splint removal after 48 hours, thereby allowing the leg to rest, usually for 24 hours, before another splint (if needed) is applied. Occasionally an older chick is diagnosed with curled toe. The same theory of splinting the leg is appropriate; however, two wooden applicator sticks will be needed on each side of the toe for the older animal.

Fractures in chicks under 5 weeks of age are very rare because the bones are primarily cartilaginous at this stage. Those fractures that do occur are often 'greenstick' fractures and coaptation splints are sufficient for bone healing. The splint may have to be changed every 4–7 days, on the rapidly growing chick. Usually the bone heals in a minimal time, and the splint may be removed in as little as 3 weeks. Wing-bone fractures that occur at a young age often cause severe disruption of the normal growth pattern, which may lead to a permanently crippled bird.

Adult orthopaedics

Many of the fractures and orthopaedic injuries that occur in other avian species are also diagnosed in cranes. **Figure-of-eight bandages have been used successfully to treat fractures of the wing distal to the elbow.** However, if additional stabilization is required, intramedullary (IM) pins and external skeletal fixation (ESF) are recommended, with the techniques for application being the same as described in most avian orthopaedic articles (Olsen 1994, Olsen et al 2000). Fractures of the femur usually require IM pinning. Historically, wing fractures in captive cranes respond favourably to treatment. In one study, all cranes treated for wing fractures had a successful outcome (the fracture healed; however, as these were all captive birds, the full flight function of the fractured wings was never tested) (Olsen 1994).

Orthopaedic problems in the pelvic limb have a more guarded prognosis because of the crane's reliance on two functional legs to survive. Any severe injury to a pelvic limb that renders the crane unable to stand may cause the animal to violently struggle, to the point where it becomes exhausted or injures the bones of the other leg or wings. Repair of the fractured bone can be accomplished using standard orthopaedic techniques such as coaptation splints, IM pins or ESF, with the goal being for the crane to stand immediately after the surgery. **If the crane patient is unable to stand after surgical repair, it may be necessary to place the bird in a temporary sling.** Crane slings have been constructed using a framework of PVC water pipes to which heavy fabric is secured (Olsen et al 1996a). Any crane placed in such a sling must be monitored carefully to determine how well the bird tolerates the device. Giving small doses of a tranquillizer such as diazepam (0.5 mg/kg) may help during the adjustment period.

Joint luxations are rarely seen in cranes. Elbow luxations can be reduced if diagnosed early; however, there is a high probability of reduced function of the affected joint. The author has treated two cases of coxofemoral luxation in cranes, and with both birds, the injury could not be reduced and maintained in a normal position. Surgery to remove the femoral head and neck was very successful in one case, but in the second case the crane never returned to a normal gait. The inability of one bird to recover was possibly related more to the severe muscle damage that had occurred in the coxofemoral area.

Ultrasonographic imaging was used to diagnose the complete avulsion of the cranial tibial tendon from its insertion in a sandhill crane, and a lateral reticular tear with medial displacement of the gastrocnemius tendon and tibial cartilage in a Siberian crane (Linn et al 2003). However, because of ossification of tendons in most of the pelvic limb muscles, ultrasonographic interpretation anywhere other than joints is difficult due to acoustic shadowing (Linn et al 2003). Because of this tendon ossification, radiography of the pelvic limb may be a useful technique for evaluating soft tissue injuries in cranes (Linn et al 2003).

One serious complication occasionally noted in cranes is necrosis of the leg when a fracture occurs below the hock. There is very little soft tissue in this area, and any vascular trauma can result in ischaemia.

However, it is possible to amputate the leg at or just above the fracture site and build a prosthetic leg for the crane. The prosthesis can be made from a thin-walled PVC pipe 2.54 cm in diameter, with an inside diameter of 2.38 cm. The prosthesis is held onto the stump of the leg using adhesive tape (Fig. 10.14), which is usually wrapped up around the hock to avoid slipping. The tape and the prosthesis must be changed every 30–60 days. One Mississippi sandhill crane lived for 20 years with such a device (Fig. 10.15, Olsen 1994).

Neoplasia

Neoplasms are generally very rare in most crane species, and those reported include renal carcinoma and adenocarcinomas (Montali 1977, Decker & Hruska 1978), lymphocytic and granulocytic leukaemias (Montali 1977,

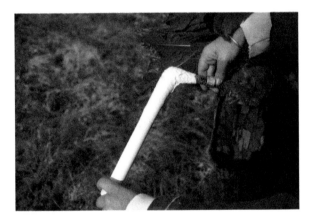

Fig 10.14 Artificial limb made from thin-walled PVC pipe and attached just below the hock on a sandhill crane with an amputated tarsometatarsus.

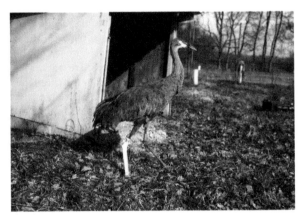

Fig 10.15 Endangered Mississippi sandhill crane with a PVC artificial leg. This crane lived for 20 years with this leg.

Wei 1986) and metastatic cholangiocarcinoma (Allen et al 1985). There has been a high incidence of adenocarcinoma found in the wild population of Mississippi sandhill cranes, with no corresponding cases identified within the captive flocks of this species.

Exertional myopathy

Exertional myopathy (also called capture myopathy or exertional rhabdomyolysis) occurs in crane species after capture or restraint. Reported cases have occurred in East African crowned cranes (*Balearica rugelorum gibbericaps*) (Brannian et al 1981), greater sandhill cranes (Windingstad et al 1983), Mississippi sandhill cranes (Carpenter et al 1991) and whooping cranes (Hanley et al 2005). **The presenting signs of exertional myopathy include pain on movement, stiff movements, swollen hard muscles, trauma to limbs associated with struggling, and peracute death from cardiac failure.** One diagnostic aid is to detect high serum concentrations of creatine kinase, lactic dehydrogenase, aspartate aminotransferase (Windingstad et al 1983, Businga et al 2007) and an elevated alanine aminotransferase (Hanley et al 2005). If the crane does not succumb immediately to cardiac failure, the kidneys may fail due to increased myoglobinuria, uric acid production or dehydration associated with inability to walk properly. **Prevention of capture myopathy is important, and can be accomplished by minimal and proper handling of all cranes.** Treatment is supportive; intravenous fluids, corticosteroids (dexamethasone 1–2 mg/kg q12h subcutaneously or intramuscularly for 1–2 days), vitamin E and selenium (0.06 mg/kg selenium IM, MU-SE, Schering, Union, NJ, USA; Hanley et al 2005) and sodium bicarbonate (4–6 mmol/kg) for a physiological acidotic condition (Olsen & Carpenter 1997, Businga et al 2007). Additional supportive therapy of lactated Ringer's solution 60–180 mL q12h subcutaneously for days 2–5 and nutritional support such as Emeraid Nutri-Support (Lafeber Company, 24981 N 1400 East Road, Cornell, Illinois 61219) 60–120 mL q12h orally by red rubber feeding tube is recommended until the crane is eating and drinking on its own.

Cranes that are unable to stand on their own or are unable to eat must be watched for possible progression of exertional myopathy. The prognosis is grave if the crane fails to improve or continues to decline. If no improvement is seen by day 12 post onset, the prognosis for return to normal function should be considered poor and euthanasia considered (Hanley et al 2005).

On gross pathological examination muscles may appear diffusely to completely pale or pale streaked. Some muscles may have fine white chalky streaks. Histopathological findings include widely dispersed to frequent necrotic myofibrils in the pectoral and leg muscles.

The affected fibres appear swollen and have suffered hyaline or flocculent degeneration (Hanley et al 2005).

Intraspecific aggression

The leading cause of trauma in cranes is intraspecific aggression. At Patuxent Wildlife Research Center, 7.3% of whooping crane deaths over a 15-year period were caused by intraspecific aggression. This aggression is often associated with the formation of pair bonds in the spring (breeding season), and it is occasionally seen with dominance hierarchy formation in a group of cranes. The latter often occurs when a new crane is moved into a pen, and it is recommended that a new social unit (pair or group) should be formed in a pen new to all the cranes to decrease the possibility of intraspecific aggression. If this is not possible, the next best scenario is to introduce the new crane into an adjacent pen until the established cranes have the opportunity to accept it. The third type of aggression that occurs among cranes is termed 'divorce', and is seen when an established pair begins fighting. In spite of the ornithology books stating that cranes mate for life, not all pair bonds last that long.

Aggression is usually directed toward the head and neck, causing extensive soft tissue injuries and even skull fractures (Fig. 10.16). The crane losing the engagement is often in deep shock when presented. Treatment consists of corticosteroids (dexamethasone 2–4 mg/kg or prednisolone sodium succinate 30 mg/kg intravenously initially), intravenous lactated Ringer's solution, and antibiotics. Radiographs and any extensive wound treatment are performed after the crane is stabilized. One result of aggression to the head is permanent scarring of the red skin on top of the head. The injured crane should never be reintroduced into the same social grouping.

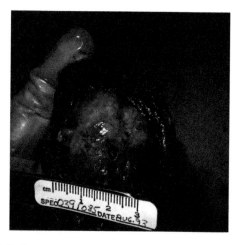

Fig 10.16 Deep wound penetrating skull and into brain caused by pen mate aggression.

HANDBOOK OF AVIAN MEDICINE

References

Allen J L, Martin H D, Crowley A M 1985 Metastatic cholangiocarcinoma in a Florida sandhill crane. Journal of the American Veterinary Medical Association 187:1215

Atyeo W T, Windingstad R M 1979 Feather mites of the greater sandhill crane. Journal of Parasitology 65:650–658

Bailey T A, Toosi A, Samour J H 1999 Anaesthesia of cranes with alphaxolone-alphadolone. Veterinary Record 145(3):84–85

Balis G, Munroe R 1964 The pharmacology of chloralose. Psychopharmacologia 6:1–30

Bowman M R, Waldoch J A, Pittman J M et al 2004 Enrofloxacin and ciprofloxacin plasma concentrations in sandhill cranes (Grus canadensis) after enrofloxacin administration in drinking water. Journal of Avian Medicine and Surgery 18(3):144–150

Brannian R E, Grahm G L, Creswell J 1981 Restraint associated myopathy in East African crowned cranes. In: Fowler M E (ed) Proceedings of the American Association of Zoo Veterinarians. American Association of Zoo Veterinarians, p 21–23

Businga N K, Langenberg J, Calson L 2007 Successful treatment of capture myopathy in three wild greater sandhill cranes (Grus canadensis tabida). Journal of Avian Medicine and Surgery 21(4):294–298

Carpenter J W 2003 Gruiformes (cranes, limpkins, rails, gallinules, coots, bustards), Chapter 20. In: Fowler M E, Miller R E (eds) Zoo and wild animal medicine, 5th edn. Saunders, St Louis, MO, p 171–180

Carpenter J W, Spraker T R, Novilla M N 1980 Disseminated visceral coccidiosis in whooping cranes. Journal of the American Veterinary Medical Association 177:488–845

Carpenter J W, Novilla M N, Fayer R et al 1984 Disseminated visceral coccidiosis in sandhill cranes. Journal of the American Veterinary Medical Association 185:1342–1346

Carpenter J W, Thomas J J, Reevers S 1991 Capture myopathy in an endangered sandhill crane (Grus canadensis tabida). Journal of Zoo and Wildlife Medicine 22:488–493

Carpenter J W, Novilla M N, Hatfield J S 1992 The safety and physiologic effects of the anticoccidial drugs monensin and clazuril in sandhill cranes (Grus canadensis). Journal of Zoo and Wildlife Medicine 23:214–221

Carpenter J W, Mashima T Y, Rupiper D J 1996 Exotic animal formulary. Greystone Publications, Manhattan, KS

Carpenter J W, Novilla M N, Hatfield J S 2005 Efficacy of selected coccidiostats in sandhill cranes (Grus canadensis) following challenge. Journal of Zoo and Wildlife Medicine 36(3):391–400

Clark G C, Dein F J, Crabbs C L et al 1987 Antibody response of sandhill and whooping cranes to an eastern equine encephalitis virus vaccine. Journal of Wildlife Diseases 23:539–544

Decker R A, Hruska J C 1978 Renal adenocarcinoma in a sarus crane (Grus antigone). Journal of Zoo Animal Medicine 9:15

Dein F J, Carpenter J W, Clark G C et al 1986 Mortality of captive whooping cranes caused by eastern equine encephalitis virus. Journal of the American Veterinary Medical Association 189:1006–1010

Di Somma A, Bailey T, Silvanose C, Garcia-Marinez C 2007 The use of voriconazole for the treatment of aspergillosis in falcons (Falco species). Journal of Avian Medicine and Surgery 21(4):307–316

Doeherty D E 1987 Inclusion body disease of cranes. In: Friend M (ed) Field guide to wildlife diseases. US Department of Interior Fish and Wildlife Service, p 129–134

Dusek R J, Spalding M G, Forrester D J, Greiner E C 2004 Haemoproteus balearicae and other blood parasites of free-ranging Florida sandhill crane chicks. Journal of Wildlife Diseases 40(4):682–687

Forrester D J, White F H, Simpson C F. 1976 Parasites and diseases of sandhill cranes in Florida. In: Lewis J C (ed) Proceedings of the International Crane Workshop. Oklahoma State University, p 284–290

Hanley C S, Thomas N J, Paul-Murphy J et al 2005 Exertional myopathy in whooping cranes (Grus americana) with prognostic guidelines. Journal of Zoo and Wildlife Medicine 36(3):489–497

Hartman L M 1983 Summary of mortality of 14 species of cranes at the International Crane Foundation, 1972–1982. In: Archibald G W, Pasquier R F (eds) Proceedings of the International Crane Workshop. International Crane Foundation, p 555–570

Hayes M A, Hartup B K, Pittman J M, Barzen J A 2003 Capture of sandhill cranes using alpha-chloralose. Journal of Wildlife Diseases 39(4):859–868

Jones K L, Krapu G L, Brandt D A, Ashley M V 2005 Population genetic structure in migratory sandhill cranes and the role of Pleistocene glaciations. Molecular Ecology 14(9):2645–2657

Joseph V, Pappagianis D, Reavill D R 1994 Clotrimazole nebulization for the treatment of respiratory aspergillosis. In: Kornelgen M J (ed) Proceedings of the Association of Avian Veterinarians. Association of Avian Veterinarians, p 301–306

Kepler C B 1978 Captive propagation of whooping cranes: a behavioral approach. In: Temple S A (ed) Endangered birds: management techniques for preserving threatened species. University of Wisconsin Press, p 231–241

Linn K A, Templer A S, Paul-Murphy J R et al 2003 Ultrasonographic imaging of the sandhill crane (Grus canadensis) intertarsal joint. Journal of Zoo and Wildlife Medicine 34(2):144–152

Lukert P D, Saif Y M 2003 Infectious bursal disease. In: Saif Y M (ed) Diseases of poultry, 11th edn. Iowa State Press, Ames, IA, p 161–179

Maeda Y, Tohya Y, Nakagami Y et al 2001 An occurrence of Salmonella infection in cranes at the Izumi Plains, Japan. Journal of Veterinary Medicine Science 63(8):943–944

Montali R J 1977 An overview of tumors in zoo animals. Journal of the American Veterinary Medical Association 171:531

Novilla M N, Carpenter J W, Jeffers T K et al 1989 Pulmonary lesions in disseminated visceral coccidiosis of sandhill and whooping cranes. Journal of Wildlife Diseases 25:527–532

Olsen G H 1994 Orthopedics in cranes: pediatrics and adults. Seminars in Avian and Exotic Pet Medicine 3:73–80

Olsen G H, Carpenter J W 1997 Cranes. In: Altman R B, Clubb S L, Dorrestein G M, Quesenberry K E (eds) Avian medicine and surgery. W B Saunders, Philadelphia, PA, p 973–991

Olsen G H, Gee G F 1996 Causes of Mississippi sandhill crane mortality in captivity, 1984–1995. Proceedings of the North American Crane Workshop 7:249–252

Olsen G H, Carpenter J W, Gee G F et al 1995 Mycotoxin-induced disease in captive whooping cranes (Grus americana) and sandhill cranes (Grus canadensis). Journal of Zoo and Wildlife Medicine 26:569–576

Olsen G H, Carpenter J W, Langenberg J A 1996a Medicine and surgery. In: Ellis D H, Gee G F, Mirande C M (eds) Cranes, their biology, husbandry, and conservation. US Department of Interior, p 137–174

Olsen G H, Taylor J A, Gee G F 1996b Whooping crane mortality at Patuxent Wildlife Research Center, 1982–1995. Proceedings of the North American Crane Workshop 7:243–248

Olsen G H, Turell M J, Pagac B B 1997 Efficacy of eastern equine encephalitis immunization in whooping cranes. Journal of Wildlife Diseases 33:312–315

Olsen G H, Redig P T, Orosz S E 2000 Limb dysfunction. Manual of avian medicine. Mosby., St Louis, MO, p 493–526

Olsen G H, Miller, K J, Docherty, D, Sileo, L, 2003 West Nile virus vaccination and challenge in sandhill cranes (Grus canadensis). In: Proceedings of the Association of Avian Veterinarians. Association of Avian Veterinarians, p 123–124

Pagac B B, Turell M J, Olsen G H 1992 Eastern equine encephalomyelitis virus and Culieta melanura activity at the Patuxent Wildlife Research

Center, 1985–1990. Journal of the American Mosquito Control Association 8:328–330

Peirce M A, Anderson M D 2002 Haematozoa in southern African cranes. Ostrich 73:179–180

Roffe T J, Stroud R K, Windingstad R M 1989 Suspected fusariomy-cotoxicosis in sandhill cranes (*Grus canadensis*): clinical and pathological findings. Avian Diseases 33:451–457

Serafin J A 1980 Influence of dietary energy and sulfur amino acid levels upon growth and development of young sandhill cranes. In: Proceedings of the American Association of Zoo Veterinarians. American Association of Zoo Veterinarians, p 30

Serafin J A 1982 The influence of diet composition upon growth and development of sandhill cranes. Condor 84:427–434

Snyder S B 1996 Avian tuberculosis in a whooping crane: treatment and outcome. Proceedings of the North American Crane Workshop 7:253–255

Swengel S R, Carpenter J W 1996 General husbandry. In: Ellis D H, Gee G F, Mirande C M (eds) Cranes, their biology, husbandry, and conservation. US Department of Interior, p 31–43

Wei Y C 1986 Three cases of granulocytic leukemia in the red-crested crane. Chinese Journal of Zoology 21:32–33

Wellinton M, Burke A, Nicolich J M, O'Malley K 1996 Chick rearing. In: Ellis D H, Gee G F, Mirande C M (eds) Cranes, their biology, husbandry, and conservation. US Department of Interior, p 77–104

Windingstad R M, Hurley S S, Sileo L 1983 Capture myopathy in a free-flying greater sandhill crane (*Grus canadensis tabida*) from Wisconsin. Journal of Wildlife Diseases 19:289–290

Windingstad R M, Richard J C, Nelson P E et al 1989 Fusarium mycotoxins from peanuts suspected as a cause of sandhill crane mortality. Journal of Wildlife Diseases 25:38–46

Young L A, Citino S B, Seccareccia V et al 1996 Eastern equine encephalitis in an exotic avian collection. In: LaBonde J (ed) Proceedings of the Association of Avian Veterinarians. Association of Avian Veterinarians, p 163–165

Ratites

Thomas N. Tully, Jr

11

Introduction

Ratites are classified into four different orders and five families. The common ratite species include ostriches, emus, rheas, cassowaries and kiwis. Ratites are native to most of the continents and a few large islands of the southern hemisphere (ostriches in Africa, rheas in South America, emus in Australia, cassowaries in Australia and New Guinea, kiwis in New Zealand; see Chapter 17). The birds are similar in being flightless, but each one is a different avian species with diverse physiological and anatomical features.

Historically ratites have been very popular animals in zoological collections, but recently there has been a worldwide interest in farming these birds. South Africa has been the major exporter of ostrich products and a leading ostrich producer for over 100 years. Ostriches are native to South Africa, thereby giving farmers the advantage of proper environmental conditions for optimum production. The South African farmer alone has maintained this market and generated a demand for ostrich skin and meat, but other countries have now seen the potential of ratites (including emus and rheas) as an alternative livestock commodity that can thrive in small unproductive areas of farm or ranch land. Currently, ratite producers around the world are working to develop a niche for the meat, hide and by-products of these avian species.

Anatomical features

This chapter will focus on the two ratite species commonly raised for production purposes; the emu and the ostrich. It will include some information regarding the rhea, but the number of rheas being raised in captivity at this time is relatively small.

The ostrich averages 2.5–3 m in height, and weighs approximately 150 kg. The emu averages 1.7 m in height and weighs about 45 kg. The male ostrich is larger on average than the female, while the female emu is generally larger than the male. Ratites as a group receive their name from their sternum, which is devoid of a keel (Fig. 11.1). The sternum in flighted birds has a prominent keel from which the large pectoral muscles originate, but ratites do not need the large pectoral muscles

to fly and therefore do not need a keel. **Since ratites do not have large pectoral muscles, the injection sites of choice are the epaxial muscles or the large upper leg muscles.**

One of the most medically significant differences between ostriches, emus and rheas concerns their digestive tracts (Table 11.1). The variations manifest themselves in common gastrointestinal disorders, especially in mismanaged ostriches. Ostriches and rheas primarily utilize their hindgut to digest their food, and animals that primarily use their caudal intestinal tract to digest food take a long period of time for the passage of digesta (Fig. 11.2). **The average length of time for the passage of digesta through the gastrointestinal tract is 48 hours in an ostrich, 18 hours in a rhea and 7 hours**

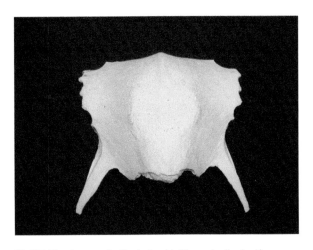

Fig 11.1 The sternum of ratites is devoid of the protruding keel bone prevalent in other avian species.

Table 11.1 Comparative length of ratite intestines (cm) (Fowler 1996)

	Ostrich	Emu	Rhea
Small intestine	36	94	62
Caeca	7	2	21
Rectum	57	4	17

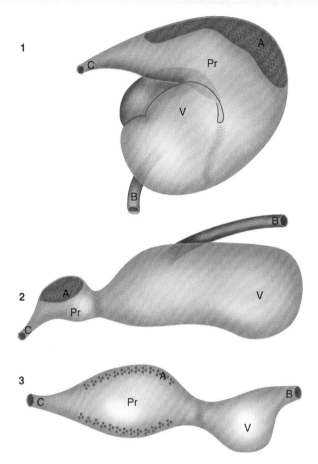

Fig 11.2 Diagrams of the stomach of ratites. **1**, Ostrich; **2**, rhea; and **3**, emu and cassowary. A, glandular area of the proventriculus; B, duodenum; C, oesophagus; Pr, proventriculus; V, ventriculus.

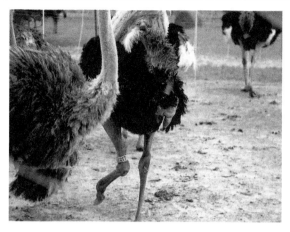

Fig 11.3 Protruding phallus of an ostrich which protrudes from the ventral floor of the proctodeum.

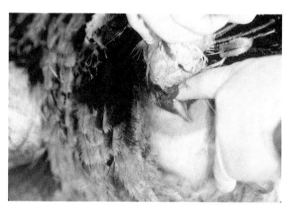

Fig 11.4 Digital presentation of the phallus of a 6-month-old male ostrich.

in an emu. The long period of time that is noted in the ostrich predisposes these birds to impaction problems and colic, whereas emus rarely develop a gastrointestinal blockage or impaction due to mismanagement or stress. The ostrich's digestive system does, however, appear to benefit the producer raising the birds as an agricultural enterprise, since feed conversion is better with longer gastrointestinal transit times.

Ostrich, rhea and emu males have protruding phalluses (Fig. 11.3). All ratites are monomorphic when hatched and at birth, and vent or DNA blood sexing and feather colour characteristics may be used to sex the young birds. It does help to have experience in sexing young ratites, and the veterinarian's skill will increase with such experience (Fig. 11.4).

The respiratory system of ratites is similar to other avian species with the exception of the emu. A tracheal cleft is located midway down the length of this anatomical structure in the emu. The cleft interfaces with a cervical 'air pouch' (Figs 11.5 and 11.6). To prevent

inflation during an anaesthetic procedure, an elastic non-adhesive bandage material (Vetwrap®, Animal Care Products – 3 M, St Paul, Minnesota, USA) may be applied around the midcervical region (Fowler 1996).

Husbandry

Nutrition

Ratite species are typically omnivores, but the birds can survive on just about any animal diet formulation. To achieve reproductive success and fast market growth, species-specific diets are required – ostrich food for ostriches, emu food for emus, breeder food for breeders, and growth diets for young birds. The nutritional requirements are simple; for success, feed a formulated diet. Although simple, it benefits the veterinarian to understand some of the basic requirements for optimum ratite growth. Water is a nutrient that is often overlooked as an important component of a bird's dietary intake. **Reduction of growth, poor feed efficiency, and impaired reproductive activity are consequences of inadequate**

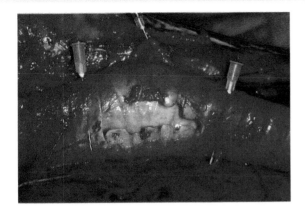

Fig 11.5 The tracheal cleft found in emus is a normal anatomical structure.

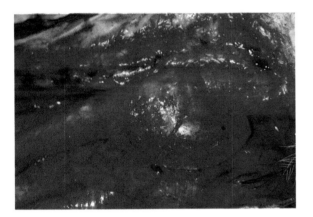

Fig 11.6 'Air pouch' surrounding the tracheal cleft.

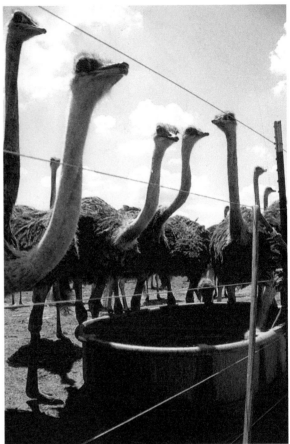

Fig 11.7 A large group of ostriches with adequate exposure to clean fresh water.

water intake (Kienholz 1978). In a study where ostriches were deprived of water for 24 hours their food intake was reduced by 45% with a further decline to 67% after 48 hours of water deprivation (Levy et al 1990). Ratites should receive adequate quantities of fresh clean water in receptacles that are easy to access. It is also important to have water available in areas where all birds can drink with minimal spillage to prevent mud pits from forming (Fig. 11.7). Ostriches consume approximately 2 to 3 times as much water as feed, on a weight basis, ranging from 1.8 to 2.6 water-to-dry matter intake for 1-year-old birds (Angel et al 1996, Degen et al 1991).

The nutrient requirements for ratites are still being investigated but there have been scientific studies performed that have determined basic energy and protein needs (Angel et al 1996). A 45.5 kg adult emu was determined to require maintenance levels of 1303 kcal metabolizable energy/day and 10.9 g protein/day based on an Australian study (Dawson 1983). Ostrich nutritional information is more readily available due to their long-term use as a production animal in South Africa. Tables 11.2–11.7 provide nutritional data for various ostrich ages and breeding states that have been scientifically

Table 11.2 Predicted energy and amino acid requirement of ostriches

Days of age	10	30	100
Intake (kg/day)	0.11	0.29	1.2
Energy metabolized (kcal/kg)	3080	2630	2390
Lysine (%)	1.2	1.0	0.86
Methionine plus cystine (%)	0.8	0.68	0.57

established in South African nutritional studies (Cilliers & Van Schalkwyk 1994, Du Preez 1991).

Adult emus will decrease food consumption by 50–75% during the breeding season, especially the male birds (Angel et al 1996). After the breeding season there is a subsequent increase in food intake for 10–20 days before returning to the normal levels of 0.9 to 1.8 kg/day (Angel et al 1996). The specific dietary requirements for age and breeding status should be considered when selecting feed to obtain optimum health in all ratite species (Table 11.8).

Table 11.3 Nutrient recommendations for South African ostriches (Du Preez 1991)

Diet	Age (months)	Body weight (kg)	Energy (kcal/kg)	% Crude protein	% Lysine	% Total sulphur amino acids
Pre-starter hatch	2	0.77–24	3150	25.0	1.25	0.70
Starter	2–4	11.36–28.2	3015	21.5	1.07	0.60
Grower	4–6	28.64–52.3	2915	17.0	0.90	0.50
Finisher	6–10	52.73–90.9	2600	13.5	0.84	0.46
Post-finisher	10–20	91.36–106.82	1950	8.5	0.63	0.35
Maintenance	Mature	–	1550	8.0	0.30	0.32
Breeder	Laying	–	2200	14.0	0.68	0.70

Table 11.4 Estimated recommendations for energy in laying ostriches (Du Preez 1991)

	Energy requirements (kcal ME) for maintenance and activity Body mass (kg)			Energy (kcal ME) requirements for egg production Egg mass (kg)		
	100	104.55	109	1.18	1.36	1.59
Maintenance	3259	3375	3490			
Activity	327	337	349			
Egg lipid				550	640	734
Egg protein				855	999	1140
Shell (18% of egg mass)				62	72	84
Total	3586	3712	3839	1467	1711	1958

Table 11.5 Estimated amino acid requirements (g/day) for mature ostrich hens (Du Preez 1991)

	For maintenance of body mass (kg)			For egg production including shell (kg)		
	100	104.55	109	1.18	1.36	1.59
Protein (g)	67	69	72	119	138	158
Amino acid (g[a])						
Arginine	5.70	5.87	6.12	3.56	4.15	4.74
Lysine	5.78	5.95	6.21	6.41	7.48	8.55
Methionine	1.86	1.90	2.00	2.67	3.10	3.56
Histidine	2.54	2.61	2.73	1.91	2.20	2.50
Threonine	3.54	3.64	3.80	6.85	8.00	9.13
Valine	4.32	4.46	4.65	5.50	6.40	7.30
Isoleucine	3.50	3.60	3.76	4.55	5.30	6.10
Leucine	6.90	7.14	7.45	9.00	10.50	12.00
Tyrosine	2.33	2.40	2.50	3.70	4.30	4.90
Phenylalanine	3.82	3.90	4.10	4.06	4.67	5.30
Cystine	0.89	0.92	0.96			
Tryptophan	0.73	0.75	0.78			

[a]*Daily requirements of dietary amino acids per gram egg produced. A female ostrich weighing 109 kg and consuming 2000 g/feed/day, producing a 1.18 kg egg at 2-day intervals will require:* $\dfrac{(6.21\,g + 6.41\,g)}{2000\,g\,feed} \times \dfrac{100}{1} = 0.63\%\ lysine\ in\ the\ diet.$

Table 11.6 Macromineral recommendations for South African ostriches (starter, finisher, maintenance, and layer diets) (Cilliers & Van Schalkwyk 1994)

	Total calcium (%)	Available phosphorus (%)	Total sodium (%)
Prestarter, starter and grower diets	1.2–1.5	0.4–0.45	0.2–0.25
Finisher and post-finisher diets	0.9–1.0	0.32–0.36	0.15–0.30
Maintenance diet	0.9–1.0	0.32–0.36	0.15–0.30
Layer diet	2.0–2.5	0.35–0.4	0.15–0.25

Table 11.7 Trace element and vitamin supplementation used in South African ostrich diets (Cilliers & Van Schalkwyk 1994)

	Units or quantity per ton		
	Grower diets (hatch–6 months)	Grower and finisher diets (6 months–slaughter)	Breeder diets
Vit A (IU)	12 000 000	9 000 000	15 000 000
Vit D$_3$ (IU)	3 000 000	2 000 000	25 000 000
Vit E (IU)	40 000	10 000	30 000
Vit K$_3$ (g)	3	2	3
Vit B$_1$ (g)	3	1	2
Vit B$_2$ (g)	8	5	8
Niacin (g)	60	50	45
Calc. panth. A (g)	14	8	18
Vit B$_{12}$ (mg)	100	10	100
Vit B$_6$ (g)	4	3	4
Choline chloride (g)	500	150	500
Folic acid (g)	2	1	1
Biotin (mg)	200	10	100
Magnesium (g)	50	–	40
Manganese (g)	120	80	120
Zinc (g)	80	50	90
Copper (g)	15	15	15
Iodine (g)	0.5	1	1
Cobalt (g)	0.1	0.3	0.1
Iron (g)	35	20	35
Selenium (g)	0.3	0.15	0.3

The digestive system in ratite species is, in general, similar to that of other birds. There are differences between the ratite species in regard to the gastrointestinal tract and this is primarily a result of their dietary intake. Ratites do not have a crop, and a gall bladder is not present in ostriches (Fowler 1996). The proventriculus is found cranial to the ventriculus in most avian species. **In the ostrich the ventriculus is cranial to the caudal half of the proventriculus.** Knowing the correct location of the proventriculus is important for the avian surgeon performing a proventriculotomy on an ostrich patient.

Young birds require growth diets, but if they eat too much too fast they may develop musculoskeletal leg abnormalities (Fig. 11.8). These abnormalities include rotation of the tibiotarsal bone and angular limb deformities. Once young ratites develop leg abnormalities, it is very difficult to treat the problem. Young birds should have exercise, access to grass and regulated feed intake.

Restraint

Ratites (especially ostriches, emus and rheas) are very dangerous to handle, and it is important that veterinarians respect their ratite patients and use proper restraint techniques to examine and treat them. Experienced handlers

Table 11.8 Nutrient ranges in practical diets for ratites

Nutrient	Starter	Grower	Breeder	Maintenance
Ostrich				
Protein (%)	17–28	17–24	15–24	10–20
Metabolizable energy (kcal/g)	2.1–3.2	1.9–2.9	1.6–2.5	1.4–2.3
Lysine (%)	>0.77	>0.75	>0.70	>0.4
Methionine	>0.38	>0.36	>0.34	>0.28
Linoleic acid (%)	>0.75	>0.75	>1.0	>0.4
Fibre (%)	>4.0	>4.0	>6.0	>8.0
Emu				
Protein (%)	17–25	16.5–23	15–25	12–20
Metabolizable energy (kcal/g)	2.0–2.8	1.9–2.7	2.0–2.8	1.7–2.6
Lysine (%)	>0.77	>0.75	>0.80	>0.45
Methionine	>0.38	>0.36	>0.40	>0.28
Linoleic acid (%)	>0.75	>0.75	>1.0	>0.4
Fibre (%)	>4.0	>4.0	>4.0	>4.0

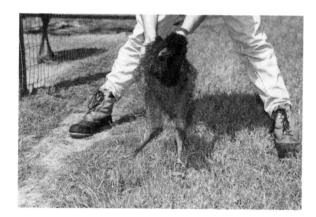

Fig 11.8 Musculoskeletal abnormalities are directly correlated to improper diet and husbandry.

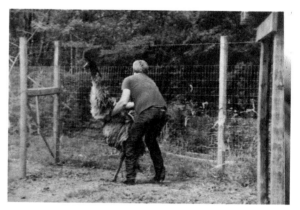

Fig 11.9 An experienced emu handler grabbing a large bird from behind.

should be the only people around adult ratites that are being captured (Fig. 11.9).

Young ostrich and emu chicks should be supported in a sternal position with the legs tucked under the bird in the arms of the handler, thereby reducing their struggles (Raines 1998). Young birds should never be carried upside down by the legs because of their susceptibility to musculoskeletal damage. Ostriches of any age can be sedated by 'hooding' – placing a cloth bag or sleeve over the bird's eyes. For larger birds, the handler may wear a sweatshirt sleeve that can be removed once the beak is captured, and placed over the bird's head. Young birds can be transported in large pet carriers that have substrates with traction to prevent leg injuries.

Juvenile and adult birds are captured and restrained in a similar manner. Emus should be captured by using a swing gate or by running the birds into a narrow chute.

Once the bird is captured the holder should stay behind it, using one hand to grab the chest and resting the other on the dorsum of the back. Adult emus are strong, and kick hard and high. Using emu wings as handles may be effective, but these vestigial wings fracture easily during restraint and, although not life-threatening, the wing fractures affect the general appearance of the bird. It is important that handlers always stay behind captured ratites, to protect both themselves and the birds. Ostriches are very big and may be aggressive during the breeding season. A head hook has been manufactured to aid in moving and capturing ostriches quickly, and is extremely useful (Fig. 11.10). This hook may cause injury, as an ostrich's first instinct when captured is to back up; if the head is pulled at the same time, muscle damage may occur. Ostriches may be captured in appropriate catch pens or chutes by grabbing the head with a

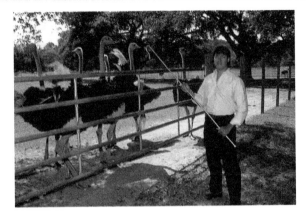

Fig 11.10 An ostrich hook can be used to grab an adult ostrich's head for capture and restraint.

Table 11.9 Tranquillizer/sedative dosages used in ratites (Cornick-Seahorn 1996)

Drug	Dosage (mg/kg)
Acepromazine	0.1–0.2 i.v.
	0.25–0.5 i.m.
Azaperone	0.5–2.0 i.m.
Diazepam	0.1–0.3 i.v.
	0.22–0.44 i.m.
	0.5–1.0 i.m.
Midazolam	0.15 i.m.
Xylazine	0.2–1.0 i.m. (sedation)
	1.0–2.2 i.m. (immobilization)
	0.4–0.9 i.m.
	1500 mg (total dose for adult ostrich)
Detomidine	1.5 i.m.
Medetomidine	0.1 i.m.

Table 11.10 Ratite normal physiological values (Cornick-Seahorn 1996)

Parameter	Ostriches	Emus
Body temperature (°C)	37.2–40.0	37.8–39.8
Heart rate (per min)	57–103	152–192
Respiratory rate (per min)	9–22	13–21

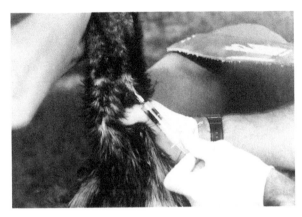

Fig 11.11 The right jugular vein is the recommended site for blood collection and intravenous catheter placement. Blood is being collected in this bird.

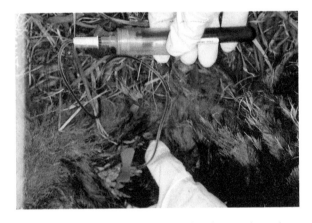

Fig 11.12 A vacutainer system using a butterfly catheter can be used to collect blood from ratites. This is a young ostrich from which a blood sample is being collected.

hook or the hands. If the head is controlled, then the animal is controlled. **A bird with its head captured will back up in order to kick forward, and the bird should therefore be led by the head with one or two people pushing from behind.**

Large ratites should be transported in a well-maintained stock trailer that provides adequate ventilation. Surfaces within the trailer must provide enough traction to prevent injury due to slippage.

Sedation

Once restrained, large aggressive birds have to be sedated with chemical agents (Table 11.9). The patient's vital signs should be monitored throughout the procedure if sedatives are used as an adjunct to restraint (Table 11.10). Ratites should be fasted for 12 hours

if there is a planned anaesthetic procedure (Cornick-Seahorn 1996). There are three main venous access locations in ostriches: the right jugular, the basilic and the medial tarsometatarsal veins (Figs 11.11 and 11.12). Emus do not have an adequate basilic vein for blood collection or catheter placement.

If the birds have to be placed under general anaesthesia, isoflurane is the agent of choice. Isoflurane is used at 4.0–5.0% for induction, and the birds are maintained at 2.0–3.0% (Cornick-Seahorn 1996). A circle rebreathing system is used for birds over 7 kg, and respiration must be

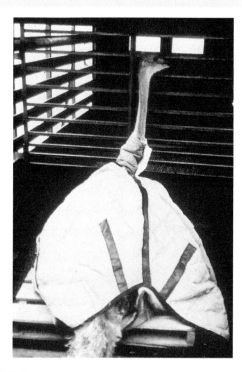

Fig 11.13 An ostrich recovering from anaesthesia with a body wrap to prevent trauma.

monitored closely because of the respiratory depressive effects of isoflurane. A padded recovery stall is recommended for large ratite patients that have been sedated. If a padded stall is not available, wrapping the bird in a heavy cloth or tarpaulin and placing in sternal recumbency will allow for a controlled recovery process (Fig. 11.13).

Health examinations

Veterinary communication and information is critical whether evaluating a single ratite or a flock. It is more likely today that veterinarians will be called for flock management at production units, and, as with many large agricultural ventures, money is made or lost on a very small margin. This small margin means that all areas are open for examination and improvement. When evaluating a ratite facility, the following factors are important criteria relating to production, health and growth: pen size; number of birds per pen; shelter; pen construction (durability); access to feed and water; pen topography; environment surrounding the pen; and stress associated with the surrounding environment (Tully 1998). **Birds should not be placed in overcrowded pens or in pens with birds that are not of the same age and/or size. Overcrowding and mismatching of birds results in injuries and in poor growth and reproduction.** Good management of the production facility means good bird health.

Prior to or during a physical examination, a veterinarian will benefit from taking a proper history regarding the bird in question. The following questions should be answerable by a ratite owner if the facility is being correctly managed (Tully 1998):

1. How long have you owned the bird or cared for it at this facility?
2. Has the bird been recently transported?
3. Has the bird had previous problems, treatments or vaccinations?
4. Is the animal properly identified with proper papers (health certificate, interstate/international transfer, microchip certificate)?
5. What is the health status and history of the flock or farm, including past disease problems and deaths?
6. What is the previous history concerning congenital abnormalities, medication and surgery?
7. What is the sex and reproductive status of the animal?
8. How long has the patient been ill?
9. Has this bird (or any other) been examined by another veterinarian?
10. What food is available, and what does the bird consume?
11. What type of water is used (well or city supply)?
12. Have any pesticides or poisons been used around the cage?
13. Is there a quarantine procedure in place?

Once the bird has been captured and restrained, a 'hands-on' physical examination can take place. The bird should be evaluated from the tip of the beak to the tail. A symmetrical head and beak is normal, and any deviation must be examined more closely to determine the cause of the problem. The ocular examination should include conjunctival, corneal, retinal and anterior and posterior chamber examinations (Tully 1998), and the dehydration status of the bird may be determined through the ocular examination by globe placement in the orbit and hydration of the cornea. Palpation and examination of the skin and feathers may reveal healed injuries, lacerations, abscesses or tumours (Tully 1998). The left ventral aspect of the ostrich body cavity, caudal to the keel, should be palpated for proventricular impactions; if enlarged, gastrointestinal problems may be present (Tully 1998). Wings and legs should be examined for developmental abnormalities, joint swellings, trauma and fractures. Toes should have normal placement and not be 'rolled', a common ostrich developmental abnormality where the toes deviate to the point where the medial or lateral surface of the digit contacts the ground. This is a potentially life-threatening injury if not corrected early in life (Fig. 11.14). **Ratites less than 1 year of age have a number of developmental problems because of their rapid growth**

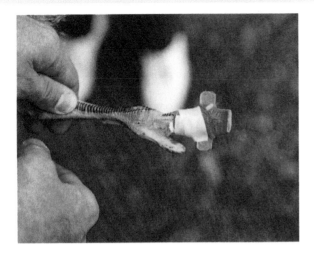

Fig 11.14 Corrective splint used to treat rolled toe in a young ostrich.

Table 11.11 Young ratite diseases

Hatching birds	Malposition/improper incubation
	Iatrogenic drug/supplement toxicity
	Yolk sac infection/retention
Musculoskeletal disorders	Neck deformities at hatch
	Tumbling chick syndrome in emus
	Spraddle leg
	Angular leg deformities
	Rickets
	Osteochondrosis
Gastrointestinal disease	Rolled toes in ostriches
	Slipped gastrocnemius tendon
	Impaction
	Intussusception
	Intestinal torsion
	Cloacal prolapse

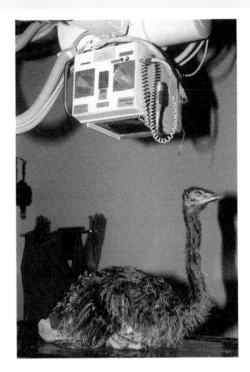

Fig 11.15 A small ostrich in sternal recumbency prepared for full body radiographs.

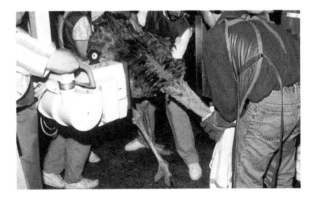

Fig 11.16 Large ostriches require equine or mobile radiographic units to obtain full body radiographs.

and dependence on legs for mobility after hatching (Table 11.11). Musculoskeletal and gastrointestinal disease often require radiographic images to aid in diagnosing a disease process. Smaller ratite patients can be placed in sternal recumbency on a radiograph cassette for full body images while larger birds require mobile units for diagnostic results (Figs 11.15 and 11.16).

The veterinarian must advise the ratite owner that, if any bird dies of unknown circumstances, a necropsy examination is recommended. To have a proper necropsy examination performed by a pathologist usually takes 10–12 days, and the sooner an animal is examined the quicker the owner will receive the results. There are a number of infectious diseases that affect ostriches, emus and rheas (Table 11.12).

Aspergillosis

Aetiology and occurrence Aspergillus *fumigatus* and other *Aspergillus* spp. Most commonly diagnosed in emus, rheas, and ostriches that have been maintained in enclosed, dusty environs (Shane 1998, Perez et al 2003, Copetti et al 2004). High morbidity and mortality at farms where this disease has been diagnosed.

Clinical signs Affected birds show signs of respiratory distress within the first few days after hatch. Birds that recover are stunted and have delayed development.

Table 11.12 Ratite infectious diseases and parasites (Shane 1998)

System	Disease	Treatment
Respiratory	Mycoplasmosis – prevent through adequate biosecurity and quarantine of new birds	Tylosin or a fluoroquinolone
	Coryza (*Haemophilus* spp.) – prevent through biosecurity	Trimethoprim-sulfa or penicillin
	Aspergillosis – prevent through hygiene and proper management	Itraconazole
	Respiratory helminths (*Syngamus* spp., *Cyanthostoma* spp.)	Ivermectin, fenbendazole or mebendazole
Gastrointestinal	Salmonellosis – prevent through biosecurity and management to reduce transmission	Fluoroquinolone
	Campylobacteriosis – prevent by chlorinating water supply	Erythromycin
	Clostridial enteritis	Zinc bacitracin
	Necrotizing typhlocolitis of rheas – prevent through proper management	Metronidazole combined with parenteral lincomycin
	Viral enteritidis – prevent through biosecurity	No treatment
	Zygomycosis	Ketoconazole or nystatin
	Candidiasis	Nystatin in combination with fluconazole
	Endoparasites	
	• *Libiostrongylus douglassii*	Ivermectin, fenbendazole and levamizole
	• *Trichostrongylus tenuis, Houttuynia struthionis*	Praziquantel
Integument	Pox	Supportive care
	Dermatomycosis – prevent through biosecurity and hygiene	Griseofulvin in drinking water
	Ectoparasites	Carbaryl (Sevin) dust (3–5%)
Systemic	Anthrax	No treatment
	Erysipelas	Parenteral penicillin or fluoroquinolone antibiotics
	Tuberculosis – prevent by disposing of affected birds	None recommended
	Chlamydophila psittaci	Doxycycline
	Pasteurellosis – prevent through high level biosecurity	Tetracyclines in drinking water
	Colibacillosis – prevent through chlorinated water	Fluoroquinolone antibiotics
	Viscerotropic eastern equine encephalitis – prevent with vaccine – prevent with vaccine	
	Avian influenza	None recommended for highly pathogenic strains
	Adenovirus	None
Central nervous system	Western equine encephalitis – prevent with vaccine	Isolation and support
	Newcastle disease – prevent with vaccine or, if Newcastle-free, quarantine	Isolation and support
	Borna disease – prevent with inactivated vaccine	Hyperimmune serum
	Baylisascaris encephalitis – prevent by reducing exposure to intermediate host	No treatment
	Chandlerella encephalitis – prevent through ivermectin treatment at the susceptible age (<1 year)	No treatment

Pathology 1–3 mm, yellow to white granulomas in lung tissue or adherent to air sacs and viscera (Fig. 11.17).

Treatment and prevention Treatment with itraconazole provides variable results and is not cost-effective for large groups of birds. Reducing exposure to the *Aspergillus* spp. spores is the key to prevention through hygiene of the hatchery and young bird production area.

Respiratory ascarids

Aetiologya ndo ccurrence *Syngamus trachea* (ostriches) and *Cyanthostoma variegatum* (emus) (Shane 1998).

Transmission Ingestion of the intermediate host or direct infection through ingestion of mature ova in soil (Shane 1998).

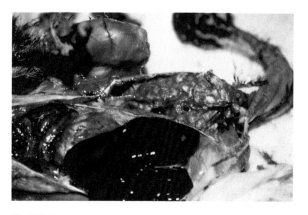
Fig 11.17 Aspergillosis granulomas in the lung tissue of a young emu.

Clinical signs Head shaking, dyspnoea, blood froth around mouth.

Pathology and diagnosis Faecal flotation to identify ova; mature worms may be seen in trachea. Bloody foam around the mouth may contain ova of the parasites.

Treatment Ivermectin, fenbendazole, mebendazole.

Salmonellosis

Aetiologya ndo ccurrence A variety of paratyphoid *Salmonella* spp. have been isolated from ratite species (Shane 1998).

Transmission Direct contact with infected carriers and indirect transmission with contact of contaminated fomites (Cooper 2005). Rodents and free-living birds are commonly considered the most likely reservoirs for this disease organism.

Clinicalsig ns Depression and acute death.

Pathology No specific pathological lesions.

Diagnosis Appropriate microbiological sampling of suspect tissue including, gastrointestinal, reproductive, heart, liver, and eggs.

Treatment Fluoroquinolone antibiotics and supportive therapy. Treatment may induce a carrier state in a recovered bird.

Prevention Strict biosecurity measures and protocol.

Ostrich pox

Aetiology ando ccurrence Ostrich pox has been diagnosed in Israel, South Africa and the United States (Shane 1998).

Transmission Mosquitoes transmit the virus, and lesions are commonly found on the featherless areas of young birds.

Clinical signs Cutaneous lesions around the face (Fig. 11.18).

Pathology and diagnosis Histopathological examination of biopsy samples of the lesions reveals intracytoplasmic inclusion bodies (Bollinger bodies).

Treatment Systemic and topical antibiotic therapy along with supportive care will save the less severe cases.

Prevention Treat unaffected birds with fowl or pigeon pox vaccine and isolate affected birds. Reduce exposure to mosquitoes.

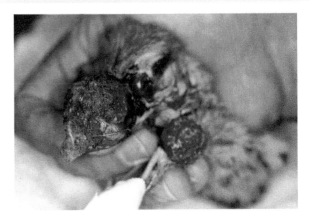

Fig 11.18 Cutaneous pox lesions cover the face of this young ostrich.

Newcastle disease

Aetiology and occurrence Paramyxovirus type 1.
Transmission Wind and fomites.

Clinical signs Torticollis, ataxia, and diarrhoea affecting 100% of exposed animals resulting in 50% mortality (Shane 1998).

Pathology No specific gross lesions have been described for birds diagnosed with Newcastle disease.

Prevention Vaccination where allowed.

Viscerotropic eastern equine encephalitis (EEE)

Aetiology and occurrence Infection with an alpha togavirus results in viscerotropic infection in emus.

Transmission Mosquito vectors feed on reservoir passeriform avian species. Once exposed, the mosquito then feeds on susceptible hosts (e.g. emus, horses).

Clinical signs Depression, sternal recumbency, blood-stained diarrhoea and terminal emesis of blood-stained ingesta are characteristic clinical signs of an EEE-infected bird (Shane 1998).

Pathology and diagnosis Petechial and ecchymotic haemorrhages are noted on the serosa of viscera and beneath the pericardium (Fig. 11.19). The intestinal lumen may contain up to 500 mL of unclotted blood.

Prevention Reduce exposure to mosquitoes and swampy, low lying areas. Vaccination of emus using an equine EEE vaccine is an effective preventive measure against this deadly virus (Tengelsen et al 2001).

Avian influenza

Aetiology and occurrence A mild H5N2 virus has been isolated from rheas and emus in the United States, with the rheas being more affected by the disease (Shane 1998). The avian influenza serotype H10N9 was isolated

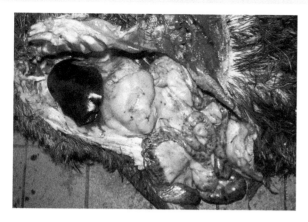

Fig 11.19 Gross pathological examination of an emu that died of Eastern equine encephalitis virus. The serosal surface of the intestinal tract has petechial and ecchymotic haemorrhages.

from wild waterfowl in an ostrich-producing area from which avian influenza outbreaks had occurred in the past (Verwoerd et al 2000). Emus were experimentally infected with avian influenza viruses of varying virulence and were shown to have minimal clinical response to either of the serotypes used (e.g. pathogenic H7N7, low pathogenic H5N3) (Heckert et al 1999).

Transmission Exposure to the avian influenza virus can occur through direct contact with free-living and migratory birds and indirect contact through contaminated fomites (Shane 1998).

Clinical signs An avian infl unza outbreak (H7N1) affecting young ostriches in South Africa showed a 100% morbidity and 80% mortality of birds exposed. Affected ostriches in the South African outbreak had diarrhoea, copious green-coloured urine, and dyspnoea (Shane 1998). Emus and rheas diagnosed with avian influenza in the Texas outbreak showed respiratory (e.g. ocular and nasal discharge) and gastrointestinal (e.g. diarrhoea) clinical signs associated with the infection. There are no specific clinical signs linked with avian influenza infection in ratite species (Shane 1998).

Treatment For birds infected with low pathogenic strains supportive care may be an effective treatment protocol. Birds infected with highly pathogenic strains are subject to depopulation procedures.

Prevention Biosecurity measure should be in place to prevent exposure. Experimental vaccine studies are currently under investigation for efficacy in avian species, including ratites.

West Nile virus

Aetiology and occurrence West Nile virus is an arbovirus that has not seriously affected ratite species to date.

Transmission Mosquito vectors feed on reservoir passeriform avian species. Once exposed, the mosquito then feeds on susceptible hosts (e.g. emus, horses).

Clinical signs Depression, but in general ratites due not appear very susceptible to the virus.

Pathology and diagnosis Serological testing and DNA isolation utilizing PCR-based testing.

Prevention Reduce exposure to mosquitoes and swampy, low lying areas. Vaccination of ratites using an equine West Nile virus vaccine has not been proven to be an effective preventive measure against this virus but it may elicit a protective immunity.

Once the veterinarian makes a correct diagnosis regarding an infectious disease, the proper management and treatment can be initiated to prevent further loss (Fig. 11.20; Tables 11.13, 11.14).

Surgery

The surgical techniques used on ratite species are similar to those used for other avian species, only the patients can be much larger. Figs 11.21 to 11.30 illustrate common orthopaedic procedures used to treat ratite injuries (Gilsleider 1998). For any ratite surgical procedure, sedation, anaesthesia, and recovery are important for a successful treatment response. If the proper facilities or veterinary expertise are not available to handle these large avian patients the case should be referred.

Proventriculotomy

Under general anaesthesia the bird is positioned in right lateral recumbency, with the left leg extended and positioned caudolaterally, in abduction (Gilsleider 1998) (Fig. 11.31). The proventriculus should be palpated in the left paramedian quadrant over the xiphoid (Gilsleider 1998). All feathers within and around the surgical site should be plucked and the area surgically prepared. **It should be remembered in ostriches that the proventriculus is located caudally to the ventriculus when making the incision into the coelomic cavity.** Once the skin incision is made, a suction hose should be placed into a stab incision in the proventriculus to aspirate any fluid prior to extending the incision into the gastrointestinal organ (Gilsleider 1998). After fluid has been removed from the proventriculus the surrounding coelomic cavity should be packed with wet surgical towels, and stay sutures or Allis tissue forceps used to evert the incision edges so that impacted material can be removed with a spoon, sponge forceps, or hands. Once all of the impacted material has been removed, the proventriculus should be flushed with warm saline.

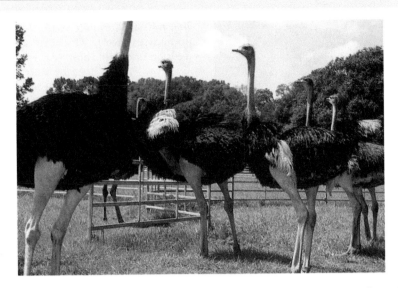

Fig 11.20 Large pen of ostriches, typical of growing production facilities. Large pens that concentrate ratite species predispose large numbers of birds to exposure of infectious disease organisms.

Table 11.13   Ostrich blood values (Fudge 1995)

	Ostrich adult	
	Mean	Range
WBC × 1000	18.65	10–24
Heterophil (%)	72.9	58–89
Lymphocyte (%)	24.2	12–41
Monocyte (%)	2.64	0–4
Basophil (%)	0.2	0–2
Eosinophil (%)	0.035	0–2
Hematocrit (%)	45	41–57
Aspartate transaminase (AST) (IU/L)	447.9	226–547
Lactic dehydrogenase (LDH) (IU/L)	970	408–1236
Creatine kinase (CPK) (IU/L)	3702	800–6600
Uric acid (mmol/L)	512.72	59.48–871.38
Calcium (mmol/L)	2.68	2–3.4
Glucose (mmol/L)	12.05	9.1–18.32
Creatinine (μmol/L)	22.98	8.84–61.88
Phosphorus (mmol/L)	1.72	0.94–2.49
Cholesterol (mmol/L)	2.66	1.01–4.45
Bile acids (μmol/L)	21	2–30

Table 11.14   Emu blood values (Fudge 1995)

	Emu adult	
	Mean	Range
WBC × 1000	14.87	8–21
Heterophil (%)	78.8	54–88
Lymphocyte (%)	19.8	10–44
Monocyte (%)	0.1	0–1
Basophil (%)	0.2	0–1
Eosinophil (%)	2.58	0–6
Hematocrit (%)	47.4	39–57
Aspartate transaminase (AST) (IU/L)	227.2	80–380
Lactic dehydrogenase (LDH) (IU/L)	778.1	318–1243
Creatine kinase (CPK) (IU/L)	428.8	70–818
Uric acid (mmol/L)	374.72	59.48–814.88
Calcium (mmol/L)	2.78	2.2–3.13
Glucose (mmol/L)	7.44	5.61–13.49
Creatinine (μmol/L)	19.45	8.84–35.36
Phosphorus (mmol/L)	1.84	1.23–2.32
Cholesterol (mmol/L)	3.15	1.76–4.4
Bile acids (μmol/L)	18	2–34

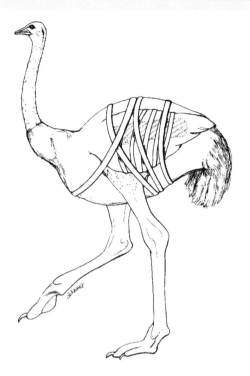

The proventriculus incision should then be closed in two layers, the first a simple continuous pattern, followed by a layer of simple continuous Cushing's pattern using a monofilament absorbable suture material (Gilsleider 1998). The muscle and skin layers should be closed separately using a simple continuous pattern after the surrounding tissue has been thoroughly lavaged with sterile saline.

Removal of the yolk sac

General anaesthesia is required to perform a yolk sacculectomy on a young ratite. The general anaesthetic agent of choice is isoflurane (Gilsleider 1998). A ventral midline incision is made on the patient positioned in dorsal recumbency. The length of the incision is cranial to the umbilicus to just beyond the limits of the yolk sac (Gilsleider 1998). The umbilical stump should be excised as the peritoneum is incised adjacent to the skin incision (Gilsleider 1998). Once the yolk sac is carefully lifted from the body to prevent tearing and spilling the contents into the coelom, the duct should be ligated (Gilsleider 1998). If the yolk sac contents enter the body cavity copious lavage with warm saline is required to reduce the incidence of coelomitis and infection. The body wall can be closed with the skin using a simple continuous or simple interrupted suture pattern. The

Fig 11.21 An ostrich with its wing taped to its body after a wing fracture. Only the injured wing is taped. A yucca board splint may be taped to the fractured wing itself to supply additional immobilization. (From Gilsleider 1998, with permission.) D K Haines © 1994 The University of Tennessee.

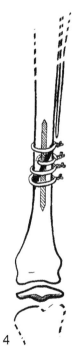

Fig 11.22 Fracture repair in tibiotarsus fractures may be accomplished with normograde intramedullary pins and stainless steel cerclage and hemicerclage wires. (From Gilsleider 1998, with permission.) D K Haines © 1994 The University of Tennessee.

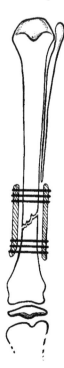

Fig 11.23 Fractured tarsometatarsus repaired with transverse pins encased in a fibreglass cast that completely encompasses the leg. (From Gilsleider 1998, with permission.) D K Haines © 1994 The University of Tennessee.

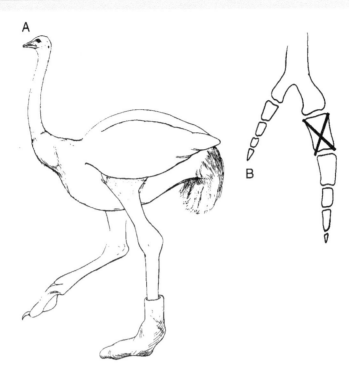

Fig 11.24 **A** Adult ostrich P_1 transverse fracture repaired with rush pins. After padding both toes and foot, a cast is applied to immobilize the foot. **B** Position of rush pins to stabilize P_1 fracture. (From Gilsleider 1998, with permission.) D K Haines © 1994 The University of Tennessee.

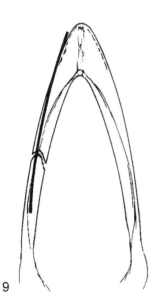

Fig 11.25 Mandibular fracture repaired with intramedullary pin drilled normograde across the fracture site. (From Gilsleider 1998, with permission.) D K Haines © 1994 The University of Tennessee.

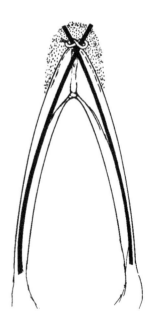

Fig 11.26 Mandibular symphyseal luxation cross-pinned and strengthened with cerclage wire interwoven with the pins. Acrylic compound overlay protects the exposed pins and wires and strengthens the surgery site. (From Gilsleider 1998, with permission.) D K Haines © 1994 The University of Tennessee.

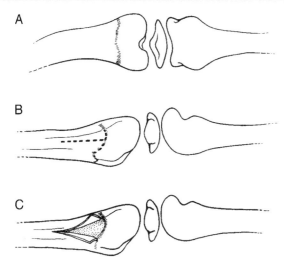

Fig 11.27 A Tarsal valgus showing bowing of tarsometatarsal (TMT) bone. **B** Site for T-shaped incision in proximal TMT. **C** Periosteal flaps created and not sutured. (From Gilsleider 1998, with permission.) D K Haines © 1994 The University of Tennessee.

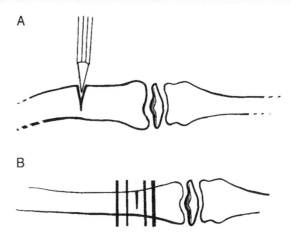

Figure. 11.29 A Modification of the tarsometartarsal wedge osteotomy allows bending of the bone so only one cortex is incised. **B** Transverse pins drilled after osteotomy and normal alignment. In small ratite chicks, the width of the bone chisel may be all that is needed to wedge the near cortex. (From Gilsleider 1998, with permission.) D K Haines © 1994 The University of Tennessee.

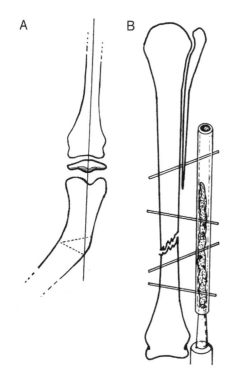

Fig 11.28 A An imaginary line is shown bisecting the tibiotarsus and hock joint. **B** Realignment and repair using acrylic compound in a plastic tube. (From Gilsleider 1998, with permission.) D K Haines © 1994 The University of Tennessee.

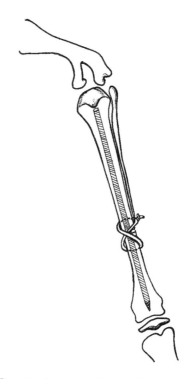

Fig 11.30 Derotational osteotomy at the mid-tibiotarsus using a single intramedullary pin and hemicerclage wire. (From Gilsleider 1998, with permission.) D K Haines © 1994 The University of Tennessee.

bird should be placed in an incubator to prevent hypothermia and on an antibiotic treatment protocol to prevent infection. Pain medication is also recommended for all surgery patients including those that have had their yolk sac removed.

Treatment

Ratite production facilities are getting larger in size and are holding more birds.

The emphasis on production has reduced the need for ratite surgery. Although not often performed at present,

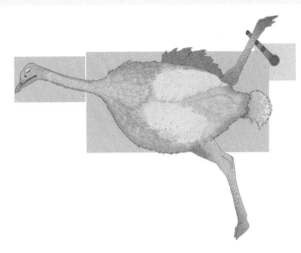

Fig 11.31 Proper positioning of the ostrich for a left paramedian approach to the abdomen. D K Haines © 1994 The University of Tennessee.

surgical techniques are based mainly on large animal and equine procedures. As the ratite producers intensify and integrate production, there will be a continuing need for veterinary care and expertise.

References

Angel R C, Scheideler S E, Sell J L 1996 Ratite nutrition. In: Tully T N, Shane S M (eds) Ratite management, medicine and surgery. Krieger Publishing, Malabar, FL, p 11–30

Cilliers S C, Van Schalkwyk S J 1994 Volstruisproduksie Klien Karoo Landboukoopserasie. Oudtshoorn, South Africa

Cooper R G 2005 Bacterial, fungal and parasitic infections in the ostrich (*Struthio camelus* var. *domesticus*). Animal Science Journal 76(2):97–106

Copetti M V, Segabinazi S D, Flores M L et al 2004 Pulmonary aspergillosis outbreak in (*Rhea americana*) in Southern Brazil. Mycopathologia 157(3):269–271

Cornick-Seahorn J L 1996 Anesthesiology of ratites. In: Tully T N, Shane S M (eds) Ratite management, medicine and surgery. Krieger Publishing, Malabar, FL, p 79–93

Dawson T J 1983 Digestion in the emu: low energy and nitrogen requirements of this large ratite bird. Comparative Biochemistry and Physiology 75A:41–45

Degen A A, Kam M, Rosenstrauch A, Plavnik I 1991 Growth rate, total body water volume, dry matter intake and water consumption of domestic ostriches (*Struthio camelus*). Animal Production 52:225–232

Du Preez J J 1991 Ostrich nutrition and management. In: Farrell D J (ed) Recent advances in animal nutrition in Australia. University of New England, Armidale, p 278

Fowler M E 1996 Clinical anatomy of ratites. In: Tully T N, Shane S M (eds) Ratite management, medicine and surgery. Krieger Publishing, Malabar, FL, p 1–10

Fudge A 1995 Ratite reference ranges. Californian Avian Laboratory, Citrus Heights, CA

Gilsleider E F 1998 Anesthesia and surgery of ratites. Veterinary Clinics of North America 14(3):503–524

Heckert R A, McIsacc M, Chan M, Zhou E-M 1999 Experimental infection of emus (*Dromaiius novaehollandiae*) with avian influenza viruses of varying virulence: clinical signs, virus shedding and serology. Avian Pathology 28(1):13–16

Kienholz E W 1978 Why is water so important to animals? Feedstuffs 50:17–18

Levy A, Perelman B, Grevenbroek M et al 1990 Effect of water restriction on renal function in ostriches (*Struthio camelus*). Avian Pathology 19:385–393

Perez J, Garcia P M, Mendez A et al 2003 Outbreak of aspergillosis in a flock of adult ostriches (*Struthio camelus*). Veterinary Record 153(4):124–125

Raines A M 1998 Restraint and housing of ratites. Veterinary Clinics of North America 14(3):387–399

Shane S M 1998 Infectious diseases and parasites of ratites. Veterinary Clinics of North America 14(3):455–483

Tengelsen L A, Bowen R A, Royals M A et al 2001 Response to and efficacy of vaccination against eastern equine encephalomyelitis virus in emus. Journal of the American Veterinary Medical Association 218(9):1469–1473

Tully T N 1998 Health examinations and clinical diagnostic procedures of ratites. Veterinary Clinics of North America 14(3):401–419

Verwoerd D J, Gerdes G H, Labuschagne A E et al 2000 Newcastle disease and avian influenza A virus in wild waterfowl in South Africa. Avian Diseases 44(3):655–660

Waterfowl

Andrew Routh and Stephanie Sanderson

12

Introduction

The term waterfowl is generally used to refer to waterbirds of the family Anatidae (ducks, geese and swans). These occur throughout the world in a wide variety of aquatic habitats. They are commonly kept in zoological and ornamental collections and are the origin of the breeds kept commercially for agricultural purposes.

This family is diverse in anatomy, physiology and behaviour. Its members are adapted to live in a wide range of habitats usually (but not exclusively) associated with water. The majority of species are instantly recognizable as Anatidae, with their dense, waterproof plumage, webbed feet and short tarsometatarsi, which produce a waddling gait on land.

Typically the Anatidae moult twice a year. In winter they moult body and head feathers to acquire their breeding plumage. After the breeding season, in the summer, they undergo a full moult including a simultaneous moult of all the primary flight feathers. This is followed by a flightless period when birds are particularly vulnerable to predators until the primaries regrow. Many species will flock together on safe waters during this period. In sexually dimorphic ducks, the summer body feathers of the male are drab and resemble the female. This is called the 'eclipse' plumage. Its nondescript nature may make species identification more difficult. The winter moult of body feathers brings birds back into full breeding plumage.

Taxonomy

This taxonomical description follows that of Johnsguard (1978) and Livezey (1986), quoted in Madge & Burn (1988).

Waterfowl are placed in the order Anseriformes. The order contains three families:

1. The family Anhimidae (screamers) are gamefowl-like birds and are not considered in this chapter.
2. The family Anseranatidae contains only one species, the magpie goose (*Anseranas semipalmata*).
3. The family Anatidae contains the true waterfowl (ducks, geese and swans) and is divided into seven subfamilies

Examples are listed in Table 12.1.

Anseranatidae

The sole representative of this family, the magpie goose, has a number of features intermediate to the true wildfowl and the Anhimidae (screamers).

It has a long hind toe and half-webbed feet to facilitate perching in trees. There is a gradual moult progression and no flightless period. It breeds in trios of one male and two females. An elongated trachea forms subcutaneous coils over the pectoral muscles, enabling it to produce a very low-pitched resonant call.

The magpie goose is native to tropical Australasia and grazes on both land and in water. During the dry season it may form large flocks and travel long distances to find suitable grazing.

Anatidae

These are the true waterfowl of which there are seven subfamilies (Table 12.1).

Subfamily Dendrocygini

This subfamily includes the whistling ducks. These ducks are tropical waterfowl, often referred to as tree ducks although many of the species do not perch. They are typically sexually monomorphic, long-legged, long-necked and short-bodied and are equally at home on land or water. They are gregarious, forming large flocks, but pair bond for life.

They range extensively across the tropics through four continents and feed mainly on aquatic fringe vegetation, dabbling and upending in shallow water.

Subfamily Thalassorninae

This subfamily contains only one species, the white-backed duck (*Thalassornis leuconotus*).

Subfamily Anserini

These are the swans and true geese. They are large, long-necked waterfowl and are typically sexually monomorphic. Some species perform long migrations.

Tribe Anserini

These are the true geese. An example would be the barnacle goose (*Branta leucopsis*). They are migratory species with three separate Arctic breeding populations,

Table 12.1 Taxonomy of waterfowl

Order Anseriformes (43 genera, 152 species)

Family	Subfamily	Tribe	
Anhimidae			Screamers: 6 species
Anseranatidae			Magpie goose (*Anseranas semipalmata*)
Anatidae	Dendrocygnini		Whistling ducks: 1 genus, 4 species
	Thalassorninae		White-backed duck (*Thalassornis leuconotus*)
	Anserini	Anserini	Geese: 3 genera, 16 species
		Cygnini	Swans: 2 genera, 8 species
	Stictonettini		Freckled duck (*Stictonetta naevosa*)
	Plectoropterinae		Spur-winged goose (*Plectropterus gambensis*)
	Tadornini		Shelducks and allies: 5 genera, 14 species
	Anatini	Anatini	Dabbling ducks: 4 genera, 40 species
		Aythyini	Pochards, diving ducks: 2 genera, 15 species
		Mergini	Mergansers, eiders, other sea ducks: 7 genera, 18 species
		Oxyurini	Stifftails: 3 genera, 8 species

each with separate wintering grounds. The Greenland population winters in western Scotland and Ireland, the Svalbard population winters in the Solway Firth in the Scottish Borders and the Novaya Zemblya population winters in the Netherlands. Barnacle geese breed on islands and coastal cliffs and have been reported to nest in association with gyrfalcons (*Falco rusticolus*) as protection from other predators. They graze on coastal grassland, with a strong preference for a short sward.

Tribe Cygnini

These are the swans, an example being the mute swan (*Cygnus olor*). This species is indigenous to Europe and Central Asia. Many populations derive from historical introductions and thrive in close association with humans. They are gregarious except during the breeding season, when males are territorial and notoriously aggressive. Swans are found on a wide range of lakes, rivers and estuaries. They feed on waterweed within reach of their long neck, up-ending when necessary, and graze on land.

Subfamily Stictinettinae

This subfamily includes the freckled duck (*Stictonetta naevosa*).

Subfamily Plectropterinae

This subfamily includes the spur-winged goose (*Plectropterus gambensis*).

Subfamily Tadorninae

This subfamily includes the shelducks and sheldgeese. It is a large and varied subfamily. All the members are equally at home in water or on land though some are primarily terrestrial in habit. These birds are often seen as being intermediate between true geese and typical ducks.

An example species from this subfamily would be the common shelduck (*Tadorna tadorna*). This species is widespread in Europe. They are large, monomorphic ducks. Common shelduck are gregarious, gathering into large flocks during the flightless period of the summer moult. They favour muddy estuaries, where they filter-feed on algae and invertebrates in the mud by walking slowly forwards, swinging their heads from side to side through the surface layer, filtering food particles from the mud with their beak lamellae. Common shelduck usually breed in old rabbit holes and newly hatched chicks are then led to the water, which may be a considerable distance away. Chicks from a number of broods will form a crèche under the care of a few adults.

Subfamily Anatini

These are the true ducks.

Tribe Anatini

The Anatini are the dabbling ducks. This is a large tribe and contains most of the typical and familiar duck species. They are typically strongly sexually dimorphic, with bright and attractive males. This feature, along with relatively undemanding husbandry requirements, makes this tribe popular in aviculture. Ducks feed by dabbling food from the water surface and by up-ending in shallow water. They also graze and feed on stubble and root crop waste after the harvest. They are mainly ground nesting, but will use a wide variety of sites.

An example of the tribe would be the mallard (*Anas platyrhynchos*). These are the most familiar ducks and are the ancestors of many domestic breeds. They range throughout the northern hemisphere, with several distinct races, and are found in a wide range of lowland habitats including sheltered coasts. Human introductions have led to an artiÞcial extension of their range and they are a threat to a number native species through hybridization. They become very tame in parks and busy waterways and mix freely with other species.

The perching ducks, for example the wood duck or Carolina duck (*Aix sponsa*), were formerly classiÞed in a separate tribe, the Cairinini. They are widely distributed on wooded lakes and marshes in North America. Elsewhere feral populations derived from escapees are common. They feed on aquatic vegetation by dabbling, but also graze on waterside grassland and are often seen standing in small groups on partially submerged branches or branches overhanging the water. They nest in holes in trees.

Tribe Aythini

This includes the pochards, for example the canvasback (*Aythya valisineria*).

These are diving ducks with short, rounded bodies and are from freshwater habitats, although greater scaup (*A. marila*) can be found coastally in the winter. The largest of the true pochards, canvasback are widespread throughout North America and are ducks of open marshes and estuarine lagoons. They feed on aquatic vegetation and invertebrates by diving and favour relatively deep water. Nests are usually built ß oating in shallow water. These species are sexually dimorphic.

Tribe Me rgini

These are sea ducks and are mainly associated with coastal waters although some species are found on freshwater, especially during the breeding season. Many species have short, dumpy bodies with legs placed far caudally and all are ungainly on land, spending most of their time on the water. Most species inhabit high latitudes and have remarkably thick down to provide adequate insulation for an aquatic lifestyle in cold climates.

The Mergini include the red-breasted merganser (*Mergus serrator*), which is a long-bodied, long-necked duck with a long, thin, serrated ÔsawbillÕ adapted for catching Þsh (see Fig. 16.1). It superÞcially resembles a grebe (*Podiceps* spp.) more than a typical duck, and is

distributed throughout the northern hemisphere, breeding close to water in rock crevices, burrows or tree holes. Mergansers are generally found on rivers, lakes and estuaries in the summer, but in the winter they generally remain on estuaries and the coast. They feed by diving for Þsh.

The Mergini are often classiÞed with the eiders of the genera *Polysticta* and *Somateria*, though the latter may be placed in a separate tribe. An example would be the common eider (*Somateria mollissima*). This species is widely distributed on northern Atlantic coasts and estuaries. They are sexually dimorphic but as full adult plumage is not attained until the third winter there are many confusing intermediate plumages. Eider nest colonially on the ground, usually on offshore islands, and line their nests thickly with down. This is ÔeiderdownÕ and it is still commercially harvested. Eider feed on molluscs and invertebrates by diving and pulling them from the seabed.

Tribe O xyurini

This includes the stiff-tailed ducks, for example the ruddy duck (*Oxyura jamaicensis*).

These birds are freshwater diving ducks, although they are occasionally found on brackish water. They have short bodies with their legs placed far caudally and have large feet, making them ungainly on land. Their long, stiff tail feathers are typically held erect when resting on the water.

They are widely distributed in North and South America. Escapee feral populations of ruddy duck in Europe have hybridized with the endangered white-headed duck (*Oxyura leucocephala*).

The ruddy duck is a gregarious small duck that rarely leaves the water and nests at the waterÕs edge, often on a ßoating platform of vegetation. Although it migrates considerable distances by ßying, it prefers to swim and dive rather than ßy when threatened. It is sexually dimorphic and feeds, mainly by diving rather than dabbling, on aquatic weed and invertebrates.

Husbandry

Housing

Waterfowl are among the most common exhibits in zoological collections. Many species are relatively tolerant of environmental conditions and cope with overcrowded environments with highly contaminated land and water. However, in a survey of deaths in a zoological collection waterfowl were the commonest fatalities and bacteriological disease of environmental origin was the commonest cause of death (Kaneene et al 1985). Good management and disease control requires attention to all the three media Ðair, land and water Ðthat make up the captive environment.

Air

Waterfowl may be kept ßightless, either temporarily by cutting the ßight feathers of one wing or permanently by surgical amputation of the terminal phalanx of one wing (pinioning). This removes the need for netting an airspace in the enclosure. However, this means that wild birds are free to ßy in and these can act as vectors for a range of diseases. Netted enclosures allow birds to be kept free-ßying and keep out wild birds. A soft, preferably knotless, nylon mesh is durable yet unlikely to result in trauma to birds colliding with it.

Land

Most enclosures consist mainly of earth and vegetation. Grazing species can gain a considerable proportion of their nutrition from well-managed grassland and management of grazing follows the same principles as for domestic livestock. Overgrazing can result in poaching and the sward can be overtaken by coarse, unpalatable grass species. Unpalatable grass species are sometimes deliberately cultivated to provide a dense green covering to the enclosure that will not become overgrazed. Ova of nematode parasites *Amidostomum* spp., *Syngamus* spp. and *Cyathostoma* spp. can, depending on their life cycle, survive over winter either on grass or in invertebrate transport hosts (earthworms). **Grazing cannot be considered clean unless it has been resown and rested for over 12 months. Juveniles grazing unclean areas are particularly at risk from parasitic infestation and should be treated regularly with anthelmintics (Lloyd 2003).**

Trees and bushes can provide habitat variety, roosting sites, shelter and shade, but dense cover can produce damp, shaded areas where bacteria, such as *Mycobacterium avium*, can survive and build up in numbers to give high levels of environmental contamination.

Natural pool surrounds are prone to erosion whereas artiÞcial surrounds, such as stone or concrete, may have an abrasive Þnish that can predispose to foot trauma and pododermatitis. Swans and geese will peck from the water at any soil within reach. Therefore surrounds should be wider than the length of a birdÕs neck. Erosion at the junction between a pool surround and the earth substrate will produce a damp, muddy area and thus a potential environment for the build-up of pathogenic bacteria such as *M. avium*.

In colder climates basic shelters can be provided for protection in winter. Tropical species may require supplementary heating.

Water

Some pools may be managed on a ÒdumpÓ and ÞllÓ regimen and enclosed recirculating systems using sand Þltration can be utilized, but the most commonly used systems depend on a through-ßow of fresh water from a natural source. If there are a number of pools supplied from the same source parallel, rather than series, ßow avoids the spread of contamination or infection between pools. Before water ßows back into a natural watercourse measures should be taken to prevent environmental pollution. These measures can vary from simple sedimentation pools to modern reed-bed (*Phragmites* spp.) technology. The water ßea (*Daphnia pulex*) acts as an intermediate host for the life cycle of *Acuraria uncinata* and increased water ßows through enclosures can be used to reduce the numbers of water ßeas in an area (Lloyd 2003).

The required water depth depends on the species kept. Dabbling ducks favour shallow water, swans favour water of a depth equal to the length of their necks and diving ducks require a depth of about one metre.

Feeding

Maintenance

Dabbling ducks, geese and swans can be maintained on natural grazing and aquatic vegetation supplemented with grain. The contribution of naturally grown food will depend on climate and stocking density and will vary with season. Wheat, barley or a mixed grain containing wheat, cracked maize, barley and oats can be used as the supplement. Alternatively, a proprietary pellet designed for maintenance feeding can be used. Shell or limestone grit provides substrate material for the grinding action of the gizzard and is a source of calcium.

Diving ducks can be fed on proprietary pellets designed for this purpose. Many diving ducks such as eiders will adapt to eating grain Ð although this is an unnatural diet Ðand thrive.

Specialized Þsh eaters such as sawbills are best fed whole Þsh of a suitable size. Such natural food may have inherent deÞciencies and attention should be paid in particular to vitamin E and thiamine levels.

Intensive care and convalescence

Inappetent birds will need feeding by stomach tube. A mix suitable for all species, containing highly assimilable protein and high energy, is:

- 500 mL Lectade Plus (SmithKline Beecham) Ðoral rehydration ßuid
- two tins of A/D Diet (Hills Pet Nutrition) Ð a canine/feline convalescent diet
- 100 mL Ensure Plus (Abbott Laboratories) Ð a human liquid nutrition product
- ½ Aquavit (International Zoological Veterinary Group) Ða vitamin supplement high in B₁ and E
- one 200 mg ferrous sulphate tablet.

As a guide a mallard should receive 60 mL b.i.d. and a mute swan 150 mL b.i.d.

Fully-grown, rehabilitating wildfowl will frequently be underweight, with varying degrees of emaciation and loss of muscle mass. A diet high in both protein and energy is desirable to promote the replacement of both muscle mass and fat reserves prior to release. For geese, swans and dabbling ducks a mixture of grain (wheat is approximately 12% protein) and poultry layer pellets (17% protein) provides a higher level of protein and energy and is a source of vitamins. (Whilst commercial layer pellets should contain no therapeutic agents this should be confirmed before feeding.) The high calcium content of the layer pellets is offset by the low calcium-to-phosphorus ratio of the grain. Layer pellets should not constitute more than 50% by weight of the diet.

To tempt swans to eat, green food such as natural duckweed, chopped lettuce or other green vegetables should be offered. Floating food on water will often stimulate feeding. Swans will also eat sprats or other small fish. Ducks will sometimes start feeding if offered commercial softbill foods or an insect mix. Live food such as mealworms may tempt an inappetent duck.

Seaducks will eat chopped or whole oily fish such as sprats, shrimp or de-shelled shellfish. Care must be taken because the fat from this diet can coat the lamellae of the beak and then be spread on the feathers during preening, resulting in a loss of waterproofing. It is generally recommended that fish eaters should receive a supplement of 25 mg thiamine/kg of fish fed, but in practice this may not be necessary (see Chapter 16).

High fat and protein diets should be withdrawn once birds have gained adequate weight and body condition and the birds returned to a maintenance diet. This is to avoid the potential risk of kidney damage and gout associated with excess protein intake, or of obesity and a fatty liver associated with excess energy intake.

Reproduction in Anseriformes

Sexing

Most adult ducks are sexually dimorphic. Even in monomorphic duck species many adult males have 'drake feathers' three feathers that curl forward from the tail. All Anseriformes can be accurately sexed by direct visualization of the phallus in males. The procedure is simple, and with practice can be used successfully even on young birds. The bird should be held with its head down between the knees of the person sexing the bird, so that the belly can be seen. By placing the thumbs on either side of the cloacal lips and exerting firm but gentle pressure downwards and outwards the phallus can be everted. It may take some time to overcome the strong cloacal sphincter. Females have two small labia-like structures.

Sexual maturity and breeding strategies

Ducks become sexually mature at 1 year of age. They are polygynous. In many species males will defend their mates until the start of incubation, but play no part in incubating and rearing the ducklings. Ducks show no mate loyalty. There are also parasitic species, notably the redhead (*Aythya americana*), in which the female will sometimes lay in a host nest and show no parental care.

Geese mature at about 2 years and swans at about 5 years. There is little morphological difference between the sexes and, unlike ducks, they show strong pair bonding and often pair for life. The female is still exclusively responsible for incubating the eggs but the male remains close by and defends the nest against predators. After hatching he will also aid in herding and brooding the young chicks.

Anseriformes copulate in water and exhibit a ritualized pre- and post-copulatory display. Most species show a marked change in behaviour during the breeding season, with many becoming highly aggressive both to each other and to other species. In ducks severe feather picking and bruising along the neck and back ('rape' injuries) are common amongst both sexes. Females are sometimes drowned by mobs of rival males during mating.

Prolapse of the phallus or penis does occur (see Fig. 3.13). Initial therapy may be limited to cleaning the organ, application of emollient creams, systemic antibiosis and manual replacement of the organ. In some instances a reduction in swelling occurs and there is no further prolapse but recurring prolapse is a common presentation. A slack purse-string suture of the cloaca may retain the phallus long enough for it to assume normal morphology but re-prolapse often occurs on suture removal after several days. The waterfowl phallus is an organ of insemination and, unlike the mammalian penis, does not have an excretory function. Thus surgical amputation of the severely traumatized or repeatedly prolapsing phallus is an option, though it will prevent the bird from breeding in the future. Though it may be assumed that a prolapsed phallus is the result of excessive sexual activity and/or trauma there are a number of conditions in which, through weakness and debility, the phallus may prolapse and these conditions should be ruled out. These include avian TB, non-specific weakness and emaciation and infection with duck viral enteritis.

Waterfowl have a wide range of preferred nesting sites with some species nesting in crevices, some in thick vegetation and some out in the open. Most species do not actively collect nest material, but merely pull anything within reach round their preferred site to form the nest. They then line it with a thick layer of down (Humphreys 1986).

Clutch size is generally inversely proportional to bird size – typically three to six eggs in geese and swans, and six to twelve or more in ducks. Females of smaller species tend to lay one egg a day and the larger species lay every other day, usually early in the morning. As the clutch size increases the female spends more and more time on the nest. Incubation is generally around 25 days for ducks, 30 days for geese and 35 days for swans and muscovy ducks (*Cairina moschata*) (Forbes & Richardson 1996). Hatching is synchronized by the acoustic stimuli of brood mates and is usually complete within 16–24 hours.

Persistent egg-laying can occur in waterfowl though it is not as common as in, for example, the smaller psittacines. Though most birds may have sufficient reserves for an extended lay these reserves may eventually become exhausted. Documented therapies for waterfowl are uncommon and in many instances the examples of hormone therapy regimens are for those directed at the management of skin disease and feather-plucking in psittacines. Bennett (1997) proposes a regimen where human chorionic gonadotrophin is given at a dose of 500–1000 i.m. on days 1, 3 and 7 of a regimen that may need to be repeated every 3 to 6 weeks. The synthetic gonadotrophin-releasing hormone agonist leuprolide acetate is an alternative (Carpenter 2005), but it is expensive per dose. Due to its severe side-effects the use of the long-acting progesterone medroxyprogesterone acetate is no longer recommended.

Wildfowl have nidifugous young. They are downcovered and capable of walking, swimming, diving and eating immediately after hatching. Maternal care consists of protection, brooding the young chicks and leading them to food, water and safety.

Captive breeding

The following is intended as an overview of waterfowl breeding. There is a wealth of information on the subject, both published and available through consultation of those active in the field.

Group size and composition

Gregarious ducks will breed successfully in mixed species groups. Hybridization is a risk, and subspecies should not be kept together. Strongly territorial species, such as swans, require separate enclosures or very large areas to avoid inter- and intra-species aggression (Forbes & Richardson 1996).

Environment

Optimum breeding will occur when the individual species are provided with an environment similar to their natural habitat. For example, photoperiod is an important trigger for breeding in polar waterfowl. This may require the provision of artificial light in lower latitudes (Humphreys 1986).

Birds should be provided with suitable nest-sites free from disturbance and predators, with nesting material readily available. Artificial islands with nest-boxes are ideal.

Artificial rearing

Most captive Anseriformes will raise a brood successfully with minimal human intervention. Some active ducks will lose or exhaust their brood. These species or individuals benefit from being confined to smaller enclosures. Artificial incubation and rearing can potentially increase brood size and decrease losses due to predation and abandonment. The main disadvantages are that specialized equipment and expertise are required and with artificial rearing there is a risk of imprinting.

Egg collection and storage

By the regular removal of eggs a female can often be persuaded to lay more than the normal clutch number. A dummy egg can be left in the nest to encourage her to continue laying. However, she should not be chased off the nest to allow egg collection as she may not return to finish the clutch. In geese it is often more successful to wait until the clutch is complete and then to remove the eggs. Some keepers will then destroy the nest to induce a new lay.

Eggs can be collected at one of two stages, either as soon as possible after laying is complete or after the eggs have been 'set' (i.e. after the hen has incubated them for the first 5 to 7 days). The latter leads to increased fertility, but potentially also to increased egg contamination from the nest. The eggshells of waterfowl are particularly porous and the contents are easily invaded by pathogenic bacteria such as *Staphylococcus* spp., *Salmonella* spp. and *Escherichia coli*. These are all common causes of fetal and neonatal death (Humphreys 1986). Any cracked, grossly contaminated or deformed eggs should be discarded. The remainder should be washed, dried and disinfected before storage. A variety of disinfection methods are currently used. These include dipping in 1% formalin, fumigation with potassium permanganate and exposure to ultraviolet light. Eggs may be stored blunt end up at 15–21°C for up to 14 days before incubation (LaBonde 1992).

Incubation

Foster hens provide a simple method of incubation. This method requires the least expertise, but runs the risk of infectious disease transmission from the foster hens. It is important to remove the eggs at pipping to avoid imprinting and later problems with mate recognition.

There are many brands of incubator commercially available. Successful incubation requires accurate control of temperature and humidity. Incubators must be easy to disinfect. The exact requirements of the different species vary. The advice of experienced breeders should be sought regarding optimum temperature and humidity. As a general guide Humphreys (1986) found that incubating at 37.7¡C and at 50% humidity until pipping then transferring the eggs to a hatching incubator kept at 37.5¡C and 70% humidity produced good results.

Regular ÔhandlingÕ (the viewing of the egg contents via transmitted light) from the Þrst week onwards is a useful procedure for assessing egg viability during incubation. It can help to identify causes of poor hatchability and allows the prompt removal of cracked, infected and sterile eggs. Fetal death before 5 days is most likely to be due to incorrect incubator temperature, jarring of the eggs during handling or inbreeding. Late deaths are often due to incorrect temperature and/or humidity or inappropriate turning (Forbes & Richardson 1996). Deaths due to bacterial contamination at laying or during incubation can occur at any stage.

Brooding

After hatching and drying the young chicks should be transferred into brooder accommodation. The key factors in duckling rearing are good hygiene and the provision of a thermal gradient, allowing individuals to select their preferred temperature zone. This is usually achieved by the use of a heat lamp that can be raised and lowered as appropriate. Heat lamps should be selected with care. Ceramic lamps are preferable as they do not produce light in the visible spectrum and are more resistant to breakage should they be splashed by water. As a guide the heated area of the brooder accommodation should initially be 37.2¡C (99¡F) with the temperature then lowered gradually over a period of 3 weeks to 21.1¡C (70¡F) or to ambient temperature (Olsen 1994). In temperate climates most ducklings can survive without artiÞcial heat from 2 weeks of age. Should the weather turn cold supplementary heat should be provided, especially at night, until they have grown a complete covering of contour feathers.

As down feathers have an open structure lacking barbs or barbules, soiling of the plumage of newly hatched chicks rapidly results in a failure of waterprooÞng. Access to water then results in soaking and hypothermia.

Chicks of dabbling ducks and geese can be reared in relatively simple, unspecialized accommodation. They may be kept away from water on a dry substrate until they have developed a full layer of contour feathers. Vinylized wire or plastic mesh, stippled rubber matting, synthetic turf, newspaper or wood shavings can all be used as ßooring. Hay and straw are a source of spores of *Aspergillus* spp., and should not be used. Use

of poultry drinkers or a shallow dish filled with pebbles allows unrestricted access to water without allowing chicks to become soaked.

Conversely species highly adapted to an aquatic lifestyle, such as the stifftails, require access to water from an early age. Rearing such chicks is more difÞcult and requires specialized facilities. An area of water must be provided which should have a constant ßow draining from the surface (surface skimming). A dry brooding area should consist of mesh or stippled rubber matting and be equipped with an overhead heat source. Food should be provided in containers that will not easily spill and contaminate the pen. Placing food containers directly over the surface drain ensures that all spilt food is immediately removed.

Food and water should be provided to all young within 24 hours of hatching, but many birds will not start feeding for at least 48 hours. A starter crumb of about 20% protein is suitable for most ducks during the Þrst 2 to 3 weeks of life, after which a grower ration with 16% protein can be used until 4 to 6 months of age. Swans and geese are predominately grazers and are adapted to a low protein diet. **Consequently cygnets and goslings are particularly prone to growth deformities exacerbated by excessive growth due to high protein rations. The most common condition seen follows carpal rotation and is known by a number of terms including 'angel wing'. Therefore they should be restricted to a diet of 16% protein or less and provided with greens from hatching onwards.**

Fostering of young Anseriformes is possible, particularly in swans and geese. Cross-species fostering should be avoided because this may lead to imprinting and later problems with mate selection. Fostering must be done at the egg stage as parents will usually kill a strange gosling or cygnet, even if introduced straight after hatching. Particular care should be taken to avoid the cross-fostering of polar and temperate species of swans, e.g. whooper swans (*Cygnus cygnus*) and mute swans (*Cygnus olor*). The former tend to brood their cygnets on land whilst the latter brood their cygnets on their backs while still on the water. Whooper swan cygnets fostered onto mute swan parents will come out of the water when they wish to be brooded while the foster swan may stay on the water, resulting in the cygnets becoming fatally chilled.

Conditions of neonate and growing waterfowl

Chilling

Most young wild birds seen in general practice will be abandoned or orphaned and suffering from hypothermia and hypoglycaemia. Treatment is symptomatic. Olsen (1994) described a syndrome of death a few days after rewarming. The aetiology is poorly understood but mortality may be decreased by the repeated use of high doses of rapidly metabolized corticosteroids during the initial stabilization. (Indiscriminate use of corticosteroids is to be avoided due to their potentially deleterious effects on the liver.)

'Starve Out'

'Starve out' is a term coined by poultry pathologists to describe a condition where young birds fail to start to eat. This is recognized in waterfowl and is one of the most common causes of neonatal death in artificially brooded waterfowl. Death typically occurs between 7 and 14 days after hatching. On post-mortem examination the gastrointestinal tract is empty and contracted, the gall bladder is distended and the liver is shrunken and yellow. Hatchlings are not expected to start eating for the first 24–48 hours of life, until their yolk sac is absorbed, but if they remain inappetent steps should be taken to encourage feeding. Some specialized species such as harlequin ducks (*Histrionicus histrionicus*) and scoters (*Melanitta* spp.) may be particularly difficult and require hand-feeding for some time. Mimicking the conditions normally encountered by a wild hatchling seems to be very effective at initiating self-feeding. Some of the stimuli used include:

- colour – yellow and green foods, such as grass or crumbled boiled-egg yolk, can be mixed with the food
- company – the presence of other ducklings, especially if these are already eating well
- physical stimuli – in the wild the young of off-the-ground cavity nesters, such as mandarins and wood ducks, would fall 20 m or more when first leaving the nest. Simulating this by tossing them into the air and letting them fall to the ground has been reported to stimulate feeding behaviour (Kear 1986).

Yolk sac problems

These fall into three interrelated categories; yolk sac retention, yolk sacculitis/omphalophlebitis and yolk sac rupture.

Yolk sac retention

The yolk sac provides nourishment and a source of maternal immunoglobulin. Most of it is resorbed in the first week and its presence beyond 2 weeks is considered abnormal. The aetiology and pathogenesis of yolk sac retention are unknown. Untreated birds will usually die. Clinical signs include abdominal distension, dyspnoea, exercise intolerance, inability to stand, inappetence and general failure to thrive. Surgical removal is the only effective treatment (Kenny & Cambre 1992).

Yolk sacculitis/omphalophlebitis

Yolk sacculitis and omphalophlebitis are due to bacterial contamination of the umbilicus, either through damage to or excessive soiling of the egg or poor incubator and brooder sanitation. Low incubator humidity also seems to be associated with increased rates of infection (Olsen 1994). The two conditions can occur concurrently or independently. Omphalophlebitis is characterized by oedema and inflammation of the abdominal wall in the area of the umbilicus. An infected yolk sac is enlarged, hyperaemic, and contains brown or yellow coagulated yolk. Gram-negative bacteria such as *Salmonella* spp. and *E. coli* are the most common isolates. Treatment is generally impractical but control by good hygiene and incubation techniques is effective.

Yolk sac rupture

Yolk sac rupture occurs either as a result of trauma in the first 2 to 3 days of life or secondary to yolk sac retention or infection. Rupture leads to shock and a rapidly fatal peritonitis. Treatment is generally impractical.

Other miscellaneous infectious diseases are discussed later in this chapter.

Developmental/nutritional disease

Though more common in captive birds, developmental musculoskeletal disease is also seen in free-living birds (Fig. 12.1, Table 12.2).

Clinical techniques

In general waterfowl are easy to handle, make good patients and are rewarding to treat. The basic principles of examination, clinical testing, imaging and nursing

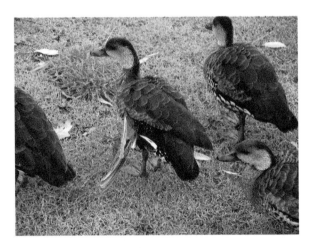

Fig 12.1 'Angel wing' deformity in a goose.

Table 12.2   Common developmental syndromes of waterfowl (based on Olsen 1994)

Condition	Pathogenesis/clinical signs	Comments and therapy
Valgus reverse (angel wing, or tilt, crooked, spear, slipped, healed over, sword, aeroplane or rotating wing)	Relative weight of rapidly growing flight feathers on a poorly mineralized skeleton produces excessive stress on the weak muscles of the carpal joint, leading first to drooping of the wing at the carpus and then, if untreated, to irreversible outward twisting, rendering the bird flightless	Proposed aetiology includes excessive growth rates induced by overfeeding and high protein diets (>16%), vitamin D and E deficiency, manganese deficiency, genetic predisposition. Most common in Anseriformes with slow natural growth rates. Unknown in fast-growing Arctic species such as the snow goose (*Anser caerulescens*)
		Taping the wing tip onto itself for 3–5 days may reverse angel wing during the early stages
		Restrict feeding of slow-growing species
		Encourage exercise (swimming, etc.)
Perosis (slipped tendon)	Cartilage deformity at hock joint leading to medial Achilles tendon luxation, swelling and non-weight-bearing	High protein diet (>16%), manganese deficiency, may be exacerbated by calcium supplementation
		Splinting usually unsuccessful, swimming exercise and dietary restriction may be helpful during early stages, surgical correction possible

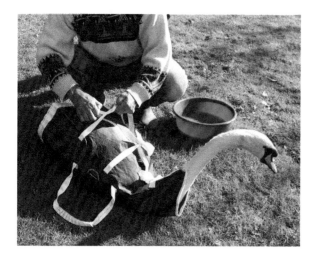

Fig 12.2 Swan being released from a 'swan bag' – a simple rectangle of canvas or tough plastic which is wrapped around the bird and held with three strips of Velcro or tape ties.

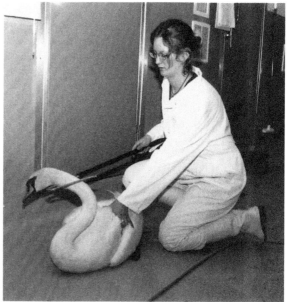

Fig 12.3 Use of swan hook. The head and neck are restrained with the hook for long enough for the wings to be restrained. Here the handler holds the humeri together over the back with one hand.

have been discussed in detail in previous chapters. The aim of this section is to mention only those aspects peculiar to waterfowl.

Handling and restraint

Various equipment has been developed for the capture and restraint of the large Anseriformes, notably the swan bag and hook (Figs 12.2, 12.3).

Examination and radiology

Physical examination and survey radiography (Figs 12.4, 12.5) can be carried out using a combination of manual restraint, swan bags and light sandbags. For

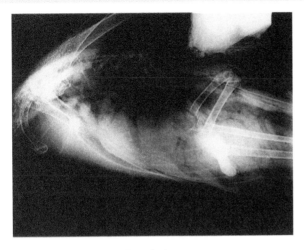

Fig 12.4 A normal lateral radiograph of a mute swan.

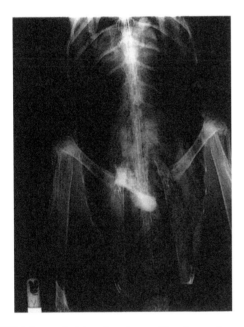

Fig 12.5 A dorsoventral view of a mute swan. There is a small penetrating foreign body in the wall of the gizzard. This is a common incidental finding.

diagnostic radiography, in particular of the appendicular skeleton, general anaesthesia is recommended.

Features of radiographic anatomy peculiar to Anseriformes include the following:

1. The thoracic vertebrae are separate – they are not fused to form a notarium.
2. Male ducks, with the exception of stifftails, have a syringeal bulla. This can be seen radiographically at the thoracic inlet.
3. Trumpeter (*Cygnus buccinator*), whooper and Bewick (*Cygnus bewickii*) swans have a loop of

their trachea coiled into an excavation in their sternum. This is often more prominent in the male (see Chapter 5).

Anaesthesia

Waterfowl ingest large quantities of water whilst feeding, hence oesophageal reßux and subsequent inhalation is a signiÞcant risk during general anaesthesia. Starving and removal of water for between 2 and 6 hours before induction and the use of a well-fitting endotracheal tube significantly reduces the risk. (In the larger species a cuffed tube can be used but care should be taken with any endotracheal tube placement, cuffed or uncuffed, and cuff insufflation to avoid focal pressure-necrosis of the trachea.)

Waterfowl produce copious tracheal secretions during anaesthesia. These can block the endotracheal tube, particularly the narrower gauges used in smaller species. Use of atropine leads to thickening of the secretions and is contraindicated. The anaesthetist should check the patency of the tube at regular intervals. The authors suggest replacing the tube every 20 minutes throughout the procedure to ensure tube patency.

Removal of a minimal number of contour feathers during the preparation for surgery will enable retention of a complete waterproof layer and the bird will be ready for an early return to the water.

Both injectable and volatile agents have been used successfully for induction of anaesthesia in Anseriformes. Some of the more common injectable agents and their dose rates are listed in Table 12.3. Ease of restraint, easy venous access via the medial metatarsal vein and a relatively large body weight make waterfowl excellent candidates for induction of anaesthesia using injectable agents. Delivery of the agent via a syringe-driver facilitates anaesthetic maintenance. Cracknell (2004) documents the use of propofol at 0.5Ð 3 mg/kg/minute for total intravenous anaesthesia (TIVA). In all instances where only injectable agents are used there should be provision of supplementary oxygen and endotracheal intubation is recommended.

Induction of anaesthesia by inhalation of a volatile agent, such as isoßurane, can be performed. A snug-Þtting mask can be made using a latex glove and a commercially produced face-mask. Good restraint is needed and with a gas-scavenging system it is possible to achieve smooth and rapid induction with minimal environmental contamination, a factor for which mask induction is often criticized.

Maintenance solely on volatile agents can be problematic, with waterfowl sometimes oscillating between periods of apnoea and a subsequent insufficient depth of anaesthesia. This may relate to physiological adaptations relating to natural behaviours. Many species, in particular the diving ducks, have extended periods of breath-holding during feeding and are presumably more tolerant of degrees of hypercapnia. Additionally a number of species migrate at altitude, often flying over substantial mountain ranges, and thus can cope with lower oxygen partial pressures. Thus intubation and the use of intermittent positive-pressure ventilation (IPPV) can give stability to anaesthesia, particularly during lengthy surgery. Pressures of 20 cm water were demonstrated to be safe in the northern pintail (*A. acuta*) during studies on contrast radiography (Sherrill et al 2001).

Recovery should be in a quiet, dark environment and extubation carried out when the bird has regained voluntary control of its head and neck. Analgesic agents for waterfowl are listed in Table 12.4.

Venepuncture and fluid therapy

Jugular and brachial veins can be used for venepuncture (see Chapter 6). In addition, the medial metatarsal vein is particularly prominent in waterfowl (see Fig. 3.40) and

Table 12.3   Injectable anaesthetic agents for waterfowl

Agent	Dose	Route	Species	Comments	Reference
Propofol	8.0 mg/kg	i.v.	Mute swan	Very short-acting	Goulden (1995)
Alphaxolone/alphadolone	4.2 mg/kg	i.v.	Mute swan	Coles (1997) believes this drug has been superseded in waterfowl by safer alternatives	Cooke (1995)
Ketamine + xylazine	12.5 mg/kg (7.2–24.0) + 0.28 mg/kg (0.16–0.53)	i.v.	Mute swan	Using a 9:1 mixture of ketamine 100 mg/mL: xylazine 20 mg/mL, the average swan dose is 1.0 mL. Used with less success in other species of waterfowl	Authors' unpublished data
Medetomidine + ketamine	200 µg/kg + 10 mg/kg	i.m.	Waterfowl	Induction takes 2–3 minutes after i.m. injection	Coles (1997)
Diazepam + ketamine	1.0–1.5 mg/kg + 10–30 mg/kg	i.m. or i.v.	Avian – not specified	Smoother induction than with ketamine alone (see text)	Lawton (1996)

Table 12.4   Analgesic agents for waterfowl

Agent	Dose	Route	Species	Comments	Reference
Carprophen	4 mg/kg s.i.d.	s.c.	All waterfowl	Have used on three successive days	Authors' unpublished data
	2 mg/kg	i.m.	Not specified	Postoperative	Coles (1997)
	5–10 mg/kg	Not specified	Not specified	Proposed synergy when combined with buprenorphine	Lawton (1996)
Meloxicam	0.2 mg/kg s.i.d.	p.o.	All waterfowl		Authors' unpublished data
	0.2–1.0 mg/kg s.i.d. or b.i.d.	p.o.	Unspecified birds		S. Forster, Boehringer Ingelheim Ltd, personal communication (2006)
Ketoprofen	1 mg/kg s.i.d. 1–10 days	i.m.	All waterfowl		Forbes & Harcourt-Brown (1996)
	5–10 mg/kg	i.m.	Not specified		Lawton (1996)
Flunixin	1 mg/kg s.i.d.	s.c.	All waterfowl	Have used on three successive days	Authors' unpublished data
	1–10 mg/kg	i.m.	Not specified		Lawton (1996)

is a convenient site both for routine venepuncture and, because it is relatively immobile, for the placement of indwelling catheters for ßuid therapy (see also Chapter 6 for description of jugular and intraosseous catheter placement). Fluid therapy has an active role to play in the management of sick and injured captive waterfowl and, in particular, of the wild bird casualty (Cousquer 2005). Some normal haematological and serum chemistry values are given in Tables 12.5 and 12.6.

Infectious diseases

Waterfowl are susceptible to a wide range of infectious diseases, and these are summarized in Table 12.7.

Some of the more signiÞ ant diseases will be discussed below.

Bacterial diseases

Avian cholera

Avian cholera is an important disease responsible for annual die-offs of thousands of over-wintering wild birds in North America. Though the causal organism is found in Europe it does not seem to cause such dramatic or frequent mortalities. Avian cholera is caused by *Pasteurella multocida* and Anseriformes are uniformly highly susceptible. Mass mortalities in waterfowl are often accompanied by deaths in other species also

(coots, raptors, rodents), in contrast to duck viral enteritis (DVE) where mortality tends to be restricted to Anseriformes (Friend & Franson 1999).

The bacteria are shed in vast quantities in the faeces and oronasal discharge of affected birds, and can persist for 3 to 4 weeks in water and up to 4 months in the soil (Olsen 1994). Bacteria persist in carcasses for several weeks and the disease will also affect avian scavengers, (e.g. eagles, vultures and corvids). Transmission is by direct contact or through environmental contamination.

Clinical signs can vary from peracute death, where birds can literally Ġall out of the skyǪto a chronic wasting disease sometimes seen in older birds and characterized by dyspnoea and diarrhoea. Most waterfowl show an acute syndrome with anorexia, profuse mucoid oronasal discharge, diarrhoea and loss of balance, leading birds to walk or swim in circles. Birds dying peracutely often show no gross pathology. Those with acute disease show pathology consistent with an acute septicaemia, petechial and ecchymotic haemorrhages on the myocardium and mesentery, a swollen copper-coloured liver with pinpoint white spots of necrosis throughout the parenchyma and sometimes a catarrhal haemorrhagic enteritis. In subacute and chronic cases, thoracic lesions predominate. There is pulmonary haemorrhage and areas of consolidation, Þbrinopurulent pleurisy, pericarditis and air sacculitis.

Differential diagnoses should include duck viral enteritis, infection due to *Escherichia coli*, *Erysipelas* spp. and, in the chronic form, duck septicaemia (new

Table 12.5 Haematology

Parameter	Units	Mute swan (n = 18)	Mallard		Snow goose (mean only; n = 10–14)	Canada goose (mean only; n = 10–14)
			Pre-remige moult (n = 7)	Post-remige moult (n = 7)		
Total haemoglobin (Hb)	g/dL	10.6–16.1	16.6–16.8	13.3–13.5	14.5	14.3
Red blood cell count (RBC)	10¹²/L	1.85–2.76	3.00–3.04	2.42–2.48	2.24	2.01
Packed cell volume (PCV)	L/L	0.350–0.500	38.8–38.2	38.6–39.6	0.457	0.454
Mean cell volume (MCV)	fL	169.1–194.6	126.5–128.5	159.4–161.6		
Mean cell haemoglobin (MCH)	pg	51.2–63.0	55.0–55.6	54.2–56.2		
Mean cell haemoglobin concentration (MCHC)	g/dL	30.3–36.0	43.2–43.6	33.9–34.5		
Total white cell count (WBC)	10⁹/L	8.8–35.0	26.0–27.0	6.8–7.5	20.1	20.8
Heterophil count	10⁹/L	4.31–17.25	12.8–13.8	2.4–2.8		
Lymphocyte count	10⁹/L	0.66–19.25	9.9–11.0	3.8–4.2		
Monocyte count	10⁹/L	0.26–2.64	0.5–0.6	0.1–0.1		
Eosinophil count	10⁹/L	0.23–3.50	0.8–1.1	0.3–0.4		
Fibrinogen	g/L		13.6–17.0	11.9–14.3		

Table 12.6 Biochemistry

Parameter	Units	Mute swan (n = 17)	Mallard Pre-remige moult (n = 8)	Post-remige moult (n = 7)
Urea	mmol/L	0.2–1.2		
Sodium	mmol/L	135.9–144.6		
Potassium	mmol/L	3.2–4.9		
Total protein	g/L	42.7–52.8	44.0–45.8	40.5–41.9
Albumin	g/L	14.9–20.0	21.0–21.8	20.1–20.8
Globulin	g/L	25.7–34.7		
Alb/glb ratio		0.43–0.68		
Calcium	mmol/L	2.22–2.86		
Inorganic phosphate	mmol/L	0.81–1.26		
Urate	μmol/L	137.0–1444.0	398.5–422.3	317.2–339.0
Alkaline phosphatase	IU/L		67.3–74.7	95.5–114.5
Alanine transaminase (ALT)	IU/L	10.1–55.3		
Gamma glutamyl transferase (GGT)	IU/L	0.1–82.1	41.3–46.7	40.2–55.8
Aspartate transaminase (AST)	IU/L	5.6–99.5		
Creatine kinase (CK)	IU/L	137.7–3577		
Iron	μmol/L			
Cholesterol	mmol/L	2.8–7.0		
Glucose	mmol/L	3.5–13.1	15.0–15.5	13.0–13.3
LDH	IU/L	190.4–876.7		

Sources: Driver (1981); RSPCA/Grange Laboratories' own data; Williams & Trainer (1971).

duck disease) due to infection with *Riemerella anatipestifer* (Table 12.8).

Staining of heart-blood smears with methylene blue, Giemsa or Wright's stain will reveal vast numbers of bacteria as bipolar rods. Diagnosis is confirmed on bacterial culture. Treatment with penicillin and tetracycline has proved effective. In large, free-living colonies prompt carcass removal followed by incineration, liming or burying is the main method of control. It is contentious whether driving birds from the affected area is beneficial or merely acts to spread the disease. Vaccines developed for Galliformes have been tried but several different strains of *P. multocida* exist and the killed vaccine does not seem to be effective in waterfowl. The modified-live vaccine has been implicated in a disease outbreak when used in pheasants and at present its use is discouraged (Jessup 1986).

Pasteurella multocida infections in humans are not uncommon; however, the strain responsible for waterfowl die-offs appears to be poorly infectious to humans and other non-rodent mammal species. It is recommended,

however, that workers wear gloves and wash thoroughly after handling birds that have died from avian cholera (Friend & Franson 1999).

Avian tuberculosis

Avian tuberculosis (avian TB), caused by *Mycobacterium avium*, is endemic worldwide. Due to its preference for damp conditions, waterfowl are particularly at risk. Those species feeding on or by fresh water are most frequently affected. Spread is by the faeco-oral route. Avian TB is particularly prevalent in long-established captive collections for two reasons:

1. The persistence of bacteria in the environment (up to 4 years).
2. The slow, insidious onset of disease leading to birds being infective many months before they show clinical signs.

The disease is characterized by a syndrome of weight loss and muscle atrophy, though many birds often retain

Table 12.7 Infectious diseases of waterfowl

Disease	Agent and transmission	Susceptible species	Relative occurrence	Clinical signs and lesions	Diagnosis and differentials	Treatment and control	Zoonotic importance
Bacteria							
Avian tuberculosis	*Mycobacterium avium*	All	Common especially in long-established waterfowl collections	See text	See text. Pseudotuberculosis (possibly *E. coli* or *Salmonella* spp. at post-mortem)	See text	Significant in immunosuppressed individuals
Pseudotuberculosis	*Yersinia pseudotuberculosis.* Through a break in the skin or mucous membranes or by ingestion. Rodents and wild birds may act as carriers infecting food supplies. Many soil invertebrates act as mechanical vectors. Organism can propagate outside the host at low temperatures if organic nitrogen available	All	Rare	Weight loss, anorexia, dyspnoea, diarrhoea, enteritis. In acute disease, enlarged liver and spleen. In chronic disease, nodules in liver, lungs, spleen and breast muscles	Bacterial isolation may take up to 2 weeks to grow, may need to store culture in fridge first. TB. *E. coli*	Improve sanitation, no reliable vaccine, mostly refractory to antibiotics	Minimal
Erysipelas	*Erysipelothrix rhusiopathiae.* Unknown, possibly wound infection or ingestion, can propagate outside the host even in seawater and reservoirs, carried by rodents and pigs	All. May cause 30% mortality in ducklings	Not uncommon. Can cause epidemics in winter	Acute death, lesions consistent with acute septicaemia	Bacterial isolation. Culture from spleen, liver and bone marrow. Acute septicaemia	Antibiotics, penicillin drug of choice, improve hygiene	Wound infection, erysipeloid
Avian cholera	*Pasteurella multocida*	All	See text	See text	See text	See text	None

New duck disease (anatipestifer; infectious serositis)	Riemerella anatipestifer; similar to Pasteurella spp. (also known as Cytophaga or Moraxella or Pfeifferella anatipestifer)	All, sporadic outbreaks in the wild, more common in captive collections. Acute form in ducklings <6 weeks of age. Chronic, localized form seen in older birds	Acute form is not uncommon and has approx. 75% mortality; chronic form is rare	Listlessness, ocular discharge, diarrhoea, CNS signs, air sacculitis, pericarditis, meningitis, fibrinous membranes on viscera	Bacterial isolation, ELISA test. E. coli septicaemia, duck viral hepatitis (DVH), DVE, Salmonella spp.	In early stages antibiotic therapy according to sensitivity	None
Colibacillosis	Escherichia coli – many species of varying pathogenicity. Primary or secondary invader. Ingestion, wound infection	All	Common	Acute septicaemia, air sacculitis, fibrinous pericarditis, enlarged necrotic spleen, caseous peritonitis. Common isolate from mucoid sinusitis, salpingitis and bumble foot	Bacterial isolation on histology serofibrinous inflammation with plasma cells in liver and kidney. Other causes: acute septicaemia, TB, Salmonella spp.	Antibiotics according to sensitivity, improve sanitation	None
Salmonellosis	Salmonella spp. (over 2000 spp.) commonly S. typhimurium. Ingestion; carriers common; human carriers may be source of infection	All	Common	Vary from acute septicaemia and sudden death to chronic non-specific illness. Enteritis, meningitis, focal hepatic necrosis, caseous caecal plugs, arthritis and infertility	Bacterial isolation, serology. E. coli, other enteric pathogens and causes of acute septicaemia	Antibiotics according to sensitivity, improve sanitation	Gastroenteritis
Other Enterobacteriaceae	Pseudomonas aeruginosa and Aeromonas hydrophilia. Both organisms may be incidental post-mortem findings. Usually secondary pathogens producing potent	All	Common	Both have similar clinical signs, localized respiratory tract infection, dyspnoea, diarrhoea. Sometimes acute septicaemia and death	Bacterial isolation	Antibiotics according to sensitivity, improve sanitation	None

(continued)

Table 12.7 continued)

Disease	Agent and transmission	Susceptible species	Relative occurrence	Clinical signs and lesions	Diagnosis and differentials	Treatment and control	Zoonotic importance
Bacteria							
	extracellular toxins. Ingestion, can propagate in cool water contaminated by organic waste, also contaminated food						
Campylobacter spp. (common isolate from the guts of healthy animals)	Pathogenic strains of *C. jejuni*. Dogs and other mammals may act as carriers. Ingestion of food or water contaminated by human sewage. Not stable in the environment	All	Not uncommon	Subacute or chronic illness. Lethargy, weight loss, anorexia, diarrhoea (often yellow), hepatitis. Enlarged liver with prominent lobules and focal necrosis, mucoid haemorrhagic enteritis. Common cause of chronic hepatitis	Bacterial isolation from faeces and affected tissues. Must use transport medium for swabs. Other pathogens causing hepatitis together with enteritis	Antibiotics according to sensitivity, improve sanitation	Gastroenteritis
Goose gonorrhoea	*Neisseria*-like organism. Direct cloacal contact and vertical transmission	Captive geese. 10% mortality in ganders	Uncommon	Cloacitis, inflammation and ulceration of the phallus	Clinical signs suggestive	Antibiotics according to sensitivity	None
Avian mycoplasmosis	*Mycoplasma* spp. *Acholeplasma* spp. Colonizers of respiratory and urogenital tract, require a breach in the mucosa to allow invasion. Transmission requires close contact egg transmission and long latent periods can also occur. Very unstable in	All	Not uncommon	Signs can include chronic conjunctivitis, rhinitis, sinusitis, tenosynovitis, arthritis and stunted growth. Marked serofibrinous, cell-mediated inflammatory response. Haematogenous spread especially to joints, brain and egg	Culture and isolation. Intracytoplasmic inclusion bodies in Giemsa-stained impression smears. Serology often not useful though has been used in poultry. Common secondary pathogens include *Staphylococcus* spp., *Streptococcus* spp. and *E. coli*, *Chlamydophila* (*Chlamydia*) *psittaci*, other	Aminoglycosides are the most useful antibiotics. Oxytetracycline may have some efficacy. Decrease stocking density, careful sanitation before disinfection	None

Disease	Aetiology	Species	Occurrence	Clinical signs	Diagnosis	Treatment	Notes
	the environment, can survive 2–4 days in drinking water			follicles. These often become colonized by secondary invaders, producing a wide range of pathology	pathogens causing upper respiratory signs		
Ornithosis	*Chlamydophila psittaci*. Inhalation, airborne contaminated faecal material. Frequent asymptomatic carriers, no identifying test presently available	Ducks, geese and possibly other Anseriformes. 20–70% mortality in infected ducklings	Common carriers. Clinical syndrome rare	Purulent conjunctivitis, rhinitis, sinusitis, lethargy. greenish diarrhoea. Serofibrinous pericarditis and air sacculitis, splenomegaly. hepatomegaly	Isolation, Giemsa-stained impression smears. Serology. Mycoplasmas, other pathogens causing upper respiratory signs	Tetracyclines daily or weekly for 6 weeks or enrofloxacin for 14 days	Important: fever with respiratory involvement
Secondary bacterial invaders	*Staphylococcus* spp.. *Streptococcus* spp.. *Proteus* spp.. *Pseudomonas* spp.. *Corynebacterium* spp.	All	Very common	Secondary invaders not normally prime cause of disease	Isolation	Antibiosis according to culture and sensitivity. Seek cause of primary insult	Minimal
Viruses							
Duck viral enteritis (duck plague)	Herpesvirus	See text	See text	See text	See text	See text	None
Goose viral hepatitis (goose influenza. goose plague. Derzsy's disease)	Parvovirus. Lateral transmission. oral and nasal exudate	Domestic geese. Canada geese, muscovy ducks	Mortality 100% under 20 days of age. resistant after 70 days o.d. Common in Europe, undocumented in USA	Diarrhoea, ataxa. coryza, fibrinous plaques under tongue. Signs consistent with acute viraemia or septicaemia. ascites, serofibrnous pericarditis	Virus isolation. serology VN and ELISA tests. DVE. acute bacterial/viral septicaemias, gosling reovirus (primarily respiratory signs)	Vaccination of stock 3–6 weeks prior to breeding	None
Duck viral hepatitis	Type 1: picorna virus	Duck type 2: astrovirus	Ducklings from 1 to 28 days of age. mallard infected but do not show clinical signs	Not uncommon. mortality up to 100%	Sudden death. Some may show terminal opisthotonus	Vaccinate breeding stock (maternal immunity will protect hatchlings)	None
	Type 2: astrovirus probably spread by gulls	Only in east of England	Mortality 10–50%	Hepatomegaly and splenomegaly with petechiae	DVE, acute bacterial septicaemia, coccidiosis, mycotoxicosis	None	

(continued)

Table 12.7 continued)

Disease	Agent and transmission	Susceptible species	Relative occurrence	Clinical signs and lesions	Diagnosis and differentials	Treatment and control	Zoonotic importance
Viruses							
	Type 3	Only in USA. mallards and domestic ducks	Mortality up to 30%	Often secondarily infected with *Salmonella*, spp. or *Chlamydia* spp.			
Avian encephalomyelitis (epidemic tremor)	Picornavirus. Vertical transmission	Ducklings 1-6 weeks old	Occasional	CNS signs, tremors, incoordination. paralysis (decreased egg production in adults)	Inoculation embryonated chicken eggs. ID and ELISA test. Histopathology of brain. Vitamin E/selenium deficiency. Newcastle's disease	None, prognosis usually hopeless. vaccination available	None
Eastern equine encephalitis and other encephalomyelitis arboviruses	Togavirus. Transmission by insect vectors, mainly in the Americas	All. Often silent infection	Rare (more common amongst non-indigenous bird species)	Up to 80% mortality. CNS signs, sometimes haemorrhagic enteritis	Virus isolation from brain homogenate. HI and ELISA tests	None. Horse vaccine has been used in ratites and pheasants	Encephalitis
West Nile virus	Flavivirus. Transmission by *Culex* mosquito vectors. High path strains in Israel and North America. Endemic strains Africa and Eurasia	All (species and strain variable)	Dependent on strain. Increasing in North America	CNS signs. Meningo-encephalitis	Virus isolation. PCR, serology. NB very similar to St Louis encephalitis virus and Japanese encephalitis viruses	Vector control. Inactivated vaccine developed for horse may provide protection	Encephalitis
Newcastle disease (notifiable disease in the UK)	Paramyxovirus serotype group 1. Faeco-oral route. Anseriformes not very susceptible	All	Rare, often latent infection	Usually mild but sometimes severe including respiratory signs, diarrhoea. CNS signs: wing drooping, torticollis, opisthotonus, paralysis	Virus isolation. HI test. Faecal and respiratory tract swabs, chilling and special transport media required	Vaccination	Severe conjunctivitis

Disease	Cause	Species	Incidence	Clinical signs	Diagnosis	Control	Zoonotic potential
Avian influenza (fowl plague, fowl pest)	Orthomyxovirus, influenza 'A'	All (susceptibility depends on subtype/strain and bird species)	Up to 5% wild waterfowl infected; however, clinical signs rare unless particularly virulent strain (cf. H5N1 epidemic)	Ranges from a subclinical sinusitis to severe respiratory disease and sudden death	PCR. Virus isolation and serology	Prevent stress especially over-crowding and severe weather conditions	Important, may lead to human pandemics
Avian pox (avian diphtheria, contagious epithelioma)	Pox virus – many distinct viruses identified, may be species-specific. Biting arthropod vectors. mosquitoes can retain virus for up to 8 weeks	All	Mild cases common	Typical wart-like lesions on feet, rarely in pharynx or around eyes	Clinical signs, virus isolation	Self-limiting. control insect vectors, may be more prevalent in birds with hypovitaminosis A	Efficacy/safety of fowl pox vaccine undetermined
Fungal							
Aspergillosis	Aspergillus spp. Over 200 species all of which are normally saprophytic and found in damp environments. Spores ubiquitous. Inhalation of spores. Clinical syndrome varies with immunocompetence and pathogenic load	All, particularly sea and diving ducks and swans	Common, especially following a stressor such as capture, transportation, oiling, concurrent disease. Injudicious use of antibiotics and steroids. Hypovitaminosis A	Three main syndromes: 1. Acute: sudden death, neurological signs initially in respiratory system then haematogenous spread to viscera, especially CNS and cardiac muscle. 2. Upper respiratory tract (URT) obstruction, localized plaques around syrinx and tracheal bend in swans. Change in voice common presenting sign; 3. Chronic air sacculitis, lethargy, gradual weight loss. May be precursor to acute form	History and clinical signs often suggestive, isolation from tracheal swab. fungal colonies usually visible on Sebouard's medium after 48 hours, bronchoscopy, laparoscopy, radiography. Post-mortem lesions include granulomas, yellow miliary nodules in lung parenchyma, grey/white fungal plaques. Serology. ELISA test, titres increase during disease and fall during remission. Causes of sudden death, syngamus, trichomoniasis, candida, tuberculosis, paratuberculosis, E. coli, salmonellosis	Prevention, avoid stressors, prophylaxis in at-risk birds. Early detection by serological monitoring (QIA) of at-risk populations. Wide variety of antifungal agents used. Izole antifungals show good penetration but slow onset of action so usually used with initial short course of amphotericin B. Amphotericin B has poor penetration and is best delivered by nebulizer or intra-air sac	Minimal

(continued)

Table 12.7 *continued*

Disease	Agent and transmission	Susceptible species	Relative occurrence	Clinical signs and lesions	Diagnosis and differentials	Treatment and control	Zoonotic importance
Fungal							
						route: treatment suspended once antibody levels fallen to background (usually 4–6 weeks) Surgical removal of tracheal form followed by systemic and topical antifungals	
Candidiasis	*Candida* spp. Usually secondary opportunist; may occur as part of normal gut flora. Predisposing factors include: concurrent disease, poor diet, poor hygiene and injudicious use of antibiotics	All. Particularly common in captive sea ducks denied access to salt water. Secretions from the salt glands seem to inhibit yeast growth	Not uncommon	Listlessness inappetence, weight loss. In sea ducks lesions often in mouth, conjunctiva and nictitating membrane. At post-mortem, oesophageal mucosa thickened, overlaid by soft white cheesy deposits. Occasionally also proventriculus, cloaca, respiratory tract and skin	Smear from mucosa stained with lacto phenol blue or Diff Quick to demonstrate organism. Trichomoniasis, aspergillosis, tuberculosis, paratuberculosis, differentiate oesophageal plaques from DVE	Avoid predisposing factors. Topical treatment with nystatin 100000 units per 300 g bird b.i.d. for 7–14 days (not absorbed from alimentary tract, care when stomach tubing not to miss lesions proximal to delivery site)	None
Protozoa							
Trichomoniasis	*Trichomonas gallinae.* Direct transmission. contaminated food source	All	Uncommon	Listlessness. inappetence, weight loss, occasionally dyspnoea if lesions obstruct larynx. At post-mortem, yellow/white cheesy deposits anywhere from pharynx to ventriculus	Immediate microscopic examination of mucosal smear in warm saline will reveal highly motile trichomonads. Candidiasis, tuberculosis, aspergillosis, renal coccidiosis paratuberculosis. Differentiate oesophageal plaques from DVE	In severe cases usually unsuccessful. debridement followed by treatment with dimetridazole or metronidazole. treat in contact birds for 12 days	None

Haematozoa	*Plasmodium* spp.	All	Rarely diagnosed	Often asymptomatic. May cause anaemia. subcutaneous bleeding, swollen eyelids, sudden death. Hepatosplenomegaly	Stained blood smear, pigmented parasite found in leucocytes and erythrocytes. Leucocytozoon	Antimalarials	None
	Leucocytozoon spp. Simuliidae (black flies) principal vector	All. Only in black fly areas. young, stressed birds most susceptible	Common. Heavy mortality and regular die offs in the wild, may be main factor limiting population size in some areas	Anaemia, inappetence, weakness, Hepatosplenomegaly	Blood smear, parasite found in leucocytes but only during first period of infection. Schizonts found in impression smears of viscera, malaria	Where possible avoid contact with black flies	None
Sarcocystis	*Sarcocystis ridleyi*	Ducks, especially dabblers, more common in adults	Rare in UK. common in USA	Usually non-pathogenic; can cause muscular weakness and lethargy. White rice grain-type lesions within muscle	Gross pathology	Usually unnecessary. 30-day course of pyrimethamine	Possible
Renal coccidiosis	*Eimeria truncata*. Localize in kidneys	All. Especially young geese	Not uncommon	Leg weakness, tendency to tip forwards, listlessness, inappetence, weight loss, diarrhoea. Kidneys grossly swollen with white pinpoint foci made up of urates and cellular debris	Gross pathology. Lead poisoning, botulism, trichomoniasis, candidiasis, tuberculosis, aspergillosis, paratuberculosis	Clazuril or sulphonamides	None
Enteric coccidiosis	*Eimeria* spp. *Tyzzeria* spp., *Wenyonella* spp. Many species-specific. Occasionally *Cryptosporidium* spp.	All	Not uncommon	Varies from acute death, mucosanguineous diarrhoea to asymptomatic	Faecal flotation, histopathology: enteric lesions contain merozoites	Improve hygiene. Amprolium	None

(continued)

Table 12.7 *continued*

Nematodes, cestodes and trematodes

Disease	Agent and transmission	Susceptible species	Relative occurrence	Clinical signs and lesions	Diagnosis and differentials	Treatment and control	Zoonotic importance
Proventricular worms (*Acuaria*)	*Echinuria uncinata* and *Echinuria autralis* (less pathogenic) *Daphnia* spp. intermediate host. Each may carry up to 20 infective larvae. Adults possess an array of spikes to anchor themselves in proventriculus wall. The posterior ends of females protrude into the lumen and shed their eggs into the gut	Ducks, swans, occasionally geese. Of most significance in young birds, can cause high mortality in cygnets on shallow water in hot summers	Not uncommon in birds with access to slow moving water. Seasonal. *Daphnia* spp. more common in warm weather	Stunted growth, anorexia, starvation, anaemia. Severe damage to proventriculus wall and excessive mucus production. Nodules containing parasites may impair passage of food	Demonstration of eggs in faeces. Small elliptical egg containing single larva. Post-mortem lesions. Thorny-headed worms, gizzard worms	Increase water flow through ponds to discourage build-up of *Daphnia* spp. Treatment with anthelmintics rarely effective in clinical cases as scarring and fibrosis remain. repeated dosing of young birds may prevent infection from becoming pathogenic	None
Gizzard worms	*Amidostomum* spp. Direct life cycle. eggs hatch in water. larvae ingested. Small hair-like worms living beneath horny gizzard lining	Mainly geese and ducks. diving ducks rarely affected. Most significant in young birds	Not uncommon	Stunted growth, anorexia, erosion and necrosis of koilin leading to ventricular dysfunction	Demonstration of egg in faeces: oval, thin-walled, embryonated, slightly larger than ascarid egg. Post-mortem lesions. *Acuaria*, thorny-headed worms	Anthelmintics. Removal from or drainage of infected water courses	None
Heartworm of swans and geese	*Sarconema eurycerca*. Filarial worm transmitted to the bird by a biting louse	Swans and geese	4–20% apparently health swans in one study North America. Further research required	Clinical significance unclear. Can be found in both healthy and chronically debilitated animals	Cardiomegaly. Adult worms visible to naked eye under epicardium or in myocardium. Blood smears reveal microfilarial stages	Anthelmintics	None
Thorny-headed worms (Acanthocephala)	*Filicollis anatis* and *Polymorphus* spp. Invade intestinal mucosa: cylindrical non-segmented parasites found in the lower small intestine.	All. Especially swans and eiders	Uncommon. Can be common in geographically localized areas. High mortality in young birds	Rapid weight loss, enteritis. May cause gut rupture and peritonitis	Demonstration of parasite on post-mortem. Spindle-shaped embryonated egg in faeces containing embryo with rostral circlet of hooks. Gizzard worms, *Acuaria*	Anthelmintics. Removal from or drainage of infected water courses	None

		Hosts	Prevalence	Clinical signs	Diagnosis	Treatment	Zoonoses
	often bright yellow or orange. Crustacea intermediate hosts						
Goose gapeworms	*Cyanthostoma bronchialis.* Direct life cycle. carrier adults contaminate pasture. earthworm may act as a vector. Worms found in bronchi and trachea	Geese. Most mortalities in young birds	Not uncommon. Seasonal. rare in prolonged dry weather	Unthriftiness secondary to anaemia. blood tinged tracheal mucus, soft cough. yawning. rarely dyspnoea	Eggs and adults in tracheal mucus and faeces. Worms in bronchi and trachea	Avoid grazing young goslings on land contaminated by adults. Regular use (every 10 days) of anthelmintics in at-risk birds	None
Gapeworms	*Syngamus trachea.* Direct life cycle. snails. slugs and earthworms may act as vectors	All	Rare	Dyspnoea. coughing. unthriftiness	Bi-operculate eggs in faeces. adults in trachea. sometimes causing total obstruction	Anthelmintics	None
Avioserpens taiwana	*Avioserpens taiwana.* Cyclops intermediate host	Ducks. Taiwan. Indo-China. North America	Common in areas with high numbers of cyclops	Tumours containing parasites on underside mandibles and chin. occasionally on thighs and shoulder	Clinical signs	If required. excision	None
Flukes	Multiple trematode species. Most species Non-pathogenic. Molluscs and crustacea act as intermediate hosts	All	Not uncommon. Occasional enzootics	Range from haemorrhagic enteritis to emaciation and hepatic fibrosis depending on species	Fluke eggs in faeces	Control difficult. praziquantel. chlorsulon. levamisole 25–50 mg/kg p.o.	None
Dwarf tapeworm	Numerous species. *Hymenolepidae* spp. common isolate. Freshwater intermediate hosts	All freshwater species	Not uncommon. Large numbers in debilitated birds	Usually asymptomatic. Found throughout GI tract. Catarrhal enteritis. diarrhoea. emaciation	Faecal flotation. proglottids in faeces. Adult sometimes seen on cloacal examination	Niclosamide (toxic to geese). Praziquantel	None
Ectoparasites							
Lice – chewing	*Mallophaga* spp. Most species host-specific. Direct contact life cycle 2–3 weeks. Feed off feather debris	All, especially common in swans	Very common	Usually asymptomatic. some local irritation. Numbers increase dramatically in debilitated animals	Black or brown and cigar-shaped. 2–8 mm in length. seen scuttling around feather vane	5% carbaryl powder. ivermectin. In heavy infestations investigate underlying cause	Enjoy patrolling human hair. local irritation only

(continued)

Table 12.7 *continued*

Disease	Agent and transmission	Susceptible species	Relative occurrence	Clinical signs and lesions	Diagnosis and differentials	Treatment and control	Zoonotic importance
Ectoparasites							
Shaft lice (wet feather)	*Holomenopon leucoxanthom*. Feed on contents of soft feather quills	Most	Not uncommon	Destruction of normal feather structure leading to loss of waterproofing and moist appearing feathers. Severe irritation	Direct visualization. Examine a freshly plucked feather with a hand lens. Other causes of loss of normal feather structure: lack of preening, soiling of feathers, chemical contaminants, physical damage	Topical acaricide. Avoid oily preparations as they will themselves cause a loss of waterproofing	None
Leeches (*Hirudinea*)	*Theromyzon* spp. Over 20 species recorded in waterfowl	Most	Common	Head shaking, continual sneezing, conjunctivitis, bloody nasal discharge, nasal obstruction. Anaemia, often fatal in ducklings, sporadic deaths in adults	Direct visualization. Found in nasal passages, sinuses, mouth and periorbital region	Drainage and disinfection of affected pond or suspend use for 1–2 years. Physical removal using ivermectin 200 µg/kg single dose p.o., i.m. or s.c.	None

Sources: Benyon et al (1996), Coles (1997), Fowler (1986), Ritchie et al (1994), Hess & Paré (2004), Friend & Franson (1999).

Table 12.8a–c Differential diagnosis. These tables are intended as an aid in differential diagnosis during disease investigation. The more common diseases of wildfowl are listed, with the major organ systems affected

a. Large die-offs of all ages, characterized by sudden death

Avian cholera

Duck viral enteritis

Leucocytozoon

Erysipelas

Botulism

Mycotoxins

Phytotoxins

b. Disease that can lead to acute mortality

Disease	Age	Systemic	Gastrointestinal (GI) tract	Central nervous system (CNS)	Respiratory system	Cardiovascular system (CVS)	Musculoskeletal system
DVH (duck viral hepatitis)	0–4 weeks		+	+	+		
Encephalomyelitis	1–6 weeks			+			
Cyanostoma	Fledgling/ juveniles		+			Anaemia	
Acuaria	Fledgling/ juveniles		+			Anaemia	
Amidostomum	Fledgling/ juveniles		+				
Renal coccidiosis	Fledgling/ juveniles						
Leeches	Mostly juveniles					Anaemia	
NDD (new duck disease)	Acute ducklings (chronic adults)		+	+	+		
Avian influenza	More common <1 year	+		+	+		
Avian cholera	Any	+					
Aspergillosis	Any				+		
DVE (duck viral enteritis)	Any	+	+				
Salmonella spp.	Any		+	+			
E. coli spp.	Any	+					
Erysipelas spp.	Any	+					
Pseudotuberculosis	Any		+		+		
Botulism	Any		+	+	+		+

(continued)

Table 12.8 (*continued*)

b. Disease that can lead to acute mortality

Disease	Age	Systemic	Gastrointestinal (GI) tract	Central nervous system (CNS)	Respiratory system	Cardiovascular system (CVS)	Musculoskeletal system
Mycotoxins	Any		+	+			+
Lead poisoning	Any		+	+			+
Zinc poisoning	Any		+	+			+
Electrocution	Any			+			+

c. Chronic wasting diseases

Disease	Gastrointestinal (GI) tract	Central nervous system (CNS)	Respiratory system	Cardiovascular system (CVS)	Musculoskeletal system
Avian tuberculosis	+				
Pseudotuberculosis	+		+		
Campylobacter spp.	+				
Salmonella spp.	+	+			
Ornithosis	+		+		
Aspergillus spp.			+		
Candida spp.	+				
Trichomonas spp.	+		+		
Plasmodium spp.				+	
Leucocytozoon spp.				+	
Lead poisoning	+	+			+

a vigorous appetite until the terminal stages. Other signs may include generalized weakness, lameness, plumage deterioration, diarrhoea and, in advanced cases, ascites. Ocular lesions are sometimes seen. On post-mortem examination there are caseous, necrotizing, granulomatous lesions, varying from pinpoint and miliary to several centimetres in size. These may be found in the parenchyma of any organ but most commonly the liver, spleen and gastrointestinal tract are affected. Diagnosis is usually on post-mortem examination, but lesions may be detected on endoscopic examination of the coelom. The presence of acid-fast bacilli on faecal examination is suggestive of disease, but affected animals are often intermittent shedders. An ELISA test capable of detecting subclinical infection has been developed and seems promising, though it is not presently commercially available (Forbes et al 1993). Work is also being undertaken to develop a PCR test for more accurate isolation and differentiation of *M. avium* from other acid-fast bacilli.

M. avium is very resistant to chemotherapy. Control is based on euthanasia of affected and in-contact animals, the removal and liming of topsoil, decreasing stocking densities, quarantine and serological testing of new stock and improving general levels of hygiene. *M. avium* has been recorded as causing disease in humans. This should be taken into consideration in collections where there is close contact between birds and people, particularly children, the elderly, those suffering from immunosuppressive disease or those on immunosuppressive medication.

Viral diseases

Duck viral enteritis

Duck viral enteritis (DVE or duck plague) is caused by a herpesvirus. It is an important cause of mass mortalities in captive wildfowl, and in the UK is thought to be endemic, causing sporadic deaths in the wild population.

The disease is seen at all times of year, but seems particularly prevalent in the UK in the late spring and autumn. This may coincide with the immigration of free-ßying waterfowl. The epizoology in North America may be slightly different, with the disease postulated as being an exotic infection spreading to wild birds from captive collections (Jessup 1986).

All Anseriformes can be affected but, in contrast to avian cholera, other bird and mammal species are not susceptible. This can be useful in differentiating these two important causes of mass mortalities (Friend & Franson 1999).

Amongst the Anseriformes there seems to be a wide range of susceptibility both between species and individuals as well as with viral strain. As a general rule, muscovies (*Cairina moschata*), wood ducks (*Aix sponsa*) and teal (*Anas crecca*) seem most susceptible to DVE, while mallard (*Anas platyrhynchos*), domestic Pekin ducks (*Anas platyrhynchos*) and pintails (*Anas acuta*) are more resistant. Symptomless carrier wild mallard are often blamed for disease outbreaks in collections in the UK. Transmission from contaminated feed and water can occur via oral, nasal and cloacal routes, and incubation is 3Ð7 days.

Birds are typically found dead. Those exhibiting clinical signs may be photophobic, lethargic, anorexic, ataxic, and have a serosanguineous nasal discharge and watery or bloody diarrhoea. Most die within 24 hours, showing terminal convulsions and, in males, a prolapsed phallus. Pathology is due to acute viral damage to the endothelial lining of small blood vessels, lymphoid tissue and selected epithelial tissues. Gross pathology is consistent with an acute septicaemia (see ÔAvian choleraÕ for a description). Inconsistent but more speciÞc Þndings include exanthematous plaques under the tongue and around the cloaca and in longitudinal rows in the oesophagus. In species with well-organized and distinct gastrointestinal lymphoid tissue these may become haemorrhagic and later necrotizing; forming annular bands in some species of ducks and button-like structures in geese. Intraluminal haemorrhages and mucosal ecchymoses are also common. Herpesvirus inclusion bodies are often (but not always) seen on histopathological examination of the liver, reticuloendothelial system and the mucosa underlying any oesophageal or cloacal lesions (Wobeser 1981, Jessup 1986, Brown & Forbes 1996).

Typical post-mortem signs are suggestive of DVE but, due to their variability, a deÞnitive diagnosis by virus isolation should be sought. There is no treatment for DVE, and the condition is often self-limiting. Immunity is thought to occur in recovered animals, but this is not reliable. In an open population, each outbreak may last for several weeks and frequently the disease recurs with new susceptible arrivals or as carriers ßy on. A modiÞed live vaccine is available in many countries. Care

should be taken when using live vaccines in species in which they have not been tested in case of reversion to virulence.

Non-infectious diseases

Toxicoses

Lead poisoning

Aetiology

Lead poisoning is caused by the ingestion of lead shot used as anglersÕ weights or shotgun pellets from wetlands that have been hunted. More uncommonly there may be the ingestion of soil or sediments contaminated with high lead levels (e.g. from mining or smelting activity). Lead shot in the proventriculus and gizzard is dissolved by the digestive acid. The process is enhanced by the grinding action of the gizzard and the lead is then absorbed into the blood. Lead shot in other tissues, e.g. from gunshot wounding, is not a cause of systemic lead toxicosis.

Pathogenesis and clinical signs

The absorbed lead ions inactivate enzymes in major metabolic pathways. Tissues affected include kidney, bone, central nervous system (CNS) and the haemopoietic system. The clinical signs produced are wideranging and include anorexia, anaemia, a green diarrhoea, weakness and weight loss. Muscular weakness in swans leads to a characteristic ßaccidity of the neck, which falls caudally to rest on the birdÕs back. There is a ßaccid paralysis of the oesophagus, frequently resulting in impaction with food material. Vocalization may change. CNS signs include ataxia which, in geese and ducks in particular, often results in a high stepping gait and a tendency to fall over backwards. Eventually there is collapse, coma and death. Post-mortem Þndings include an emaciated carcass, a dark-coloured liver (which may be enlarged or shrunken) with greenish bile staining, an enlarged gall bladder with viscous bile, dark-coloured caeca, watery green faeces, enlarged spleen and kidneys and deposits of urates in tissues.

Confirmation of diagnosis

Two tests are regularly used to conÞrm a diagnosis of lead poisoning in live birds; radiography of the gastrointestinal (GI) tract and analysis of whole blood (Fig. 12.6). Both need interpretation and are best used in conjunction with each other and with reference to the clinical condition of the bird (Routh 2000).

A dorsoventral radiograph of the abdomen can be taken in the conscious bird, using restraint with sandbags or with the bird in a swan-bag. The X-ray beam should be centred in the midline at the level of the

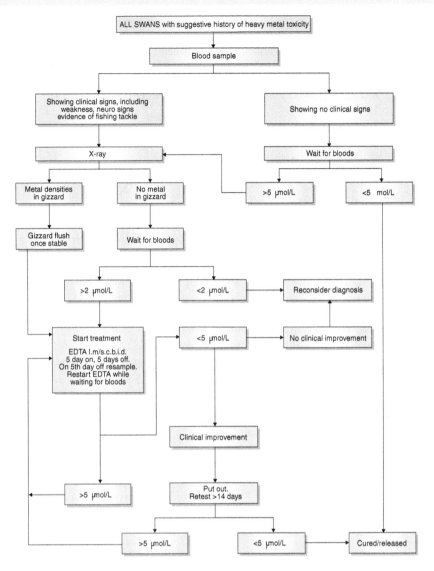

Fig 12.6 Diagnostic flowchart for determining lead exposure in waterfowl.

elbows and the view should include the gizzard, proventriculus and caudal oesophagus. The presence of strongly radiodense material is suspicious of lead, but it may not be distinguishable from modern lead-free shot (Figs 12.7, 12.8). Degernes et al (1989) found that 25% of birds diagnosed as suffering from lead poisoning had no radiographically visible lead but this does not preclude a diagnosis of lead poisoning as the particulate lead may have been completely absorbed or may have been voided from the GI tract.

Heparinized blood or blood in lithium heparin (minimum 1 mL) can be analysed for blood lead concentration. There appears to be no consistent toxic threshold and, as mentioned, the result must be interpreted in the light of the clinical and radiological Þndings. The

authors use the procedure represented in Figure 12.6, which uses 2 μmol/L in the presence of and 5 μmol/L in the absence of clinical signs as a threshold for practical decision-making.

Treatment

Particulate lead can be removed from the gizzard of an anaesthetized bird by the method described by Forbes (1993). With an endotracheal tube in place the anaesthetized bird is tilted, on a table, head-down to an angle of more than 45 degrees. A stomach-tube is passed into the gizzard and copious quantities of warmed water are flushed through by means of gravity or using a hand-pump. It is important to ensure that the oesophagus

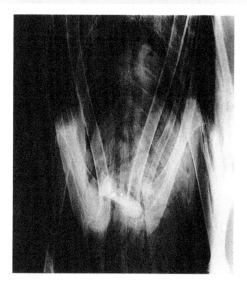

Fig 12.7 Dorsoventral radiograph of a mute swan showing lead shot in the gizzard. This swan has been radiographed in a normal resting position with the wings folded. The elbow joints obscure the view of the gizzard. There is a sharp penetrating foreign body as an incidental finding.

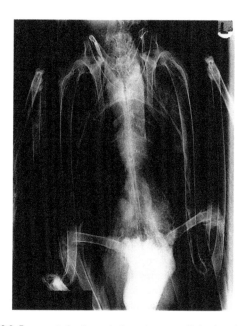

Fig 12.8 Dorsoventral radiograph of a mute swan suffering from lead poisoning. The lead shot is visible, together with a dilated gizzard and proventriculus and a dilated and impacted oesophagus.

is not obstructed with vegetable matter or other food material cranial to the tube end. If water cannot escape, pressure can build up and rupture the proventriculus. Removal of lead is confirmed by repeat radiography and examination of the flushed-out material. The whole of the head and neck should be radiographed to ensure no pellets remain in the upper oesophagus or pharynx.

On occasion pieces of lead may be trapped in the koilin folds of the gizzard. Sometimes these can be dislodged by gently rolling the bird but it is better to repeat the procedure several days later rather than extend the procedure excessively. Individual large pellets may be removed by endoscopy using a grasper. Occasionally large pieces of lead may become embedded in the koilin layer of the gizzard and ventriculotomy may be required to remove them.

Sodium calcium edetate (EDTA) is the most commonly used drug for the treatment of lead toxicosis and recommended doses range from 12 to 40 mg/kg s.c. or i.v., b.i.d. or t.i.d. The authors' treatment of choice is EDTA at 35 mg/kg s.c. b.i.d. for 5 days, followed by 5 days with no treatment. The bird is resampled and treated again for 5 days until the blood lead is below 5 µmol/L and the bird is clinically improving. A higher initial dose, e.g. 100 mg/kg b.i.d. on the first day, with subsequent dose reduction can be used (Forbes, personal communication, 2006) but this protocol must be accompanied by vigorous fluid therapy. A lower protein, higher fibre diet may reduce lead absorption from the gut but affected birds are often in poor physical condition and require a higher plane of nutrition. A high-calcium oyster or cockleshell grit should be provided throughout the treatment period to, again, reduce lead absorption from the gut and to offset any potential EDTA-induced calcium deficiencies (though these have not been seen by the authors).

The use of oral D-penicillamine at a dose of 55 mg/kg b.i.d. for 7 to 14 days has also been recommended (Forbes & Harcourt-Brown 1996). This has the advantage that it can be administered to free-living birds but in the authors' experience it produces a poor response. Its use in conjunction with EDTA has been recommended (Olsen 1994), but an apparent adverse reaction to this protocol has been reported (Keeble 1997), so caution is recommended.

Meso-2,3 dimercaptosuccinic acid (DMSA) is a water-soluble heavy metal chelating agent that has been used in the USA, but it is currently not available in the UK.

Prognosis and prevention

Simpson et al (1979) reported a poor prognosis for birds with a haematocrit of below 29%. Severe emaciation or evidence of liver or kidney damage on blood test carry a poor prognosis. In absolute terms the prognosis is not dictated by the blood lead level in isolation and birds with initially very high levels can make spectacular recoveries.

In the UK the ban on the use of lead in fishing weights of under 28 g has drastically reduced the incidence of lead poisoning in mute swans but Kelly & Kelly (2004), using a threshold of 1.21 µmol/L, diagnosed lead poisoning in 74% of all swans admitted to a Royal

Society for Prevention of Cruelty to Animals (RSPCA) wildlife hospital over a 3-year period. Lead used up to two decades ago can be found intact in the environment but the most recent contamination lying in the surface soil and sediment layers is the most frequently ingested. Older deposits become less accessible over time and thus a ban on use of lead by anglers and hunters is effective in reducing the incidence of lead poisoning.

It is presumed that lead is inadvertently picked up in heavily contaminated environments by birds seeking out grit to facilitate digestion. In grit-free habitats lead shot may be picked up selectively and the provision of grit may reduce ingestion of lead shot (O'Halloran et al 2002). Birds are often site-faithful and thus may return to a heavily contaminated habitat but birds that have recovered from lead poisoning may develop a pica and selectively ingest lead shot. Birds treated and released once are more likely to be affected a second time (Sears 1988).

The significance of high lead levels in relation to birds suffering from other conditions is difficult to determine, although it is possible that debility due to subclinical lead poisoning increases the incidence of collision with power lines and other traumatic injuries (O'Halloran et al 1988). Swans bullied by conspecifics, ones involved in road traffic accidents or that have crash-landed often have evidence of lead toxicosis (Routh 2000).

Botulism

Botulism is a paralytic disease that affects birds and mammals. It is caused by the toxin of the anaerobic bacterium *Clostridium botulinum* but is an intoxication rather than an infectious disease. It is contracted only by the ingestion of toxin preformed in suitable media. Type C toxin causes sporadic deaths in birds worldwide, but type E toxin is largely restricted to the Great Lakes of North America. *C. botulinum* cannot survive or its toxin persist in environments with a salinity equivalent to that of seawater but deaths of birds in brackish water environments have occurred. High temperatures, shallow, still or slow-moving water and decaying organic matter create a nutrient-rich anaerobic environment that predisposes to outbreaks of botulism from the germination of *C. botulinum* spores found naturally in soil. Carcasses of botulism casualties increase the bacteria numbers in the environment as they putrefy and the maggots feeding on them are rich sources of toxin and will cause further deaths if ingested.

Clinical signs are an acute progressive flaccid paralysis of voluntary muscles. Wings, legs and neck are affected first. Classic clinical signs are ataxia and 'limberneck', a weaving motion with the head and neck, leading to eventual collapse of the neck as paralysis progresses. Early signs may be as little as a single drooping wing or an inability to swallow. Birds often show respiratory distress with open-mouth breathing before the head carriage becomes affected. The prognosis has been linked to the severity of clinical signs (Forbes 1996) but, in the authors'experience, is often unpredictable. Once birds are unable to stand and hold their heads resting on their backs the prognosis is poor. Death is due to respiratory arrest, cardiac arrest or drowning.

Treatment consists of supportive management and aggressive fluid therapy, both oral and parenteral. Oral fluids are used to flush out or dilute any toxin present and are followed by the administration of intestinal adsorbents (activated charcoal and/or bismuth). Specific antitoxins, manufactured for the treatment of horses, are available but are reported to be ineffective (LaBonde 1996).

Confirmation of diagnosis can be made by detection of toxin in serum or stomach contents. The authors have found that samples from birds showing classical clinical signs frequently fail to reveal the presence of toxin. Once ingested toxin is rapidly bound to nerve endings and disappears from the gut and circulation. The time elapsed since ingestion of toxin is usually unknown and this interval may be the reason for the unreliability of treatments, unreliability of disease prognosis and the difficulties with toxin identification.

Control measures include management of affected environments through the removal of carcasses, drainage or oxygenation of affected water. Captive birds may be physically removed from the affected environments but the use of bird-scarers to drive potentially-affected wild birds away from affected areas is controversial. A vaccine produced commercially for use in mink has been reported successfully to prevent disease in groups of waterfowl at high risk (Cambre & Kenny 1993).

Algal toxins

Eutrophic freshwaters exposed to warm temperatures and long hours of sunlight can suffer explosive blooms of toxin-producing phytoplankton of a range of species, usually referred to as blue-green algae. Very high concentrations of toxins can result. These toxins can be neurotoxic, hepatotoxic and locally irritant. Clinical signs include irritation of the skin and eyes, salivation, regurgitation, collapse and death. Diagnosis is often based on circumstantial evidence, presence of toxic blooms and clinical signs or sudden death in a wide range of species of different taxa, including both birds and mammals. Waterfowl were amongst the species affected by a cyanobacterial bloom in a national park in Spain (Alonso-Andicoberry et al 2002). It was postulated that previously uninvestigated deaths in the same national park could have had a similar aetiology and this may indicate that the condition is possibly overlooked in some die-offs. Treatment is symptomatic. The toxins will affect humans and care must be taken when handling affected birds or carcasses, or if there is contact with affected water.

Toxic algae in the marine environment are discussed in Chapter 16.

Various other toxicities

Other toxicities that occur in wildfowl but do not differ significantly from disease seen in other species include:

- Mycotoxicosis, due to fungal toxins in mouldy food. Most are hepatotoxic. Ingestion of toxic plants can occur in captivity, but is rarely seen in the wild.
- Zinc toxicity, which can occur from ingesting galvanized metal or some coins. Clinical signs include weight loss, lethargy, anorexia and posterior paresis.
- Environmental contaminants and oil pollution. These are discussed in Chapter 16.

'Downer-duck' syndrome

A frequent presentation, in particular for general practitioners, is the severely lame or collapsed individual adult duck, often one of a small 'back-yard' flock.

As with any case a full history should be taken. This should include the age of the individual, its gender, the flock size and the individual's status in the flock. The bird's plumage and general body condition should be assessed along with any signs of infectious disease.

In a female bird there may be exhaustion through harassment by over-vigorous males or reproductive pathology including over-production of eggs, being 'egg-bound' or suffering from egg peritonitis.

The emaciated bird may have a heavy parasite burden or be suffering from avian TB or aspergillosis.

Conversely birds that have lived in a cosseted environment may be obese and this may be coupled with arthritis, which may be septic in origin or the result of degenerative joint disease in the older bird. With non-septic arthritis pain management is essential. A variety of drugs can be used for short-term, peri-operative and longer-term management (Cracknell 2004, Cousquer 2005, Machin 2005). Non-steroidal anti-inflammatory drugs (NSAIDs) have a role to play, in particular as there are oral preparations suitable for long-term administration, but specific circumstances and possible species idiosyncrasy may present as unexpected toxicities. Mulcahy et al (2003) reported mortalities due to renal failure several days after general anaesthesia and surgery on free-ranging spectacled eiders (*Somateria fischeri*) and king eiders (*Somateria spectabilis*) where ketoprofen had been used for postoperative pain management at accepted dose rates.

Collapse through cardiac disease, e.g. pericardial effusion (Straub et al 2001) or cardiomegaly (Fischer et al 2005), may be under-diagnosed and must be ruled out.

Lameness or paresis may be neurological in origin. Back injuries should be considered but more local neurological effects may be due to pressure on the sacral nerve plexus from renal pathologies such as coccidiosis and space-occupying masses including neoplasia and polycystic disease (Sanchez et al 2004).

Irrespective of cause this presentation requires a thorough, and often complex, clinical work-up with the resulting diagnosis often having a guarded prognosis.

Fishing tackle injuries

Sports fishing is popular all over the world and takes place in most aquatic habitats. It is Britain's most popular participation sport and it is therefore not surprising that there is interaction between waterfowl and fishing tackle. On crowded waterways close to centres of human population fishing tackle entanglement or ingestion (see previous comments on lead toxicity) is a major cause of injury or illness. Over a 3-year period Kelly & Kelly (2004) recorded fishing tackle injuries in 17% of all mute swans admitted, the single highest cause for rescue as diagnosed on admission to a wildlife hospital. They believed that the majority of these birds would not have survived without intervention.

Modern monofilament nylon line is strong, elastic, persists in the environment and is almost invisible in water. Line may be accidentally lost or carelessly discarded either on its own or attached to hooks, weights or lures. It may be left loose on the ground or entangled in vegetation or round obstructions such as branches or roots above or below the water. Line entangled around extremities will restrict circulation and gradually penetrate tissues, eventually severing muscles, tendons and blood vessels and even bone. Care must be taken to remove all nylon which may be deeply embedded in (or even overgrown by) granulation tissue and healing skin, especially when very fine line is wrapped repeatedly around a leg. Even after line removal, annular scar tissue can contract to restrict circulation. Wounds should be carefully debrided to remove hard scar tissue and kept moist and supple with cellulose gel (Intrasite – Smith & Nephew Medical Ltd) or petroleum jelly until healed. Wounds to the propatagium are prone to severe contraction of the wound edges. Longstanding wounds often result in permanent flightlessness. Ducks may sometimes survive the amputation or loss of function of a leg, but heavier geese and swans almost invariably develop pressure necrosis over the keel and protrusion of the keel bone. Hooks can tear skin – again the propatagium is vulnerable – or become embedded in muscle, tendons or joints, resulting in physical damage and secondary infection.

Birds presenting with line hanging from the mouth should first be checked for tackle entangled externally or around the beak, tongue or glottis. Radiography of head, neck and body caudally as far as the gizzard will reveal the presence of ingested hooks, weights or lures (Fig. 12.9). If no hooks are present, the line can be cut and allowed to be ingested and work its way out naturally. If one end of the line has entered the gizzard it is usually difficult to extract and there is a danger of 'cheesewire' cuts if excess traction is applied. Once in the gizzard line is ground into pieces and it is very unusual for intact line to pass on into the intestine. It is important to be alert for loops of line wrapped around the upper or lower beak, tongue or larynx. In these cases the line will be gradually pulled caudally, the situation exacerbated by ingested food building up and impacting cranially to the distal line. With increasing tension on the looped line there is restriction of extension of the neck and a palpable tense band in the oesophagus, followed by the rapid development of 'cheesewire' cuts. In some instances the greater damage is to the head where the line has looped over the beak: 'chinstrap' injuries (Cracknell 2004). General anaesthesia

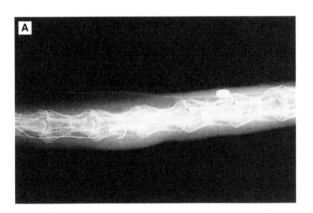

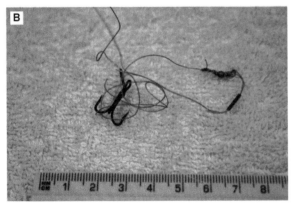

Fig 12.9 A Radiograph of a swan's neck showing two hooks and a wire trace in the oesophagus. The airgun pellets are an incidental finding. **B** Fish hook.

should be induced and radiography performed to ensure no hooks are involved in the entrapment. The loop of line over the beak should then be isolated and two pairs of artery forceps attached to it. The line is sectioned between the forceps and they are then manipulated, individually or together, to gently retract the line back through the mouth.

Radiography is invaluable in identifying the type, size and site of any ingested hook. Hooks can be barbed or barbless, single or multiple. They may be attached direct to the line or to a lure in various combinations. Large treble hooks are particularly traumatic. If traction has been applied to the hook it can become deeply embedded or cause tearing of the oesophagus. Embedded barbed hooks can be difficult to remove and create considerable damage. It is important to check for small hooks embedded in the tongue or upper pharynx. Single hooks can be removed from the pharynx with long-handled forceps. Further down the oesophagus hooks can be 'disgorged' by passing the attached line through a 'fisherman's' disgorger or, for longer-necked species, a suitable semi-rigid rod such as a bovine uterine irrigation catheter. With the line gently taut, the disgorger is slid over the shank of the hook, which is pushed away from the direction of penetration. Barbless hooks will often disengage easily and can be withdrawn. Barbed hooks may be more firmly embedded and excessive pressure should not be applied. Visualization of the site with a flexible endoscope and inflation of the oesophagus can facilitate disgorging.

Large hooks can sometimes be manipulated to protrude through the skin. The bend of hook can then be cut with pincers, allowing the shank to be easily removed by traction (Cracknell 2004).

Surgery is indicated when hooks are deeply embedded or when there is a sizeable tear in the oesophageal wall. Surgical approach is routine, but careful debridement and removal of any necrotic tissue is essential. Closure of the oesophagus is best achieved using a synthetic absorbable monofilament material (Monocryl, Ethicon) on a swaged atraumatic needle, using a continuous inverting suture pattern. Postoperative antibiotic cover should be provided and, if necessary, feeding carried out by careful gavage for the first 3 days.

Hooks are usually made of bronzed or stainless steel, both of which will rust and eventually disintegrate in the digestive tract. The remains of hooks, surrounded by necrotic material and walled off by foreign body reaction, are not uncommon incidental post-mortem findings in the upper GI tract. Small, deeply embedded hooks causing no clinical signs may not warrant surgical intervention. Occasionally large hooks are encountered deeply embedded and far caudal to the thoracic inlet, making surgical approach difficult. **These birds may display no clinical signs once the excess line has been removed. The authors have managed such birds** without treatment, with no signs of inappetence or discomfort, suggesting that conservative treatment may produce a natural resolution without resorting to high risk surgery. Monitoring and assessment through regular haematology, radiography and possibly coelomic endoscopy is appropriate and prudent.

Power line injuries

Large birds such as swans require space to manoeuvre in the air and are prone to collision with overhead power cables as these may be difficult for birds to see and avoid. Birds suffer physical trauma due to the collision and subsequent crash landing. Moreover, if a bird's extremities touch or are close to two differently charged wires an electrical discharge can result, causing added electrical trauma.

Birds may immediately show clear signs of electrical shock or burning, including large open wounds with charred or coagulated flesh and a smell of burning. In some instances there are often no signs of electrical injury but over the following days a progressive wing or leg lameness may be noted. On examination there are often cold oedematous areas, especially the wing distal to the carpus, the ventral abdomen or thigh muscles. These are the result of irreversible coagulative necrosis and these areas of tissue will slough. Prognosis is poor (Cooper 1996). There is no evidence that therapy is effective, the damage having been done at the time of the initial injury, and euthanasia is indicated unless the affected area is small. Post-mortem examination often reveals the presence of additional areas of electrical coagulation in internal organs. Some birds show paralysis of one or more limbs without associated signs of either physical or electrical trauma. Such paralysis is usually unresponsive to treatment and permanent.

As some birds known to have hit power lines show no immediate evidence of electrical trauma but develop the clinical signs later it is recommended that all birds having collided with power cables be hospitalized for a minimum of 5 days. Injuries due to physical trauma should be treated as appropriate. If there is no evidence of electrical trauma after the 5 days, it can be presumed that electrocution did not occur.

Cables sited on regular flight paths into a feeding or roosting area can be marked with large, brightly coloured lightweight plastic spheres. These are effective in reducing bird-strikes. The incidence of bird-strikes can be greatly increased in foggy weather when flocks may repeatedly circle regular landing sites unable to see well enough for their final approach.

Gout

Other than in cases of lead toxicosis, visceral and articular gout are unusual in waterfowl. Discrete swellings seen in tendon sheaths and containing glistening white paste-like solids are aggregations of urate crystals caused by gout.

Bumblefoot (Pododermatitis)

Hard or excessively abrasive surfaces can cause swelling, skin erosion and secondary infection of any of the joints on the plantar surface of the foot. Early or mild signs may be treated conservatively by providing soft floor surfaces (rubber matting, natural grass, Astroturf or wood shavings) and encouraging time spent on water. Application of steroid and antibiotic in dimethylsulphoxide (DMSO) has been recommended (Olsen 1994). More severe cases may require surgical debulking and antibiotic therapy, preferably based on bacterial culture and sensitivity testing. Post-surgical dressing is achieved by cutting a template of the extended foot from a semi-rigid material such as plastic or stiff card. Soft dressings are applied to the plantar surface of the foot, which is then extended and stuck to the template with zinc oxide tape applied to the dorsal surface. The whole is then covered with a water-repellent dressing.

Acknowledgements

The authors wish to acknowledge the contribution of Ian Robinson to this chapter, both in this edition and in the first edition of the book. For the first edition he was a co-author of the chapter and was credited as such in the final proofs though his name, inexplicably, did not appear in the published text.

References

Alonso-Andicoberry C, Garcia-Villada L, Lopez-Rodas V, Costas E 2002 Catastrophic mortality of flamingoes in a Spanish national park caused by cyanobacteria. Veterinary Record 151(23):706–707

Bennett R A 1997 Medical and surgical management of avian reproductive disorders. Proceedings of the Mid-Atlantic States Association of Avian Veterinarians Conference, p 40–44

Benyon P H, Forbes N A, Harcourt-Brown N H (eds) 1996 Manual of raptors, pigeons and waterfowl. BSAVA Publications, Cheltenham

Brown M J, Forbes N A 1996 Respiratory diseases. In: Benyon P H, Forbes N A, Harcourt-Brown N H (eds) Manual of raptors, pigeons and waterfowl. BSAVA Publications, Cheltenham, p 315–316

Cambre R C, Kenny D 1993 Vaccination of zoo birds against avian botulism with mink botulism vaccine. In: American Association of Zoo Veterinarians Annual Proceedings, p 383–385

Carpenter J W 2005 Exotic animal formulary, 3rd edition. Elsevier Saunders, St Louis, MO, p 215

Coles B H 1997 Avian medicine and surgery. Blackwell Science, Oxford

Cooke S W 1995 Swan anaesthesia. Veterinary Record 136(18):476

Cooper J E 1996 Physical injury. In: Fairbrother A, Locke L N, Hoff G L (eds) Non-infectious diseases of wildlife. Manson Publishing, London, p 163–165

Cousquer G 2005 First aid and emergency care for the avian casualty. In Practice 27:190–203

Cracknell J 2004 Dealing with line and hook injuries in swans. In Practice 26:238–245

Degernes L A, Frank R K, Freeman M L, Redig P T 1989 Lead poisoning in trumpeter swans. In: Proceedings of the Association of Avian Veterinarian Annual Conference. AAV, Boca Raton, FL, p 144–155

Driver E A 1981 Haematological and blood chemical values of mallard (Anas platyrhynchos) drakes before, during and after remige moult. Journal of Wildlife Diseases 17(3):413–421

Fischer I, Christen C, Scharf G, Hatt J-M 2005 Cardiomegaly in a whooper swan (Cygnus cygnus). Veterinary Record 156(6):178–182

Forbes N 1993 Treatment of lead poisoning in swans. In Practice 15(2):90–91

Forbes N A 1996 Nervous conditions. In: Benyon P H, Forbes N A, Harcourt-Brown N H (eds) Manual of raptors, pigeons and waterfowl. BSAVA Publications, Cheltenham, p 317–321

Forbes N A, Harcourt-Brown N H 1996 Appendix formulary – waterfowl. In: Benyon P H, Forbes N A, Harcourt-Brown N H (eds) Manual of raptors, pigeons and waterfowl. BSAVA Publications, Cheltenham, p 352

Forbes N A, Richardson T 1996 Husbandry and nutrition. In: Benyon P H, Forbes N A, Harcourt-Brown N H (eds) Manual of raptors, pigeons and waterfowl. BSAVA Publications, Cheltenham, p 289–298

Forbes N A, Cromie R L, Brown M J et al 1993 Diagnosis of tuberculosis in wildfowl. In: Proceedings of the Association of Avian Veterinarians Annual Conference. AAV, Boca Raton, FL, p 182–186

Fowler M E (ed) 1986 Zoo and wild animal medicine. W B Saunders, Philadelphia, PA

Friend J, Franson J C 1999 Field manual of wildlife diseases: general field procedures and diseases of birds. US Geological Survey

Goulden S 1995 Swan anaesthesia. Veterinary Record 136(17):448

Hess J C, Paré J A 2004 Viruses of waterfowl. Seminars in Avian and Exotic Pet Medicine 13(4):176–183

Humphreys P N 1986 Ducks, geese, swans and screamers (Anseriformes): reproduction. In: Fowler M E (ed) Zoo and wild animal medicine. W B Saunders, Philadelphia, PA, p 355–357

Jessup D A 1986 Ducks, geese, swans and screamers (Anseriformes): infectious diseases. In: Fowler M E (ed) Zoo and wild animal medicine. W B Saunders, Philadelphia, PA, p 342–352

Kaneene J B, Flint Taylor R, Sikarskie J G, Meyer T J 1985 Disease patterns in the Detroit Zoo: a study of the avian population from 1973 through 1983. Journal of the American Veterinary Medical Association 187(11):1129–1131

Kear J 1986 Ducks, geese, swans and screamers (Anseriformes): feeding and Nutrition. In: Fowler M E (ed) 1986 Zoo and wild animal medicine. W B Saunders, Philadelphia, PA, p 335–341

Keeble E 1997 Suspected allergic reaction to penicillamine in mute swans. Veterinary Record 140(17):464

Kelly A, Kelly S 2004 Fishing tackle injury and blood lead levels in mute swans. Waterbirds 27(1):60–68

Kenny D, Cambre R C 1992 Indications and techniques for the surgical removal of the avian yolk sac. Journal of Zoology and Wildlife Medicine 23(1):55–61

Labonde J 1992 The medical and surgical management of domestic waterfowl collections. In: Proceedings of the Association of Avian Veterinarians Annual Conference. AAV, Boca Raton, FL, p 223–233

Labonde J 1996 Private collections of waterfowl. Proceedings of the Annual Conference and Expo, Association of Avian Veterinarians 6:215–223

Lawton M P C 1996 Anaesthesia. In: Benyon P H, Forbes N A, Harcourt-Brown N H (eds) Manual of raptors, pigeons and waterfowl. BSAVA Publications, Cheltenham, p 79–88

Lloyd C 2003 Control of nematode infections in captive birds. In Practice 25:198–206

Machin K L 2005 Controlling avian pain. Compendium on Continuing Education for the Practicing Veterinarian April: 299–309

Madge S, Burn H 1988 Wildfowl, an identification guide to the ducks, geese and swans of the world. A&C Black Publishers, London

Mulcahy D M, Tuomi P, Scott Larsen R 2003 Differential mortality of male spectacled eiders (Somateria fischeri) and king eiders (Somateria spectabilis) subsequent to anesthesia with propofol, bupivacaine and ketoprofen. Journal of Avian Medicine and Surgery 17(3):117–123

O'Halloran J, Myers A A, Duggan P F 1988 Lead poisoning in swans and sources of contamination. Ireland Journal of Zoology 216:221–223

O'Halloran J, Smiddy P, Xie Q I, O'Leary R, Hayes C 2002 Trends in mute swan blood lead levels: Evidence of grit reducing lead poisoning. Waterbirds 25(Special Issue 1):363–367

Olsen J H 1994 Ansiformes. In: Ritchie B W, Harrison G J, Harrison L R (eds) Avian medicine: principles and application. Wingers, Lake Worth, FL, p 1237–1275

Ritchie B W, Harrison G J, Harrison L R (eds) 1994 Avian medicine: principles and application. Wingers, Lake Worth, FL

Routh A 2000 Veterinary care in the mute swan. In Practice 22:426–443

Sanchez C, Bush M, Montali R 2004 Polycystic kidney disease associated with unilateral lameness in a northern pintail (Anas acuta). Journal of Avian Medicine and Surgery 18(4):98–106

Sears J 1988 Regional and seasonal variations in lead poisoning in the mute swan (Cygnus olor) in relation to the distribution of lead and lead weights, in the Thames Area, England. Biology Conservation 46:115–134

Sherrill J, Ware L H, Lynch W E et al 2001 Contrast radiography with positive-pressure insufflation in the northern pintail (Anas acuta). Journal of Avian Medicine and Surgery 15(3):178–186

Simpson V R, Hunt A E, French M C 1979 Chronic lead poisoning in a herd of mute swans. Environmental Pollution 18:187–202

Straub J, Pees M, Krautwald-Junghanns M-E 2001 Diagnosis of pericardial effusion in birds by ultrasound. Veterinary Record 149(3):86–88

Williams J I, Trainer D O 1971 A haematological study of snow, blue and Canada geese. Journal of Wildlife Diseases 7:258–265

Wobeser G A 1981 Diseases of wild waterfowl. Plenum Press, New York

Galliformes

13

Brian H. Coles

Introduction

The order Galliformes (fowl-like birds), in line with the most up-to-date taxonomic information derived from DNA and other biochemical techniques (Sibley & Ahlquist 1990), is now divided into three families:

1. Phasianidae
2. Numididae
3. Odontophoridae.

These families, showing various representative species and the general characteristics, are listed in Table 13.1.

Until comparatively recently, taxonomists included within the order Galliformes two other avian families, the Cracidae (i.e. guans, chachalacas and curassows) and the Megapodiidae (megapodes, scrub fowl and brushturkeys). However, the latest taxonomic information now places these families in a separate order, the Craciformes. Both Galliformes and Craciformes are now included in the superorder Gallomorphae (or Gallomorphs). Within this super order there are some 283 species, the original representatives of which were found in all the world's continents except Antarctica, and on many islands except those of Polynesia and New Zealand.

Although the Galliformes range in size from the relatively small Chinese painted quail (body length 13 cm) to the much larger turkeys and peafowl (approximately 117 cm), most are medium-sized birds similar in size, body form and behavioural characteristics to domestic chickens. The Galliformes are considered to be rather primitive, unspecialized birds that probably evolved early in the evolutionary cycle. They all have relatively large stout legs and feet, with three forward-pointing digits and a smaller hind digit. Many of these birds are mostly terrestrial, and are incapable of prolonged sustained flight. In most species within the order the mode of flight is a short but rapid take-off, and then gliding or fluttering for short distances. The majority of these birds are non-migratory. However, both grouse and guinea fowl can fly quite strongly, and the Old World quail and some species living in high altitudes do undergo a partial migration to better feeding grounds in winter.

Veterinary anatomy and physiology

The skeleton

This is similar in all Galliformes to that of the domestic chicken, with well-developed muscular legs consistent with the relatively stout legs needed for a terrestrial lifestyle and scratching the ground in search of food. Some species (e.g. turkeys) have ossified leg tendons. All Galliformes have an anisodactyl foot with three cranially directed digits and a fourth, the hallux, situated somewhat higher up the tarsometatarsus and directed caudomedially. In some families or subfamilies (e.g. jungle fowl, turkeys, pheasants) the cock birds have an extra osseous sharp-pointed spur situated above the hallux and directed medially, which is used for fighting and territorial dominance. In the common pheasant (*Phasianus colchicus*), annual rings are formed at the base of the spur and can be used for ageing the bird. Care must be taken when handling such birds, since they can injure the handler. The green peacock will make a positive attack on humans and other animals using the spurs, and turkey cocks will fight to the death.

Some breeds of domestic chicken (e.g. Chinese silks, Dorkings and Houdans) have five digits, with the extra digit situated medial to the hallux.

The skull of the sand grouse (*Pteroclidae* spp.) has a well-developed fossa that contains the large salt gland, which acts as a supplementary excretory organ in these species. The helmeted guinea fowl (*Numida meleagris*) carries a spongy bone extension situated at the junction of the nasal and frontal bone, which is covered by pigmented skin. This structure, together with the wattles, is better developed in male birds.

In Galliformes, there are two deeply and cranially directed non-ossified incisions covered in fibrous sheets on each side of the sternal plate. **It should be noted that these leave the underlying liver exposed and vulnerable to deep intramuscular injection if due care is not exercised.** The furcula (i.e. the 'wishbone') in the crested and plumed guinea fowl and in the capercaillie (*Tetrao urogallus*) is cup-shaped to receive the elongated trachea.

The integument

The most obvious characteristic of the Galliformes is the presence of well-developed eye combs, wattles and 'beard' (in the common turkey), all of which are highly coloured (usually red) and inflatable. Some grouse also have inflatable coloured cervical air sacs. In some species (jungle fowl, pheasants, turkeys and some grouse) the tail feathers are well developed for display purposes, but the tail of the peacock is not formed of true rectrices but of elongated coverts. Most Galliformes moult

Table 13.1a–c Families, genera and representative species within the order Galliformes. The following are most likely to be encountered by the veterinarian, as they are often kept in captive collections

a. Family: Phasianidae

i. Subfamily Phasianinae (pheasants); 8 genera containing 21 species

In most species the male bird has highly coloured plumage whilst the female is more dowdy. Most cock pheasants have exceptionally long tails which are vaulted, i.e. in cross-section they are like an inverted V. The tail is used by the cock bird for display purposes when courting. The fourth digit (the hallux) is located more proximally on the metatarsus than the three forward-directed digits. In many species there is a pointed spur placed proximal to this fourth digit on the metatarsus. This appendage is used by the male birds for fighting to gain territory. Some species of pheasant have coloured facial skin on the head. Most pheasants make a whirring wing noise during territorial display and are also quite vocal.

Genus	Species	Characteristic	Size	Global distribution and normal habit
Gallus	G. gallus	The red jungle fowl: like the domestic chicken. From this species all the numerous breeds of domestic fowl have originated. The red jungle fowl will hybridize with domestic chickens. The species was probably first domesticated during the Bronze Age, and was originally kept for cock fighting. Unlike other pheasants, it has a more longitudinally arched tail and the cock has well-developed comb and wattles	66 cm (body) 28–30 cm (tail)	SE Asia (Kashmir, central India, Burma, Thailand, Malaysia, Sumatra and Java). Inhabits tropical rain forest, secondary growth scrub and rice stubble
	G. sonneratii	The grey jungle fowl: Sonnerai's jungle fowl: a somewhat larger, more dowdy bird than the red jungle fowl. Will hybridize with above species	76 cm (body) 41 cm (tail)	Western and southern India. Habitat: forest scrub, bamboo
Lophura	L. nycthemera	The silver pheasant: male bird, marked comb and red facial skin, silver grey wings and tail, black under parts. Will hybridize with above species	122 cm (body) 61–66 cm (tail)	South China, Burma, Thailand, Laos, Vietnam. Habitat: forest
	L. swinhoii	Swinhoe's pheasant: Formosan pheasant: marked comb and wattles, white neck, brown and dark blue/green plumage, dorsal tail white	150 cm	Taiwan. Habitat: mountainous up to 2800 m
	L. diardi	Siamese fire-back pheasant: male has crest, grey mantle, golden back patch, black tail	81–86 cm (body)	Burma, Thailand, Indo-China
Phasianus	P. colchicus	Common pheasant: two varieties: the white ring-necked form and the dark-necked form	60–90 cm (body) 52 cm (tail)	Eurasia, China, Taiwan. Introduced to North America, Hawaii, New Zealand. UK. Habitat: grass scrub, temperate woodland
Syrmaticus	S. reevesii	Reeves's pheasant, bar-tailed pheasant: body plumage golden with feathers edged with black. Tail long, silver banded with dark brown	86 cm (body) 101–152 cm (tail)	North and central China. Habitat: open woodland with pine, cypress and oak, tall grass and bushes
Chrysolophus	C. pictus	Golden pheasant: red under neck and breast, head and back golden, wings green, red, blue and brown, tail brown	39 cm (body) 76–79 cm (tail)	Central China, introduced locally in UK. Habitat: bushy slopes, bamboo, terraced fields
	C. amherstiae	Lady Amherst's pheasant: body plumage shows patches of green and white, silver, golden. Very long silver and brown tail	55 cm (body) 76–117 cm (tail)	SE Tibet, SW China, Burma. Habitat: wooded slopes, bracken hillsides, bamboo thickets

The eared pheasants – all have exceptionally long, rather bushy tails

| Crossoptilon | C. crossoptilon | The white eared pheasant: Tibetan eared pheasant | 91 cm (body) | SE Tibet to NE Yunan and central Szechwan. Habitat: coniferous and mixed forest, rhododendron scrub, grassy slopes |

	Species	Description	Size	Distribution/Habitat
	C. manchurian	The brown eared pheasant. Manchurian eared pheasant. Body brown, red facial skin with white collar and ear tufts	99 cm (body)	NE China. Habitat: stunted conifer or birch, rocky open shrub, coarse grass
	C. urium	The blue eared pheasant, Mongolian eared pheasant	97 cm (body)	W China. Habitat: conifer and mixed forest, bushy alpine meadow
ii. Subfamily Tragopinae: 5 species				
Tragopan	T. satyra	Satyr tragopan or crimson horned pheasant: white-specked orange and crimson plumage, back and tail base olive brown. Scapulars crimson but wing otherwise brown. Head, crest and throat black, tail reddish brown barred black and rather truncated	69 cm body which looks plumpish	Eastern Palaearctic, central and eastern Himalayas. Habitat: high forests. Migrates downhill in winter
iii. Subfamily Lophophorinae: 3 species				
The monal pheasants: heavy-bodied birds with a shorter, more square-shaped tail rather like a turkey. The cock birds have an iridescent plumage.				
Lophophorus	L. impeyans	The Himalayan monal or Impeyan: male has an upright crest, white lower back and lower rump. Upper tail coverts dark glossy blue-green, tail reddish-brown. Body and wings dark metallic green to purple, underparts black	71 cm (body)	Afghanistan Himalayas, SE Tibet. Habitat: open forest up to 3000 m
iv. Subfamily Argusianinae: 3 genera, 8 species				
Argusianus	A. argus	The great argus pheasant: male bird rusty brown plumage with black circled eye spots and mottling. Long tail with two central tail feathers broad and very long. Head bare, blue skin	72 cm (body and tail)	Indochina, Sumatra, Borneo. Habitat: primary tropical rain forest up to 1500 m
Polyplectron	P. bicalaratum	The grey peacock pheasant, Burmese peacock pheasant: male greyish brown, light-coloured throat and underparts. Large violet ocelli on back and tail. Crest, yellowish facial skin	30 cm (body) 41 cm (tail)	Central and southern Burma, Thailand, Laos, North Vietnam. Habitat: humid forest lowlands and mountains up to 1800 m
	P. empharum	Palawan peacock pheasant, Napoleon peacock pheasant: male darkish brown with iridescent blue-green plumage and large blue-green pointed crest. Tail has large blue-green eye spots. Facial skin reddish, white cheek patch	26 cm (body) 25 cm (tail)	The island of Palawan in the Philippines, north of Borneo. Habitat: humid forest lower elevation tropical rain forest
v. Subfamily Parvoninae: 2 genera, 3 species				
Peafowl: all have well-developed spurs.				
Parvo	P. cristatus	Common peafowl, Indian peafowl, blue peafowl: it is only the cock bird, the peacock, which develops the spectacular train and this does not develop until the third year. The long ornamental feathers of the tail are not true rectrices but elongated covert feathers	198–229 cm	India, Sri Lanka. Habitat: moist dry deciduous lowland forest up to 1500 m
	P. muticus	Green peafowl, Javanese green peafowl, Green necked peafowl: large bird, long train, brilliant green plumage, blue and yellow facial skin	213–244 cm	SW China, Assam, Burma, Thailand, Vietnam, Laos, Malaysia, Java. Habitat: open forest, riverbanks, forest edge, sometimes found up to 1000 m

(continued)

Table 13.1 *(continued)*

Genus	Species	Characteristic	Size	Global distribution and normal habit
Afropavo	*A. congesis*	The African peafowl: male dark glossy green and bronze on back rump. Underside dark green, violet iridescent back of neck and sternum. Crown white and black spots. Facial skin blue	60–68 cm	Zaire (Congo Basin). Habitat: dense lowland tropical rain forest

vi. *Subfamily Tetraonidae: 6 genera, 17 species*

The grouse: birds in this subfamily have feathered external nares as well as feathered tarsi and sometimes feathered digits, particularly the ptarmigan, which inhabits colder regions. Grouse do not have tarsal spurs. During the breeding season some species (e.g. the prairie chicken, black, sharp-tailed and sage grouse) gather at traditional display arenas or *lecks*, where the males carry out an intricate repetitive dance to hold territory and attract females. All grouse are powerful fliers.

Genus	Species	Characteristic	Size	Global distribution and normal habit
Lagopus	*L. lagopus*	Willow grouse. Willow ptarmigan in North America: a stout, short-winged bird, reddish brown in colour with white wings. Wedge-shaped tail with darker outer feathers. Moults three times yearly. White in winter except tail. Male has inflatable red skin combs above eyes. Will burrow under snow for food and shelter	38 cm	Northern Palaearctic, temperate and subarctic. Introduced to Belgium. Habitat: tundra and taiga, heather moorland, willow, birch and juniper scrub, peat bog. Migrates to lower ground in winter
	L. lagopus subspecies *scoticus*	Red grouse: the same species as above but moults completely to red brown in summer without retaining the white wings		Scotland. West Norwegian population is intermediate between red and willow grouse
	L. mertus	Ptarmigan, rock ptarmigan in North America: a similar species to willow grouse, retains white wings, belly and legs throughout year. In breeding season plumage blackish brown mottled. In winter completely white except outer tail feathers. Red eye combs. Smaller than above species	33 cm	Holarctic as for willow grouse. Habitat: tundra but higher altitudes than *L. lagopus* and more barren rocky slopes
Lyrus	*L. tetrix*	Black grouse: black cock and grey hen, male plumage blue/black. Unusual lyre-shaped tail in male also white wing bar and pronounced red eye combs	Male 50 cm, female 38 cm	Palaearctic, UK, Eurasia, NE Siberia and eastern China. Habitat: peat bog with rushes and scrub with some trees. Rocky heather moorland up to 2000 m
Dendragapus	*D. canadensis*	Spruce grouse, Franklin grouse, fool-hen: male has dark head and neck, flecked white on breast otherwise brownish. Pronounced red eye combs, when erected with fan-shaped tail looks like small turkey cock	41 cm	Canada. Habitat: coniferous forest with dense undergrowth
	D. obscurus	Blue grouse: not unlike spruce grouse but cock bird greyer and larger. Male displays yellowish or red skin covered inflatable oesophagus	51 cm	Western North America to California. Habitat: open mixed woodland and conifer. Lowland and mountain slopes, dry sage brush. Will roost under snow
Centrocercus	*C. urophasianus*	Sage grouse: male a very large bird (female smaller) mainly brownish in colour with white ruff on breast. Inflatable oesophagus, yellow eye combs. Pointed tail feathers	71 cm	Western North America. Habitat: sage brush, foothills and plains

Genus	Species	Size	Description	Distribution and habitat
Bonasa	B. umbellus	43 cm	Ruffed grouse: plumage reddish brown to grey. Dark edge to fan-shaped tail. Dark ruff around neck. No eye combs	Canada, Alaska and North America. Habitat: deciduous and mixed woodland
Tympanuchus	T. cupido	43 cm	Greater prairie chicken – similar species, lesser and Attwater's prairie chicken: plumage buff-coloured markedly barred with dark brown. Male has large yellow eye combs and inflatable yellow skin covered oesophagus. Small rounded tail. Male shows prominent forwardly directed ruff of upper neck feathers which could be mistaken for a head crest	Mid-West to southern USA. Habitat: tall grass prairie, open and scrubby grassland. Will burrow in snow to roost.
Tetrao	T. urogallus	79-84 cm	Capercaillie: a huge grouse. Male slate grey, wings brown, head and throat dark. Small red eye combs. Black tail flecked white, also on abdomen. Hens may hybridize with blackcock	Palaearctic and temperate western Europe to USSR. Habitat: coniferous and mixed forest. Taiga

vii. *Subfamily Meleagrinae: 2 genera, 2 species*

Turkeys: large powerful grouse-like birds in which the male bird carries on the head and neck coloured erectile caruncles (wattles) over bill, used during courtship. The cock turkeys have tarsal spurs and will fight to the death. There is a square-ended fan-shaped tail. Rattle wing quills during courtship.

| Meleagris | M. gallopavo (5 distinct races) | 94 cm | Wild turkey: slightly smaller than the domesticated varieties. First domesticated by the Mexican Indians in the sixteenth century | North America to Mexico. Habitat: woodland and open forest thickets |
| Agriocharis | A. ocellata | 86 cm | Ocellated turkey: has eye spots on the tail. No expandable crest wattles as in common turkeys. Skin of head more blue than red of common turkey | Yucatan in Guatemala. Habitat: subtropical lowland |

viii. *Subfamily Perdicinae: 20 genera, 106 species*

The Old World quails, francolins, partridge and snowcocks: all tend to be rather small, rotund birds with much shorter tails than pheasants. The Old World quails are all small birds with almost non-existent tails. The genus *Coternix* contains the only migratory Galliformes.

Coternix	C. japonica	15 cm	Japanese quail: dull, grey/brown with light coloured streaks and eye stripes. Domesticated by the Japanese	SE Asia, Burma, Thailand, Laos to Hong Kong and Japan. Taiwan. Introduced to North America. Habitat: grassland and cultivated areas
	C. delegorguei	15 cm	Harlequin quail. Delegorgue's quail	Senegal to Ethiopia and South Africa. Habitat: savannah and grassland
	C. coromandelica	15 cm	Rain quail, black-breasted quail	India, Sri Lanka, Burma
	C. coturnix	16 cm	Eurasian quail: Rather like Japanese quail with black throat and rufous upper breast. Migrated in huge numbers in Biblical times and collected by the Children of Israel in the Sinai	Southern UK, Europe: migrate across Mediterranean to North Africa. Habitat: rough grassland, cropland with grass tussocks
Excalfactoria	E. chinensis	13 cm	Chinese painted quail, king quail, blue breasted quail: female, like other female quail, brownish, but male brilliant blue eye stripe, neck and flank. Black neck and white collar	SE Asia and Australia. Habitat: grass and scrub

(continued)

Table 13.1 *(continued)*

The partridges, francolins and snowcocks – all medium-sized birds with fairly short tails. A few species have tarsal spurs.

Genus	Species	Characteristic	Size	Global distribution and normal habit
Rollulus	*R. rollulus*	The Roul Roul partridge, crested green wood partridge, crowned wood partridge, green partridge: upper parts of body bright green. Only male has pronounced chestnut crest with iridescent black/blue breast and wing coverts. Female mostly green with brown wings	28 cm	Malaysia, Sumatra and Borneo. Habitat: dense tropical forest but prefers drier more open clearings. Up to 1500 m elevation
Perdix	*P. perdix*	Common or grey partridge: upper parts brown streaked black and white, brownish wing coverts. Face and throat orange/brown. Male has brown inverted horseshoe markings on breast	28 cm	UK, most of Europe except southern Spain, Sicily and Sardinia, across to central Asia. Introduced to North America. Habitat: pastures, moorland, cultivated land, wasteland, sand dunes, semi-desert, shingle
Alectoris	*A. rufa* subspecies *A. graeca*	Red-legged partridge: distinguished from above species by white eye stripe, white throat, mottled black 'bib'. Red bill and red legs	34 cm	SW Europe, southern UK, introduced to UK, Azores, Madeira, Canary Isles and North America as a game bird. Habitat: lowland scrub, drier land and heath. Dry cultivated land
	A. chukar	Chukar partridge: upper parts grey brown, flanks noticeably barred black and white	36 cm	Asia and Asia Minor. Introduced to North America as a game bird. Habitat: similar to *A. rufa*
Francolinus (circa 41 species)	*F. francolinus*	Black francolin: a brownish bird, the male has black under parts markedly white flecked, also white cheeks	36 cm	Cyprus, Syria, Iran to Pakistan, India and Assam. Introduced to Louisiana and southern Florida. Habitat: grass and cropland
Tetraogallus	*T. himalayensis*	Himalayan snowcock: all snowcocks (5 species and many subspecies) are very large partridge-like birds	71 cm	Himalayas up to 6000 m, Afghanistan, India, western China. Introduced to mountainous areas of North America. Habitat: steep stone-covered slopes with sparse vegetation, alpine meadow
Lerwa	*L. lerwa*	Snow partridge: body form like other partridge but slightly longer. Tail plumage grey brown faintly barred white. Breast deep chestnut streaked white	35 cm	Himalayas up to 5000 m, Pakistan, India, Tibet, western China. Habitat: alpine meadow, rocky slopes above tree line

b. Family: Odontophoridae (9 genera, 31 species)

The New World quail. Small compact birds with a short bill that shows a serrated or toothed mandible. The fourth digit (the hallux) is above the level of the other digits. There are no tarsal spurs. Many species have a prominent plume on the forehead. Generally somewhat larger than Old World quail, to which they are quite unrelated.

Genus	Species	Size	Description
Lophortyx	*L. californicus*	25 cm	Californian quail, valley quail, crested quail: small pigeon-sized bird. Brownish grey upper breast, under parts flecked white, black throat, white collar, prominent teardrop-shaped plume	Western North America, West of the Rockies to southern California. Introduced New Zealand, Chile, Hawaii, Canada. Habitat: low tree shrub, open ground with low cover, city parks, sage brush
Callipepla	*C. squamata*	24 cm	Scaled quail, blue quail: greyish brown. Tinge of blue from scaled breast and neck. Crest not typical quail type, more triangular and white tipped	SW North America and Mexico. Introduced to Washington State and Nevada. Habitat: barren semi-desert and scrubby grassland
Colinus	*C. virginianus*	23-27 cm	Bobwhite quail: brownish with distinct white flecking and scaling on breast and flanks, white throat, white eye stripe, crest not well developed	SE Canada to Mid West and eastern North America to Mexico and Central America. Introduced to Britain and New Zealand. Habitat: scrub, open farmland, cities, road sides, derelict land

c. Family: Numididae (4 genera, 7 species)

The guinea fowl: there are four genera and seven species, all of which are found only on continental Africa and the adjacent island of Madagascar. All are medium-sized birds tending to be rather plump and heavy bodied with a fairly long neck, which together with the head is naked and the skin variously coloured. Some species have casques (e.g. helmeted and tufted guinea fowl) or occipital feather crests or wattles. Their plumage is mostly dark or grey. The tail of guinea fowl is small and drooping. Although mainly terrestrial birds that tend to run rather than walk, the guinea fowl can fly quite strongly.

Genus	Species	Size	Description
Acryllium	*A. vulturinum*	58 cm	Vulturine guinea fowl, so-called because it looks rather like a vulture with an almost vulturine bill. Black spotted white, underparts cobalt blue. Marked cape around neck of streaked black and white feathers	Southern Somalia, eastern Uganda, Kenya, NE Tanzania. Habitat: desert, thorn scrub, occasional forest
Numida	*N. meleagris* subspecies *N. meleagris mitrata*	56 cm	Tufted guinea fowl, helmeted or hooded guinea fowl: 20 subspecies occur regionally. Very noisy birds which often have been used as good watchkeepers. Domesticated by the Romans circa fourth century BC	Most of Africa from Cameroon to Central Africa, Chad, Sudan, Ethiopia, Kenya, Tanzania, Zaire, Angola, South Africa. Habitat: dry thorn, bush, grassland and cultivation

annually after the breeding season, but ptarmigan moult three times yearly in line with the changes in colour of their sub-Arctic habitat (Jones 1998). They also moult the claws. The capercaillie and ptarmigan also fractionally moult the horn of the beak. When handled, grouse tend to shed some feathers as a normal defence reaction against attack. Most Galliformes have a bilobed preen gland with an associated wick of feathers, but its presence in grouse and turkeys is variable. Sand grouse have modified breast feathers during the breeding season for carrying water to the chicks left in desert nest sites.

The respiratory system

In some species the trachea is elongated into loops, particularly in the male bird. This occurs in crested and plumed guinea fowl and in the capercaillie. The extended section of the trachea lies subcutaneously over the thorax and abdomen. The presence of an extended trachea may be important for the anaesthetist, because if respiration becomes depressed these birds may require assisted positive pressure ventilation in a much shorter time span than where a similar situation occurs in other species.

Normal respiratory rates in the common turkey (28–49 per minute) are approximately twice the rate in the domestic fowl (12–37 per minute); also, the common turkey has no caudal thoracic air sac.

Heart rates in the domestic turkey (93–163 per minute), in contrast to respiratory rates, are much lower than in the domestic fowl (220–360 per minute). Respiratory and cardiac rates are not documented for other species.

The alimentary canal

In the grouse, the beak is more robust than in most other Galliformes, being adapted to dealing with coarse vegetation. The New World quail have a 'toothed' lower beak. All Galliformes except snowcocks have a well-developed crop, which is, of course, an expansion of the oesophagus; in snowcocks its absence is compensated for by a dilatable oesophagus. Some male North American grouse (sage grouse, *Centrocercus urophasianus*; blue grouse, *Drenragapus obscurus*; prairie chickens, *Tympanuchus cupido*) have an inflatable diverticulum of the oesophagus covered with featherless, brightly coloured skin (red or yellow), and this is used during courtship and territorial displays.

The ventriculus (gizzard) is well developed muscularly in all Galliformes except for the sage grouse, which consumes softer food. Muscular development of the ventriculus is particularly pronounced in most other grouse because of their coarse vegetable diet. Also, certainly in the red grouse (*Lagopus lagopus scoticus*), the length of the intestine changes seasonally in line with the seasonal change in diet and its digestibility, a physiological adaptation also recorded in species other than Galliformes.

A gall bladder and well-developed caeca are present in all Galliformes, and the latter organs are commonly involved in infectious processes, especially coccidiosis.

Reproductive system

Although usually white or buff in colour, the testicles of some Galliformes such as the capercaillie and some breeds of poultry are pigmented a darker colour. The cock birds in all Galliformes have a non-intromittent phallus formed by two lateral folds (the lymphatic phallic bodies) situated on the ventral lip of the vent. During ejaculation, which is very rapid, the lymphatic bodies are momentarily engorged with lymph and the protruding vent is quickly applied to the protruding oviduct of the female. Semen is channelled between the two dilated lateral lymphatic phallic bodies.

Young wild turkeys are sexually mature at 2 years of age. New World quail are sexually mature at 1 year, although amongst the Old World quail (and certainly the Japanese quail, *Coternix japonica*), some are developed and able to breed at 6 weeks! Grouse mature at 1 year. The male peafowl is not sexually active until 3 years, whilst the hen is mature at 2 years. The common pheasant (*Phasianus colchicus*) is sexually mature at 1 year; in the golden pheasant (*Chrysolophus pictus*) the male bird is not mature until 2 years whilst the hen breeds at 1 year. Differential sexual maturity between the sexes may be an adaption to limit breeding between siblings and so disperse the gene pool.

Hybridization occurs between some species. The grey jungle fowl (*Gallus sonneratii*) hybridizes with the red jungle fowl (*G. gallus*), and of course the latter will breed with domestic chickens. The grey hen (*Lyrus tetrix*) will hybridize with the male capercaillie. Some other hybrids may occur between some species of wild grouse.

Basic biology

The Galliformes are mainly terrestrial birds, and are found in a variety of habitats (Table 13.1). However, all these birds feed mainly on the ground, searching for food by scratching with the feet (except for the eared and monal pheasants, which prefer to use the beak for digging) for seeds, fallen fruit, nuts, roots and invertebrates. The latter are particularly important for growing chicks. Some adult birds are more specialized feeders, such as red and willow grouse, which eat freshly growing shoots of heather (*Calluna* spp.); the spruce grouse, which consume pine shoots; or the sage grouse, which feed on sage tips (*Artemisia* spp.).

Although spending much of their time on the ground, Galliformes, except for those species inhabiting tree-less landscape (tundra, moorland, prairie or desert), all prefer to roost in trees.

In all cases the nest is simple, with the grouse, guinea fowl and quail being satisfied with a scrape in the ground. Pheasants and turkeys will embellish the scrape with a few leaves or twigs. In all cases, the eggs are white or mono-chrome. Average clutch size and incubation times are indicated in Table 13.2. The downy chicks are nidifugous and able to feed themselves from the time of hatching. In all cases the remiges of the chicks grow rapidly, and all chicks can fly before they are fully grown. Quail fly at 7 days and grouse at 10 days of age, whilst wild turkey chicks are 2 weeks old before they fly.

Husbandry

Housing

All Galliformes need dry frost- and weatherproof shelters or huts placed away from prevailing wind and direct hot sunshine. Some species, such as the Siamese fireback pheasant, are particularly liable to frostbite. For some species the birds need to be indoors in more substantial buildings supplied with supplementary heating during the winter months: this applies to bobwhite and Chinese quail and also to Palawan peacock pheasants. Some guinea fowl and francolins also need good winter protection, although the helmeted guinea fowl, a domesticated bird, is fairly tough provided it has frost protection. In contrast, some of the pheasants (such as Swinhoe's, silver, golden, Lady Amherst's and monal pheasants) are much more hardy and need only an open-fronted shelter with high off-the-ground perches, situated away from direct wind and hot sunshine. The common peafowl is also a hardy bird, in contrast to the green peafowl and the Congo peafowl, both of which need good protection and supplementary heat in severe winter weather.

All shelters and housing should provide appropriate perches, which, in the case of Reeves's and argus pheasants and peafowl, need to be well above ground level so that the long tail feathers do not become damaged. Also, all such shelters and housing should be attached to suitably sized and spacious aviaries. These should provide a minimum of 2–3 square metres of floor space per bird for birds the size of pheasants. About half this floor space should be provided for shelter accommodation. Outside aviaries should be on dry and well-drained ground and preferably have a concrete base, which can be covered with a good layer of sand or peagravel that can periodically be cleared out. However, some species (such as the eared and monal pheasants) like to dig with their beaks in the ground in search of roots and invertebrates. This activity helps to maintain the beak to the correct length, and if these birds cannot dig the bill tends to become overgrown.

The mesh of aviaries should be small enough to prevent the entry of rodents and small predators such as rats and weasels. Loose nylon fish netting placed across the top of an aviary (height approximately 2 m) instead of the more rigid wire netting may help to prevent startled birds that suddenly take off from injuring themselves by collision with an unyielding obstruction.

Galliformes do not require water in which to bathe, but most species appreciate a dust bath. Dust baths are particularly important for francolins and Roul Roul partridge.

The aviary can be provided with suitable plants, shrubs and grasses, preferably planted in tubs or shallow pots. These will give some shade and security, enabling birds to hide if they feel the need. This facility is particularly appreciated by such species as Bob White, harlequin and rain quail.

Mixed species aviaries

In general it is not good avicultural practice to mix species, although with experience and foreknowledge large mixed aviaries can successfully be maintained. In mixing species there is always a risk of inter-species aggression. There is also the danger of the transmission of infectious disease from a species that is relatively resistant and a latent carrier of a pathogen to a species that is much more susceptible (e.g. turkeys can be latent carriers of *Histomonas*, to which other species are more susceptible).

Intra- and inter-species aggression

Jungle fowl usually mix well with any of the pheasants, and most pheasants and the blue and California quail are safe with arboreal Passeriformes. In contrast, bobwhite quail, Japanese quail and partridges are not safe with any other birds. The Chukar partridge will even attack larger species. The male green peafowl is a particularly aggressive bird which not only attacks other birds but also mammals and even humans, using its spurs with devastating effect. In some species the male birds are not safe even to members of their own species, especially to the chicks when the cock bird is in breeding condition. This applies to blue, Californian and Chinese painted quail, and also to the monal pheasants. The cock silver pheasant will try to fight through the wire of an adjoining aviary, and some monogamous grouse will even attack the female bird if the two are confined in too small an aviary. Breeding pairs of some species need to be housed out of sight and sound of similar pairs. In contrast to these aggressive species, all species of guinea fowl do much better if kept in family groups.

Table 13.2 The breeding biology of representative species of Galliformes

Genera/species	Mono- or polygamous	Clutch size	Incubation time in days	Particular characteristics and any special requirements
PHASIANIDAE	With few exceptions (where indicated) mostly polygamous in captivity: one male to four or five females			Most pheasants do not make good mothers. They tend to scatter the eggs. Many semi-domesticated species have lost their normal breeding behaviour and the eggs have to be artificially incubated
Gallus sp. (jungle fowl)		5-10	20-21	
Lophura sp.			22-27	
(silver pheasant)		6-12		
Swinhoe's pheasant		8-12		
Siamese pheasant		5-8		
Crossoptilon sp. (white, brown and blue eared pheasants)		4-12	24-28	
Syrmaticus sp. (Reeves's pheasant)		8-12	24-25	
Chrysolophus sp. (golden and Lady Amherst's pheasant)	In the wild monogamous, in captivity one male to three or four females	6-12	23-24	Good mothers: the female matures at 1 year, the male at 2 years. Both sexes quite aggressive during breeding season
Tragopinae: e.g. Satyr tragopan	Monogamous	4-10	27-37	Often nests in trees. May need to incubate the eggs artificially
Lophophorinae: e.g. Himalayan monal pheasants	Monogamous	4-6	27-28	Male bird aggressive to female and needs a large aviary
Argusianinae: e.g. peacock pheasants		2	18-23	All species can be difficult breeders. Both male and female pheasants will defend breeding territory
Argus pheasants		2	24-25	It is wiser to restrict the time the male is left with the female
Parvoninae: Parvo sp. (common peafowl)		3-8	28-30	Male matures at 3 years, female matures at 2 years
Green peafowl				Male green peafowl are very aggressive
Afropavo sp. (Congo peafowl)	Monogamous	3-4	26-27	Nest in trees
Tetraonidae. grouse: willow/red grouse, ruffed, hazel, spruce and blue grouse, rock ptarmigan	All are monogamous	All species a minimum of 9 with some species laying up to 30	21-24	The wild species will hybridize if a male of the same species is not available but that of a related species with similar plumage and behavioural characteristics is at hand, e.g. female capercaillie will mate with a male blackcock

Species	Mating system	Clutch size	Incubation (days)	Notes
Black grouse, sharp-tailed and sage grouse, capercaillie, prairie chicken	All are polygamous and associate in lecking grounds	5–15	24–29	
Meleagridinae: common turkey, ocellated turkey	Polygamous	8–15	28	Wild hen birds normally associate in a flock in winter. Males will fight to the death. Only the female rears the young, but both male and female guard them
Perdicinae: *Coturnix* sp. (Japanese, harlequin, rain quail)	May be polyandrous in the wild	6–14; if eggs pulled will go on laying up to 200 in a year	16–20	Female birds not good brooders. May need to incubate artificially
Exafacteria sp. (Chinese painted quail)		5–12	16	Male bird can be aggressive to the chicks, which are extremely small and can escape through small-gauge wire mesh
Partridges: *Rollulus* sp. (Roul Roul, crested green and wood partridge)		2–4	18–20	Can be a difficult species to breed and may need artificial incubation or the use of a bantam hen
Alectoris sp. (red-legged and Chukar partridge)	Monogamous	8–16	24–26	The male can be aggressive. The hens may not incubate the eggs and a bantam hen may have to be used, but not if the young are to be released for game shooting
Galloperdicine: *Francolinus* sp. (black francolin)		4–8	19–23	Eggs incubated by the female but tend to be rather erratic breeders
Odontophorinae: *Callipela* sp. (blue quail)		10–12	22–23	Both the male and female live together in large groups (coveys) outside the breeding season. The cocks become aggressive to young male birds at the start of the breeding season. Females may not brood eggs and artificial incubation may be necessary
Lophortyx sp. (Californian quail)		10–15	22–23	A very easy species to hatch and rear artificially
Colinus sp. (bobwhite quail)	Captive varieties are partially polygamous: one male to two females	6–30	22–25	The female bird is an erratic sitter and artificial incubation may have to be used
NUMIDIDAE: *Acryllium* sp. (vulturine guinea fowl)	Polygamous	8–20	23–28	
Numida sp. (helmeted guinea fowl)		8–20	24–28	

Diet and feeding

The diet provided for captive birds should be as near to their natural diet as possible. However, apart from the domesticated species (domestic chickens, turkeys and, to some extent, guinea fowl, quail and reared pheasants and partridge) for which commercial diets at various age ranges, etc. are available, little scientifically based information is documented. Much of the following data is derived from the practical experience of aviculturists (Woolham 1987) and the staff of the North of England Zoological Society.

For Galliformes the following general principles apply:

1. Birds should not be overfed. Obese birds do not breed. Captive grouse species do better if the diet has plenty of roughage during the winter non-breeding period.
2. Protein needs to be increased during the breeding season and for growing chicks, then gradually reduced.
3. Any changes to the diet should be made gradually, since all birds tend only to accept food that they recognize.
4. Commercial poultry foods containing coccidiostats may upset the caecal autochronous flora of some species for which they were not designed, and may even prove toxic.
5. Growing chicks need abundant live food. For instance, in the wild, Chukar partridge and grouse will take many kinds of invertebrates such as small snails, slugs and earthworms, and the larvae or pupa of a variety of insects. As the chick grows it gradually changes from a protein-dominated diet to one containing more energy-producing constituents, which again reduces as the bird reaches adult weight. As an alternative to live food, some aviculturists use cottage cheese or hard-boiled egg for growing chicks.

The following give an indication of suitable diets for more specific groups of Galliformes.

Diet A – suitable for adult pheasants, monals, guinea fowl, wild turkeys, jungle fowl and peafowl

Equal parts of cereal grains composed of wheat, maize, corn and barley together with game bird pellets. It is probably best to feed late in the day and let the birds actively search the ground for food early in the day. Some green food such as spinach, cabbage, lettuce, diced carrot, dandelion leaves, clover, chickweed, chives and wild berries (e.g. rowan and bilberry) should be included.

Diet B – suitable for Californian, blue, bobwhite and Japanese quail

Four parts of plain canary seed (i.e. mixed millet), four parts of chick starter crumbs, three parts of wheat, three parts of split or kibbled maize (i.e. corn) and one part groats (i.e. crushed oats). Some fresh green food such as cress, spinach leaves and a little lettuce should also be included. A vitamin–mineral supplement *manufactured for avian species* should also be given.

This diet can also be used for Chukar and red-legged partridge, francolins and peacock pheasants if some live food and wild berries (when available) are added. Live food, either by itself or mixed with a commercial live food substitute (e.g. Nekton Products), can be used. Suitable live food includes mealworms reared on a bran diet, wax moth larvae (these are soft bodied and easily digestible), crickets, locusts and fruit flies. Note that both mealworms and maggots pupate and eventually produce adult insects and, if maggots are fed to birds kept inside, the flies will infest the building. Maggots are probably best avoided because of the danger of botulism, especially if they have been cultured on carcasses. If they are used, let the maggots pupate and then feed the pupae to the birds; however, it may take birds some time to recognize these pupae as food.

Diet C – suitable for harlequin and Japanese painted quail (i.e. the smallest Galliformes)

Three parts of each of canary seed, yellow millet, white millet and panicum millet. Green food and a vitamin–mineral supplement should be included as in Diet B.

This diet is also suitable for the Roul Roul partridge if some mixed fruit (for example, four parts diced pear or apple together with three parts sliced tomato and one part sliced grape) is included. Live food should also be provided as in Diet B.

Diet D – suitable for tragopans, captive grouse species and snowcocks

All these birds feed almost entirely on fairly coarse vegetation. They can be fed on branches of willow and birch (catkins and leaves), raspberry plants (leaves and berries), grass, berries, fresh vegetables, fruit (apple), spinach, lettuce and cucumber. A little grain (e.g. oats) or commercial game bird pellets can be added.

General

All species need an adequate supply of mixed composition grit of a size suitable for the particular species concerned. This should regularly be completely changed, as the birds tend to select the parts they require. Mixed grit should be composed of limestone chips, oyster shell and cuttlefish bone.

The management of red grouse on grouse moors

Unlike pheasants and partridge, grouse for game shooting cannot be reared and subsequently successfully released onto the moor. Numbers of grouse for shooting have to be encouraged by the management of their natural habitat. Red grouse feed predominantly on heather (*Calluna vulgaris* and *Erica* spp.), but will also eat the shoots and flower heads of other plants and the berries of bilberry (*Vaccinium* spp.). The flower heads of cotton grass (*Eriophorum* spp.), which is really a sedge and not a grass, are particularly important for the egg-laying female bird, as the plant contains twice the amount of crude digestible protein as heather.

To encourage the new growth of heather for the grouse to feed on, controlled burning of the plant takes place in the late winter or early spring. The top growth is burnt off, leaving the root stock unharmed. The heather is fired in strips approximately 40 m wide, and this is carried out on a 12–15-year cycle so that a patchwork of varying growth is produced. Fresh nutritious shoots are produced in the spring, whilst taller stands of heather are left for cover in which the grouse can nest. Mammals, especially sheep, carry ticks (*Ixodes ricinus*), and these arthropods carry louping ill virus, which affects both sheep and grouse. The population density of ticks varies regionally, and is affected by moisture, temperature and the underlying vegetation. In some regions louping ill in grouse can be reduced by vaccinating the sheep. In other areas the ticks are maintained at too high a density by feeding on deer, hares and other small mammals.

Another important factor affecting the numbers of grouse on the moor is predation. Predators have traditionally been controlled by gamekeepers, but this activity is now limited in the UK by the Wildlife and Countryside Act 1981. Principal among the predators is the fox, the numbers of which tend to be influenced by the availability of rabbits. The peregrine falcon (*Falco peregrinus*) is also an important predator, as is the occasional hen harrier (*Circus cyaneus*). Both bird species are fully protected by law in the UK.

Grouse numbers are influenced by the nematode *Trichostrongylus tenuis*, which infects the birds' caeca and can prove fatal in heavy infections – or at least reduce fertility in female birds. Heavily parasitized birds are also more liable to predation. Survival of the parasite is favoured by warm, moist conditions, and its numbers tend to rise as the grouse population increases. The larvae of the worm crawl up the heather plants and are ingested by the grouse.

In conclusion, it can be appreciated that the numbers of grouse on the moor can be affected by a complex web of influences. These include the many single-interest human activity groups such as sheep farmers, foresters, deer stalkers, hill walkers, bird protection societies interested in the protection of falcons and hen harriers and, of course, the gamekeepers.

Pheasant and partridge management on shooting estates

During the nineteenth century large numbers of grey partridge (*Perdrix perdrix*) were shot as game birds on big private estates in the UK, and hand rearing of some birds occurred up to the beginning of the Second World War. However, with the reduction in the numbers of gamekeepers employed together with the legal restrictions of the Wildlife and Countryside Act 1981 (amended by the Countryside and Rights of Way (CRoW) Act 2000 in England & Wales and the Nature Conservation – Scotland – Act 2004), there has been a consequent increase in the numbers of natural predators such as foxes, stoats, weasels and aerial raptors. This change has occurred simultaneously with changes in farming practice, such as the removal of hedgerows and the marginal land surrounding arable crops, and the intensive use of selective herbicides to control weeds – which has at the same time reduced insect food suitable for partridge chicks. Furthermore, all types of insect life have been reduced by the use of pesticides on crops. The net result is fewer and less-suitable cover and nesting sites for partridge, with little, if any, insect larvae for growing chicks.

Grey partridge are not an easy species to rear in captivity and release successfully. On the other hand, the red-legged partridge (*Alectoris rufa*) is in some ways less vulnerable to these changes and easier to hand rear. The chicks are much less dependent on insect food from the time of hatching, and will eat grass and search for weed seeds. Red-legged partridge hens will lay two separate clutches of eggs, one of which she will incubate whilst her mate, the cock bird, simultaneously incubates the second clutch. Productivity is therefore doubled. In the wild, however, red-legged partridge are not so good at hiding their nests, so they are more susceptible to predation. Up until 1992, red-legged partridge were crossed with the related Chukar partridge (*Alectoris chukar*) and the hybrids were very successfully released; however, this practice has now been stopped because it was having a detrimental effect on wild-bred red-legged partridge.

Undoubtedly the most important game bird to be hand reared in large numbers is the common pheasant (*Phasianus colchicus*). These birds can be reared intensively using the techniques of the commercial poultry industry, with artificial incubators and large hatchers dealing with up to 1500 eggs at a time. The newly hatched chicks can then be placed in heated brooders and gradually given access to outside runs. They are subsequently placed in release pens at 6–7 weeks, where they can familiarize themselves with the surrounding habitat. Eventually the birds are released into suitable woodland and game crops. Throughout this period the chicks will be fed on a variety of commercially developed diets, and some feeding often continues after release to retain birds on the estate. Many pheasants still breed in the wild on shooting estates, particularly where farming practices are such that suitable cover for nesting birds is provided and the ground living predators controlled, and where modern farming procedures have not devastated the insect life.

A suitable balance between hand-reared and wild-bred birds has to be maintained, as evidence suggests that artificially reared birds are not so viable for the following reasons:

1. Truly wild birds are more alert and will react quicker to predators.
2. Wild birds take and survive better on a greater range of wild foods.
3. Hand-reared birds are less resistant to the parasite *Heterakis* spp.
4. Muscle development in hand-reared birds is heavier and take-off flight is therefore less rapid and at a shallower angle.

In the past game birds' eggs have been incubated and hatched under bantam hens, but it has been shown that the behavioural responses to predator attack learned from the bantam hen may be inappropriate to the game bird chick; hence mortality rates were higher.

When investigating disease in all game birds, it is essential that the veterinarian takes a broad holistic view and is aware of the complexity of environmental influences on the overall health of these birds.

Breeding and sexing Galliformes

Most species of Galliformes are markedly sexually dimorphic, with the male having more colourful plumage, often a larger body size, a longer tail and the presence of combs or wattles. In a few species of Phasianidae, which are not so easy to distinguish, the cock birds have spurs on their legs. In guinea fowl that are not sexually dimorphic the male usually has a voice with a greater range of sound, and in the helmeted and plumed guinea fowl the appendage on the head is slightly larger. In many Old and New World quail, the sexes are similar in appearance but have behavioural differences. Most galliform chicks are not sexually dimorphic and can only be sexed, like domestic poultry, by the meticulous examination of the cloaca by a skilled technician. However, grouse chicks are distinguishable, the males being slightly larger.

Some species of Galliformes are monogamous, whilst in other species a cock bird can be kept with several hens. In some species the cock birds are particularly aggressive during the breeding season, not only to other species of birds but also to their own hen birds – particularly if they can see or hear another cock.

Some general principles when breeding Galliformes

1. When introducing a new cock bird to an unfamiliar hen, always place the hen in the aviary first.
2. Many male birds will chase the female during normal courtship behaviour, but the female does need a sufficiently large aviary to escape if she so desires. It also may be helpful to clip the cock bird's wings. If there is a definite difference in size between male and female, the two sexes can be kept in adjoining aviaries with a connecting passage only just large enough for the hen bird to pass through. This system can be used for capercaillie.
3. Most Galliformes lay their eggs in a primitive nest on the ground but some species are tree nesters, and these should be provided with a flat wooden tray or basket containing hay, moss and dried leaves and situated approximately 1–2 m above the ground level. Typical tree-nesting species include the Congo peafowl, bronze-tailed peacock pheasant and crested argus pheasant. All nesting sites, whether in trees or on the ground, should be provided with visual security.
4. In some species, greater breeding success is achieved if the eggs are incubated artificially. Such species include the New World quail, blue quail, Californian quail, bobwhite quail and also Japanese quail from the Old World.
5. Fostering using a broody bantam or Japanese silky hen to incubate and rear the chicks is a practice used by many aviculturists when a particular species is difficult to breed in captivity. If the foster hen is sitting quietly and tight, her eggs are exchanged for those to be hatched after 3 days. Species where this technique has been used include the common pheasant, partridges (Chukar, red-legged, Roul Roul and green wood), tragopans and Palawan peacock pheasants, and grouse.
6. After the chicks have hatched and dried, they should be placed in boxes approximately 50 × 100 cm with a heat source so as to maintain a floor temperature of 40°C. A 150 W infrared lamp can be used. Damp cloths can be used on the sides of the box to maintain a relative humidity of 60%. Placing the chicks on towels (changed frequently) spread on the floor will help to prevent splayed legs. After 8–12 days, the chicks can be placed in a large rearing pen outside if the weather is suitable. This is best provided

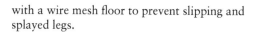

with a wire mesh floor to prevent slipping and splayed legs.

The investigation of infertility in a breeding pair of birds

1. In some birds, particularly grouse, the hen chooses the cock bird with which to mate. If the male bird provided is not of her choice or is incompatible, mating will not take place even though infertile eggs may be laid.
2. If male or female have recently been acquired from different countries which are at different latitudes so influencing the number of daylight hours, even if the birds are of the same species, their breeding cycles may not be synchronized so that they may not breed.
3. If two cock birds spend all their time fighting through the wire of their adjoining aviaries, they may not have time to mate with their hens.
4. The age and general condition of the bird should be considered. Aged and particularly obese hens do not breed.
5. Finally, infectious disease should be ruled out.

Disease in Galliformes

The important infectious diseases of Galliformes are listed in Table 13.3 and organized according to their presenting clinical signs. Each disease in these notes has been numbered to make cross-referencing easier.

Considerations when investigating disease

First consider whether the problem is primarily management related or a serious epizootic disease of birds. The latter, particularly viral infection, is usually seen in birds kept in flocks through which disease can spread rapidly

Rarely is any disease syndrome entirely due to a single pathogen. Often bacteria isolated and identified on a culture may not be the primary pathogen but are only secondary invaders. Usually the condition originates from a multiplicity of causes, some of which may be management related. It is essential to consider all possible predisposing factors.

Standards of hygiene are not always high, nor is prophylactic vaccination or regular systemic control of parasites always routinely carried out. However, it should be noted that current thinking by some workers is that an ongoing *low* level of parasitic infection may be conducive to a healthy immune system in the host.

Management problems

Inadequate housing, hygiene and diet can predispose to disease.

Inadequateh ousing

Housing must be suitable for the species. Some species require supplementary heating in winter. Overcrowding of birds in a corner of a house in cold weather not only results in smothering but can also lead to a localized build-up of ammonia fumes, causing coryza, corneal ulceration, blindness and a predisposition to respiratory problems. Accommodation should be completely wind- and weather-proof. Perches must provide adequate space between perched birds, be periodically renewed and be the correct height from the ground. There should be sufficient floor space and space in the outside aviaries. Overcrowding leads to increased stress, aggression, feather picking and cannibalism, which in some cases may need to be controlled by plastic spectacles or beak clipping. Overcrowding in aviaries can also result in an unsustainable parasite load. However, in cases with low parasite levels and in otherwise healthy stock this can sometimes confer a degree of resistance to parasitism.

Hygiene

Before new stock is introduced the housing should be thoroughly cleaned out and disinfected and the outside aviaries sufficiently rested so they become free of living parasites or their eggs. Very many pathogens (see disease Nos. 3, 4, 6, 7, 10, 12, 18, 19 20, 21, 22, 23, 25, 27, 28, 29, 30, 35, 38, 44, 45, 48, 70, 76 and 77 in Table 13.3) are environmentally persistent in dirty wooden buildings with faeces, exudate and fomites. Water supplies and food containers easily become contaminated, particularly by some pathogens (e.g. disease Nos. 2, 4, 6, 10, 17, 22, 23, 37, 38, 52, 54 and 70). Invertebrate vectors may help in maintaining disease in empty enclosures by either transmitting or themselves causing disease (e.g. disease Nos. 12, 15, 34, 47, 49, 66, 67, 70 and 77). Vermin and wild free-living wild birds may carry disease, and can infect an aviary with their faeces or exudate if these are allowed to enter the bird enclosure (e.g. disease Nos. 4a, 6, 20, 23 and 39).

Diet

This must be adequate in quantity and properly balanced, particularly for the growing stage of chicks or in relation to the breeding cycle. Food should be stored properly so that it is not mouldy or contaminated with the droppings of vermin or with forage mites (note: some mycotoxins, besides being overtly poisonous, can be immunosuppressive). A sudden increase in the number of cases of visceral gout in a flock may be the result of a faulty water supply or dietary imbalance. All fresh vegetables must be adequately washed (they may be contaminated by wild bird faeces, very small minute molluscs, industrial aerial pollution, pesticides or herbicides used during cultivation).

Table 13.3 Avian diseases

Diseases primarily exhibiting respiratory signs (i.e. sneezing, wheezing, coughing, rattling with each respiration, gasping for air, dyspnoea and often ocular or nasal discharge together with anorexia)

No.	Disease	Primary cause	Species susceptible	Particular disease characteristic	Diagnosis
1.	Mycoplasmosis ('roup')	*Mycoplasma* spp. Many species and strains, primary spread by close contact. Latent carriers. Turkeys are infected venereally	All species of Galliformes	May be an asymptomatic infection. This is often a secondary infection but may govern the severity of the disease process. Usually the infraorbital sinuses are swollen, but the bird's joints may also be affected	PM, histopathology, serology, culture (use special transport media)
2.	Chlamydophilosis Ornithosis. **Important zoonosis**	*Chlamydophila* sp. Several strains. Intermittently shed in faeces	All Galliformes but particularly turkeys	Respiratory signs may be accompanied by diarrhoea. Some birds may exhibit only a vague debility	PM, note particularly an enlarged spleen, histopathology, serology, cytology, culture
3.	Infectious laryngotracheitis	Herpesvirus carried by latently infected birds. Can persist in fomites for at least 3 months	Mainly chickens and peafowl but also pheasants and turkey poults	Can be a mild or subclinical to a severe infection with birds having extended head and neck, gasping for air. May die in 2–3 days. The sinuses may be swollen (compare to No. 1) and the birds may cough a bloody mucus. Oropharynx and trachea may show diphtheritic membranes	PM, histopathology, virus isolation
4.	Newcastle disease (fowl pest) **Zoonosis**	Group I paramyxovirus. Virus is contained in infected faeces	All species of Galliformes, particularly backyard fowl. All grouse tend to be fairly resistant and in partridges the infection may be asymptomatic	Respiratory signs may be accompanied by a greenish, watery diarrhoea and some birds exhibit CNS signs. Grouse may only show a conjunctivitis together with loss of weight	PM, serology, virus isolation
4a.	Pigeon paramyxo disease	Group I paramyxovirus (pigeon variant)	Can affect chickens, pheasants and peafowl	In UK many wild pigeons are carriers. Signs similar to Newcastle disease	
5.	Turkey rhinotracheitis ('swollen head syndrome')	Pneumonovirus. Related to the paramyxoviruses	Principally turkeys but also pheasants, chickens, guinea fowl. Can cause egg drop in chickens	Upper respiratory signs with swollen sinuses (compare to Nos 1 and 3) and conjunctivitis. Morbidity and mortality can be high	PM, serology, virus isolation
6.	Avian influenza (fowl plague of the 1890s; also known as 'fowl pest') **An important zoonosis, strains such as H5N1 may cause pandemics after occurrence of antigenic shift primarily occurring after virus has infected pigs**	Influenza A viruses. Many strains (varying combinations of the 16 haemagglutinin binding factors and the 9 neuraminidase characters) of the virus. Environmentally stable in faeces and static water. Free-ranging domestic and wild waterfowl act as a reservoir of the virus	All Galliformes but particularly farmed poultry also pheasants, and Japanese quail. May also infect a number of mammalian species including domestic cats, dogs horses, cetaceans, mustelids (e.g. otters, pine marten), fox and possibly other fur-bearing animals	The subtypes (H and N) of the virus are continually changing so that morbidity and mortality (high and low pathogenic types) vary together with secondary infections. Massive sudden die-offs can occur. Respiratory signs vary from mild to severe. Oedema of the head and neck may occur (compare to Nos. 1,3 and 5) as well as egg drop syndrome	PM, virus isolation

7.	**Fowl adenovirus** ('vent gleet')	Group I fowl adenovirus. A number of serotypes. Birds may be latently affected	Chickens, particularly backyard fowl, also guinea fowl and Japanese quail and pheasants	Infection can be subclinical to a moderately severe respiratory disease accompanied by mucoid pasty white droppings causing an offensive smell and adherent to the vent. Mortality can be 10–30%. There may be an egg drop syndrome. Guinea fowl can develop a pancreatitis or marble spleen-like disease (No. 9). Pheasants may die suddenly with no premonitory signs	Serology, virus isolation, PM, histopathology (oviduct)
8.	**Quail bronchitis**	Group I adenovirus	Bobwhite quail	100% of very young chicks under a week old may suddenly die. Older chicks up to 6 weeks show severe respiratory signs with greenish diarrhoea and the occasional dropped wing and die in 24–48 hours	Serology
9.	**Marble spleen disease**	Group II adenovirus	Pheasants, guinea fowl, chickens	This is not primarily a respiratory infection but the grossly enlarged spleen may cause dyspnoea through pressure on the air sacs (see No. 27 for more detail)	See No. 28
10.	**Infectious bronchitis** (blue comb of turkeys')	Coronavirus. Virus shed in faeces, spreads in contaminated water and food or from poultry-manured fields. Different serotypes in chickens, pheasants, guinea fowl. Japanese quail, turkeys	All Galliformes but particularly pheasants	Respiratory signs may be mild with only a drop in egg production. Pheasant chicks (8–10 weeks) may sustain a 40% mortality. Guinea fowl may develop an enteritis and pancreatitis and chicks as young as 3 days old may die but are usually protected by maternal antibody	PM, serology
11.	**Aspergillosis** ('brooder pneumonia')	*Aspergillus fumigatus*	All Galliformes, particularly turkey and pheasant	Usually seen in chicks up to 4 weeks old. Can vary from sudden death to a chronic wasting disease with some respiratory signs. Occasional paralysis in older birds	PM, serology, culture
12.	**Syngamiasis** ('gapes')	*Syngamus* spp. Transport hosts, e.g. earthworms, slugs and beetles	All Galliformes particularly those in overstocked grass aviaries	Typical gasping for air (compare to No. 3) cough, head shaking, anorexia and loss of condition. Usually individual birds affected sporadically	Faecal exam, visual exam
13.	**Trichomoniasis**	Protozoan	All Galliformes but particularly pheasants	Dyspnoea may result from exudate obstructing the airway (see No. 36)	See No. 36

(continued)

Table 13.3 *(continued)*

No.	Disease	Primary cause	Species susceptible	Particular disease characteristic	Diagnosis
14.	Crytosporidiosis	A coccidial protozoan parasite which grows on all mucosal epithelia. Ingestion or inhalation of sporulated oocyst. Resistant to many disinfectants	Recovered from the respiratory tract of many Galliformes	May be a primary pathogen but often a secondary invader of immunosuppressed birds causes inflammation and typical upper respiratory signs also diarrhoea (see No. 32).	PM, faecal exam (Giemsa stained)
15.	Avipox	Fowl pox virus infects pheasants and peafowl. Quail pox distinct virus but can infect chickens and turkeys. Biting insects may act as transport vectors	All Galliformes	Lesions on skin dry. Diphtheritic lesions on respiratory mucosa. May cause severe respiratory signs and death. May be egg drop. Can cause up to 30% mortality in quail	Culture, cytology
16.	Infectious coryza	*Haemophilus* spp.	All Galliformes but usually chickens, turkeys and pheasants	Often cultured as a secondary infection from other primary disease. Signs include rhinitis, sinusitis, air sacculitis and pneumonia	PM, culture
17.	Turkey coryza	*Alcaligenes* spp. *Bordetella* spp. Shed in faeces and contaminate water and food supply	Usually turkeys	Opportunistic pathogens, sometimes occurring as secondary invaders associated with turkey rhinotracheitis (see No. 5)	Culture
18.	Cryptococcosis, torulosis, blastomycosis, histoplasmosis. A zoonosis	Saprophytic fungi which may occur in old wooden and insanitary aviaries. Inhalation of spores	All Galliformes	Can cause gelatinous granulomatous lesions on the mucous membranes of respiratory and gastrointestinal tracts. Also systemic lesions in the viscera. Individual birds affected sporadically	Faecal exam, culture, histopathology
19.	Avian mycobacteriosis A zoonosis particularly in immunosuppressed humans	*Mycobacterium avium*	All Galliformes	Peafowl are documented as having been presented with rattling sounds due to granulomas in the trachea (see No. 69)	Culture, histopathology

Many commonly known bacteria such as *Staphylococci* spp.. *Streptococci* spp.. *E. coli* and *Klebsiella* spp. act as secondary invaders of avian respiratory disease

	Diseases primarily presented with signs of alimentary disorder (i.e. diarrhoea in varying forms) occasionally vomiting accompanied sometimes by malaise and loss of condition				
20.	Salmonellosis. Zoonosis	*S. typhimurium*, *S. enteritidis*. Faecal dust carriers: wild birds, rodents. Vertical transmission and latently infected birds	All Galliformes, particularly backyard fowl	Depression and diarrhoea, resulting in death but death may occur without any premonitory signs	PM, culture
21.	Pullorum disease, bacillary white diarrhoea	*S. gallinarum*, *S. pullorum*. Latent carrier birds. Poor hygiene	All Galliformes, but common in backyard fowl	Enteritis, malaise. In pullorum disease malformed ovules occur in the ovary, also enlarged liver and spleen	PM, culture, serology

22.	**Coli bacillosis. Some strains of *E. coli* are zoonotic, particularly the 0157 strain**	*Escherichia coli*. Ingestion and inhalation of faecal dust. Some strains produce a potent toxin. Can be a primary or secondary pathogen	All Galliformes, but particularly backyard fowl. Also turkeys, peafowl, partridge and capercaillie	Coliform septicaemia may cause acute deaths or a brownish diarrhoea with stunted growth and poor feathering. Birds may develop coliform granulomas in the liver and spleen and a peritonitis and air sacculitis due to coli septicaemia	PM, culture
23.	**Campylobacteriosis. Zoonosis**	*Campylobacter* spp. Many serotypes shed in faeces, which contaminate food and water supplies. Poor hygiene	All Galliformes	Weight loss, yellowish, sometimes bloody, diarrhoea (caused by hepatosis) and eventual death. At PM, focal necrosis of the liver. Spontaneous recovery and relapse are not uncommon. Spread through a flock is often slow	PM, culture (special transport media)
24.	**Clostridial enterotoxaemia**	*Clostridium perfringens*	All Galliformes but particularly game birds, i.e. grouse and New World quail	In young birds (10 days and over) a haemorrhagic enteritis leads to bloody diarrhoea with polydipsia and death. In older birds the infection is more chronic with gradual weight loss before death. At PM, hepatomegaly and necrotic enteritis	PM, culture, toxin identification
25.	**Chlamydophilosis. Zoonosis**	*Chlamydophila* sp. Intermittently shed in faeces	All Galliformes, but only well documented in turkeys	Diarrhoea, respiratory signs, unthriftiness (see No. 2)	See No. 2
26.	**Newcastle disease. Zoonosis**	Group I paramyxovirus, also Group I paramyxovirus (pigeon)	All Galliformes	May be a greenish diarrhoea together with or without respiratory and CNS signs (see Nos. 4 and 4a)	See No. 4
27.	**Fowl adenovirus disease** (vent gleet)	Group I fowl adenovirus. In faeces. Persistent in the environment. Hygiene important	Chickens, guinea fowl, Japanese quail	An enteritis with white pasty mucoid droppings adherent to the vent and causing an offensive smell (see No. 7)	See No. 7
28.	**Turkey haemorrhagic enteritis**	Group II adenovirus. Shed in faeces. Very environmentally persistent	Turkeys, chickens, pheasants	Only documented in domesticated birds, not in wild birds. Affects young birds from 4 to 12 weeks causing up to 60% mortality. Can be asymptomatic or cause severe and haemorrhagic enteritis	Serology
29.	**Pheasant marble spleen disease**	Group II adenovirus. Virus may persist in the environment for months. Good hygiene is imperative, particularly in rearing pens	Primarily pheasants, but can also affect guinea fowl and chickens, and blue grouse	Mostly documented in captive birds, not in wild free-living birds but has been documented in blue grouse. Affects young birds 3–8 months old causing highest mortality (i.e. 20%) in young birds. Pheasants may die suddenly or become anorexic, depressed and show diarrhoea and dyspnoea (see No. 9)	PM, serology

(continued)

Table 13.3 *(continued)*

No.	Disease	Primary cause	Species susceptible	Particular disease characteristic	Diagnosis
30.	Coccidiosis	*Eimeria* spp. Protozoan parasites generally host-specific so cross-species infection does not usually take place. Can be environmentally persistent	All Galliformes, particularly young birds circa 3 weeks. Adults may act as latent carriers	Disease may be exhibited as anything from a vague pathogenic syndrome causing listlessness to a severe enteric disease with mucoid bloody faeces dependent on parasite load and other predisposing causes	Faecal exam
31.	Crytosporidiosis. Zoonosis	*Crytosporidium* spp. A coccidial protozoan.	All Galliformes	Invades the whole of the alimentary tract, causing diarrhoea and malabsorption (see No. 14)	See No. 14
32.	Hexamitiasis	*Hexamita* spp.	Turkeys	Can cause heavy loss in turkey poults around 3 weeks of age, causing diarrhoea and unthriftiness	Faecal exam
33.	Quail herpes or Colinus disease	Herpesvirus	Bobwhite quail under 4 weeks	Depression, anorexia and diarrhoea and death in 3-4 days. Focal necrosis of enlarged liver and spleen	PM, serology
34.	Histomoniasis (blackhead)	*Histomonas meleagridis*. A protozoan carried by the ova of caecal worms *Heterakis* spp. Earthworms may act as vector	All Galliformes but particularly turkeys, pheasants. Partridge if in close contact with chickens	Yellowish diarrhoea (because of hepatopathy). Sometimes birds just unthrifty. Particularly common without regular deworming	PM, faecal exam
35.	Helminth worm infestation	*Ascaridia* spp., *Capillaria* spp. *Heterakis* spp. Ova persist in environment	All Galliformes	All helminths may cause a mucoid diarrhoea or just general unthriftiness. Occasional sudden death	PM, faecal exam
36.	Candidiasis	*Candida albicans*. Opportunistic yeast	All Galliformes, especially young turkeys, partridge and captive grouse	Primary or secondary pathogen of upper alimentary tract results in delayed crop emptying and vomiting with sporadic death	Cytology
37.	Trichomoniasis	*Trichomonas gallinae*. A flagellated protozoan. Thrives in poor hygiene	All Galliformes, but particularly pheasant chicks in crowded conditions	Causes cheesy exudate in oropharynx resulting in vomiting, diarrhoea, dyspnoea. Unthriftiness and sporadic death, particularly in chicks	Cytology
38.	Gumboro disease (infectious bursitis')	A birna virus disease so called from first identification at Gumboro, USA. Very environmentally persistent in contaminated faeces	Chickens 3-6 weeks old. Pheasants (up to 80% mortality), turkeys	Necrotic bursa of Fabricius results in severe immunosuppression resulting in secondary infection. Affected chicks may be anorexic with watery diarrhoea and die	PM, histopathology, virus isolation
39.	Spirochaetosis	*Borrelia gallinarum*. Transport host, ticks. Also sometimes mosquitoes	All Galliformes. Young chicks 4-8 days reared on rough pasture inhabited by ticks	May be sudden death or dullness with yellow diarrhoea, ataxia and then death. Mortality up to 100%. Hepatomegaly with necrotic foci	PM, serology, stained blood smear
40.	Tagoviruses	See disease No. 47	All Galliformes	Sometimes cause diarrhoea (see No. 47)	Virus isolation

41.	**Stunting and runting syndrome** (viral enteritis)	Reo- and rotaviruses	All Galliformes	Infection sometimes results in diarrhoea (see No. 64)	Virus isolation
42.	**Reticuloendotheliosis**	Reticuloendothelial virus	All Galliformes	Infection occasionally exhibits signs of an enteritis (see No. 65)	Virus isolation
43.	**Helminth worms in grouse**	*Trichostrongylus tenuis*. Worm thrives in warm moist heather	Grouse	Worm invades and severely damages the caecal mucosa causing a haemorrhagic enteritis. Birds usually found dead. May be unthrifty with bloody diarrhoea	PM, faecal counts not reliable
43a.	**Vitamin C deficiency in grouse chicks**	Young growing chicks up to 4 weeks do not produce sufficient endogenous vitamin C. Need to obtain it from wild berries, etc.	Only documented in willow ptarmigan, but may be a factor in other grouse chicks	Weight loss, petechiae in muscles, weakness, enteritis, fractures and bone dystrophia, death	PM
Diseases presented with clinical signs related to either the nervous or locomotor systems (i.e. torticollis, opisthotonus, dropped or trailing wings, paralysis, lameness, etc.)					
44.	**Marek's disease**	Herpesvirus. Very environmentally persistent in feather debris. Latently infected chickens maintain infection. Tends to be geographically localized	All Galliformes. Mortality in adults 10–15%, in chicks up to 40%	Young chicks under 3 weeks rarely affected. Usually affects female birds 6–12 weeks up to time of laying. Lymphoid thickening of peripheral nerves and visceral tumours. Results in lameness, dropped wing, paralysis, emaciation, death. Vaccine breakdowns occur. Compare Nos. 67 and 45	PM, histopathology, serology, virus isolation
45.	**Avian sarcoma leucosis syndrome**	Caused by a number of RNA viruses. Very environmentally stable. Disease may flair up in periods of stress. Latently infected birds	All Galliformes, especially chickens and pheasants. In contrast to Marek's disease (No. 44) usually affects birds over 14 weeks old	Note: partridge and quail affected by a distinct species–specific virus. Female birds more susceptible. Multiple tumours seen throughout body. Clinical signs similar to Marek's (No. 44) but vary with site of neoplasm. Tumours may cause thickening of legs	PM, histopathology
46.	**Newcastle disease ('fowl pest'). Zoonosis**	Group I paramyxovirus, also pigeon variant	All Galliformes, particularly backyard fowl	A variety of CNS signs, together with respiratory and enteric disease signs (see Nos. 4 and 4a)	See No. 4
47.	**Eastern and western equine encephalitis and similar infections. Zoonotic diseases**	Togaviruses. EEE and WEE virus. Currently restricted to USA. Similar viruses occur in other parts of the world. Transmitted by biting insects, e.g. mosquitoes, therefore a seasonal disease	All Galliformes. Mortality in turkeys 6%, pheasant 5–8%, quail 40–90%, partridge 30–90%	Can be asymptomatic. Mortality is highest in those species non-indigenous to a region. A variety of clinical signs of CNS as well as anorexia, ruffled feathers, diarrhoea and sudden death	Histopathology, virus isolation

(continued)

Table 13.3 (continued)

No.	Disease	Primary cause	Species susceptible	Particular disease characteristic	Diagnosis
48.	**Specific avian encephalomyelitis** (epidemic tremor)	An enteropicorna virus shed in faeces. Can persist in litter for years. Both vertical and horizontal transmission	All Galliformes, but not in free-living wild birds	Young birds up to 16 weeks, particularly 2-4 weeks old. Acute epidemic with variety of CNS signs. Survivors exhibit persistent eye lesions. Adult birds show drop in egg production. Note: folic acid deficiency can be responsible for paralysis of the neck in turkey poults	Serology
49.	**Louping ill** (so called because infected sheep 'loup' or stagger). **Zoonosis**	A flavirus, transport host ticks. Restricted to British Isles	Grouse and pheasants on tick-infested rough pasture and woodland also grazed by mammals	Produces a variety of CNS signs. A serious problem on some grouse moors. May be asymptomatic, birds just found dead	Serology
50.	**Turkey meningio-encephalitis virus**	A flavirus, only so far documented in Israel and South Africa. Vector unknown	Turkeys over 10 weeks, mortality 10-80%, also in Japanese quail and chickens	Virus recovered from free-ranging wild birds, causes paralysis and a drop in egg production	Serology
51.	**Fowl adenovirus infection**	Group I fowl adenovirus	Chickens, particularly backyard fowl, guinea fowl, Japanese quail	In addition to other clinical signs, may cause CNS signs (see No. 7)	Virus isolation
52.	**Botulism**	Clostridium botulinum. Toxin, may be contained in maggot-infested carcasses or in sewage	All species, particularly backyard fowl	Not nearly so common in Galliformes as in waterfowl. May cause paralysis, usually found dead	Serology
53.	**Bacterial encephalitis**	A variety of pathogens and resulting from a systemic infection	All Galliformes	A variety of CNS signs usually with accompanying other clinical signs. Possibly also signs of trauma	Histopathology, PM, culture
54.	**Toxins**	A great variety of agricultural and industrial chemicals may pollute water supplies or the atmosphere. Misused chemotherapeutics	All species	Free-ranging wild birds may be affected at the same time. A variety of CNS and other clinical signs are seen, often just found dead	Deep frozen, separately wrapped tissues
55.	**Reovirus** ('stunting and runting' syndrome)	Reo- and rotaviruses	All Galliformes, particularly chicks	Infection may produce a tenosynovitis and arthritis with enlarged hocks and ruptured gastrocnemius tendons (see No 64)	See No. 64
56.	**Reticuloendotheliosis**	Reticuloendothelial virus	All Galliformes, particularly chickens 3-8 weeks	Apart from other clinical signs may show lameness, dropped wings and other CNS signs (see No. 65)	See No. 65
57.	**Bumblefoot**	A pododermatitis caused by a variety of pathogenic bacteria invading a traumatized foot in unhygienic conditions	All Galliformes, but particularly backyard fowl kept in unhygienic conditions	Swelling of the foot and occasionally the hock. Lameness and loss of condition. Old birds on worn out or unsuitable perches	

No.	Disease	Cause / Spread	Species affected	Signs / Notes	Diagnosis
58.	Fractures	Usually caused by rough handling or accident	All Galliformes	Lameness, paralysis, dropped wing	
Diseases that may show few, if any, premonitory signs but which may cause unthriftiness and loss of condition					
59.	Pullorum disease	See disease No. 20			
60.	Colibacillosis	See disease No. 21			
61.	Spirochaetosis	See disease No. 39			
62.	Ornithosis	See disease No. 2			
63.	ILT	See disease No. 3			
64.	Marek's disease	See disease No. 44			
65.	Avian sarcoma leucosis syndrome	See disease No 45			
66.	Pox virus infection	Avipox virus may be spread by biting insects. Virus in faeces. Fowl pox virus infects only chickens, grouse and pheasants. Turkey pox, quail and pheasant pox and peafowl pox viruses infect chickens	All Galliformes. Common in unvaccinated flocks of pheasants. Some free-living wild bird pox viruses infect chickens, e.g. sparrow pox, starling pox, magpie pox, some pigeon pox. Free-ranging wild turkey pox infects domestic birds	Sometimes an apparently asymptomatic subacute to chronic infection. Yellowish brown scabs on skin of head and legs. Diphtheritic lesions in oropharynx and trachea cause dysphagia and asphyxia (see No. 15). Compare to disease Nos. 3, 11, 35 and 36. Tends to occur seasonally when biting insects (mosquitoes, mites) are abundant. Morbidity in wild free-ranging New World quail is quite high. Mortality in captive quail can up to 40%	Histopathology, virus isolation, faecal exam. by electronic microscopy, culture, serology
67.	Stunting and runting syndrome (viral enteritis)	Reo- and rotaviruses. Adult birds may act as latent carriers. Biting insects may spread viruses, which are environmentally stable	All Galliformes, the young being more susceptible: chickens 4–10 days, partridge 6–56 days	An immunosuppressive disease affecting alimentary mucosa causing malabsorption. May also be abnormal feathering. May have diarrhoea, secondary infection produces other signs	PM, virus isolation, faecal exam. by electronic microscopy, serology
68.	Reticuloendothelial virus	Reticuloendothelial virus	All Galliformes, particularly chickens 3–8 weeks. Mortality may be 100%	Weight loss, anaemia, growing feathers fail to exsheath. Subcutaneous nodules on head and oral mucosa or sinusitis. Multivisceral neoplasms. Compare to diseases Nos. 44 and 45	Histopathology, virus isolation, serology
69.	Aspergillosis	*A. fumigatus*	All Galliformes	Can be presented as a chronic wasting disease (see No. 11)	Culture, serology

(continued)

Table 13.3 *(continued)*

No.	Disease	Primary cause	Species susceptible	Particular disease characteristic	Diagnosis
70.	**Avian tuberculosis and paratuberculosis.** **Zoonosis (see No.19 above)**	*Mycobacterium avium.* 3 subspecies. Infected birds shed large numbers of organisms in faeces. Environmentally persistent. Ectoparasites act as a vector	All Galliformes, particularly backyard fowl	Chronic wasting disease. Birds often quite alert, appetite unaffected. Anaemia, dull plumage. Possibly sporadic diarrhoea and occasional lameness. May be granulomas in oropharynx or in conjunctival sac. Compare to disease Nos. 3, 11, 35, 36 and 65	PM, culture, histopathology
71.	**Coccidiosis**	See disease No. 29			
72.	**Cryptococcosis**	See disease No. 18			
73.	**Histoplasmosis**	See disease No. 33			
74.	**Hexamitiasis**	See disease No. 31			
75.	**Leucocytosis**	A haemoprotozoan parasite. *Leucocytozoon* spp. transmitted by biting flies *Simulium* spp. and *Culicoides* spp.	All Galliformes, particularly young birds	Can cause anaemia, unthriftiness and anorexia	Haematology
76.	**Helminthiasis**	*Ascardia* spp. Proventricular and gizzard worms, capillariasis, heterakis (caecal worms), trichostrongyliasis (in grouse)	All Galliformes	All these helminth infections may cause loss of condition without any other clinical signs	Microscopy
77.	**Ectoparasitosis. All may act as mechanical vectors of other pathogens**	(1) Lice	All Galliformes	Only heavy infection important, usually species-specific therefore cross-species infection unlikely. Whole life cycle carried out on the host	
		(2) Fleas, a number of types		Not so species-specific as lice but eggs and larvae environmentally persistent	
		(3) *Dermanyssus* spp. (red mite, roost mites)	**Feed nightly.** **Zoonosis** A human contact can quickly become covered in the mites	Can cause severe anaemia, unthriftiness and death in young. Environmentally persistent	Diagnosis, examination of birds and environment using a shaded light at night
		(4) *Ornithonyssus* spp. (fowl mites)	As above	Signs as for *Dermanyssus* spp. but parasite never leaves host, therefore more pathogenic. High mortality	
		(5) *Trombicula* spp. (harvest mites)	As above	Seasonal, causing pruritus and damage to plumage	
		(6) *Knemidocoptes* spp. (scaly leg)		Causes pruritus. Compare to disease No. 65	
		(7) Ticks (*Ixodes* spp. and others)		Pruritus, anaemia, occasional fatal toxin kills chicks	

PM, post-mortem

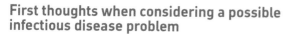

First thoughts when considering a possible infectious disease problem

Age group affected

First consider whether the problem is confined to a certain age group of birds.

Chicks from hatching up to approximately 10 days of age

Some of these chicks may be weak, not feeding properly and failing to thrive. This can be due to faulty incubation (humidity may be wrong), or they may just be genetically small. Small chicks easily get chilled (or can overheat) if in the brooder or with a bad hen. The artificial brooder ventilation may be faulty; there may be a build-up of fumes (ammonia, possibly carbon monoxide). All these predisposing causes may be presented as an *E. coli* or aspergillosis infection. Alternatively, poor incubator hygiene may be seen as umbilical or yolk sac infection.

Chicks in this age group that fail to thrive may be affected by an acute form of runting syndrome (see disease No. 67 in Table 13.3). Sudden death in very young quail chicks may be caused by an adenovirus (disease No. 8). Sudden death in young chicks of all species in outside aviaries could be due to spirochaetosis (disease No. 39).

Disease in older chicks from about 10 days to approximately 11 weeks

These birds are also liable to Runting syndrome (disease Nos. 67 and 68), Marek's disease (disease No. 44) and Gumboro disease (disease No. 38). **All these diseases are immunosuppressive, so the clinical signs may be caused by a secondary infection.** Other disease problems in this age range include coccidiosis (disease No. 30), necrotic enteritis (disease Nos. 24 and 28) and infectious bronchitis (disease No. 10). Hexamitiasis can be a problem in turkey poults (disease No. 23). The possibility of mycotoxins should always be considered.

Conditions affecting older growing birds over about 11 weeks of age

This age group may also be affected by Marek's disease (disease No. 44), particularly if they are female birds coming up to lay. However, they are more likely to be affected by the avian sarcoma leucosis virus (disease No. 45). Pheasants in this age group are often severely affected with marble spleen disease (disease No. 29). Both candidiasis (disease No. 36) and trichomoniasis (disease No. 37) can be a problem in young growing birds, particularly turkeys, pheasants, partridge and captive grouse.

Mixed species collections

Mixing widely different taxa of birds is never a good idea because some species are much more susceptible to certain diseases, whilst others can be asymptomatic and act as latent sources of infection (e.g. disease Nos. 4, 7, 10 and 34).

Quarantine

Owners of backyard flocks often purchase their stock from a variety of sometimes dubious sources – markets, pet shops or poultry shows – or acquire them from friends or relations. Most of these birds will be unvaccinated, and many will be carrying parasites. Some will be sero-positive for adenoviruses and mycoplasma, and may be latent carriers of disease. All new stock should be adequately quarantined from the main flock for at least 90 days. When newly acquired chicks are all obtained from one source, a period of 30 days may sufficient.

Use of vaccines

Appropriate prophylactic vaccination is good practice, but some live vaccines may exacerbate a problem if given to birds infected with an immunosuppressive virus. A vaccine administered in the water supply may be inactivated by chlorine. The vaccine used should always be licensed for the particular species concerned.

Seasonal occurrence of disease

Some diseases, particularly those transmitted by biting insects, only occur or are prevalent when the weather and/or the presence of nearby standing water is conducive to an increase in the number of insects (for instance the mosquito *Simulium* spp.), e.g. disease Nos 39, 47, 49, 52, 66, 67, 75 and 77.

Specific diseases according to clinical signs

To make differential diagnosis easier, these diseases are listed in Table 13.3 according to their commonly presented clinical signs. Zoonotic diseases and suggested diagnostic routines for each disease are also indicated.

Egg drop syndrome

The following causes can be responsible for a drop in egg production and production of malformed eggs:

1. Specific egg drop syndrome adenovirus – affects many species besides Galliformes; environmentally persistent in faeces
2. Infectious bronchitis virus – see disease Nos. 4 and 4a (Table 13.3)
3. Newcastle disease virus – see disease Nos. 4 and 4a
4. Influenza A virus – see disease No. 6
5. Fowl adenovirus Group I – see disease No. 7
6. Pullorum disease – see disease No. 20

7. Specific avian encephalomyelitis Picorna virus – see disease No. 48

8. Turkey meningio-encephalitis virus – see disease No. 49

9. Turkey rhinotracheitis pneumovirus – see disease No. 5

10. Diet – take into account the nutritional content of the diet

11. Husbandry – is the husbandry, housing, etc. satisfactory? Are stressors operative?

12. Egg stealing – always note the possibility of egg stealing, particularly in backyard flocks

13. Neoplasms and torsions – in single birds, note the possibility of neoplasms and torsion of the oviduct and other causes of egg binding.

References

Jones A K 1998 The normal moulting process in birds. Proceedings of the Annual Conference of the Association of Avian Veterinarians, 26–28 August 1998

Sibley C G, Ahlquist J E 1990 Galliformes. In: Phylogeny and classification of birds. Yale University Press, New Haven, CT

Woolham F 1987 The handbook of aviculture. Blandford Press, Poole, UK

Ramphastids

Amy B. Worell

14

Introduction

Toucans are members of the family of birds Ramphastidae, which is part of the order Piciformes. These colourful and interesting birds are further subdivided into six different genera, encompassing approximately 42 species. An additional division into three general categories, the larger toucans, the smaller toucanettes and the small, slender aracaris, is also useful for descriptive purposes.

Toucans as a group are considered tropical birds, encompassing a range that extends from southern Mexico to Bolivia and northern Argentina. Most species inhabit lowland rain forests, although some of the species can be found in mountainous regions.

The most prominent and distinguishing feature of the family Ramphastidae is the presence of the large protruding bill. Bills vary in colour from black to bright or multicoloured, and are actually quite lightweight, being composed of a thick outer covering of keratin with an intricate inner network of trabeculae. The prominent bill is thought to function in species recognition, in procuring food items that might otherwise be beyond their reach, and possibly in courtship rituals.

Toucans are not commonly kept as aviary or pet birds. While there are several large collections of ramphastids in the world, and a few birds are maintained as pets, the relative numbers are quite small when compared to captive psittacine species. Toucans that are hand-fed make the best pets/companion birds. Though toucans are unable to talk, these energetic birds are able to vocalize, and produce a variety of interesting sounds. The most common species found in captivity are the toco toucan (*Ramphastos toco*) and the sulphur-breasted (also commonly called the keel bill toucan or rainbow bill toucan) (*Ramphastos sulfuratus*) (Fig. 14.1).

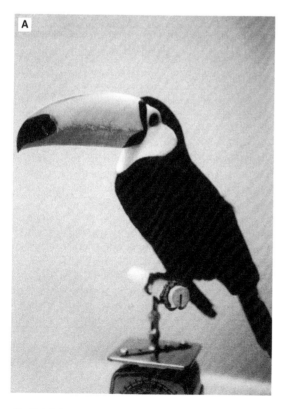
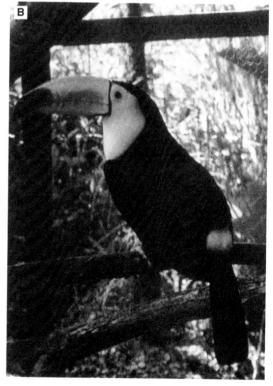

Fig 14.1 A Toco toucan. **B** Keel bill toucan.

Table 14.1 Anatomical variations found in ramphastids

Grossly visible anatomical characteristics:

- Lack of a discernible crop
- Presence of a gall bladder that is elongated in shape
- Frequent presence of pigmented gonads
- Keratinized bill with an inner intricate pattern of trabeculae
- Slender and elongated fibrous tongue

Radiographically visible anatomical characteristics (Smith & Smith 1992):

- Ventral deviation of the trachea at the thoracic inlet (this characteristic is present in Piciformes)
- Reticulated pattern in the protruding bill

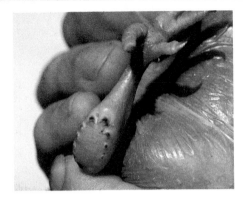

Fig 14.2 Heel pads on a young toucan.

Anatomical considerations

Toucans have several noteworthy anatomical features that differ from those commonly observed in psittacine species, with the most obvious being the large prominent bill (Table 14.1). **Toucans do not have crops, rather an oesophagus that is somewhat distensible. These birds can still be gavage fed and basically have the same capacity as a similarly sized parrot.** The gall bladder is elongated and generally retains a dark pigmented appearance. The trachea deviates ventrally, cranial to the thoracic inlet, which can be easily observed on lateral radiographs.

Biology and husbandry

Ramphastids have been noted to be relatively gregarious birds, but unlike psittacines, which fly in compact formations, toucans regularly fly in a more staggered formation (Grimes 1985). Like many birds, ramphastids prefer high treetops for security. Toucans prefer to remain in a cluster of trees, hopping from branch to branch, instead of flying over long distances for food and shelter.

Ramphastids are cavity nesters, utilizing holes made by other birds or animals or naturally occurring decay holes. They may enlarge the nest spot with their beaks, but do not usually line their nests with gathered materials such as grasses and twigs. The incubation period for ramphastids is 16 days. The larger species often lay three and occasionally four white eggs, while the smaller species average four eggs; clutches of three or five eggs have also been noted. As with other altricial species, toucans are born featherless and sightless. Although altricial, ramphastids have developed an interesting anatomical adaptation for additional body support during this critical life phase, in the form of a temporary heel-pad on the caudal aspect of the hock (Fig. 14.2). It is present at birth, and gradually regresses at 4 weeks of age. Depending on the species, toucans fledge between 44 and 50 days of age.

Housing

Toucans that are kept as companion animals thrive in large, horizontally oriented cages (Fig. 14.3). **As these colourful birds move about by hopping, it is preferable to have a large cage with several perches that allow for hopping back and forth both as exercise and to aid psychological wellbeing.** Toucans need food bowls that will allow easy access with their large bill to the food items. As they drink by scooping up water with their bill, the water bowl must accommodate the large bill. There should be at least three bowls in the cage: one for water, one for dry food, and one for daily diced fresh fruits.

Toucans that are housed as aviary birds, or those pets maintained in large cages, benefit from being kept in the largest cage that is practical within the confines of the compound. Aviaries 3–6 m in length, 2–4.5 m wide and 2–3 m in height are preferable for housing these active birds in captivity. Aviary birds are generally kept as pairs, but several combinations of birds are possible for a holding cage or in a mixed aviary. This practice is possible for all species of ramphastids presently in captivity except the emerald toucanette (*Aulacorhynchus prasinus*). **Toucans are aggressive and territorial birds that will often attack and kill other birds that are introduced into their environment.**

Two females may be placed together but, as with males of many animal species, two mature toucan males may show aggression towards one another when housed in the same enclosure.

In each aviary there should be at least two perches positioned high in the cage and at opposite ends of the flight. The diameter of the perches should be based on the bird's foot position while resting; the foot should not extend more than halfway around the perch circumference (Fig. 14.4). Ideally, perches should be of different diameters to aid in the prevention of plantar foot lesions (pododermatitis).

Toucans in the wild nest in excavated tree holes, and in captivity most toucans prefer nest logs over

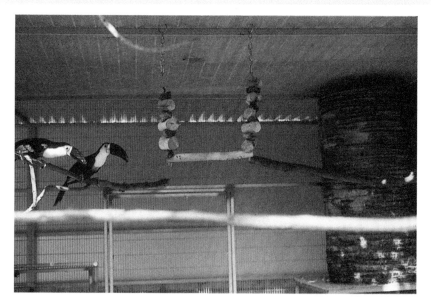

Fig 14.3 Ramphastid caging consists of large, horizontally oriented cages.

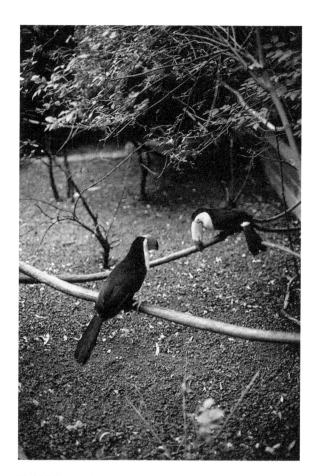

Fig 14.4 Perches for toucans.

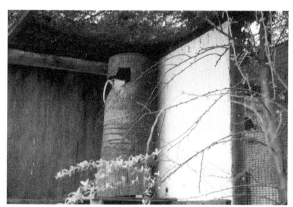

Fig 14.5 A palm tree nest box.

traditional psittacine-type nest boxes. There are, however, well-documented cases in which toucans have successfully laid eggs and fledged young in psittacine nest boxes. Although any species of tree may be utilized for captive nesting sites, the most commonly used is the palm log. Palm tree sections can be hollowed out with a chain saw and an entrance hole placed near the top of the log (Fig. 14.5). Nest logs should be securely anchored in the aviary and placed as high in the enclosure as possible.

The aracaris generally will sleep in their nest log, while the toucans prefer to sleep standing on a perch with their tail extended upwards. Aracaris kept as pets also seem to feel more secure hiding in a nest box at night.

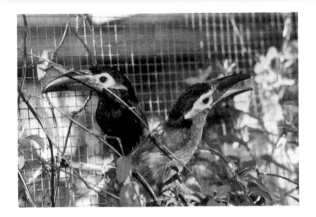

Fig 14.6 A planted toucan flight.

Both cement floors and natural dirt floors have been used for toucan aviary flooring. Cement is easier to keep clean, but dirt is more aesthetically pleasing. Toucan aviaries can be extensively planted with foliage, as these birds do not destroy growing vegetation (Fig. 14.6). The ramphastids appear to feel more secure in moderately planted aviaries than in those left barren and devoid of vegetation. Plants in the flight should be non-toxic to the resident birds in case ingestion does occur.

Diet

Dietary recommendations for captive ramphastids focus on concern about a life-threatening condition called iron storage disease (ISD) which affects many of the ramphastid species commonly maintained in captivity. Iron storage disease, which will be discussed in greater detail later in this chapter, potentially results in an abnormal absorption and resulting deposition of iron in a variety of tissues in the body. Even though the aetiology of iron storage disease is not presently known in ramphastids, there are concerns about iron levels in the diets of captive toucans. As a general note, it should be pointed out that human medicine has concluded that dietary iron does not contribute to or augment the deposition of iron in the human body (Dambro 1996). How this human finding relates to ramphastids is not known at this time.

Present dietary recommendations for captive toucans include one of the commercially available pelleted low iron softbill diets and a variety of fresh fruits. Any ramphastid diet should ideally meet the recommendation for poultry with regard to dietary iron levels (40–60 ppm) (Kincaid & Stoskopf 1997). Practically speaking, and considering the products currently available commercially, the author suggests using a product that contains less than 100 ppm of iron, and most likely greater than 50 ppm (G P Olsen et al, unpublished work, 2006).

The dry component of the diet should be offered on an *ad lib* basis. A variety of fresh, diced fruits should be offered daily in a separate bowl. As ramphastids swallow their food items whole rather than separately, the fruit must be chopped into bite-sized pieces. Fruits that have a high moisture content, such as grapes, berries, melons and papaya, are readily accepted by toucans. Other fruits such as apples, pears, bananas and peaches are also acceptable. Fruits high in vitamin C, such as oranges, actually enhance the absorption of iron, and should therefore not be included in the diet of these birds (Worell 1997).

Neonatal and young toucans that are hand-fed may be offered a variety of hand-feeding diets. As ramphastids do not have a discernible crop, food items should be offered in small quantities on a frequent basis. One option for feeding toucans utilizes commercially available psittacine hand-feeding formulas. This type of mixture can be fed alone, or with the addition of finely diced or pureed fruits. These diets can also be gavage-fed into the mid-oesophagus region, or offered free choice to be ingested voluntarily through normal eating mechanisms. As stated earlier, because small ramphastids cannot store food, babies need to be fed frequently (i.e. once an hour). When the chick is full it will turn its head, or more commonly regurgitate the offered food items.

Sex determination

It is important to determine the sex in birds that are to be used for breeding purposes, and surgical sexing is a commonly used method for sex determination in monomorphic ramphastids. Additionally, some commercial laboratories are able to determine the sex of these birds through DNA methods on a small sample of submitted blood.

The surgical sexing procedure is similar to that in psittacines. Fasting for 4 hours is recommended prior to surgical procedures. Because of their enlarged bills, anaesthetic masks must be extended to accommodate the entire structure. Gonads in toucans may be dark green in coloration.

Several of the species of toucan that are currently in captivity are dimorphic, and thus can be visually sexed. All of the larger toucans are essentially monomorphic, while two of the smaller toucans currently in captivity, the tetes, are monomorphic (spot bill toucanette (*Selenidera maculirostris*), Guyana toucanette (*Selenidera culik*)). In the aracaris grouping, several captive species are dimorphic (e.g. black neck aracari (*Pteroglossu aracari*), green aracari (*Pteroglossus viridis*), ivory bill aracari (*Pteroglossus flavirostris*), many banded aracari (*Pteroglossus pluricinctus*)). In these species, the feather coloration of the head or neck is markedly different in the males as compared to the females.

Additionally, many ramphastids demonstrate visible, but often subtle, bill length differences. Males often will have longer, narrower bills than females of the same species. The females' bills, generally, are shorter and broader. These bill differences can be quite clear or sometimes non-existent in many bird species. Determining bill differences can be helpful in an initial visual inspection of ramphastids, in particular if a group of the same species is present.

Breeding ramphastids

Ramphastid reproduction is similar to that of psittacine species, in that the smaller species of psittacines (e.g. budgies and cockatiels) generally reproduce more readily in captivity than do the larger species (e.g. certain species of cockatoos, many species of Amazon parrots). This trend also is noted for toucans; the smaller species (e.g. *Selenidera maculirostris*, or spot bill toucanette) breed much more readily than the larger, easily recognizable species (e.g. toco toucan (*Ramphastos toco*)).

Ramphastid reproduction is most successful in long flight cages. Visual separation of adjoining pairs enhances successful reproduction and hence is highly recommended, while vocalization of nearby or adjacent pairs appears to be less important for successful breeding. Palm nest logs are usually recommended for a nesting site, with or without bedding material. **The larger species of toucans become sexually mature around 2 years of age, and the smaller species at about 12 months. The captive life span for ramphastids is approximately 20 years, and with some of the larger toucan species productive breeding may occur well into later years.** The reproductive activity of some of the smaller rhamphastid species rapidly decreases after 5–6 years of annual breeding.

The majority of toucan species that have been captive bred in the past were parent reared rather than incubator hatched. As the value of these birds has increased tremendously through the years, many breeders now routinely incubate all eggs and hand rear the young from day one of hatch.

Potential problems encountered with parent-reared birds include mutilation, both severe and minor, to babies either shortly after birth or as late as 3–4 weeks of age. Stress to the parents or the lack of live food to feed the babies is often thought to be the reason for the abuse. Once young disappear from the nest or are found mutilated, the remaining offspring should be removed for their own safety.

Handling and restraint

The handling of ramphastids is similar to that for other types of avian species, and includes using the bill as a 'handle' for improving control over the bird. When toucans bite, they grasp and manipulate the object with their bill; if this object is a handler's arm or hand, it can be quite painful as the body part is rocked back and forth in the bird's mouth. Therefore, when removing an untamed bird from a carrier, the bird should be rapidly grasped by its protruding bill and removed from the carrier. The body is held in the same way as for other avian species.

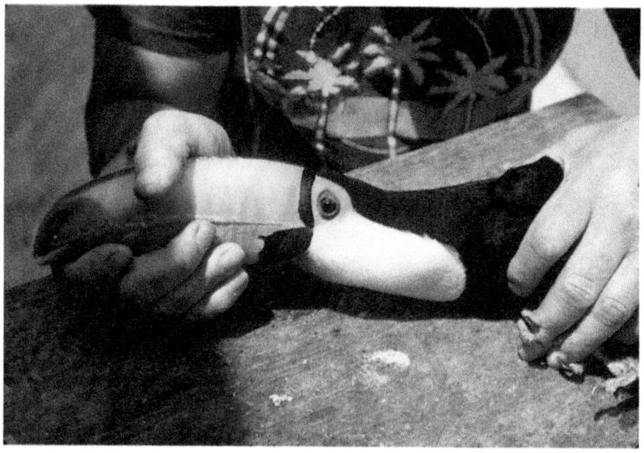

Fig 14.7 Restraint of a toucan.

Restraining toucans is easier when holding the bill than when holding the bird by the back of the head (Fig. 14.7). The technique is, of course, a matter of personal preference, but bill holding is especially preferable in the larger species of toucans, where the bill is quite formidable. Smaller species, such as some of the toucanettes, are easily held with the hand placed on the back of the bird's head.

Blood collection

The technique for blood collection is similar to that utilized in other avian species. The patient should be held in a left lateral position by the technician, with one hand on the bird's mid-bill and the other on the body. Blood is easily collected from the right jugular vein by this method. The feather tracts of ramphastids differ from those in psittacines, and feathers simply need to be moved to one side to expose a substantial section of skin so that the jugular vein can be viewed.

Basic surgery

The three most common forms of surgery performed on ramphastids are exploratory surgery, keyhole incisions or endoscopic visualization for hepatic biopsy, and laparoscopy for surgical sexing. Toucans are induced and maintained on gas anaesthesia similar to other avian species. The obvious difference for anaesthetic induction is the need for a modified mask to fit over the large bill (Fig. 14.8). Sevoflurane is the anaesthetic agent of choice for these large-billed birds. Exploratory

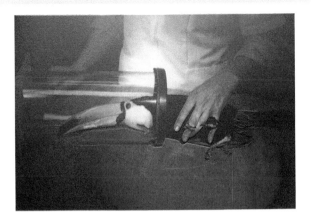

Fig 14.8 Anaesthesia of a toucan.

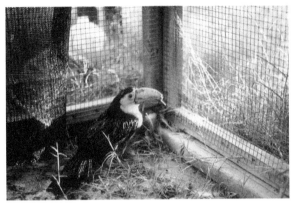

Fig 14.9 Metabolic bone disease can cause soft folds or distal tip compressions in the bills of ramphastids.

surgery generally involves exploration of the body cavity for abdominal distension, and the approach is through a ventromedial abdominal incision. The bird's feathers may not need to be pulled if feather tracts are not in the area of the incision.

Hepatic biopsy may be performed via a keyhole incision. In this case the approach is through a small, horizontal incision approximately 1.25 cm just distal to the distal ventral aspect of the sternum and to the right of the midline. The distal tip of the right liver lobe is exteriorized or visualized, and a small wedge of tissue is removed. If there is a concern over bleeding, a commercially available product such as Gelfoam or Hemablock can be placed on the bleeding liver lobe. For an endoscopic hepatic biopsy, the technique used in psittacines is applicable.

For surgical sexing by laparoscopy, the approach is the same as that utilized in other avian patients.

Metabolic and nutritional disorders

Three conditions involving metabolic and/or nutritional disorders occur with varying frequencies in ramphastids: metabolic bone disease, diabetes mellitus and iron storage disease.

Metabolic bone disease

Apparent metabolic bone disease (MBD) or nutritional hyperparathyroidism has been observed in a number of immature toucans (Fig. 14.9). Metabolic bone disease has been frequently observed involving two different scenarios and time frames of avian development. In one case, neonatal babies (e.g. crimson rump toucanettes (*Aulachorynchus haematopygus*), collared aracaris (*Pteroglossus torquatus*)) that have been incubator hatched will have affected beaks and bent or bowed legs respectively. If detected early enough, manual manipulation in addition to environmental and/or management

changes can be instituted to gain some resolution of the deformities.

Many reported cases of MBD have occurred in young but not neonatal keel bill or rainbow billed toucans (*Ramphastos sulfuratus*). The affected birds were obtained from multiple sources and had been fed various diets. These birds presented with soft folds in their bills or lateral and/or distal tip compression of the bill. Many of the bill lesions were the direct result of trauma (i.e. flying into the aviary wall) but appeared to have an underlying component of metabolic bone disease, because the bills were abnormally soft for the age and stage of development of the bird. Lesions commonly found in avian species diagnosed with metabolic bone disease (e.g. deviations in the ridge of the keel, bowing of the legs) have not been observed in cases affecting keel bill toucans.

Assessment and modification of the diet is necessary to prevent further skeletal changes. Dietary manipulation, such as addition of foods high in calcium or supplementation with a vitamin–mineral powdered supplement, may be warranted, as well as conversion to a different pelleted soft bill diet. **Covering aviary walls with some form of opaque netting may aid in preventing trauma-related bill damage to birds being treated for MBD.**

The majority of the affected birds' bills remodel to closely resemble a normal appearance following dietary and aviary modifications. Birds with a substantial amount of damage to the distal bill adjust to their condition and thrive even when the mandible, maxilla, or both are affected. One bird's bill that suffered significant damage involving compression of the distal maxilla has remodelled itself over time to become more normal in appearance.

Diabetes mellitus

Diabetes mellitus is a relatively common condition that is diagnosed in many different species of animals and birds. **There have been only two ramphastid species in which diabetes mellitus has been reported, the toco and keel bill toucans (Worell 1988).** As relatively large numbers of these two species of toucans are presently in captivity, and few individuals are affected, the overall incidence of diabetes in toucans appears to be quite low.

Birds affected with diabetes mellitus demonstrate the classic signs of the disease (e.g. weight loss, polyuria, polydipsia, polyphagia, significantly elevated glucosuria, hyperglycaemia). When measured, glucosuria will generally be 0.056 mmol/L on a urine test strip, and the blood glucose levels exceed 55.51 mmol/L. Blood glucose levels over 111.02 mmol/L have been documented in affected rhamphastid species (Murphy 1992).

As with other avian species, glucose metabolism with regard to hormonal regulation in the avian body is not yet completely understood. Diabetes mellitus is often considered to be a secondary condition in affected birds rather than a primary condition. Glucagon, as opposed to insulin, may actually be the regulating hormone for blood glucose levels. **Affected birds, including toucans, can be treated with PZI or NPH insulin injections for the regulation of diabetes.** Initial treatment should be instituted utilizing less than one unit of the selected insulin once or twice daily, with intramuscular dosages ranging from 0.06 to 3.3 U/kg having been suggested for avian species (Oglesbee 1997). The initial amount should be selected by the clinician, taking into account factors such as current blood glucose levels, body weight of the bird, physical condition of the bird, other underlying medical problems, the clinician's experience in treating diabetes in birds, and the owner's ability in treatment and monitoring the affected patient. Clinical hypoglycaemia is displayed as in mammals, and may produce signs of weakness, lethargy, ataxia and disorientation. If hypoglycaemia results, oral or injectable glucose products, or glucose-containing foods, should be administered.

Toucans, and other avian species diagnosed with diabetes mellitus, may be difficult to monitor and regulate (Cornelissen & Ritchie 1994). Insulin injections may optimally regulate blood glucose if given once daily, twice daily, or on a schedule such as every other day. One study suggests that dietary changes may be advantageous in the regulation of diabetes in toucans (Murphy 1992).

Many diabetic toucans eventually succumb to the disease. Post-mortem examinations, when permitted, have demonstrated changes including pancreatic islet cell hyperplasia (Worell 1988, Murphy 1992), and deposition of iron in the pancreas (Worell 1988).

Iron storage disease

Iron storage disease (ISD) is the most common life-threatening disease to affect captive ramphastids (Table 14.2) (Worrell 1996). Iron storage disease results when an excessive amount of iron accumulates in various body tissues.

Table 14.2 Species of ramphastids affected with iron storage disease

Channel-billed toucan (*Ramphastos vitellinus*)
Toco toucan (*Ramphastos toco*)
Keel bill toucan (*Ramphastos sulfuratus*)
Red bill toucan (*Ramphastos tucanus*)
Ariel toucan (*Ramphastos vitellinus ariel*)
Choco toucan (*Ramphastos brevis*)
Plate-billed mountain toucan (*Andigna laminirostris*)
Pale mandible toucanette (*Pteroglossus erythropygius*)
Chestnut-eared aracari (*Pteroglossus castanotis*)
Black-necked aracari (*Pteroglossus aracari*)
Spot bill toucanette (*Selenidera maculirostris*)
Saffron toucanette (*Baillonius baillioni*)
Emerald toucanette (*Aulacorhynchus prasinus*)

In affected individuals, an iron-containing pigment may be identified microscopically in diseased tissues. In those cases where iron deposition results in cellular damage, organ dysfunction, disease and death may occur.

Iron storage disease occurs in several different species of mammals and birds, including mynahs, birds of paradise, quetzals, cranes, starlings, hornbills and tanagers (Worell 1988). Although various avian species show different clinical presentations, the disease process is a progressive condition that eventually results in death.

In humans, there are two different forms of the disease. In the secondary form, excessive iron deposition is related to chronic anaemia, a variety of haemolytic disorders, and exogenous iron administration. In the primary, idiopathic or genetic form, the disease is due to a recessively transmitted autosomal disorder, which involves a defect in the mucosal cells of the intestinal tract. The defective gene is found on the short arm of chromosome six. Even though the exact nature of the defect is not presently known, it is thought that the normal controls affecting iron metabolism are lost in these individuals, and hence excessive iron is absorbed. Idiopathic haemochromatosis in humans is not thought to be related to the amount of iron in the diet (Worell 1988). There has not been any correlation found at this time between avian iron storage disease and the human forms of the disease.

Current research and present knowledge of ISD in toucans and other avian species has not identified a specific aetiology for this condition. Since there is a lack of uniformity of clinical signs, there is speculation that differing aetiologies may be the initiating cause of ISD in avian species. It has been shown that the amount of iron in the diet can affect hepatic iron levels and storage, and that iron does accumulate over time (Crissey et al 2000). Susceptible species of ramphastids should be fed diets that are compatible with poultry recommendations for dietary iron levels (50–100 ppm). To date,

13 species of ramphastids have been identified as being susceptible to iron storage disease. **The most common ramphastid species affected by iron storage disease are also the most commonly kept species in captivity, the toco, keel bill and red bill toucans.**

Other dietary components, in particular ascorbic acid (vitamin C), can increase absorption of iron from non-haem food sources but not from haem food sources. Ascorbic acid has been shown to enhance iron bioavailability from the diet. Thus, supplementation of diets with ascorbic acid containing foodstuffs is not recommended (Sheppard & Dierenfield 2002, Farina et al 2005).

Dietary recommendations:

- Low iron pelleted diet with iron level between 50 and 100 ppm
- Diced fruit offered daily
- Avoidance of foods containing ascorbic acid.

Clinical signs in affected toucans are often not apparent to the caretaker. Even though the clinical signs may be subtle and difficult to identify, depression and minor disease signs are probably present in affected birds prior to death. Often, birds affected by ISD are found dead without apparent clinical abnormalities. The lack of overt disease signs may be due to the strong instinctual preservation nature of birds or ability of the target organs to function even when severely compromised.

Iron storage disease is most accurately diagnosed through histopathological examination of biopsied liver tissue samples. Previous serology by the author explored serum iron determinations to render an ante-mortem diagnosis of iron storage disease. However, further work demonstrated that hepatic biopsy is, at this time, the gold standard for diagnosis of ISD in affected rhamphastid species (Worell 1991a, 1993). Liver samples can be obtained either by using endoscopic techniques or through a small ventral abdominal incision. The harvested sample should be analysed for characteristic histopathological changes as well as exact iron levels.

A fineneedle non-aspiration biopsy of hepatic tissue can be utilized in high risk, debilitated patients for a diagnosis of ISD. Although this method has limited sensitivity, its use may be warranted in certain patients (Olsen et al 2005).

Diagnosis of ISD:

- Hepatic biopsy
- Non-aspiration needle aspirate in very ill birds.

Once a bird has been diagnosed with ISD, the prognosis is guarded and the bird will eventually die of the disease, although the disease process may take several years. The recommended treatment for birds diagnosed with iron storage is similar to that for humans; i.e. the once- or twice-weekly removal of blood (phlebotomies) in an attempt to lower the iron level in the body, in addition to dietary modification by providing food that is low in iron content. It may take 2–3 years for human patients to achieve the anticipated endpoint where excess iron is removed, resulting in a mild anaemia. The lifetime maintenance therapy involves intermittent phlebotomies at a rate of four to six a year, which leads to normalization of the serum iron levels (Dambro 1996). Further information may be obtained by visiting the Iron Overload Diseases Association, Inc. at their web page (http://www.emi.net/~iron_od/).

The treatment of choice in toucans affected with iron storage disease is the use of phlebotomies and dietary modification. One study involving two toco toucans demonstrated decreased hepatocellular haemosiderin levels with lowered dietary iron levels alone (Drews et al 2004). In affected toucans, birds undergo weekly phlebotomies for more than a year. Birds are seen on a weekly basis, and 10% of the bird's blood volume is removed each time. Bird blood volume is calculated by taking 10% of the bird's body weight in grams. For example, if a bird's weight is 450 g, the total blood volume will be 45 mL^3. The calculated safe volume of blood that can be removed, calculated at 10% of the blood volume, is therefore 4.5 mL. To put it another way, it is safe to remove an amount of blood equal to 1% of the toucan's body weight on a weekly basis (Worell 1991b). Weekly packed cell volume (PCV) percentages should be evaluated, even though no appreciable drop in this value has been documented. In humans, if the haematocrit drops below 36% (normal range 37–47% in women), or if the haemoglobin is less than 10, then the phlebotomy is not performed. Suggested criteria for toucans would be to perform the phlebotomy if the bird's oral mucous membrane is pink and if the haematocrit is greater than 30%.

In addition to phlebotomies, several other treatment modalities have been investigated with varying results. Chelation of iron is used to induce increased excretion or inhibit its absorption. Ligands that are known to inhibit the absorption of iron include phytates, tannates, phosphates, oxalates and carbonates. Of these, tannates (tannin) are the most potent inhibitors of non-haem iron absorption. Black tea, which is rich in tannins, has been utilized to attempt to inhibit iron absorption. In one study of people affected with genetic haemochromatosis (GH) iron absorption was reduced by 70% when tea, as compared to water, was consumed with a test meal. This study confirmed the inhibitory effect of black tea on intestinal iron absorption in patients with GH (Kaltwasser et al 1998). Multiple anecdotal stories of individuals using tea in the birds' drinking water abound in the avian community. **No documented studies have shown tea water to be beneficial and effective as a treatment option for ISD affecting toucans.**

Research studies using European starlings (*Sturnus vulgaris*) have shown that addition of a phytate (inositol) and tannic acid to a high iron diet prevented an increase in stored liver iron concentrations (Olsen et al 2006a). Additional research with European starlings (*Sturnus vulgaris*), comparing four treatment regimens for iron storage disease, showed that when a low iron diet was fed, the addition of inositol and tannic acid to the diet did *not* affect the iron absorption as it did with the high iron diet (Olsen et al 2006b).

As a note regarding toucans and tannins in the wild, toucans rarely if ever come to the ground to drink. Instead, they drink water that collects in tree crotches that are thought to leach tannins into this reservoir of rain water. It has been assumed that this 'natural method' of tannin introduction in the diet is beneficial in keeping the liver iron concentrations of susceptible species in check. Tannin-impregnated rainwater in addition to choice of food items in the wild, may aid in keeping the bird's iron levels within a manageable range. This idea has been supported in part by a study analysing foodstuffs consumed by keel bill toucans in Belize, which reported that the species in question consumed foods that were shown to be generally low in iron content (Otten et al 2001).

In human haemochromatosis patients who are too anaemic for phlebotomies, an alternative treatment is attempted with the iron-chelating drug deferoxamine mesylate (Desferal, Novartis Pharmaceuticals Corp, East Hanover, NJ, USA). There have been several non-documented cases of the use of deferoxamine in toucans, and one documented study (Cornelissen et al 1995). In this study, a 4-month protocol of daily subcutaneous injections with deferoxamine (100 mg/kg) was given to a channel-billed toucan. Monthly biopsies were performed and at the completion of the 4-month study the bird was considered free of iron storage disease.

The author has utilized deferoxamine in several ramphastids that have been diagnosed with severe iron storage disease by hepatic biopsy. Injections were given once daily into the pectoral muscle mass. Initially dosages of 100 mg/kg were administered, with the latter dose being closer to 200 mg/kg. Subsequent tissue samples did not demonstrate a decrease in iron deposition in the liver. Visually, on subsequent hepatic samples, the livers have appeared more abnormal than on previous submissions. These visual changes include continuing hepatomegaly and grossly visible tissue bronzing. However, the owner of the birds perceived that the birds were clinically more alert and active. Studies with deferoxamine are continuing in order to determine its clinical effectiveness. The stress of daily handling a patient to administer this drug should be strongly considered prior to its use as a long-term treatment option for ISD.

Recent work with an oral iron-chelating agent, deferiprone, administered q12h, was conducted using domestic pigeons (*Columba livia*) and white leghorn chickens (*Gallus fallus f. domestica*) (Whiteside et al

2004). Several of the chickens succumbed during the study, suggesting that there was an acute reduction of iron available for normal enzymatic processes. It is thought that this product has treatment potential for species with ISD, especially if it could be incorporated into a low iron diet (Whiteside et al 2004).

Treatment of ISD:

- **Low iron diet if not already on a diet with an iron level between 50 and 100 ppm**
- **Weekly or biweekly phlebotomies**
- **Avoidance of ascorbic acid foodstuffs in the diet**
- **Intermittent liver biopsies to monitor progression of ISD.**

The ideal diagnostic path for ISD would be to perform a hepatic biopsy for both histopathological examination and quantitative determination of hepatic iron levels. If the hepatic tissue demonstrated iron storage disease, then serial hepatic tissue samples should be considered at intervals of 6–12 months. Assuming a response is seen in the hepatic tissue, then a maintenance protocol for phlebotomies may be instituted on a once-monthly basis. This protocol is recommended to clients with birds in which ISD has been confirmed.

Other than monitoring ISD in affected birds by serial hepatic samples, use of serial magnetic resonance imaging (MRI) has been studied (Paul-Murphy et al 2003). This modality is not readily available to most clinicians and its overall effectiveness as a diagnostic tool to quantitate ISD has not been established.

Additionally, as a screening test, whole body radiographs are useful in suggesting the presence of ISD in susceptible avian species. Both lateral and ventrodorsal views can be taken, but the most useful is the ventrodorsal view. The attending clinician must be able to distinguish a normal liver silhouette from hepatomegaly in radiographs. As this non-invasive radiographic technique is not diagnostic for iron storage disease in ramphastids, a differential diagnosis for liver enlargement should always be considered. The primary and secondary differential diagnoses of a toucan patient with significant radiographic hepatic enlargement is ISD and avian tuberculosis.

In toucans that succumb to ISD, post-mortem examinations are often performed on birds in good body condition. Gross internal changes that are noted include a markedly enlarged liver that is orange to bronze in colour. Both grossly and histologically, the liver is often the only affected organ or tissue. This is in marked contrast to the clinical effects of iron deposition seen in humans, where iron deposition commonly occurs in multiple body organs and tissues, resulting in serious complications (Worell 1988, Dambro 1996). Iron deposition may be noted in the heart, spleen, kidneys, pancreas and small intestines, although this is a less common finding.

Additionally, ascites, which is commonly seen in mynah birds with ISD, has not been documented by the author in affected toucans.

Microscopic changes in the specially stained (e.g. Prussian blue) liver tissue of birds often show varying degrees of iron deposition in both hepatocytes and Kupffer cells. Also observed in many of these tissue sections are small areas of non-affected, apparently functioning hepatic tissue.

Infectious diseases

As an avian group, ramphastids are quite hardy birds, apart from the predisposition to ISD in some species. There are a number of other disease conditions that are occasionally diagnosed in ramphastids (Table 14.3). Upper respiratory infections occasionally occur, as do generalized unspecified bacterial infections that respond to broad-spectrum antibiotics.

Viral diseases

Viral diseases in ramphastids have rarely been documented. The few isolated cases of viral infections diagnosed in toucans include Newcastle disease (paramyxovirus), an occasional herpes virus (Charlton et al 1990), and pox virus. Several cases involved lesions that resembled either proventricular dilatation disease of psittacines or psittacine polyomavirus (D. Reavill, personal experience and person communication).

Chlamydial infections

Presently, there are no documented cases of ramphastid chlamydial infections. Although no documented cases of *Chlamydophila psittaci* have been reported in toucan species these birds should be considered susceptible.

Fungal and yeast infections

Occasional *Aspergillus* spp. infections have been noted in ramphastids, but the overall occurrence appears to be very low. *Candida albicans* may frequently be diagnosed in ramphastids, and is confirmed using techniques such as gastrointestinal tract cytology or microbiology. The presence of candidiasis may be considered as normal flora or a pathogen, depending on the individual presentation. If the bird is clinically healthy and the organism has been identified from the gastrointestinal tract of an individual, the organism should be considered a normal inhabitant. If the bird is a neonate being hand-fed, or is a poor doer and losing weight, the organism should be considered a potential pathogen.

Parasitic infections

Currently the incidence of internal or external parasites in indoor captive toucans appears to be very low.

However, in those birds that are housed in outdoor flights with dirt floors, and exposed to recently imported or imported birds in general, the incidence can be significant and higher. Infection with intestinal parasites such as nematodes, *Capillaria* spp. and *Giardia* spp. still occurs in toucan species. Toucans housed outdoors have also been diagnosed on post-mortem examinations with *Sarcocystis*. As with other species, toucans are thought to be the intermediate hosts of the protozoan parasite while the opossums are considered to be the definitive hosts. Lice have also been identified externally in some birds. Imported toucans should still be closely screened for both internal and external parasites.

Bacterial infections

Although the overall incidence is low, bacterial infections are the most common microorganisms affecting ramphastids. Most bacterial infections in toucans are isolated in the upper respiratory or gastrointestinal systems. As with other avian species, most potentially pathogenic bacteria are Gram-negative organisms. An investigative study in which five species of clinically normal toucans were examined for the presence of cloacal microflora demonstrated the presence of large numbers of *Staphylococcus* spp., *Streptococcus* spp. and *Escherichia coli* (Cornelissen & Ritchie 1994). The results of the cloacal study parallel the isolates from the numerous cloacal cultures that have been performed by the author. Additionally, *Lactobacillus* spp. are commonly isolated from clinically healthy birds and should be considered normal flora in these cases. *E. coli* should be considered a potential pathogen, especially when isolated from a clinically ill patient. Since the serotypes of *E. coli* have not been explored in clinically healthy and clinically ill birds, it is unknown which serotypes are pathogenic, opportunistic pathogens, or commensals. The entire clinical picture of the individual patient should be considered when deciding pathogenicity of a bacterial isolate.

Rapid and sometimes peracute deaths have been noted in several collections of toucans from *Salmonella*. Initial contamination of the environment and food bowls by rodents has been considered as the possible source of these infections, followed by horizontal transmission of the disease to other nearby birds in an aviary.

Choanal and oesophageal cultures taken from ramphastids frequently demonstrate the presence of varying numbers of bacteria that may be considered either normal inhabitants or potential pathogens in these birds. Once again, the entire clinical picture should be assessed to determine the significance of the isolates.

Ramphastids are considered to be very susceptible to *Yersinia pseudotuberculosis*, a Gram-negative bacteria. *Y. pseudotuberculosis* infections commonly result t0030　**Table 14.3**　Diagnosis of medical problems in ramphastids with regard to clinical signs

Problem	Occurrence	Clinical signs	Aetiology	Differential diagnosis	Confirmative diagnostic tests	Treatment
Respiratory problems	Upper respiratory infections occur with a small frequency in ramphastids. Many of these are quite chronic in nature, and may never completely resolve	Congestion wheezing, and intermittent insufflation of the cervical air sacs are most commonly seen. Occasionally sneezing and a clear nasal discharge may be evident	A definitive diagnosis is not reached in most upper respiratory infections. Unretrievable bacterial and/or viral organisms may possibly be involved	Lower respiratory infections	None. Radiographs, Gram stains and choanal cultures may be helpful	Affected birds may be treated with broad-spectrum antibiotics and nasal flushes. Nebulization therapy is often useful. Treatment may be lengthy
Diarrhoea	Uncommon, or difficult to distinguish from normal loose droppings	Loose faecal component of the droppings. It should be noted that ramphastids will often pass chunks of undigested food in their droppings	Most commonly due to bacterial or parasitic infections	Polyuria; could be normal for the bird's diet or due to recently ingested food	Faecal parasite examinations. Gram stains or cloacal cultures	Broad-spectrum antibiotics or anthelmintics
Anorexia	Not common	Not eating	No specific condition	All conditions affecting toucans	Should do thorough work-up, including CBC, serum chemistries, bile acids, cultures or Gram stains, faecal parasite examination, EPH and radiographs	Broad-spectrum antibiotics, two to three times daily gavage feeding with a commercially available psittacine hand-feeding formula
Nervous signs	Not documented in ramphastids					
Polyuria/polydipsia (PU/PD)	Very few birds are affected	Drinking large amounts of water with subsequent polyuria	Most commonly due to diabetes mellitus in those affected species (tocos and keel bills)	Any condition, similar to mammals, that could cause PU/PD, such as renal or hepatic involvement in particular. Does not occur with ISD	CBC, serum chemistries and urinalysis	Insulin injections. At this time, Ultralente is the recommended insulin

(continued)

Table 14.3 *(continued)*

Problem	Occurrence	Clinical signs	Aetiology	Differential diagnosis	Confirmative diagnostic tests	Treatment
Breeding problems	Very varied. Probably depends on keeper's management style and familiarity with birds. A percentage of toucans molest and cannibalize their young. Frequency rates have not been documented. Difficulty may be encountered with getting the larger species of ramphastids to breed in captivity (similar to breeding some of the wild-caught psittacines in captivity)	Depending on the specific problem. May be disappearance of young, or finding partially ingested young. May have no breeding in larger ramphastids	Probably related to over-managing and not enough security for a pair of birds. May also be related to not enough live food. Could be related to incompatible pairs of birds	Should run diagnostic tests on non-producing pairs or modify aviary situations		
Foreign body ingestion	Potentially could occur in any ramphastid, but only documented by the author in aviary birds. Incidence is related to environment and management	Vague. May not see signs of a sick bird	Ingestion of foreign body – most commonly metal objects such as wire or nails in the author's experience	Would depend on whether clinical signs were observed	May be visualized on radiographs depending on the density of the object. Many of these are found on post-mortem examination	If the foreign body is discovered prior to death and the object cannot pass, surgery may be the treatment of choice unless the object is removable via endoscopy through entrance into the oesophagus
Damage to the bill	Incidence is low. Most commonly occurs in young, growing birds	Deformed beak due to stage of development of the beak. age of the bird and increased malleability of the bill. May also see that a distal section of either the maxilla or mandible is missing. Occasionally seen as defect on lateral surface of either bill	Trauma to the bill. Often precipitated by underlying metabolic bone disease	None	None. Could perform a CBC plus serum chemistries to rule out underlying disease	Generally not necessary. Some of the defects can be repaired. but unsuccessful in the long run

| Iron storage disease | Very high in those species known to be affected with the condition | Ranges from none to general signs of a sick bird, or finding a dead bird | Due to excessive absorption and deposition of iron in the liver. Specific cause of this condition is unknown | Avian tuberculosis, hepatic disease due to other causes, other systemic disease | Hepatic biopsy | Weekly phlebotomies for several years, monitored by intermittent hepatic biopsies, gradually adjusting to a more intermittent schedule of phlebotomies for the remainder of the bird's life |
| Ankylosis of the tarsometatarsal joint | Most commonly occurs in birds that have been imported or shipped | Swelling and decreased range of motion of this joint | Trauma to this joint in transit. May potentially involve bacterial invaders if the skin is punctured | Fractures in the distal tibiotarsus or proximal metatarsus | Radiographs. May consider joint cytology, culture if indicated | Return to normal function is generally unrewarding. Success may be related to length of time between injury and presentation. Antimicrobial therapy can be utilized if indicated. Otherwise, some relief may be obtained by topical use of DMSO and anti-inflammatory products |

in acute or peracute deaths in affected birds. Chronic infections with the bacteria also occur, but appear to be less frequent in ramphastid species. Post-mortem fi ndings of birds infected with Y. *pseudotuberculosis* typically demonstrate hepatomegaly, splenomegaly and, sometimes, the presence of granulomatous lesions in various body organs. The enlarged liver and spleen usually demonstrate the presence of small white or yellow foci (Dhillon & Shafer 1987). Transmission is thought to occur from ingestion of rats and mice or their droppings. Rodent control in an aviary experiencing infection due to Y. *pseudotuberculosis* is of paramount importance to stop the spread of the disease and control future outbreaks.

***Mycobacterium* spp. infections in ramphastids are occasionally diagnosed. Birds infected with tuberculosis may present with depression, emaciation and hepatomegaly.** Diagnosis may require biopsy samples of the liver, intestines and pancreas. Affected birds from both pet and aviary situations seem to be isolated cases, within a collection. Affected birds may demonstrate the presence of these acid-fast organisms in addition to iron storage disease on post-mortem or hepatic biopsies.

Miscellaneous conditions observed in ramphastids

Several other conditions have been observed in ramphastids with varying degrees of frequency.

Tongue damage involving the distal end of the tongue is occasionally noticed in toucans. It is assumed to be traumatic in nature. Affected birds have managed well without the presence of the distal tongue. Distal amputation can be performed if deemed necessary.

Foreign body ingestion: objects that have fallen into or been left in a bird's aviary may be ingested, with resulting 'hardware disease'. Affected birds may be presented for post-mortem examination, with discovery on the gross examination of ingestion and subsequent perforation into the coelomic cavity. Foreign bodies such as nails, wire and tacks have been identified.

Mate aggression occasionally occurs, with a male violently attacking the female in an aviary situation. Aggressive males should be removed from the present female as severe trauma and death may occur.

Articular gout that is severe, debilitating and affecting multiple joints in the body has been seen in young hand-fed toucanettes. **Affected birds diagnosed with articular gout have not done well due to the rapidly progressive and painful nature of the condition, and euthanasia is a viable options in these individuals.**

Propylene glycol sensitivity is suspected to occur in keel bill toucans. Affected birds were exposed to propylene glycol through ingestion of their formulated pelleted diet or when used as a vehicle for suspension of compounds, such as ivermectin. Even though other species of toucans were exposed to these situations, only the keel bills were affected, thus suggesting a possible species-specific sensitivity to the ingestion of propylene glycol. Hence, the use of propylene glycol in keel bills should be avoided (Worell 2000).

References

Charlton B R, Barr B C, Castro A E et al 1990 Herpes viral hepatitis in a toucan. Avian Diseases 34(3):787–790

Cornelissen H, Ritchie B W 1994 Rhamphastidae. In: Ritchie B, Harrison G, Harrison L (eds) Avian medicine: principles and application. Wingers, Lake Worth, FL, p 1276–1283

Cornelissen H, Ducatelle R, Roels S 1995 Successful treatment of a channel-billed toucan (*Ramphastos vitellinus*) with iron storage disease by chelation therapy; sequential monitoring of the iron content of the liver during the treatment period by quantitative chemical and image analyses. Journal of Avian Medicine and Surgery 9(2):131–137

Crissey S D, Ward A M, Block S E et al 2000 Hepatic iron accumulation over time in European starlings (*Sturnus vulgaris*) fed two levels of iron. Journal of Zoo and Wildlife Medicine 31(4):491–496

Dambro M R (ed) 1996 Griffith's five minute clinical consult. Williams & Wilkins, Baltimore, MD

Dhillon A S, Shafer D 1987 *Yersinia pseudotuberculosis* infection in two Toco toucans and a turaco. In: Proceedings of the 1st International Conference of Zoo and Avian Medicine. American Association of Zoological Veterinarians, p 37–38

Drews A V, Redrobe S P, Patterson-Kane J C 2004 Successful reduction of hepatocellular hemosidein content by dietary modification in toco toucans (*Ramphastos toco*) with iron-storage disease. Journal of Avian Medicine and Surgery 18(2):101–105

Farina L L, Heard D J, Leblanc D M et al 2005 Iron storage disease in captive Egyptian fruit bats (*Rousettus aegyptiacus*): relationship of blood iron parameters to hepatic iron concentrations and hepatic histopathology. Journal of Zoo and Wildlife Medicine 36(2):212–221

Grimes L G 1985 Toucans, honeyguides and boubets. In: Perrins E M, Middleton A L A (eds) The encyclopaedia of birds. Facts on File Inc, p 286–290

Kaltwasser J P, Werner E, Schalk K et al 1998 Clinical trial on the effect of regular tea drinking on iron accumulation in genetic haemochromatosis. Gut 43:699–704

Kincaid A, Stoskopf M 1997 Passerine dietary iron overload syndrome. Zoo Biology 6:79–88

Murphy J 1992 Diabetes in toucans. In: Annual Proceedings of the AAV, New Orleans. Association of Avian Veterinarians, p 253–262

Oglesbee B 1997 Diseases of the endocrine system. In: Altman R B, Clubb S L, Dorrestein G M, Quesenberry K E (eds) Avian medicine and surgery. W B Saunders, ,Philadelphia, PA, p 482–488

Olsen G P, Russell K E, Phalen D N 2005 Estimation of avian nonheme iron concentrations by cytologic and image analysis. In: Annual Proceedings AA, Monterey. Association of Avian Veterinarians, p 45–47

Olsen G P, Russell K E, Dierenfeld E et al 2006a Impact of supplements on iron absorption from diets containing high and low iron concentrations in the European starling (*Sturnus vulgaris*). Journal of Avian Medicine and Surgery 20(2):67–73

Olsen G P, Russell K E, Dierenfeld E, Phalen D N 2006b A comparison of four regimens for treatment of iron storage disease using the

European starling (*Sturnus vulgaris*) as a model. Journal of Avian Medicine and Surgery 20(2):74–79

Otten B A, Orosz S E, Auge S et al 2001 Mineral content of food items commonly ingested by keel-billed toucans (*Ramphastos sulfuratus*). Journal of Avian Medicine and Surgery 15(3):194–196

Paul-Murphy J, Maatheson J, O'Brien R et al 2003 Quantitative ultrasound analysis and magnetic resonance image analysis of iron accumulation in the liver of birds. In: Annual Proceedings, AAV, Pittsburgh. Association of Avian Veterinarians, p 137–139

Sheppard C, Dierenfield E 2002 Iron storage disease in birds: speculation on etiology and implications for captive husbandry. Journal of Avian Medicine and Surgery 16(3):192–197

Smith S A, Smith B J 1992 Atlas of avian radiographic anatomy. W B Saunders, Philadelphia, PA, p 77–81

Whiteside D P, Barker I K, Mehren K G et al 2004 Clinical evaluation of the oral iron chelator deferiprone for the potential treatment of iron overload in bird species. Journal of Zoo and Wildlife Medicine 35(1):40–49

Worell A B 1988 Management and medicine of toucans. In: Annual Proceedings, AAV, Houston. Association of Avian Veterinarians, p 253–262

Worell A B 1991a Serum iron levels in ramphastids. In: Annual Proceedings, AAV, Chicago. Association of Avian Veterinarians, p 120–130

Worell A B 1991b Phlebotomy for treatment of hemachromatosis in two sulfur-breasted toucans. In: Annual Proceedings, AAV, Chicago. Association of Avian Veterinarians, p 9–14

Worell A B 1993 Further investigations in ramphastids concerning hemachromatosis. In: Annual Proceedings, AAV, Nashville. Association of Avian Veterinarians, p 98–107

Worell A B 1996 Medicine and surgery of toucans. In: Rosskopf W J, Woerpel R W (eds) Disease of cage and aviary birds, 3rd edn. Williams & Wilkins, Baltimore, MD, p 933–943

Worell A B 1997 Toucans and mynahs. In: Altman R B, Clubb S L, Dorrestein G M, Quesenberry K E (eds) Avian medicine and surgery. W B Saunders, Philadelphia, PA, p 910–917

Worell A B 2000 Suspected propylene glycol sensitivity in keel-billed toucans. In: Annual Proceedings, AAV, Portland. Association of Avian Veterinarians, p 199–203

Pigeons

15

Peter De Herdt and Frank Pasmans

Introduction

Among the many representatives of the Columbiformes, the rock dove *Columba livia* is the most universally kept by humans on all continents. A large variety of breeds have been developed, the most famous of which, the homing pigeon, is used in races. This chapter is intended mainly for use with racing pigeons, but most of the data presented are easily applicable to other breeds.

The objective of homing pigeon fanciers is to achieve good results with their birds in competition races. What counts is the overall performance of the group rather than that of the individual pigeon, and consequently, pigeon fanciers are especially concerned about the overall health of their pigeon flock and less so about individual pigeons. For this reason, pigeon medicine focuses on infectious diseases. It is impossible to discuss all infectious pigeon diseases in this chapter, so the most important ones have been selected. The section devoted to non-infectious pigeon diseases includes only those conditions specific to pigeons, as most non-infectious diseases of pigeons are similar to those seen in other birds and referral can therefore be made to the relevant chapters dealing with these problems.

This chapter approaches the different pigeon diseases in a practical manner; nevertheless, data that may help with comprehension are included.

Handling pigeons

Pigeons are easy to handle with practice. **There is one golden rule: the bird should always be held in the hand with its chest facing the handler** (Fig. 15.1), otherwise it will invariably try to escape if the hand grip is loosened even slightly. The sternum of the pigeon rests in the palm of the hand and the thumb is placed over the tail base and the wing tips. The legs are held with the free hand between the index and the middle finger of the hand that is holding the bird.

Anatomy

As in other birds, but not mammals, the oesophagus is situated at the right side of the trachea. The narrow part is short and widens into the crop, which has a special function in pigeons. The so-called crop milk consists of rapidly desquamating crop cells (Fig. 15.2). **During the time that squabs are fed with this substance, the crop surface appears as if covered with cooked rice and the mucosa is heavily congested. This should not**

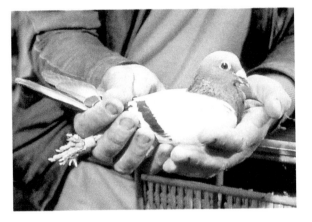

Fig 15.1 The proper restraint technique for a pigeon.

be mistaken for a pathological condition such as crop candidiasis.

The gizzard contains many stony particles. When palpating the abdomen, it should not be confused with an egg.

Although pigeons do not have a gall bladder, bile is abundantly produced. **When pigeons do not eat, the production of faeces diminishes but bile continues to be produced, resulting in slimy green droppings.** This is not a pathological condition in itself, but it may indirectly indicate clinical disease-related inappetence. Normal intestinal peristalsis also flushes bile into the stomach, resulting in a strong green aspect of the koilin layer of the gizzard.

When examining pigeon droppings, it should be remembered that urine is excreted together with faeces. **Fluid urine is generally not visible in pigeons' droppings but becomes apparent in cases of polyuria. This is often interpreted by pigeon fanciers as diarrhoea, but is in fact polyuria. Inappetent diseased pigeons defecate almost exclusively fluid urine, with one or two small flakes of greenish faecal matter. This may also be erro**neously interpreted as a sign of enteritis. Non-infectious factors such as nervousness or vitamin D_3 overdose may also lead to polyuria.

Examination procedures

The clinical examination of pigeons requires a thorough inspection and palpation from beak to cloaca, as described in the general introduction section. Additionally,

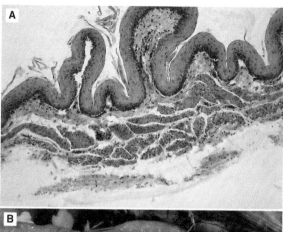

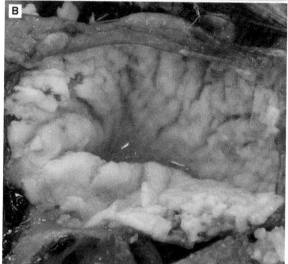

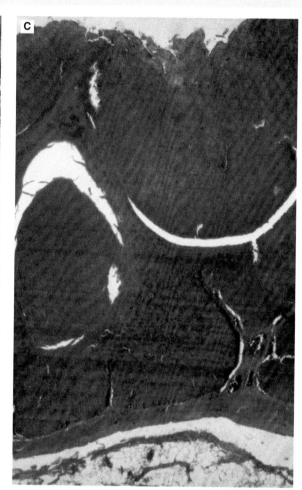

Fig 15.2 Crop lining of pigeons producing crop milk. **A** Normal crop epithelium, haematoxylin & eosin. **B** Crop producing crop milk. **C** Thickened crop epithelium, haematoxylin & eosin.

the direct microscopic examination of crop swab samples and of pooled faecal samples to detect the presence of *Trichomonas* sp. and worm eggs, respectively, should be part of the routine clinical examination procedure.

Swab samples can furthermore be taken with relative ease from the nose, the conjunctiva, the trachea and the cloaca (Figs 15.3, 15.4). Smears from these samples can be examined cytologically and in this way contribute to the diagnosis of respiratory and intestinal diseases. Of course the swabs can also be processed for bacteriological and virological examinations if necessary.

Blood can be easily collected from the metatarsal vein. Blood biochemistry reference values are given in Table 15.1. Serology can be used to monitor the serological paramyxovirus status and for the diagnosis of salmonellosis (see below).

The diagnostic value of faecal bacteriological examination for the presence of *Salmonella* can be enhanced considerably when droppings from several birds per loft and collected during a 5-day period are pooled.

It should be mentioned that the veterinary approach applied in pigeon medicine differs slightly from that in other companion birds. The maintenance of flock health to ensure optimal performance often implies the sacrifice of a live pigeon for post-mortem examination. Therefore, necropsy is a vital part of pigeon medicine. To avoid post-mortem bacterial contamination and loss of parasite viability (rendering the diagnosis of e.g. hexamitiasis and trichomoniasis more difficult), the necropsy should ideally be performed within 2 hours of the time of death.

Infectious diseases

The most common infectious diseases will be presented in a classical way: aetiology, epidemiology, pathogenesis, clinical signs and lesions, diagnosis, and control. The diseases to be discussed are viral infections (paramyxovirosis, adenovirus infections, herpesvirus infections, pox virus infections, circovirosis and avian influenza), bacterial infections (salmonellosis, streptococcosis, *Escherichia coli* septicaemia, and ornithosis (*Chlamydophila psittaci*)

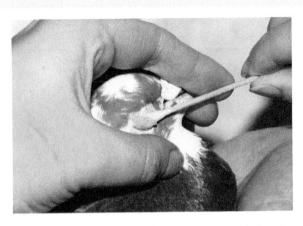

Fig 15.3 Conjunctiva swab. Cytological examination of samples from the conjunctiva may reveal *Chlamydophila* infection.

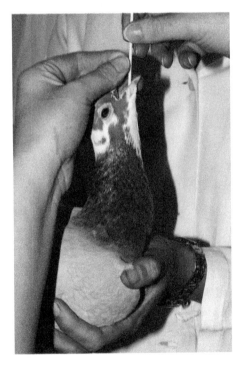

Fig 15.4 Ingluvium swab. A crop sample, examined for the presence of *Trichomonas*, is part of the routine examination of pigeons.

and respiratory disease) and the most common parasitic infections (trichomoniasis, hexamitiasis, coccidiosis, worm infestations, and ectoparasite infestations).

Viral infections

Paramyxovirosis

Aetiology

Paramyxovirosis in pigeons is caused by a serotype 1 paramyxovirus (PMV1). Pigeon PMV1 strains in most cases can be distinguished on a molecular basis from

PMV1 strains causing Newcastle disease in poultry (Alexander et al 1985, Aldous et al 2004). The virus can easily be cultivated in the allantoic sac of embryonated chicken eggs.

Epidemiology

In western Europe, paramyxovirus infections in pigeons typically occur in the late summer and autumn, predominantly from August to November. The prevalence of clinical paramyxovirosis is easily influenced by vaccination. Well-vaccinated pigeons hardly ever develop clinical disease.

Pathogenesis

The pathogenesis of paramyxovirosis in pigeons has not been thoroughly studied. Pigeons are probably infected aerogenically or orally, as in poultry (Alexander 1991). In pigeons, the viruses typically spread to the kidneys and/or the central nervous system. Following viral replication in the kidneys an interstitial nephritis arises, resulting in a diminished blood flow through the mammalian-type (medullary) nephrons and an augmented blood flow through the reptilian-type nephrons. The reptilian-type (cortical) nephrons of birds are unable to absorb water efficiently because they lack the loops of Henle. Because of this, multiplication of paramyxovirus in the pigeon kidneys results in polyuria and subsequent polydipsia. Replication of paramyxovirus in the central nervous system often leads to demyelination and perivasculitis. These lesions can be associated with central nervous disorders. The incubation period of the pigeon paramyxovirus infection is between 5 and 35 days (Viaene et al 1983).

Clinical sig ns a nd l esions

The clinical signs resulting from paramyxovirosis in pigeons seem to have evolved over the years.

Between 1983 and 1986, at the beginning of the pandemic spread of this disease, central nervous disorders were the main clinical expression of paramyxovirosis (Viaene et al 1983). These signs consist of torticollis, incoordination of head movements, trembling wings and complete or partial paralysis (Fig. 15.5). After 1 week there may already be spontaneous clinical improvement of the birds, and approximately 70% of pigeons recover completely. Lesions in affected animals consist of a non-suppurative encephalitis with perivasculitis and demyelination.

From the late 1980s onwards, nervous signs were observed far less frequently. Instead signs and lesions related to viral replication in the kidneys became prominent. At autopsy of infected pigeons, macroscopic kidney lesions can hardly be seen. Histologically, however, an interstitial nephritis is evident, which in the subacute phase evolves to cause destruction of tubular epithelium and diffuse infiltration of lymphocytes. Due to these lesions, polyuria and polydipsia will develop.

Table 15.1 Reference values for plasma biochemistry and packed cell volume (PCV) in pigeons (Vereecken et al 2001)

	Units	Average	Lower limit	Upper limit
Albumin	g/L	11	6	15
Albumin : globulin ratio		0.51	0.27	0.70
Ammonia	μmol/L	11	3	52
Cholesterol	mmol/L	7	5.4	9.8
Creatinine	μmol/L	11	0	20
Globulin	g/L	22	18	29
Glucose	mmol/L	17	12	22
Total bilirubin	μmol/L	2.2	0	9
Total protein	g/L	33	24	41
Triglycerides	mmol/L	2.1	1.2	3.7
Urea nitrogen	mmol/L	0.9	0.77	1.63
Uric acid	μmol/L	336	191	663
AST	IU/L	79	17	191
ALT	IU/L	15	11	22
Amylase	IU/L	645	384	994
AP	IU/L	292	64	1160
CK	IU/L	349	166	629
gGT	IU/L	0	0	1
LDH	IU/L	217	133	321
Lipase	IU/L	39	6	73
Sodium	mmol/L	144	128	166
Potassium	mmol/L	4.07	3.03	5.00
Chloride	mmol/L	116	106	135
Calcium	mmol/L	2.12	1.76	2.87
Inorganic phosphate	mmol/L	1.63	0.42	2.33
PCV	%	52	43	63

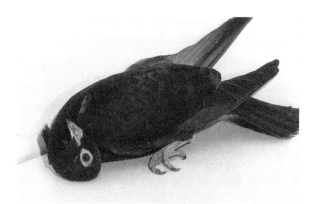

Fig 15.5 Pigeon exhibiting torticollis due to a paramyxovirus infection.

These clinical signs spread to the entire population within a few days. Polyuria and polydipsia can last for 6–8 weeks. Pigeons that are not cured within that period often suffer from irreversible lesions and show polyuria for the rest of their life. **Notwithstanding the extreme polyuria, the general condition of the pigeons remains well, and they show no or only slight weight loss.** Indeed, the intestinal tract keeps its normal absorption capacity because of the absence of lesions. Furthermore, the uric acid concentration in the blood is normal since the glomeruli and the proximal tubules are intact. Morbidity in this type of disease is usually 100%. Mortality, on the other hand, is usually less than 5%. This 5% comprises pigeons that became unable to eat or drink due to nervous disorders.

In the late 1990s the clinical features of the disease appeared to change once again. Indeed since then pigeons with paramyxovirosis have been developing gastrointestinal symptoms with vomiting (regurgitation) and diarrhoea. The mortality may be as high as 50% in some severe cases. Pigeons may be found dead without previous symptoms (mainly but not exclusively in nestlings) or after an episode of vomiting and/or diarrhoea.

When paramyxovirosis occurs during moult, the growth of replacement feathers may be interrupted and, when growth is initiated again, an indentation in the vane may remain. The younger part of the feather will grow to its normal size while the older part often breaks off.

Except for birds with irreversible brain lesions, most pigeons resume their previous racing performances after an outbreak of paramyxovirosis. Chronic polyuria does not influence racing results except during hot weather, when it results in rapid dehydration of affected pigeons. Pigeons with chronic lesions can be used for breeding without adverse effects.

Finally, it must be noted that pigeons suffering from paramyxovirosis develop little or no respiratory distress. This is clearly different to paramyxovirosis (NCD) in poultry.

Diagnosis

Torticollis as well as polyuria and polydipsia in the absence of weight loss are very indicative signs for paramyxovirosis. It may be important to distinguish between polyuria and diarrhoea; lay people often fail to make this distinction. Weight loss, diarrhoea and vomiting are less typical and might as well be ascribed to other infectious diseases such as adenovirosis, salmonellosis or hexamitiasis.

Serology, using haemagglutination inhibition (HI) of paramyxovirus with pigeon sera, can be used as a diagnostic tool (Viaene et al 1983). The test can be performed using homologous pigeon paramyxovirus and/or heterologous chicken La Sota paramyxovirus as an antigen. For a reliable serological diagnosis paired sera of multiple pigeons should be tested. Veterinary practitioners, however, often try to interpret serological results on the basis of single samplings. High titres found in unvaccinated pigeons can give a good indication of a paramyxovirus infection. The interpretation of single serological samples might be hampered by vaccination titres. After a single vaccination antibody titres are usually low or even absent. Repeated vaccinations lead to higher titres. It should be kept in mind, however, that paramyxovirosis almost never occurs in well-vaccinated pigeons, suggesting that the interpretation of titres of well-vaccinated birds mostly is of little practical importance.

Histological lesions in the kidneys and the brains can also be indicative for paramyxovirosis. However, the kidney lesions are not pathognomonic and non-suppurative encephalitis is not always present.

Pigeon paramyxovirus furthermore can easily be isolated in embryonated chicken eggs or in cell culture.

Control

Pigeons suffering from paramyxovirosis can be supplemented with vitamins and essential amino acids or fed with a low protein diet in order to relieve the function of the kidneys. Antimicrobials, electrolytes and glucose might be an aid in pigeons showing diarrhoea and vomiting. However, a therapy directed against the aetiological agent is not available.

Preventive vaccination against paramyxovirosis is advisable. Both inactivated and live vaccines are available and even legally required in many countries. Best results are obtained with inactivated adjuvanted vaccines, containing either a pigeon paramyxovirus strain or a poultry La Sota strain (Viaene et al 1983, Duchatel & Vindevogel 1986). Homologous vaccines induce the strongest protection (Knoll et al 1986). Pigeons can be subcutaneously injected with the vaccines from the age of 5–6 weeks. If possible, they should be vaccinated during the late winter or early spring. Protective immunity develops between 1 and 3 weeks after vaccination. After a year, pigeons should be revaccinated. In the past (when inactivated vaccines were not yet available), live La Sota vaccine of poultry was advised for the vaccination of pigeons (Viaene et al 1983). Recently, however, this practice has been discouraged, since only weak immunity is obtained and vaccine breaks occur very frequently unless the pigeons are vaccinated repeatedly at 4-week intervals. La Sota vaccine can be administered via eye and nose drops or drinking water. For the eye and nose drop method, 1000 La Sota vaccine doses should be suspended in 50 mL water and one drop of the resulting suspension administered into each nostril and each eye. For the drinking water method, 1000 La Sota vaccine doses should be suspended in 1–10 L of a 9:1 ratio of distilled water and skimmed milk. Vaccine-supplemented water should be consumed completely within 2 hours; therefore, drinking water should be withheld for 12 hours before administration of the vaccine.

Adenovirus infections

Adenoviruses are responsible for two clinical disease entities in pigeons; adenovirosis type I and adenovirosis type II (De Herdt et al 1995a). The postscripts I and II refer to the clinical signs and lesions caused by these adenoviruses, and not to the antigenic nature of the agents. Both types of adenovirus infections have a large impact on pigeon populations. The aetiological agents of adenovirosis type I and II in pigeons are adenoviruses, as determined by electron microscopy, and the isolation of adenoviruses from pigeons has occasionally been described (McFerran et al 1976a, Hess et al 1996). In these reports it is not always clear how the agents were cultivated, and/or if the isolation concerned adenoviruses causing type I or type II disease. Furthermore, it is not known to which antigenic type(s) adenovirus type I and II agents belong. Isolates belonging to the fowl adenovirus (FAV) types 2, 5, 6, 8, 10 and 12 have been described but other isolates could not be classified (Hess et al 1996). To date, the distinction between the two agents and disease entities is based mainly on disease course, epidemiology in Europe and histological lesions.

Adenovirosis type I

Epidemiology

Adenovirosis type I, first diagnosed in the 1970s (McFerran et al 1976b), occurs worldwide in pigeons younger than 1 year. Pigeons over 1 year old are not affected (Coussement et al 1984). **In western European countries, the disease has a typical seasonal appearance from March to July**, peaking in frequency in June (Uyttebroek & Ducatelle 1991) In the second half of the year, only sporadic cases are noted.

Pathogenesis

To date, the pathogenesis of adenovirus type I infections has not been studied sufficiently. Most outbreaks of adenovirosis type I occur after the initial races of the young pigeons (Coussement et al 1984, Uyttebroek & Ducatelle 1991), and it is supposed that these pigeons are orally infected with adenoviruses by cross-contamination in the common baskets. The viruses replicate in the nucleus of epithelial cells of the intestinal tract, resulting in severe intestinal damage. As a result, proteins and ions are lost via the intestinal tract. This alteration of the intestinal environment often leads to mass multiplication of facultative pathogenic agents that are part of the normal intestinal flora, predominantly *E. coli*, and these bacteria may aggravate the intestinal lesions and even cause septicaemia. Viruses are spread via the droppings, thereby infecting all other young pigeons in the loft within a period of 4–5 days. Morbidity is generally very high, 100% of the pigeons being infected within a few days, but mortality is generally low. **It is remarkable that only pigeons less than 1 year of age develop clinical signs, while older pigeons remain clinically healthy.** This may indicate age-related resistance or a strong acquired immunity in these animals. The adenoviruses may spread from the intestinal tract to the internal organs, predominantly the liver, where replication will also take place.

Clinicalsig nsa ndl esions

Macroscopically, adenovirosis type I lesions are characterized by catarrhal enteritis in young pigeons.

Histologically, there is an atrophy of the villi and intranuclear inclusion bodies can be observed in the epithelial cells of the small intestine. Pigeons suffering from such lesions show poor general condition, watery diarrhoea, vomiting and weight loss. These clinical signs usually disappear within 1 week, since the adenoviruses are apparently eliminated very quickly, and the epithelium of the intestinal tract regenerates within a few days. Secondary *E. coli* infections may, however, lead to a more severe and prolonged disease. In such complicated cases, pigeons suffer from a green and foul diarrhoea, emaciation and severe weakening, eventually resulting in death. Furthermore, some pigeons die peracutely from *E. coli* septicaemia.

After the recovery of diseased pigeons, racing performances remain low for several weeks. This may be due to slowly healing liver lesions following multiplication of adenoviruses in the hepatocytes. During this hepatic replication phase intranuclear inclusion bodies are formed with degenerative lesions. Affected pigeons will therefore acquire less racing experience and may drop behind non-infected contestants.

Diagnosis

In most cases, adenovirosis type I can be strongly suspected on a clinical basis: sudden appearance in the entire group; typical signs of diarrhoea and vomiting; young pigeons only affected; and a typical seasonal appearance. However, the disease should not be confused with paramyxovirosis, salmonellosis or hexamitiasis, and these three diseases should be excluded and/or the adenovirus infection itself demonstrated. The definite diagnosis of adenovirus type I can be made by the demonstration of intranuclear inclusion bodies in the liver or in the intestinal epithelium using histology and/or cytology (Fig. 15.6). Hepatic inclusion bodies are

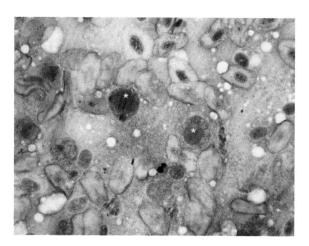

Fig 15.6 Cytology of the liver showing adenovirus intranuclear inclusion bodies (*) Hemacolor © stain 100×.

usually numerous and large, and extensive necrosis is not present (Coussement et al 1984). These criteria can be used to differentiate adenovirosis type I from type II histopathologically. Alternatively for at least some of the strains, PCR can be applied to demonstrate the presence of adenoviral DNA in organs (Raue et al 2002).

Control

No preventive vaccines or therapeutic drugs are available at the moment. However, clinical improvement can be obtained by rehydration of affected pigeons and the control of complicating bacterial infections. In the authors' experience, spectacular results can be obtained in most cases by the administration of 200 mg trimethoprim, 100 mg ronidazole and 20 g glucose per litre of drinking water for 5 days. An antibiogram of complicating bacteria can be useful when pigeons do not respond to this treatment.

Adenovirosis type II

Epidemiology

Adenovirosis type II was first recognized in Belgium in October 1992 (De Herdt et al 1995a). Later, the disease was diagnosed not only among the Belgian pigeon population but also in pigeons originating from neighbouring countries. Seasonal variations in the prevalence of the disease are not seen, strongly contrasting with the situation in adenovirosis type I.

Pathogenesis

Only very few data on the pathogenesis of adenovirus type II infections are available. The viral agent is able to induce extensive hepatic necrosis, which may result in sudden death of the pigeons. *E. coli* secondarily invades the liver and other internal organs in approximately 15% of cases (De Herdt et al 1995a), and *Staphylococcus intermedius* and *Streptococcus gallolyticus* are occasionally observed as a complicating factor in adenovirosis type II. However, the authors believe that these secondary bacterial infections do not essentially influence the course of the disease.

Clinicalsig nsa ndl esions

The disease in pigeons suffering from adenovirosis type II always follows a characteristic course (De Herdt et al 1995a). Clinical signs are always minimal, since all affected pigeons die within 24–48 hours. The only clinical signs occasionally seen are vomiting and production of yellow, liquid droppings (Fig. 15.7). Sudden deaths can continue for 6 weeks, with new cases occurring intermittently. Mortality in affected pigeon lofts is usually about 30%, but in some cases amounts to 100%. It is remarkable that in colonies where acute deaths due to adenovirosis type II occur, pigeons that do not die

remain completely normal and show no clinical signs. Sometimes nestlings even grow up completely normally (provided they are already able to feed themselves or are raised by other pigeons) after one or both of their parents have died of the disease. Adenovirosis type II has been observed in pigeons between 10 days and 6 years of age. No correlation exists between the occurrence of the disease and the pigeons' physiological condition, sex or obvious stressing factors.

The most typical necropsy finding in pigeons that have died from adenovirosis type II is a yellow, pale and swollen liver with a red sheen. Histological and cytological examination of such livers reveals extensive focal or diffuse hepatic necrosis and eosinophilic or amphophilic intranuclear inclusion bodies.

Diagnosis

Adenovirosis type II can be suspected from the owner's complaint of acute deaths in pigeons of all ages without premonitory signs except for occasional short-term vomiting and diarrhoea. Adenovirosis type II does of course have to be differentiated from other causes of sudden death, such as intoxication, streptococcosis, *E. coli* septicaemia and salmonellosis. The ultimate

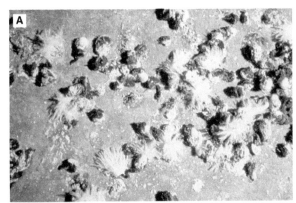

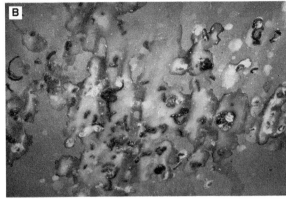

Fig 15.7 A Normal droppings of a pigeon. **B** Yellow regurgitant and droppings due to an adenovirus infection.

diagnosis can be made at necropsy on the basis of the typical macroscopic aspects of the liver, and extensive hepatic necrosis with intranuclear inclusion bodies at histological or cytological examination. These inclusion bodies are less numerous and smaller than in adenovirosis type I (De Herdt et al 1995a).

Control

Neither preventive nor curative measures are available for the control of adenovirosis type II in pigeons. The administration of antibiotics is useless; pigeons do not die from secondary bacterial infections, but from the extensive hepatic necrosis induced by the virus. The use of glucocorticoids must be discouraged since it has been proven experimentally that pigeons become more susceptible to the disease following administration of these products. Pigeon fanciers dealing with an outbreak of adenovirosis type II should always be advised to maintain excellent hygienic conditions within the loft combined with good ventilation, in order to keep infection pressure as low as possible.

Herpesvirus infections
Aetiology

Pigeon herpesviruses all belong to the same antigenic type (PHV1) (Vindevogel et al 1980). They are antigenically different from psittacine herpes types or herpesviruses from other animals. PHV1 can be isolated in chicken embryo fibroblast cell cultures or in embryonated chicken eggs.

Epidemiology

In the past more than 50% of racing pigeons possessed antibodies against PHV1 (Vindevogel et al 1981), and this usually indicates latent infections. **Clinical disease occurs rather seldom and the demonstration of herpesviruses combined with herpesvirus-associated lesions is very low.** A German study (Holz 1992) demonstrated that up to 60% of pigeon transport baskets may be positive for herpesvirus.

Pathogenesis

The majority of the pigeon population is latently infected with herpesviruses. These birds may intermittently shed the agents, especially when under stress. Stressing factors that contribute to virus excretion are breeding and transport conditions of high temperature and high occupation density. Squabs with maternal antibodies do not usually develop clinical disease following a herpesvirus infection, but they become latently infected for the rest of their lives. Clinical herpesvirus infections predominantly prevail in squabs from uninfected parents and in immunosuppressed pigeons. Herpesvirus may cause systemic disease between 2 and 10 weeks of age, while in older pigeons the agents may play a (minor) role in problems of coryza. Possibly, immune suppression caused by circovirus infection might predispose to a clinical herpesvirus infection.

Clinical signs and lesions

Systemic herpesvirus infections in nestlings cause acute deaths without clinical signs (Vindevogel et al 1975). In affected animals, the liver is enlarged and shows focal necrosis. Histologically, intranuclear herpes-type inclusion bodies are found in the hepatocytes surrounding necrotic areas (Vindevogel & Pastoret 1981). Necrosis may also be present in the spleen. The herpes-type inclusion bodies are smaller and less numerous than adenovirus inclusions.

The role of herpesviruses in outbreaks of coryza is discussed elsewhere in this chapter. Pigeons with respiratory herpesvirus infections may develop diphtheric inflammation of the larynx, oesophagus and trachea (Vindevogel & Duchatel 1978) (Fig. 15.8). Nuclear inclusion bodies can also be observed in these lesions.

Diagnosis

Herpesvirus infections can be diagnosed through isolation of the agents from lesions or through the demonstration of nuclear inclusion bodies. Herpesvirus as a cause of acute death in nestlings must be differentiated from other infectious agents that may cause similar problems, such as paramyxovirus, *Salmonella*, *Streptococcus gallolyticus*, *E. coli*, *Trichomonas* spp. and *Hexamita* spp.

Diphtheric lesions in the mouth may also originate from infections with pox viruses, *Trichomonas* spp. and *Candida albicans*. Furthermore, they should be differentiated from sialoliths, which are white

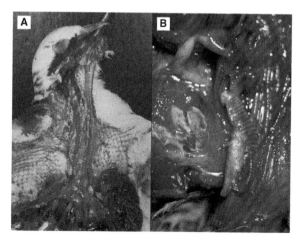

Fig 15.8 Diphtheritic membrane of the crop, larynx and trachea due to herpesvirus infection. **A** Crop. **B** Larynx and trachea.

concretions that may occur at the back of the pharynx. These plugs originate in the fundus of the salivary glands, and their aetiology and significance are unknown. Racing performances of pigeons presenting sialoliths are often poor.

Control

No preventive or curative control measures against herpesvirus infections in pigeons are available to date.

Pox virus infections

Aetiology

Two different types of clinical pox virus infections are known in pigeons. The first type is the 'typical' pox virus infection (Tripathy 1991), while the second type is 'atypical' pox or 'blood pox' infection (Hartig & Frese 1973). Viruses that cause the two diseases are probably unrelated. The typical virus is host-specific and has common antigens with fowl pox viruses. This agent can be cultivated on the chorio-allantoic membrane of embryonated chicken eggs. Isolation of atypical pox viruses has not been described. The pox virus aetiology of atypical pox disease has been demonstrated by electron microscopy.

Epidemiology

The occurrence of typical pox virus infections in pigeons is strictly correlated with the availability of vectors responsible for the transmission of the disease. Therefore, these infections may have a typical distribution in time and space. Under moderate climatic circumstances, typical pox virus infections prevail in late summer and autumn because of the large numbers of vector mosquitoes occurring at that time. Clinical outbreaks predominantly occur in young pigeons. Spread of the disease is usually very slow, and may take several weeks. **Atypical pox occurs very sporadically and, in contrast with typical pox, only one or a few pigeons in the loft are affected.** These birds are usually less than 2 years old.

Pathogenesis

Typical pox virus infections in pigeons are initiated when the aetiological agents are inoculated in skin defects (Eleazer et al 1983). After an incubation period of 10–20 days, viral replication will lead to typical epithelial pox lesions. From this primary site of entry the virus may spread to internal organs and, through a secondary viraemia, reach distant parts of the skin as well as different mucosae. This will result in further dermal diphtheroid and mucosal lesions, respectively. The virus is shed predominantly through desquamation of infected epithelial cells. Transmission of pox virus occurs through direct contact with infected birds

(e.g. during fighting) or indirectly through stinging and blood-sucking parasites (such as mosquitoes, mites and ticks) that may act as vectors. In such vectors, the virus does not replicate but retains its infectivity for life. Besides spreading the virus, vectors are important for creating dermal defects. During non-lethal infections, pox lesions will spontaneously regress after 7–21 days, when immunity is built up. The pathogenesis of atypical pox in pigeons is unknown. Blood pox spontaneously shrivel and disappear without residual lesions after 3–4 weeks.

Clinical signs and lesions

Clinical manifestations of typical pox in pigeons are extremely characteristic. Traditionally, a more common cutaneous form and a less common diphtheroid form are distinguished. In the cutaneous form, lesions consist of hypertrophic proliferation of epithelium, predominantly around the beak and on the eyelids (Fig. 15.9). Swollen eyelids can inhibit the pigeon's vision and consequently the uptake of food, resulting in starvation. In the diphtheroid form, pseudomembranous lesions are found in the anterior part of the oral cavity (Fig. 15.10). These lesions may also lead to starvation when they interfere with food intake. Histologically, typical pox viruses induce hyperplasia and necrosis of epithelial cells (Tripathy 1991). At the border of necrotic foci, eosinophilic cytoplasmic inclusion bodies, the so-called Bollinger bodies, can be found (Fig. 15.11). Inclusion bodies become particularly evident in the epidermal cells during the subacute or chronic stages of the disease.

Atypical pox are wart-like lesions that are predominantly located on the body or wings of pigeons. Usually they are solitary lesions, but sometimes several of them are present. They grow until they measure 1–3 cm, and black, bloody contents glimmer through an intact skin. When these wart-like lesions are damaged they may bleed heavily, occasionally leading to death of the

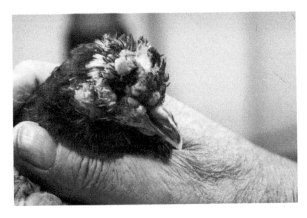

Fig 15.9 Typical cutaneous lesions associated with an avian pox virus infection.

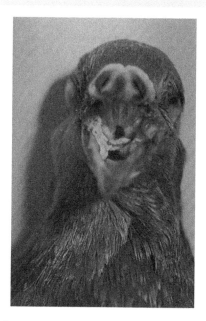

Fig 15.10 Oral diphtheritic membrane from an avian pox virus infection.

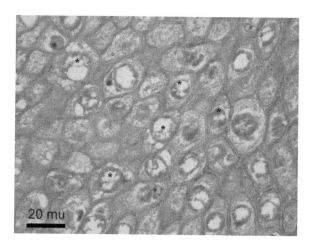

Fig 15.11 Intracytoplasmic inclusion bodies (*, Bollinger bodies)

pigeon. Pigeons with atypical pox are not visibly sick. Histologically, there is proliferation of the epithelium of the feather follicles or of the skin. The cells contain melanin and cytoplasmic inclusion bodies.

Diagnosis

Cutaneous and diphtheroid forms of typical pox as well as atypical pox can generally be diagnosed easily by the characteristic lesions. The clinical diagnosis can be confirmed by histological examination. Typical pox agents can also be isolated in embryonated chicken eggs. The diphtheroid form of typical pox must be differentiated

from trichomoniasis, candidiasis or herpesvirus infections. Atypical pox must be distinguished from melanomas.

Control

Typical pox virus infections can be prevented by vaccination with live, attenuated, homologous pigeon pox viruses. Vaccines can be administered from the age of 6 weeks, either by the feather follicle method or by subcutaneous injection. A strong protective immunity is induced within 2 weeks and lasts for at least 1 year. Vaccination can also be a useful measure during an outbreak; however, under such circumstances, care must be taken not to spread the infectious virus via the equipment used. Curative treatment of pigeons suffering from typical pox virus infections is not possible. Drugs can be used to prevent complicating infections with bacteria or *Trichomonas* spp. Forced feeding may be useful in valuable pigeons with severe beak or eyelid lesions.

Preventive vaccines or curative treatments against atypical pox in pigeons do not exist. In order to prevent mortality through bleeding of the lesions, affected pigeons are best kept in isolation until the pox lesions have fallen off. **For the same reason, no attempt should be made to remove the lesions surgically.**

Circovirosis

Aetiology

The pigeon circoviruses, together with e.g. psittacine beak and feather disease virus, canary and duck circoviruses, belong to the genus *Circovirus* in the family of the Circoviridae. These viruses are considered host specific.

Epidemiology

Circoviruses are probably widespread amongst pigeons. Clinical circovirus infections typically occur in pigeons less than 1 year of age.

Pathogenesis

The pathogenesis of circovirus infections in pigeons is not well studied. Until the age of 4 months pigeons appear to be most sensitive (Shivaprasad et al 1994). No seasonal or sex predilections have been observed. Transmission of the virus can occur both horizontally and vertically (Duchatel et al 2005, 2006). In young animals, lymphoid tissue such as the bursa and the thymus are affected but viral DNA has also been demonstrated in liver, kidney, brain, crop and intestine (Duchatel et al 2006). In older birds, the virus probably persists in the respiratory tract.

Clinical signs and lesions

In pigeons between 1 and 4 months of age, circovirus infections are associated with lethargy, weight loss, respiratory distress, diarrhoea and poor performance, a disease also known as 'young pigeon disease syndrome' (YPDS) (Duchatel et al 2005, Raue et al 2005). However, this syndrome should be considered a multifactorial disease. Indeed, in most cases, concurrent infections can be demonstrated with all possible viral, bacterial and parasitic agents hampering the assessment of the exact role of the circovirus. Tavernier et al (2000) were not able to demonstrate any clinical indications for the possible immunosuppressive effects of circovirus other than enhanced mortality in young pigeons. **Probably, most infections, especially in older birds, have a subclinical course.**

The most obvious lesion is a swollen, oedematous bursa in the acute phase of infection. However, more chronic infections result in atrophy of the bursa.

Histological lesions consist of lymphocyte depletion in lymphoid tissue and characteristic intracytoplasmic basophilic inclusion bodies (mainly in macrophages) in the lymphoid tissue.

Diagnosis

Circovirus infections can be diagnosed using histological examination of the bursa, showing the typical inclusion bodies. This diagnosis can be confirmed using electron microscopy or by PCR (Todd et al 2002).

Control

No vaccination exists today to prevent circovirosis in pigeons. The only thing that can be done is to control concurrent infections.

Avian influenza

Pigeons are officially listed as susceptible to avian influenza. Nevertheless, pigeons show a remarkably low susceptibility to avian influenza viruses. After infection with viruses belonging to the haemagglutinin subtypes H5 or H7, little or no virus replication, clinical symptoms and seroconversion are noted (Kaleta & Honicke 2004). Therefore, they probably do not play a role of significance in the spread of the H5 and H7 subtypes.

Bacterial infections

Salmonellosis

Aetiology

In pigeons, salmonellosis means infection with pigeon-specific pathogenic *Salmonella* strains, notably *Salmonella enterica* subspecies *enterica* serovar Typhimurium variant Copenhagen phage types 2 and 99 (*Salmonella* Typhimurium; Pohl et al 1983, Pasmans et al 2004), which is a Gram-negative, facultative intracellular bacterium belonging to the family Enterobacteriaceae. These phage types can be considered host-restricted (Pasmans et al 2003).

The bacteria can be cultured from internal organs on non-selective Columbia agar with 5% bovine blood, or from intestines or faeces on selective agars such as Brilliant Green agar. Enrichment media for the selective isolation of *Salmonella* from contaminated materials are also available, e.g. tetrathionate broth.

Epidemiology

Salmonella Typhimurium (together with *Streptococcus gallolyticus*) is the most important bacterial disease in pigeons. Feral pigeons constitute a source of infection. Infected pigeons often are not able to eliminate the bacterium, resulting in long-term carriers that excrete the bacterium intermittently with the faeces. Although infections of humans with pigeon-associated *Salmonella* strains are rare, these strains are able to cause severe disease in mice (Pasmans et al 2004).

Pathogenesis

Pigeons suffering from salmonellosis excrete the bacteria in the droppings, thereby effecting horizontal spread of the disease. Pigeons are infected by oral uptake of the agent from contaminated food, drinking water, baskets, etc. *Salmonella* first colonizes the pigeon's intestinal tract, and from this primary site of replication often invades the bloodstream, causing bacteraemia. During haematogenic spread the bacteria reach different parts of the body, such as the lungs, liver, spleen, testis, ovary, brains, muscles, eyes, skin and joints, where they also multiply. Localization of *Salmonella* in the gonads, as well as eggshell contamination, may eventually cause vertical spread of the disease.

Pigeons can clinically recover from a *Salmonella* infection, either spontaneously or following antibiotic treatment. Some of these pigeons, however, do not manage to eliminate all the bacteria, and become asymptomatic carriers. *Salmonella* bacteria may survive inside different cell types, such as macrophages, or within necrotic lesions. Carriers play an important role in the pathogenesis of pigeon salmonellosis, since they intermittently shed the bacteria and thereby infect other pigeons. Because of this, salmonellosis is often chronically present in pigeon lofts.

Replication of *Salmonella* generally induces lesions and clinical signs, but lesions may also arise in the absence of bacteria. Typical in this respect is an extreme swelling of the elbow joint that may develop months to years after the bacteria were eliminated from the loft. The pathogenesis of this type of lesion is unknown. Fluid obtained from such elbows often contains large amounts of antibodies against *Salmonella*.

Clinical signs and lesions

The ability of *Salmonella* to replicate in various pigeon organs is reflected by a variety of lesions found in affected birds. Depending on the organs affected and the extent of the lesions, several specific and general clinical signs may occur either solely or simultaneously (Devriese 1986).

In acute salmonellosis, intestinal lesions with fibrinous enteritis and focal ulceration are consistently present. When septicaemia occurs, enlargement of the internal organs is seen, caused by inflammatory activity of heterophilic granulocytes and macrophages. **Clinically, this acute form of the disease generally begins with one single pigeon in the loft that refuses to eat and eventually shows a slimy green or bloody diarrhoea.** Only small amounts of droppings are produced, and they consist almost exclusively of green-stained urates. Polyuria may be present. After a few days, the affected pigeon either dies or starts to recover. Meanwhile, other pigeons generally develop similar signs.

The acute organ lesions may evolve to focal necrosis and formation of abscesses and granulomas. Pigeons suffering from such lesions show a poor general condition, until they eventually succumb. When specific organs are involved in the disease process, lesion-dependent signs may occur. Arthritis of the legs and the wings results in lameness and inability to fly, respectively. **Extensive swelling of the elbow is an almost pathognomonic sign (Fig. 15.12)**, although the shoulder joint and the canalis triosseus may also be involved. Infertility and/or embryonic death are associated with multiplication of the bacteria in the gonads, and blindness can be ascribed to *Salmonella*-panophthalmitis. Dermal lesions include small abscesses in the eyelids or in the subcutis of the neck region, as well as occasional exudative dermatitis on the lower side of the wing. Sporadically, opisthotonus occurs when the infection localizes in the brain. Respiratory signs are not associated with salmonellosis; nevertheless, necrosis and abscess formation in the lungs and air sacs are often characteristic lesions.

Sudden and virulent outbreaks of salmonellosis are seen exclusively in nestlings. Nestlings can be infected during an outbreak of acute salmonellosis in the loft, or when asymptomatic carrier pigeons are used for breeding. Carrier pigeons may infect their progeny by vertical or neonatal transmission, resulting in mass mortality of nestlings, usually starting from day 5. In less acute cases, nestlings may show retarded growth, paralysis and non-unfolding feathers.

Diagnosis

In pigeons that die from salmonellosis, the aetiological agent can be isolated from internal organs at necropsy. Bacteriological examination of the droppings can confirm the diagnosis in live animals, but the method is not very reliable for chronically affected individual pigeons since they may excrete the bacterium intermittently. It is therefore best to pool faecal samples over a period of 5

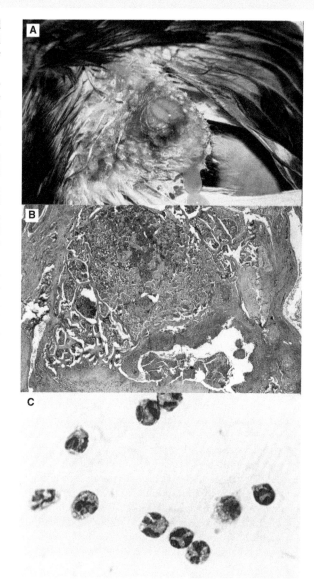

Fig 15.12 *Salmonella*-induced arthritis of the elbow. **A** Swollen elbow with mucoid discharge. **B** Histology of the arthritis; haematoxylin & eosin. **C** Cytology of the fluid showing toxic heterophils.

days. *Salmonella* should be seen both on direct inoculation of culture plates and/or following enrichment.

For a rapid diagnosis of salmonellosis, a slide agglutination test can be used (Devriese 1986). In this test, one drop of formaldehyde-inactivated *Salmonella* group B bacteria is mixed with one drop of plasma from a suspected pigeon and placed on a slide. The slide is then rocked and tilted slowly for 2 minutes, and a positive reaction demonstrates the presence of antibodies resulting from salmonellosis or possibly vaccination against salmonellosis. False negative reactions occur. **It is mainly pigeons suffering from acute salmonellosis with** severe clinical signs that react positively in the slide agglutination test. Chronically infected pigeons, as well as asymptomatic carriers, usually remain negative. The slide agglutination test can also be performed with fluid obtained from the joints of pigeons with arthritis. More sensitive serological tests have been described, but they are usually time-consuming and expensive, which make them less useful in clinical practice.

Clinical disease due to *Salmonella* infections must be differentiated from other diseases with rather similar signs, e.g. streptococcosis, adenovirosis, hexamitiasis, ascaridiosis, capillariosis and paramyxovirosis.

Control

Control of salmonellosis is possible but difficult. Eradication programmes for infected lofts include four points that must be rigorously followed: sanitation, antimicrobial treatment, vaccination and bacteriological checks of the faeces. Sanitation must be performed first (Devriese 1986), and this includes euthanasia of clinically diseased pigeons, since these animals may develop chronic lesions and become asymptomatic carriers. Valuable pigeons, which the owner refuses to sacrifice, must be treated in quarantine, and can only be reintroduced to the loft when repeated bacteriological examinations of faecal samples have proved them to be free of *Salmonella*. Further sanitary measures include thorough cleaning and disinfection of the loft. Breeding must be interrupted, and over-population avoided. After sanitation, the remaining pigeons must be treated with antimicrobials for at least 10 days. In vitro the bacteria are sensitive to a large number of antimicrobials, but in vivo the best results are obtained with enrofloxacin (200 mg/L) or trimethoprim (200 mg/L) (Uyttebroek et al 1991). The oral application of florfenicol was proven to promote *Salmonella* carriers in pigeons because intracellular persistence was not inhibited (Pasmans et al 2008). Treatment does not, however, guarantee complete elimination of the bacteria, and an inactivated vaccine for administration immediately after completion of antimicrobial treatment has been developed (Uyttebroek et al 1991). When given as preventive measure, this vaccine does not protect the pigeons from *Salmonella* colonization but reduces *Salmonella* faecal shedding and limits clinical symptoms, including mortality. When applied curatively, it stimulates the cellular immunity of infected pigeons so that they will spontaneously eliminate the infection. Following vaccination, pigeons may become serologically positive for 3–18 months. Side-effects resulting from an intense immunological response to the *Salmonella* antigens in the vaccine may occur, mainly in pigeons previously infected with *Salmonella*. Occasionally, a pigeon dies within 24 hours of vaccination. In some lofts, large subcutaneous nodules with histiocyte accumulations of the 'foreign body' type may develop at the site of injection 7–10 days after

vaccination. These granulomas cause pain, anorexia, poor general condition and eventually death. In severe cases, they have to be removed surgically. The outcome of the control programme has to be assessed on the basis of regular bacteriological examinations of pooled faecal samples, for example 1 month after treatment and subsequently every 6 months. When samples appear positive, the treatment protocol must be repeated.

Streptococcosis

Streptococcal infections were first described in pigeons in 1990 (Devriese et al 1990). Since then, streptococcosis has been recognized as an important systemic disease in pigeons (De Herdt et al 1992a).

Aetiology

The aetiological agent of streptococcosis in pigeons is *Streptococcus gallolyticus*, a Gram-positive bacterium. Within this species, different types have been recognized in pigeons: there are five biotypes, two sub-biotypes, five serotypes and six supernatant-phenotypes (De Herdt et al 1992b; Vanrobaeys et al 1996). The biotypes and sub-biotypes are determined by their haemolytic properties, polysaccharide production and carbohydrate fermentation; the serotypes are distinguished by agglutination; and supernatant-phenotypes are identified on the basis of the presence of four proteins (A, T1, T2, T3) in the supernatant of *S. gallolyticus* broth cultures.

S. gallolyticus isolates from pigeons can be cultured on non-selective media such as Columbia agar with 5% bovine blood. Slanetz and Bartley agar can be used as a selective medium. The medium needs to be boiled for at least 5 minutes for optimal recovery of *S. gallolyticus*, and the media should preferably be incubated in the presence of a 5% elevated CO_2 concentration.

Epidemiology

Approximately 40% of all pigeons carry *S. gallolyticus* in the intestinal tract without showing clinical signs (De Herdt et al 1994a). These bacteria may belong to different biotypes, serotypes and supernatant-phenotypes. The carriage rate is not related to the season or to the age of the pigeons. **Healthy carrier pigeons can be found in approximately 80% of pigeon lofts**, indicating that *S. gallolyticus* can be part of the normal intestinal flora in pigeons. **On the other hand, *S. gallolyticus* is also an important cause of bacterial septicaemia in pigeons.** Therefore, the bacterium must be considered a facultative pathogenic agent. The incidence of *S. gallolyticus* septicaemia in pigeons is higher between January and August than between September and December (De Herdt et al 1994a).

Pathogenesis

As long as *S. gallolyticus* bacteria are limited to the intestinal tract of pigeons, no clinical signs are observed.

Clinical disease problems can occur when the bacteria enter the bloodstream and cause septicaemia. *S. gallolyticus* septicaemia often occurs in pigeons held under poor hygienic conditions. The incidence of streptococcosis is also high in female pigeons during breeding (De Herdt et al 1991, De Herdt et al 1994b). Finally, *S. gallolyticus* septicaemia sometimes complicates *Salmonella* infections.

Morbidity and mortality during an outbreak of streptococcosis will depend on the virulence of the causative strain. It has been demonstrated that the supernatant-phenotypes T1, AT1, AT2 and AT3 are highly virulent, while the T3 strains are moderately virulent and the T2 isolates are almost apathogenic (De Herdt et al 1994c, Vanrobaeys et al 1997). Virulent strains have several virulence mechanisms. First, they are able to multiply intracellularly in macrophages, resulting in protection against humoral defence mechanisms and, consequently, promotion of the invasive character of the bacteria (De Herdt et al 1995b). Furthermore, *S. gallolyticus* bacteria can adhere to muscle fibres and they probably also form toxins (De Herdt et al 1994c). These two virulence factors may contribute to the formation of some specific necrotic lesions, e.g. in the pectoral muscles.

The course of an infection can of course be influenced by the immune status of the pigeons. At present, immunity against *S. gallolyticus* septicaemia is not well understood and data on this subject are scarce (De Herdt et al 1995c). It has been demonstrated that pigeons suffering from *S. gallolyticus* septicaemia with a serotype 1 or serotype 2 strain build up protective immunity against reinfection with the serotype 1 strain. However, no protection against serotype 1 septicaemia was induced after infection with a serotype 3 strain.

Clinical signs and lesions

Acute or hyperacute death in pigeons of all ages is the most constant clinical sign related to *S. gallolyticus* septicaemia, occurring in nearly half the pigeon lofts dealing with outbreaks of the disease. In pigeons that die very suddenly, an overwhelming multiplication of *S. gallolyticus* has usually taken place in different internal organs such as the liver, spleen, kidneys and myocardium. In these organs, inflammatory activity and focal necrosis can be observed. **The most typical lesion of streptococcosis consists of a large, well-circumscribed area of necrosis in the pectoral muscle. When present, this lesion can be seen through the skin.** Pigeons with pectoral muscle necrosis always die within a few hours of the lesion(s) developing.

Another typical sign is drooping of the wings and an inability to fly, which is observed in approximately 6% of affected pigeons. Lesions in affected pigeons include tenosynovitis of the tendon of the deep pectoral muscle and/or arthritis of the shoulder joint. Sometimes, large amounts of oedematous or viscous fluid, occasionally with fibrin clots, are accumulated at these sites. The lesions result from multiplication of *S. gallolyticus* around the deep pectoral muscle tendon in the canalis triosseus or the shoulder joint.

Lameness occurs in approximately 8% of cases. Lesions consist of arthritis of the stifle joint or the hock joint, as a reaction to replication of *S. gallolyticus*. In 17% of the outbreaks, pigeon owners' anamnesis includes the production of green, slimy droppings and/or polyuria. The green, slimy droppings do not result from intestinal tract lesions, but are probably due to inappetence of the pigeon. Polyuria can be explained by tubular necrosis in the kidneys.

Inappetence and emaciation are predominant signs in 9% of the lofts affected by streptococcosis. Usually, most internal organs show coagulation necrosis and inflammation resulting from multiplication of the bacteria.

Nervous disorders can also be associated with *S. gallolyticus* septicaemia (approximately 9% of cases). CNS signs include complete paralysis and leaning on the forehead in trying to stand up. Meningitis and/or encephalitis in the cerebrum and the cerebellum occurs in these pigeons.

Pigeons suffering from the clinical signs mentioned above usually show a bad general condition. However, in 7% of all diagnoses of *S. gallolyticus* septicaemia, a wasting condition is the only clinical expression of the disease. Organ lesions under these conditions are often rather mild, although live bacteria are present.

It is important to keep in mind that in lofts identified as having an outbreak of *S. gallolyticus* septicaemia, the different clinical signs may occur either simultaneously or singly (De Herdt et al 1994b).

Diagnosis

The diagnosis of streptococcosis can be suspected on the basis of the clinical signs. However, these signs are not specific to streptococcal infections. Acute death, the most constant clinical sign in *S. gallolyticus* septicaemia, is also associated with adenovirus type II infections, intoxication, *E. coli* septicaemia and acute salmonellosis. Chronic salmonellosis, trauma or hypocalcaemia may lead to an inability to fly. Lameness can be ascribed to trauma or salmonellosis. Green, slimy droppings can indicate *Hexamita* spp., adenovirus type I, paramyxovirus or *Salmonella* infections. For a final diagnosis of streptococcosis, necropsy is required. **Typical lesions have to be present, and/or the bacterium has to be isolated from affected organs. Isolation of *S. gallolyticus* from intestinal contents or droppings cannot be used for diagnostic purposes because of the occurrence of healthy carrier pigeons.**

Control

Antimicrobials can be used for the treatment of pigeons suffering from streptococcosis (De Herdt et al 1993).

In vitro, *S. gallolyticus* strains from pigeons are always (so far) sensitive to penicillin G, ampicillin and amoxicillin. Acquired resistance to macrolides, lincomycin, enrofloxacin and tetracyclines was found to occur in approximately 45%, 48%, 12% and 85% of the strains respectively (Kimpe et al 2002). All strains are intermediately sensitive to neomycin and gentamicin. Pigeon *S. gallolyticus* strains are resistant to trimethoprim or sulphonamides. In practice, the administration of ampicillin 2 g/L for at least 7 days is the treatment of choice. Doxycycline 500 mg/L and erythromycin 1 g/L are good alternatives when the infecting *S. gallolyticus* strains do not have acquired resistance to these drugs.

Antibiotics do not eliminate *S. gallolyticus* from the intestinal tract, even after an otherwise successful treatment. If the factors predisposing to septicaemia and disease are still present when excretion of *S. gallolyticus* resumes, a new outbreak of streptococcosis may occur. Since poor hygiene is often involved, antibiotic treatment should be accompanied by hygienic measures. In this respect, keeping the pigeons on wire floors is very effective. This inhibits reinfection of pigeons with *S. gallolyticus* bacteria from the droppings, thus reducing the reinoculation of the agent in the intestinal tract.

Escherichia coli *septicaemia*
Aetiology
Escherichia coli is a Gram-negative rod-shaped bacterium that belongs to the family Enterobacteriaceae. There appears to be great variety in the biochemical properties of pigeon *E. coli* strains, and the antigenic properties of pigeon *E. coli* bacteria have not yet been determined. *E. coli* isolates from pigeons can easily be cultivated on numerous media, for example on non-selective Columbia agar with 5% bovine blood, or on selective McConkey agar.

Epidemiology
E. coli bacteria are present in the intestinal tract of approximately 97% of all pigeons as a part of the normal flora (De Herdt et al 1994d). On the other hand, *E. coli* also is an important cause of bacterial septicaemia in pigeons, representing 7% of the necropsy diagnoses at Ghent University. To date, no differences have been found in *E. coli* strains isolated from healthy and diseased pigeons, indicating that *E. coli* is a facultative pathogenic agent in pigeons.

Pathogenesis
Very little is known of the pathogenesis of *E. coli* septicaemia. *E. coli* bacteria are normal inhabitants of the intestinal tract in pigeons. Factors leading to septicaemia and disease include adenovirus infections and probably numerous other conditions that are unknown. Most *E. coli* strains isolated from pigeons produce aerobactin and resist the bactericidal activity of pigeon serum

(De Herdt et al 1994d). The possible relationship between these properties and virulence is unclear.

Clinical signs and lesions
Clinical disease can occur either solely in the nestlings or in pigeons of all ages. In the first case, *E. coli* septicaemia may cause sudden death in nestlings, usually between days 3 and 5. The parents do not usually develop clinical signs. Nestlings from the same parents may suffer from *E. coli* septicaemia in successive nests.

In other outbreaks, pigeons of all ages are affected (De Herdt et al 1994d). The main clinical signs in these birds are sudden death, diarrhoea, vomiting and weight loss, which occur in 55%, 23%, 23% and 13% of cases, respectively (De Herdt et al 1994d). The lesions in the affected pigeons are caused by septicaemia, but are not typical: congestion or paleness of organs, and infiltration of inflammatory cells and bacteria in the affected organs.

Diagnosis
It is very difficult to establish the diagnosis of *E. coli* septicaemia on a clinical basis only. **Vomiting is more or less typical for *E. coli* septicaemia, but it also occurs with adenovirosis and heavy infestations of *Ascaridia* or *Capillaria*.** Acute death in nestlings can be attributed to trichomoniasis, salmonellosis, paramyxovirosis and tick infestations. Sudden death and/or diarrhoea in pigeons of all ages can also be associated with adenovirosis, intoxication, streptococcosis and salmonellosis.

E. coli septicaemia can only be diagnosed at necropsy. **Lesions indicative of septicaemia have to be present, and the bacterium has to be isolated from affected organs in pure culture. Isolation of *E. coli* from intestinal contents or droppings is not diagnostic because of the occurrence of healthy carrier pigeons.**

Control
Antimicrobials are generally used for the treatment of pigeons with *E. coli* septicaemia. The choice of antimicrobial should preferably be based on the results of antibiograms, since pigeon *E. coli* strains may have very high levels of acquired antibiotic resistance. Acquired resistance is especially high against tetracyclines, ampicillin, nitrofurans and chloramphenicol (De Herdt et al 1994d, Kimpe et al 2002). When the bacteria are sensitive, good results are obtained with enrofloxacin 150 mg/L or trimethoprim 200 mg/L.

Ornithosis (Chlamydophila psittaci) *and respiratory disease*
Aetiology
Respiratory disease in pigeons is a multifactorial problem that may include infectious and non-infectious

components. Non-infectious factors include the climate and the environment of the pigeon loft: hygiene, humidity, temperature, population density, draught, ventilation, dust, etc. The infectious agents that cause respiratory disease in pigeons have not yet been fully determined. In the literature there is much confusion and disagreement concerning the identity of respiratory pathogens in pigeons. In the authors' experience, the following agents can be primarily or secondarily involved: herpesvirus, *Chlamydophila psittaci*, *Escherichia coli*, *Staphylococcus intermedius*, *Pelistega europaea* and *Aspergillus fumigatus* (De Herdt et al 1998). Mycoplasmas such as *Mycoplasma columborale* are only rarely associated with respiratory disease in pigeons (Loria et al 2005). Yet unidentified viruses may also play a role. Although occasionally mentioned in handbooks on pigeon medicine, paramyxovirus serotype 1 and *Avibacterium* spp. are probably not respiratory pathogens in pigeons, as opposed to the situation in poultry.

Epidemiology

Respiratory disease may occur throughout the year and in all age groups. However, clinical signs are most obvious in young birds. Problems are typically seen in late winter–early spring, or in summer.

C. psittaci, *E. coli*, *P. europaea* and *S. intermedius* are the main agents that cause respiratory disease of pigeons. *A. fumigatus*, on the other hand, is seen only very rarely, and almost always affects individual cases. Herpesvirus is widely spread among pigeon populations, but only occasionally causes clinical infections.

Pathogenesis

Non-infectious factors may predispose pigeons to infection with respiratory pathogens, and unfavourable environmental conditions also contribute to the severity of infectious respiratory diseases.

The pathogenesis of herpesvirus infections is discussed earlier in this chapter. Infection of pigeons with *C. psittaci* occurs through inhalation of the bacterium (Schachter & Caldwell 1980). The agent multiplies inside epithelial cells of the respiratory and intestinal tract, and in various internal organs. This often leads to respiratory signs and generalized disease. Pigeons can become asymptomatic carriers and excrete the bacterium through nasal secretions, faeces and crop milk (Burkhart & Page 1971). The pathogenesis of *E. coli*, *S. intermedius* and *P. europaea* infections has not been studied in pigeons.

A. fumigatus is an ubiquitous fungus that occurs particularly in warm and humid environments. Pigeons may develop aspergillosis infections when they are infected with a high number of spores. High infection pressures

tend to prevail during overcrowding and under poor hygienic conditions, for example in lofts with low ventilation, putrefying droppings, contaminated litter and decayed food. Spores are easily spread by air, causing subsequent infections of air sacs and lungs. Intercurrent disease, long-term antibiotic treatment and use of corticosteroids may furthermore predispose pigeons to aspergillosis.

Clinical signs and lesions

The clinical signs associated with respiratory disease in pigeons are very diverse. In obvious cases, pigeons may produce rattling respiratory noises and nasal mucus. This condition is known as coryza. **Pigeon coryza is purely a clinical disease entity, and does not indicate an infection with specific agents.** This is different to the situation in poultry, where coryza indicates infection with *A. paragallinarum*. **An extremely valuable sign of respiratory disease in pigeons is open mouth breathing, even when this is very discrete, as healthy pigeons always breathe through their noses, except during hot weather or after heavy physical effort.** Another respiratory sign is conjunctivitis, which may occur in one or both eyes. This usually indicates a *Chlamydophila* infection. In severe cases, the third eye lid may hang down. In some pigeons, respiratory signs are less obvious. Pigeon owners often note swollen heads and insufficient patency of the pigeons' nostrils, and such pigeons often sneeze abundantly during a massage of the nostrils or larynx. Feathers next to the auditory canal are typically erected, and tracheal noises can occasionally be heard.

In lofts that suffer chronically from *Chlamydophila* infections, respiratory signs may be less pronounced. Complaints may rather include poor racing performances and intermittent production of somewhat green, pasty droppings.

In most pigeons suffering from respiratory disease, lesions are confined to rhinitis, sinusitis, conjunctivitis, tracheitis or air sacculitis. The nature of this inflammatory process is usually catarrhal, but it may become purulent in some cases. In clinical herpesvirus infections, necrotizing tracheitis with fibrin formation as well as focal hepatic necrosis can be seen. Generalized *Chlamydophila* infections lead to swelling and inflammation of several internal organs, predominantly the spleen and liver. Lesions in pigeons suffering from aspergillosis are comparable to those described in parrots.

Diagnosis

The diagnosis of respiratory disease must be made by a thorough clinical examination. In live animals, it is not always easy to identify the infectious agent that causes the problems. It is possible, however, to determine whether *Chlamydophila* spp. is involved, and this may be important with respect to the treatment. *Chlamydophila* spp. can be traced by microscopic examination of swab samples from the choanae stained with the modified Gimenéz stain (Vanrompay et al 1992). **When examining conjunctiva swabs, the results must be interpreted with care: positive samples may indicate a pigeon suffering from ornithosis as well as a *Chlamydophila* spp. carrier pigeon.** In pigeons suffering from ornithosis, numerous cells of the conjunctiva are usually positive for the bacterium; in carrier pigeons only a low number of conjunctival cells contain chlamydiae. For confirmation, samples can be examined using (RT-) PCR and/or isolation on cell cultures. **When pigeons are negative for ornithosis, it can be useful to stain a swab sample of the nose contents or trachea with a rapid blood staining technique.** Large numbers of coccal bacteria may indicate a staphylococcal infection.

Autopsy of affected pigeons may give additional information when the aetiological agent can be demonstrated in internal organs, air sacs or sinuses. Herpesvirus infections can most easily be diagnosed on the basis of the presence of intranuclear inclusion bodies in tracheal or hepatic lesions examined by exfoliative cytology or histology. Isolation of herpesvirus is also possible. Identification of most bacteria and *Aspergillus* spp. requires isolation, except for *Chlamydophila* spp., which can also be recognized cytologically.

Control

A first measure that must be taken in all outbreaks of respiratory disease in pigeons is to improve the climate in the pigeon loft. Besides that, curative therapy must be directed against the infectious cause of the disease. Infections with *Chlamydophila* spp., and *E. coli* are controlled most effectively with doxycycline (600 mg/L for at least 14 days), and enrofloxacin (150 mg/L for 5 days), respectively. Infections with *S. intermedius* and *P. europaea* respond well to treatment with amoxicillin (1.5 g/L for 5–10 days.) When an antibiogram indicates acquired resistance of bacteria to some of these products, other drugs such as trimethoprim, macrolides or sulphonamides can be used. The abuse of antimicrobial agents by pigeon fanciers is quite famous among avian veterinarians. This has probably led to the high levels of acquired antimicrobial resistance in pigeon bacterial isolates as mentioned in the literature (Kimpe et al 2002). Moreover, **yeast infections notably caused by *Candida albicans* occur frequently in overmedicated flocks. These infections mainly cause inflammation of the pharynx, oesophagus and crop.**

Control of aspergillosis in pigeons consists of the elimination of the source of infection. Treatment of individual pigeons is useless. No curative or preventive treatment exists against herpesvirus infections.

Parasitic infections

Trichomoniasis

Aetiology

Trichomoniasis in pigeons is caused by *Trichomonas gallinae*, a 5–19 μm parasite with four anterior flagella (Levine 1985a). The pigeon is the primary host, but *T. gallinae* also occurs in a number of other birds, including hawks, falcons and eagles, that feed on pigeons.

Epidemiology

T. gallinae is extremely common in domestic pigeons. However, severe lesions or clinical signs are predominantly seen in nestling and young pigeons, and not in adult birds.

Pathogenesis

Pigeons suffering from trichomoniasis shed the parasites through the saliva and the crop milk. Trichomonads have no cysts and are very sensitive to drying, so direct contamination is necessary. Pigeons are infected with the parasite by the uptake of contaminated water or oral contact with affected pigeons during fighting or feeding of squabs. The parasites colonize the upper digestive tract, predominantly the crop. In severely infected pigeons, trichomonads may descend to the oesophagus and eventually break through the intestinal wall, affecting the large blood vessels and the liver. The parasites may also multiply in the umbilical region, causing inflammation.

Clinical signs and lesions

Lesions and clinical signs due to trichomoniasis largely depend on the virulence of the infecting strain and the age of the pigeons. Most strains are of low virulence, and the majority of pigeons infected with *Trichomonas* do not show macroscopic lesions. Early lesions in the mouth consist of irregular yellow plugs and exudate on the mucosa of the soft palate. Small, yellowish, circumscribed areas can increase in number and become progressively larger, finally developing into very large, caseous masses that may invade the roof of the mouth and even extend to the sinuses (Fig. 15.13). The early lesions in the pharynx, oesophagus and crop are small, whitish to yellowish caseous nodules that may also grow to thick necrotic masses. It is very typical that these lesions can be easily removed without bleeding. In squabs, similar 'yellow button' lesions can be found in the liver and in the umbilical region when the parasites multiply in these parts of the body.

In adult pigeons, trichomoniasis is associated with poor racing performance and no manifest clinical signs. Heavily infected pigeons usually show somewhat fluid droppings with a sour odour. Rarely, adult pigeons may

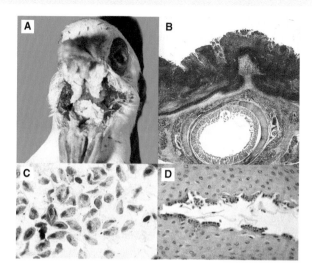

Fig 15.13 Trichomoniasis. **A** Caseous masses in the mouth. **B** Necrotic layer on the crop wall; haematoxylin & eosin. **C** *Trichomonas* sp. in cytology; Hemacolor © 100×. **D** A layer of *Trichomonas* sp. on the crop epithelium; haematoxylin & eosin.

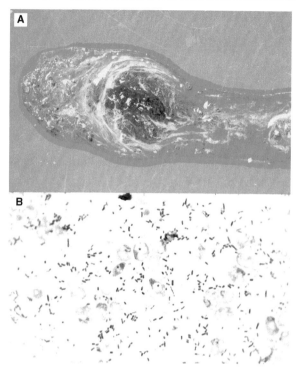

Fig 15.14 *Hexamita columbae*. **A** Diarrhoea associated with *Hexamita columbae*. **B** *Hexamita columbae* in cytology.

die acutely when the parasite affects the large blood vessels. **Sudden death and wasting are complaints associated with trichomoniasis in nestlings.**

Immunity can apparently be achieved with great difficulty, although in chronically infected lofts very old pigeons may remain consistently negative. There is usually cross-protection between virulent and less virulent strains of trichomonads.

Diagnosis

Crop samples from pigeons can easily be obtained using a swab or an inoculating loop. Contents from the crop collected in this way should be suspended immediately in a drop of phosphate-buffered saline solution on a cover slip, and observed microscopically with an objective lens of 10×. Trichomonads can be recognized as a wriggling flagellar parasite. The water used for this examination should preferably be sterile, since tap water may contain saprophytic flagellates.

Mouth lesions due to trichomoniasis should not be confused with diphtheric lesions due to a pox virus infection. The latter lesions are more voluminous, are localized in the front of the mouth and bleed if attempts are made to remove them. Furthermore, sialoliths (very small white or yellowish nodules in the roof of the pharynx) and herpesvirus-associated lesions should not be misdiagnosed as trichomoniasis.

Control

Pigeons suffering from trichomoniasis can be treated with different 5-nitro-imidazoles such as ronidazole (100–200 mg/L), dimetridazole (400 mg/L) and metronidazole (1 g/L) (Devriese 1986). Treatment is usually over

5 days using ronidazole and metronidazole, and 3 days for dimetridazole. Pigeon fanciers often give metaphylactic treatments with these products in the same dose; for example for 2–3 days at regular intervals during the racing season.

In some countries, 5-nitro-imidazoles are also registered as tablets for single administration in pigeons. These tablets are especially useful for the treatment of individual pigeons. **Therapeutic failure of nitroimidazole treatment due to acquired resistance of trichomonads is an increasing problem (Franssen & Lumeij 1992, Munoz et al 1998).** Pigeon fanciers must be educated only to use antiparasitic or antibiotic treatment based on a proper diagnosis of a parasitic or bacterial disease.

Hexamitiasis
Aetiology

Hexamita columbae, which is also called *Spironucleus columbae*, is a host-specific protozoan organism that causes hexamitiasis in pigeons (Levine 1985b). This parasite has six anterior and two posterior flagella, and it measures 5–9 μm (Fig. 15.14).

Epidemiology

Clinical signs due to hexamitiasis occur mainly in young pigeons during the spring or summer (Devriese 1986).

Pathogenesis

Pigeons are infested with *Hexamita columbae* by oral uptake of contaminated droppings, food or water. The parasite multiplies in the intestinal tract by longitudinal binary fission. This replication results in severe intestinal damage, predominantly in squabs. Bacterial invasion of the lesions may exacerbate the disease in infested birds. Hexamitiasis can occur as a primary disease, but it also constitutes an important complication in adenovirosis type I.

Clinical signs and lesions

Replication of *Hexamita* spp. in the intestinal tract results in catarrhal enteritis with small ulcerative lesions in the ileum and rectum. Due to these lesions, pigeons will develop vomiting, diarrhoea, polydipsia, weight loss, dehydration and a poor general condition. The faeces are watery or contain mucus, and have an intense green colour and a bad odour. When left untreated, infested birds may die after 1–2 weeks. In infested nestlings, wasting is observed. Following an infection, carrier birds may occur among survivors; in these birds the organism can be found in the caecal tonsils. These carriers are a source of infection for other pigeons.

Diagnosis

Hexamitiasis can be diagnosed in vivo by direct microscopic examination of fresh cloacal samples or intestinal contents of very fresh cadavers. **The organism can be recognized by its linear movement when seen microscopically, the optimal microscopic magnification being 200–400×.** This diagnostic tool allows differentiation of hexamitiasis from other agents causing similar clinical disease signs, such as *Salmonella*, *E. coli*, adenovirus and paramyxovirus.

Control

Pigeons suffering from hexamitiasis can be treated successfully with ronidazole (100 mg/L) or metronidazole (1 g/L) over 7 days. Dimetridazole (400 mg/L) is equally effective, but pigeons suffering from polyuria may ingest extremely high amounts of the product, resulting in acute toxicity.

In severe cases, it is advisable to use an antimicrobial simultaneously with the 5-nitro-imidazoles to control secondary bacterial invasion of the lesions. Trimethoprim (200 mg/L) or enrofloxacin (100 mg/L) are suited for this purpose.

Coccidiosis
Aetiology

Two species of *Eimeria* can cause coccidiosis in pigeons; *E. labbeana* and *E. columbarum* (Varghese 1980). The species can be distinguished by their morphological characteristics; *E. labbeana* measures approximately 16.5 × 15μm, while *E. columbarum* is somewhat larger at 20 × 18.7μm.

Epidemiology

In Belgium, more than 80% of pigeons suffering from coccidiosis are infested with *E. labbeana* (Devos et al 1980) and less than 20% with *E. columbarum*. **The pathogenicity of both *Eimeria* spp. is rather low.** Approximately 50% of all pigeons are infested. Infection pressure is especially high in lofts with poor standards of hygiene.

Pathogenesis

Pigeons become infested with *E. labbeana* or *E. columbarum* by the uptake of sporulated oocysts. Sporozoites are released from these oocysts, and infect the epithelial cells of the small intestine. *E. columbarum* predominantly parasitizes the jejunum and ileum, while *E. labbeana* develops in the colon. After a developmental cycle, oocysts are formed and shed in the faeces. The prepatent period is 5–7 days (Van Reeth & Vercruysse 1992). The prepatent period after a single infection is approximately 30 days. Sporulation of oocysts is promoted by temperature and humidity, and usually occurs within 4 days.

Immunity against coccidiosis is species-specific. This immunity quickly disappears in the absence of reinfection.

Clinical signs and lesions

In 10–12-day-old nestling pigeons with diarrhoea, high numbers of oocysts can often found in the faeces (Devriese 1986). It has not been proven, however, that coccidiosis is actually the aetiology of these clinical signs.

Diagnosis

Coccidiosis can be diagnosed by microscopic examination of the faeces. Usually oocytes per gram (OPGs) are less than 5000, but in winter they may be higher. Pooling of faecal samples may give misleading results, since a single shedder of oocysts may give the impression that the entire group is positive. Before the onset of important races, it may be useful to perform an individual check on the pigeons' faeces to assess the birds' general condition.

Control

To prevent coccidiosis, contact with contaminated faeces must be avoided. This can be achieved by using wire floors. Daily cleaning of the loft is also effective, since oocysts will not have the opportunity to sporulate and will die in the absence of organic materials. Survival of oocysts can be reduced by keeping the environment dry. Disinfection can only be achieved by heat (burning); oocysts are resistant to the common disinfectants.

Treatment of infested pigeons is by a single oral administration of clazuril 2.5 mg (Vercruysse 1990), or by drinking water medicated with toltrazuril (15 mg per pigeon for 2 days) (Vercruysse 1990) or sulphonamides (dose depending on the type of sulphonamide, usually administered over 7 days) (Vindevogel & Duchatel 1979). **However, the authors believe that in most cases it is unnecessary to treat pigeons with coccidiosis.**

Worm infestations
Aetiology

Pigeons can suffer from nematode, cestode and trematode intestinal infestations (Thienpont et al 1979). The main pigeon nematodes include *Ascaridia columbae*, *Capillaria obsignata* and *Capillaria caudinflata*. *A. columbae* is approximately 10 cm long, and produces oval eggs with a smooth, thick shell that measure 68–90 μm × 40–50 μm. *Capillaria* worms, on the other hand, are only 1–2 cm long and less than 1 mm in diameter, and their eggs are lemon-shaped with bipolar plugs (Fig. 15.15). *C. obsignata* eggs measure 50–62 μm × 20–25 μm, and *C. caudinflata* eggs are 43–60 μm × 20–27 μm. Occasionally, nematode species belonging to the genera *Tetrameres* and *Acuaria* are seen in pigeons.

The main cestodes in pigeons are *Raillietina* spp. and *Hymenolepis* spp. Trematodes usually belong to the genus *Echinostoma* (e.g. *E. paraulum*, *E. recurvatum* and *E. revolutum*).

Epidemiology

In racing pigeons, the genera *Ascaridia* and *Capillaria* have the highest prevalence, occurring worldwide. This can be explained mainly by the fact that these nematodes do not have intermediate hosts in their life cycles, in contrast to the tetramerial, acuarial nematodes, cestodes and trematodes (Eckert & Bürger 1992), and because racing pigeons are usually kept indoors they have little contact with intermediate hosts. Furthermore, it must be kept in mind that such parasites only occur under climatic and environmental conditions that allow survival of the intermediate hosts.

Ascaridia and *Capillaria* infestations occur most frequently in lofts with poor hygienic conditions.

Pathogenesis

A. columbae and *C. obsignata* have direct life cycles without intermediate hosts (Ruff 1991). For *C. caudinflata*, on the other hand, intermediate stages develop in the earthworm. Adult ascaridial and capillarial worms live in the intestinal tract of pigeons, and produce eggs that embryonate in the outer world. *C. obsignata* is not

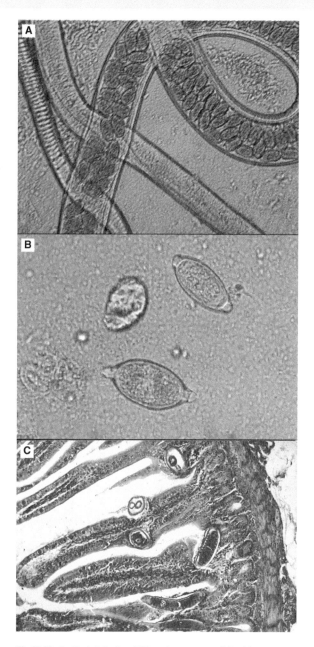

Fig 15.15 *Capillaria* infection. **A** Worm in wet mount. **B** Double operculated eggs of *Capillaria*. **C** Villi in the intestine damaged by *Capillaria* sp.; haematoxylin & eosin.

host-specific, and also parasitizes chickens, pheasants, quails and guinea fowl, which may additionally act as a source of infection for pigeons. Depending on humidity and temperature, embryonation of the eggs takes place within 16–20 days for *Ascaridia* and within 3–14 days for *Capillaria* spp. Organic materials promote survival of the eggs. Following the uptake of embryonated eggs, larvae will grow to adult ascaridial worm in 42–45 days and to adult capillarial worm in 21–28 days.

Tetrameres spp. and *Acuaria* spp. use sow bugs, which predominantly occur in tropical or subtropical areas, for intermediate development (Eckert & Bürger 1992). Pigeon cestodes have an indirect life cycle, with earthworms, beetles or snails as intermediate hosts.

The life cycle of pigeon trematodes is complex and includes intermediate stages in two different hosts, such as amphibians, water snails, mussels and insects. Pigeons are infested with these parasites at pasture or in brooks. Besides pigeons, these trematodes also infest water birds.

Clinicalsig nsa ndl esions

Capillaria spp. adhere to the villi of the intestinal mucosa and feed on epithelium and glandular secretions, causing a catarrhal or fibrinous enteritis and mild anaemia. A poor general condition and weight loss are observed, even when pigeons are infested with few of these parasites. Heavily infested pigeons show diarrhoea, vomiting and emaciation. *Ascaridia* spp. are less pathogenic. In most cases, poor racing performance is the only complaint in the owner's anamnesis. In mass infestations, the worms may migrate to the stomach and the oesophagus. Clinical signs in such pigeons are similar to those seen in capillariosis.

Tetrameres spp. and *Acuaria* spp. can be found in the proventriculus. *Tetrameres* are not very pathogenic and only lead to a poor general condition. *Acuaria*, on the other hand, cause severe anaemia and a high mortality rate.

The pathological and clinical significance of cestode infestations is minimal. *Echinostoma* spp. cause haemorrhagic enteritis in young pigeons (squabs).

Diagnosis

Nematode and trematode infestations can be diagnosed by demonstrating parasite eggs in the faeces, preferably by using flotation techniques. Enteritis resulting from worm infestations must be differentiated from adenovirosis, salmonellosis and hexamitiasis. Cestode infestations usually are found incidentally during necropsy.

Control

Treatment of pigeons suffering from ascaridiosis or capillariosis is by a single oral dose of levamisole, febantel, fenbendazole or cambendazole (Devriese 1986, Baert et al 1993). In heavily infested pigeons, treatment must be repeated after 10 days. Pigeons should be left unfed during levamisole administration, since this product induces vomiting. **Benzimidazole anthelmintics should not be used during moulting, since they can induce feather abnormalities.**

Cestodes and trematodes in pigeons can be controlled by oral treatment with praziquantel (Devriese 1986) and by eliminating contact with the intermediate hosts.

Reinfection of pigeons must be avoided by taking hygienic measures such as thorough cleaning of the loft. Embryonation of the eggs will be arrested in a dry environment without organic materials. Disinfectants are not effective against worm eggs.

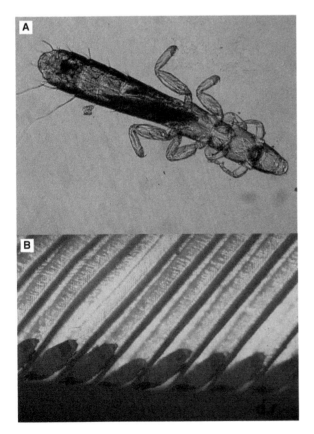

Fig 15.16 A The pigeon louse (*Columbicola columbae*). **B** Feathers infected with the louse.

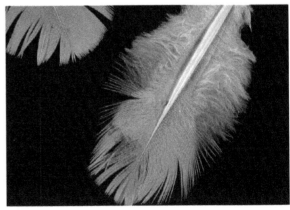

Fig 15.17 *Campanulotes bidentatus*, another common pigeon louse that parasitizes the feathers of the tail.

Ectoparasite infestations

Aetiology

Many species of ectoparasites may occur in pigeons (Kutzer 1992). *Columbicola columbae* and *Campanulotes bidentatus* are the most important pigeon lice, parasitizing the feathers of the wings and the tail respectively (Figs 15.16, 15.17). Feather mites include *Megninia columbae* and *Falculifer rostratus*. Mange of the feathers is usually induced by *Neoknemidocoptes laevis* mites, while *Cnemidocoptes mutans* is responsible for leg mange lesions. *Dermanyssus gallinae* and *Ornithonyssus sylviarum* are the main blood-sucking mites in pigeons. The tick *Argas reflexus* is also of major importance, because it feeds on pigeon blood. Hippoboscid flies are flat, and can transmit *Haemoproteus* spp. during feeding. These flies remain on the bird, darting in and out of the feathers.

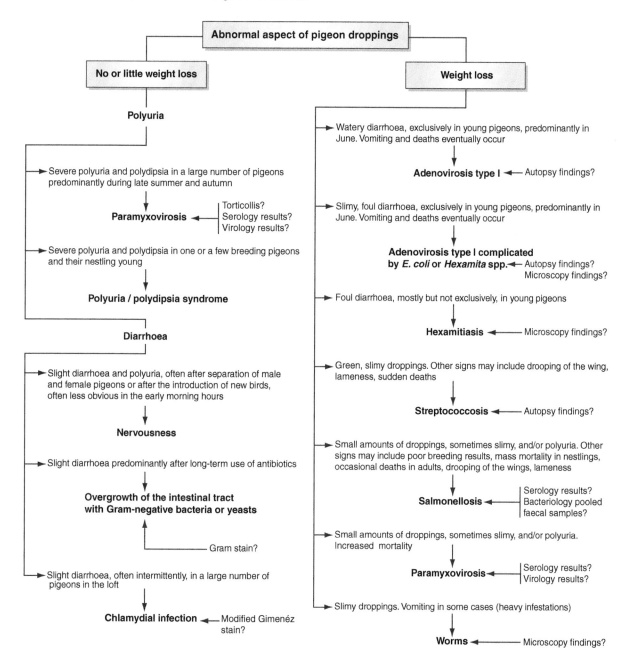

Fig 15.18 Abnormal aspects of pigeon droppings.

Pathogenesis,c linicals ignsa ndl esions

Each of the different pigeon ectoparasites has a species specific life cycle, but these are not discussed here.

Columbicola columbae, Campanulotes bidentatus, Megninia columbae and *Falculifer rostratus* feed on pigeon feather dust. **The significance of these parasites is not so much the damage to the feathers, which is minimal, but the restlessness in infested birds.**

Neoknemidokoptes laevis and *Cnemidocoptes mutans* induce typical mange lesions on the body and legs of pigeons. Clinical signs include broken feathers, scaly skin and legs, and baldness occurring predominantly in the neck region. *Dermanyssus gallinae, Ornithonyssus sylviarum* and *Argas reflexus* are temporary pigeon parasites. Most of the time they hide in the environment, and they come out only for a short time (often during the night) for a pigeon-blood meal. This may lead to restlessness, fatigue, anaemia and even death in nestlings.

Diagnosis

Most ectoparasite infestations can be seen on external inspection. **To diagnose blood-sucking parasites, it is often necessary to visit the pigeon loft during night and examine the pigeons and their environment.** Careful inspection of nest cups and the floor beneath is indicated.

Control

Different insecticides can be used to treat pigeons infested with ectoparasites. For the control of blood-sucking mites and ticks, it is also necessary to thoroughly clean and disinfect the environment. Long-acting drugs can be very useful in such cases.

Summary

Figs 15.18–15.21 summarize the paths to the diagnosis of diseases in pigeons.

Non-infectious diseases

Besides infectious agents, non-infectious factors may cause *polyuria* in pigeons. Non-infectious polyuria is often related to stress. Transport is a typical stress factor frequently associated with polyuria. Stress due to the sexual urge is predominantly seen in male pigeons kept separately from females. Polyuria may also occur when squabs are converted from crop milk to grain food. At that time, some parent pigeons ingest excessive amounts of water, leading to polyuria in both parents and squabs. Finally, vitamin D_3 overload is an occasional cause of polyuria in pigeons.

Pigeons suffering from polyuria due to stress or breeding usually produce normal droppings during the night. This information may be important for differentiation from infectious polyuria.

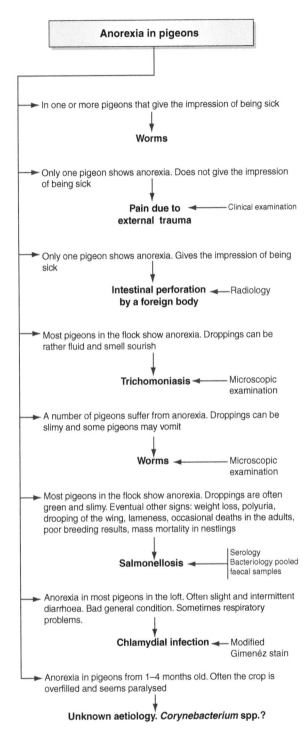

Fig 15.19 Anorexia in pigeons.

Treatment is not generally required; however, minerals should be available *ad libitum* for affected pigeons.

Rupture of air sacs may have an infectious or traumatic aetiology. Infectious causes have been described

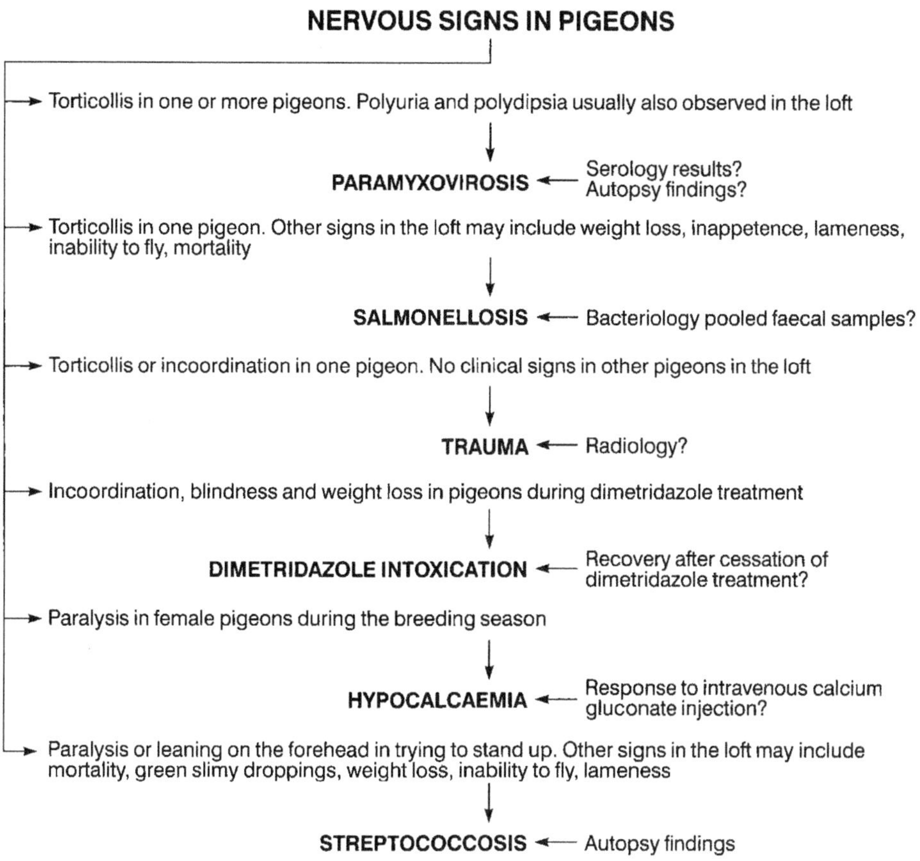

NERVOUS SIGNS IN PIGEONS

→ Torticollis in one or more pigeons. Polyuria and polydipsia usually also observed in the loft

↓

PARAMYXOVIROSIS ← Serology results?
Autopsy findings?

→ Torticollis in one pigeon. Other signs in the loft may include weight loss, inappetence, lameness, inability to fly, mortality

↓

SALMONELLOSIS ← Bacteriology pooled faecal samples?

→ Torticollis or incoordination in one pigeon. No clinical signs in other pigeons in the loft

↓

TRAUMA ← Radiology?

→ Incoordination, blindness and weight loss in pigeons during dimetridazole treatment

↓

DIMETRIDAZOLE INTOXICATION ← Recovery after cessation of dimetridazole treatment?

→ Paralysis in female pigeons during the breeding season

↓

HYPOCALCAEMIA ← Response to intravenous calcium gluconate injection?

→ Paralysis or leaning on the forehead in trying to stand up. Other signs in the loft may include mortality, green slimy droppings, weight loss, inability to fly, lameness

↓

STREPTOCOCCOSIS ← Autopsy findings

Fig 15.20 CNS signs in pigeons.

above. Trauma may be due to bone fractures (e.g. humerus) or puncture lesions resulting from injections. Air that escapes from the ruptured air sac accumulates subcutaneously, especially in the neck region, and this may lead to respiratory distress.

For treatment, subcutaneous air must be removed by puncturing the affected area with a hollow needle and repeatedly squeezing. Movement of the pigeons must be limited. Infections leading to air sacculitis must be controlled.

Egg binding or dystocia can be suspected if there is distension of the abdomen, anorexia and dyspnoea. The diagnosis can be confirmed with palpation and/or diagnostic imaging. Muscle dysfunction, usually resulting from calcium deficiency, misshapen eggs or anatomical abnormalities, is frequently involved. Eggs should be removed as soon as possible, since prolonged presence of eggs in the oviduct may cause complications to the blood vessels, nerves, kidneys and oviduct. **In most cases, the egg can be pushed out by pressure on the abdomen and inoculation of the cloaca with glycerine.** Other therapeutic options, depending on the aetiology of the problem, are intramuscular administration of

calcium gluconate up to 100 mg/kg, intravenous injection with 1 IU oxytocin followed by placing the pigeon in a quiet and dark environment, or surgical removal.

As in other birds, *feather abnormalities* can be due to nutritional deficiencies (e.g. of vitamins and amino acids). The administration of benzimidazole products during moulting may lead to various feather anomalies. In the authors' experience, febantel is safe but should never be administered to squabs under the age of 3 weeks. Translucent lines across the vane of the feathers indicate temporary growth stops, which may be due to severe physical efforts, starvation or generalized disease conditions. 'Stress lines' at regular intervals usually **indicate intermittent administration of corticosteroids.** These drugs are often misused in pigeons for doping purposes.

Organophosphates are the predominant drugs causing *intoxication* in pigeons. Clinical signs include salivation, tremor, tetany, paresis, diarrhoea, mydriasis and death. It is advisable to induce vomiting in intoxicated pigeons, for example through administration of levamisole. Atropine 1 mg/kg can also be administered, subcutaneously. Treatment must be repeated when clinical

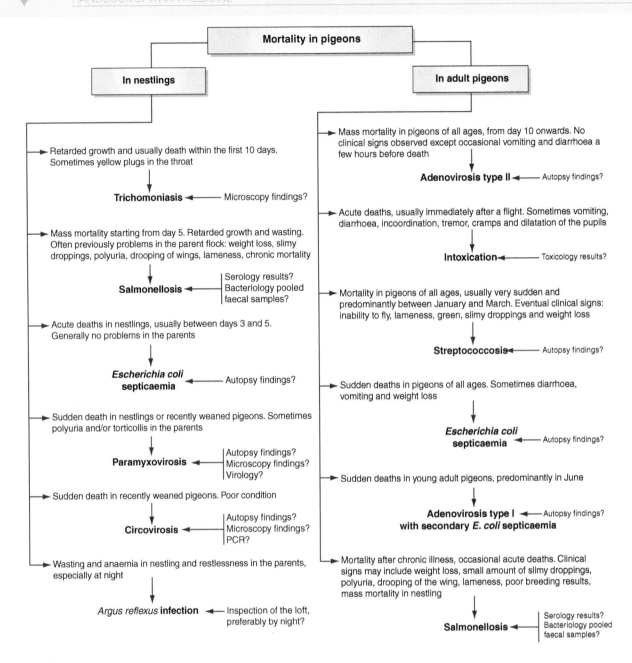

Fig 15.21 Mortality in pigeons.

signs reappear. Dimetridazole given in overdose may cause intoxication in pigeons, with clinical signs of incoordination, blindness and weight loss. Pigeons recover completely after cessation of the treatment.

Acknowledgements

The authors would like to thank Professor R. Ducatelle for his helpful advice, and C. Puttevils for the preparation of the figures.

References

Aldous E W, Fuller C M, Mynn J K et al 2004 A molecular epidemiological investigation of isolates of the variant avian paramyxovirus type 1 virus (PPMV-1) responsible for the 1978 to present panzootic in pigeons. Avian Pathology 33:258–269

Alexander D J 1991 Newcastle disease and other paramyxovirus infections. In: Calnek B W (ed) Diseases of poultry. Wolfe Publishing, London, p 496–519

Alexander D, Russel P, Parsons G et al 1985 Antigenic and biological characterization of avian paramyxovirus type 1 isolates from pigeons – an international collaborative study. Avian Pathology 14:365–376

Baert L, Van Poucke S, Vermeersch H et al 1993 Pharmocokinetics and anthelmintic efficacy of febantel in the racing pigeon. Journal of Veterinary Pharmacology and Therapeutics 16:223–231

Burkhart R L, Page L A 1971 Chlamydiosis. In: Davis J W (ed) Infectious and parasitic diseases of wild birds. Iowa State University Press, Ames, IA, p 118–140

Coussement W, Ducatelle R, Lemahieu P et al 1984 Pathologie van adenovirus infecties bij duiven. Vlaams Diergeneeskundig Tijdschrift 53:227–283

De Herdt P, Devriese L S, Uyttebroek E et al 1991 Streptococcus bovis infekties bij duiven. Vlaams Diergeneeskundig Tijdschrift 60:51–54

De Herdt P, Desmidt M, Haesebrouck F et al 1992a Experimental Streptococcus bovis infections in pigeons. Avian Diseases 36:916–925

De Herdt P, Haesebrouck F, Devriese L A, Ducatelle R 1992b Biochemical and antigenic properties of Streptococcus bovis isolated from pigeons. Journal of Clinical Microbiology 30:2432–2434

De Herdt P, Devriese L A, De Groote B et al 1993 Antibiotic treatment of Streptococcus bovis infections in pigeons. Avian Pathology 22:605–615

De Herdt P, Haesebrouck F, Devriese L A, Ducatelle R 1994a Prevalence of Streptococcus bovis in racing pigeons. Veterinary Quarterly 16:71–74

De Herdt P, Ducatelle R, Haesebrouck F et al 1994b An unusual outbreak of Streptococcus bovis septicaemia in racing pigeons. Veterinary Record 134:42–43

De Herdt P, Haesebrouck F, De Groote B et al 1994c Streptococcus bovis infections in pigeons: virulence of different serotypes. Veterinary Microbiology 41:321–332

De Herdt P, Van Ginneken C, Haesebrouck F et al 1994d Escherichia coli infections in pigeons: Characteristics of the disease and its etiological agent. In: Proceedings IX Tagung über Vogelkrankheiten, München, p 211–214

De Herdt P, Ducatelle R, Lepoudre C et al 1995a An epidemic of fatal hepatic necrosis of viral origin in racing pigeons (Columba livia). Avian Pathology 24:475–483

De Herdt P, Haesebrouck F, Charlier G et al 1995b Intracellular survival and multiplication of virulent and less virulent strains of Streptococcus bovis in pigeon macrophages. Veterinary Microbiology 45:157–169

De Herdt P, Haesebrouck F, Devriese L A, Ducatelle R 1995c Immunity in pigeons against homologous and heterologous serotypes of Streptococcus bovis after infection. Veterinary Microbiology 42:111–119

De Herdt P, Devriese L A, Vereecken M et al 1998 Bacteria associated with respiratory disease of racing pigeons. In: Proceedings XI Tagung über Vogelkrankheiten München, p 83–89

Devos A, Viaene N, Spanoghe L et al 1980 De gezondheidssituatie bij pluimvee en konijnen in 1979. Vlaams Diergeneeskundig Tijdschrift 49:414–421

Devriese L 1986 Ziekten van Siervogels en Duiven, 3rd edn. Rijksuniversiteit Gent

Devriese L A, Uyttebroek E, Gevaert D et al 1990 Streptococcus bovis infections in pigeons. Avian Pathology 19:429–434

Duchatel J, Vindevogel H 1986 Assessment of vaccination of pigeons against paramyxovirus type 1 infection with inactivated aqueous suspension or oil emulsion vaccines. Avian Pathology 15:455–465

Duchatel J P, Todd D, Curry A et al 2005 New data on the transmission of pigeon circovirus. Veterinary Record 157:413–415

Duchatel J P, Todd D, Smyth J A et al 2006 Observations on detection, excretion and transmission of pigeon circovirus in adult, young and embryonic pigeons. Avian Pathology 35:30–34

Eckert J, Bürger H J 1992 Parasitosen des Nutzgeflügels: Helminthen. In: Buch J, Supperer R (eds) Veterinärmedizinische Parasitologie. Paul Parey, Berlin, p 694–732

Eleazer T H, Harrel J S, Blalock H G 1983 Transmission studies involving a wet fowl pox isolate. Avian Diseases 18:495–506

Franssen F F, Lumeij J T 1992 In vitro nitroimidazole resistance of Trichomonas gallinae and successful therapy with an increased dosage of ronidazole in racing pigeons (Columba livia domestica). Journal of Veterinary Pharmacology and Therapeutics 15:409–415

Hartig F, Frese K 1973 Tumorförmige Tauben- und Kanariepocken. Zentralblatt für Veterinärmedizin 20:153–160

Hess M, Prusas C, Gelderblom H, Monreal G 1996 Characterisation of adenoviruses isolated from pigeons. In: Proceedings of the International Symposium on Adenovirus and Reovirus Infections in Poultry, p 122–128

Holz B 1992 Virusisolierungen aus Kotproben von Kabinenexpressfahrzeugen. In: Proceedings VIII Tagung über Vogelkrankheiten, München, p 1–6

Kaleta E F, Honicke A 2004 Review of the literature on avian influenza A viruses in pigeons and experimental studies on the susceptibility of domestic pigeons to influenza A viruses of the haemagglutinin subtype H7. Deutsche tierärztliche Wochenschrift 111:467–472

Kimpe A, Decostere A, Martel A et al 2002 Prevalence of antimicrobial resistance among pigeon isolates of Streptococcus gallolyticus, Escherichia coli and Salmonella enterica serotype Typhimurium. Avian Pathology 31:393–397

Knoll M, Lütticken D, Kösters J 1986 Zur Schutzwirkung einer homologen Ölemulsionsvakzine gegen die Paramyxovirose der Tauben. Der praktische Tierartz 3:216–218

Kutzer E 1992 Parasitosen des Nutzgeflügels: Arthropoden. In: Buch J, Supperer R (eds) Veterinärmedizinische Parasitologie. Paul Parey, Berlin, p 734–748

Loria G R, Tamburello F, Liga F et al 2005 Isolation of mycoplasmas from pigeons suffering eye lesions and respiratory disease. Veterinary Record 157:664–665

Levine N D 1985a Flagellates: the trichomonads. In: Norman N D (ed) Veterinary Protozoology. Iowa State University Press, Ames IA, p 59–79

Levine N D 1985b Flagellates: Spironucleus, Giardia and other flagellates. In: Norman N D (ed) Veterinary Protozoology. Iowa State University Press, Ames, IA, p 89–108

McFerran J B, Connor T J, McCracken R M 1976a Isolation of adenoviruses and retroviruses from avian species other than domestic fowl. Avian Diseases 20:519–524

McFerran J F, McCracken R M, Connor T J, Evans R T 1976b Isolation of viruses from clinical outbreaks of inclusion body hepatitis. Avian Pathology 5:315–324

Munoz E, Castella J, Gutierrez J F 1998 In vivo and in vitro sensitivity of Trichomonas gallinae to some nitroimidazole drugs. Veterinary Parasitology 78:239–246

Pasmans F, Baert K, Martel A et al 2008 Induction of the carrier state in pigeons infected with Salmonella enterica subspecies enterica serovar Typhimurium PT99 by treatment with florfenicol: a matter of pharmacokinetics. Antimicrobial Agents and Chemotherapy, in press

Pasmans F, Van Immerseel F, Heyndrickx M et al 2003 Host adaptation of pigeon isolates of Salmonella serovar Typhimurium var. Copenhagen PT99 is associated with macrophage cytotoxicity. Infection and Immunity 71:6068–6074

Pasmans F, Van Immerseel F, Hermans K et al 2004 Assessment of virulence of pigeon isolates of *Salmonella enterica* subsp. *enterica* serovar Typhimurium variant Copenhagen for humans. Journal of Clinical Microbiology 42:2000–2002

Pohl P, Lintermans P, Vandendriessche A, Boutiflat Y 1983 Epidémiologie de *Salmonella typhimurium* variété Copenhagen. Annales de Médecine Vétérinaire 127:279–287

Raue R, Hafez H M, Hess M 2002 A fiber-gene based polymerase chain reaction for specific detection of pigeon adenovirus. Avian Pathology 31:95–99

Raue R, Schmidt V, Freick M et al 2005 A disease complex associated with pigeon circovirus infection, young pigeon disease syndrome. Avian Pathology 34:418–425

Ruff M D 1991 Nematodes and acantocephalans. In: Calnek B W (ed) Diseases of poultry. Wolfe Publishing, London, p 731–778

Schachter J, Caldwell H D 1980 Chlamydiae. Annual Review of Microbiology 34:285–309

Shivaprasad H L, Chin R P, Jeffrey J S et al 1994 Particles resembling circovirus in the bursa of Fabricius of pigeons. Avian Diseases 38:635–641

Tavernier P, De Herdt P, Thoonen H, Ducatelle R 2000 Prevalence and pathogenic significance of circovirus-like infections in racing pigeons (*Columba livia*). Vlaams Diergeneeskundig Tijdschrift 69:338–341

Thienpont D, Rochette F, Vanparijs O 1979 Diagnose van Verminose door Koprologisch Onderzoek. Janssen Research Foundation

Todd D, Duchatel J P, Weston J H et al 2002 Evaluation of polymerase chain reaction and dot blot hybridisation tests in the diagnosis of pigeon circovirus infections. Veterinary Microbiology 89:1–16

Tripathy D N 1991 Pox. In: Calnek B W (ed) Diseases of poultry. Wolfe Publishing, London, p 583–596

Uyttebroek E, Ducatelle R 1991 Epidemiology of adenovirus infections in pigeons. In: Proceedings of the 1st Conference of European Committee of the Association of Avian Veterinarians, Vienna, p 289–292

Uyttebroek E, Devriese L A, Gevaert D et al 1991 Protective effects of vaccines against experimental salmonellosis in racing pigeons. Veterinary Record 128:152–153

Van Reeth K, Vercruysse J 1992 Coccidiose bij de duif. Pathologie, epidemiologie en behandeling. Vlaams Diergeneeskundig Tijdschrift 61:104–110

Vanrobaeys M, De Herdt P, Haesebrouck F et al 1996 Secreted antigens as virulence associated markers in *Streptococcus bovis* strains from pigeons. Veterinary Microbiology 53:339–348

Vanrobaeys M, De Herdt P, Ducatelle R et al 1997 Extracellular proteins and virulence in *Streptococcus bovis* isolates from pigeons. Veterinary Microbiology 59:59–66

Vanrompay D, Ducatelle R, Haesebrouck F 1992 Diagnosis of avian chlamydiosis: specificity of the modified Giménez staining on smears and comparison of the sensitivity of isolation in eggs and three different cell cultures. Journal of Veterinary Medicine 39:105–112

Varghese T 1980 Coccidian parasites of birds of the avian order Columbiformes with a description of two new species of *Eimeria*. Parasitology 80:183–187

Vercruysse J 1990 Efficacy of toltrazuril and calzuril against experimental infections with *Eimeria labbeana* and *E. columbarum* in racing pigeons. Avian Diseases 34:73–79

Vereecken M, Vanrobaeys M, De Herdt P 2001 Usefulness of two commercial analysers for plasma chemistry in pigeons. Flemish Veterinary Journal 70:44–49

Viaene N, Spanoghe L, Devriese L et al 1983 Paramyxovirus bij duiven. Vlaams Diergeneeskundig Tijdschrift 52:278–286

Vindevogel H, Duchatel J P 1978 Contribution à l'étude de l'étiologie du coryza infectieux du pigeon. Annales de Médecine Vétérinaire 122:507–513

Vindevogel H, Duchatel J P 1979 Les principales maladies parasitaires du pigeon. Annales de Médecine Vétérinaire 123:85–92

Vindevogel H, Pastoret P 1981 Pathogenesis of pigeon herpesvirus infection. Journal of Comparative Pathology 91:415–426

Vindevogel H, Pastoret P P, Burtonboy G et al 1975 Isolement d'un virus herpès dans un élevage de pigeons de chair. Annales de Recherches Vétérinaires 6:431–436

Vindevogel H, Pastoret P P, Leroy P, Coignoul F 1980 Comparaison de trois souches de virus herpetique isolées de psittacides avec le virus herpes du pigeon. Avian Pathology 9:385–394

Vindevogel H, Dagenais L, Lansival B, Pastoret P P 1981 Incidence of rotavirus, adenovirus and herpesvirus infections in pigeons. Veterinary Record 109:285–286

Seabirds

Ian Robinson

16

'Seabirds' is a general term used to describe birds from a wide range of taxa, all of which share a common environment – the sea. Within this generic group there is a vast diversity of morphology and behaviour, as each species is adapted to its particular range of habitats, from the poles to the tropics, from open oceans to coastal shallows. However, some adaptations are common to all.

Morphological, physiological and behavioural adaptations for survival in the marine environment

Seawater is hypertonic

Seabirds must be able to maintain their water balance in a permanently hypertonic environment.

The nasal or salt glands

Birds have a very limited capacity to produce hyperosmotic urine, and the kidneys alone are incapable of maintaining homeostasis in a marine environment. Many species are able to move between environments in which their intake of water and electrolytes varies greatly. They do this by activating excretion of a hypertonic saline solution containing Na^+, Cl^- and K^+ ions from the nasal glands (Croker et al 1974). Paired nasal glands lie dorsal to the orbit. They are usually bilobed, with a lateral and medial lobe each consisting of blind-ended secretory tubules emptying into a central canal. Each lobe has a separate duct and ostium, opening into the vestibular region of the nasal cavity, or into the oral cavity in taxa without nares. The nasal glands are capable of secreting a hypertonic saline of up to 5% concentration. This enables birds to drink seawater (approximately 3% solution) and still maintain homeostasis (King & McLelland 1984).

When moving from fresh to salt water, the rate of uptake of ingested electrolytes by the intestinal mucosa increases. This triggers secretion from the nasal glands, which continue to function as long as the bird continues to ingest hypertonic drinking water. Any disease or condition that interferes with intestinal absorption will affect the functioning of the nasal glands and the bird's ability to survive in a saltwater environment.

Water is a good thermal conductor

As most seabirds spend prolonged periods floating on or diving beneath the sea, they have plumage that provides an efficient waterproof outer layer over a thick layer of insulating down. Body temperature can further be controlled by the use of circulatory countercurrents in the extremities.

Waterproofing

Water repellency is a function of the anatomy of the feathers. The feather vane, consisting of barbs connected by interlocking barbules, creates a lattice structure with air spaces between. The size of these air spaces is such that an impenetrable air–water interface is created and the feather surface repels water. The efficiency of this lattice structure can be expressed mathematically (Rijke 1968).

The shape of the feathers can also contribute to the efficiency of the waterproof layer as a whole. In particular, the shaft curvature of the ventral contour feathers helps to maintain the continuity of the waterproof layer, and is most pronounced in aquatic birds (Mahaffy 1990). Different species vary in how effectively their plumage is waterproofed; cormorants, for example, have incompletely effective plumage (Rijke 1968), and will eventually 'wet out' as water penetrates into the air spaces. Birds are then forced to leave the water and can be observed with wings outspread, drying out.

Preening

Preening has two functions:

1. To ensure the integrity of the layer of contour feathers – feathers must be correctly aligned with all interlocking barbules in place.
2. To spread the secretions of the uropygial (preen) gland onto the feathers.

The uropygial gland secretes an oily substance consisting mainly of fatty acids, and this is spread on the feathers and skin. The water-repellent characteristics of body feathers are often, and incorrectly, attributed to this secretion; feathers are waterproof by their intrinsic structure. However, over time, feathers exposed to environmental insult, abrasion, immersion in water, ultraviolet light, etc. become dry and brittle, and tend to break. Once the structure of interlocking barbules is lost and a stable lattice no longer exists, the feathers lose their natural water repellency. Regular application of oil from the uropygial gland increases the life of

377

the feathers, which remain supple and strong from one moult to the next.

Although physical abrasion or loss of interlocking barbules will cause loss of water repellency until feathers are replaced at the next moult, there are several other circumstances under which a physically intact feather can lose its water repellency:

1. Clogging of the barbules (e.g. with oil, dirt, etc.). Contamination may not always be obvious to the naked eye.
2. Reduction of the surface tension of water. If contamination with surfactants or small particulate matter causes the surface tension of seawater to drop from the normal 720–750 μN/cm (72–75 dyn/cm) to 650 μN/cm (65 dyn/cm) or below, water will penetrate a bird's plumage and it will become waterlogged (Swennen 1977).
3. Contamination of feathers with surfactant. At a microscopic level, water will fail to form droplets and will penetrate the feather lattice structure. **Failure to remove all surfactant from feathers is the commonest cause of failure of treated oiled birds to regain waterproofing.**

Adaptation to extremes of temperature

Although their dense waterproof plumage insulates against both heat and cold, seabirds that live and nest within the tropics have a limited area of skin available to expose to cooling breezes. The rete mirabile ophthalmicum is an adaptation to maximize cooling without having large areas of exposed skin and is well developed in many taxa. A network of anastomosing arterioles arising from the external ophthalmic branch of the internal carotid artery enmeshes within a venous rete receiving cooled blood from the rostral region of the face and pharyngeal wall, where there is heat loss by evaporation. Some of the emerging arterioles anastomose with intracranial arteries and can thus supply the brain with cooled blood (King & McLelland 1984).

Adaptations for survival in cold climates include a lower body temperature (down to 38.8°C) and a countercurrent tibiotarsal rete in the legs to prevent heat loss from the distal limb.

Seabirds spend most of their time swimming on or flying over the sea

Birds that are adapted to spend much of their lives on the water surface are often ungainly on land. The sea warms slowly and is relatively flat, providing poor thermal uplift for flight, and aerial ocean wanderers therefore have extreme adaptations for soaring flight.

Limb placement and shape

In birds adapted for swimming the pelvic limbs are far caudal on the body, leading to an inability to stand on land or a tendency to an upright posture, bearing weight on the caudal surface of the whole of the lower limb below the hock. Feet are usually webbed or palmate. Surface diving birds may have reduced pneumatization of bones and absence of some air sacs to make them less buoyant. Some aerial oceanic species have long, high aspect-ratio soaring wings. In both cases birds require space free from obstacles and a water surface on which the feet can be used to gain extra speed to become airborne. Take-off from land may require launching from a cliff or a raised mound.

Some surface diving birds (divers, grebes, anhingas, auks) undergo a synchronized annual moult of flight feathers and a flightless period until new feathers grow. This flightless period may be associated with reduced appetite and increased susceptibility to disease.

Marine diets usually consist of fish and/or invertebrates

Marine diets are usually soft and high in protein and fat. Seabirds therefore tend to have a relatively simple digestive system.

Gastrointestinal tract

Beaks may be adapted for catching, holding and swallowing large fish (Fig. 16.1), or for specialized feeding on invertebrates or plankton. The crop is often a simple dilatable portion of the oesophagus, and the gizzard is often vestigial.

Taxonomic classification

(See Table 16.1.)

Gaviiformes and podicipediformes

Divers (Gaviidae) and grebes (Podicipitidae) are foot-propelled, surface diving, fish-eating birds, with a reputation for extreme shyness. They are rarely seen on land. They nest on the margins of freshwater lakes, and the nest is accessible directly from the water. Birds winter in shallow coastal waters.

Their legs are extremely caudal, resulting in difficulty in locomotion on land. The tarsometatarsi are flattened craniocaudally with a teardrop cross-section for maximum hydrodynamic efficiency. Grebes have a lobate foot. When swimming, the tibiotarsus is rotated 90° at the end of the power stroke to reduce resistance to forward motion on the recovery stroke (King & McLelland 1984).

The feather structure is primitive, with few barbs and barbules and an open structure, and birds must spend a considerable time on the water preening in order to maintain waterproofing. Feather eating is a phenomenon observed in grebes. Adults will ingest their own feathers,

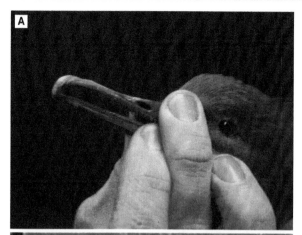

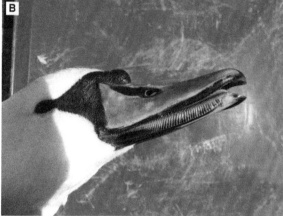

Fig 16.1 A Goosander beak showing adaptation for catching, holding and swallowing large fish. **B** Mute swan showing ridged beak adaptation for filtering sediment.

Table 16.1 Taxonomic classification of seabirds

Gaviiformes	Gaviidae	Divers, loons
Podicipediformes	Podicipitidae	Grebes
Sphenisciformes		Penguins:
	Pygoscelidae	Adelie, chinstrap, gentoo
	Aptenodyptidae	Emperor, king
	Eudyptidae	Rockhopper, macaroni
	Megadyptidae	Yellow-eyed
	Spheniscidae	African, Humboldt, Magellanic, Galapagos
	Eudypotulidae	Little blue
Procellariiformes	Diomedeidae	Albatrosses
	Procellariidae	Petrels, prions, shearwaters
Pelecaniformes	Phaethontidae	Tropic birds
	Pelecanidae	Pelicans
	Sulidae	Gannets, boobies
	Phalacrocoracidae	Cormorants
	Anhingidae	Anhingas
	Fregatidae	Frigate birds
Charadriiformes	Rostratulidae	Painted snipe
	Haematopdidae	Oystercatchers
	Recurvirostridae	Stilts, avocets
	Dromadidae	Crab plover
	Burhinidae	Stone curlews
	Glareolidae	Coursers, pratincoles
	Charadriidae	Plovers, lapwings
	Scolopacidae	Sandpipers and allies
	Stercorariidae	Skuas
	Laridae	Gulls
	Sternidae	Terns
	Rhynchopidae	Skimmers
	Alcidae	Auks

and even feed feathers to their chicks. Grebes have also been observed to regurgitate pellets of feather and bone. It has been postulated that this activity may have a function in reducing proventricular parasitic burdens (Piersma & Van Eerden 1988). Unusually for fish-eating birds, grebes have a small but distinct gizzard. Gizzard impaction with a mixture of feathers, oil and sand was considered to be a contributory factor in mortality of grebes in the Gulf War oil spill (Greth et al 1995).

In captivity, whenever these birds are on land they move by resting on their keels and propelling themselves with their back feet, resulting in keel lesions and damage to feather structure over the breast leading to waterproofing problems (Fig. 16.2). Their extreme shyness makes them difficult patients, prone to stress-associated deaths.

Sphenisciformes

Penguins (Sphenisciformes) occur only in the southern hemisphere, and in cooler waters; but this encompasses a range from the high Antarctic to the Galapagos islands on the equator. There are seventeen species of six genera recognized (see Table 16.1). Penguins are amongst the best-studied avian groups kept in zoos (Beall et al 1994), and the African penguin (*Spheniscus demersus*) is probably the only avian species for which rehabilitation has been shown to have played a major role in its conservation (Nel & Whittington 2003). Penguins are flightless, their wings have no flight feathers and are modified into stiff flippers with which they propel themselves underwater to feed on fish and squid. Long bones are not pneumatized. Feathers are not arranged in tracts; short stiff

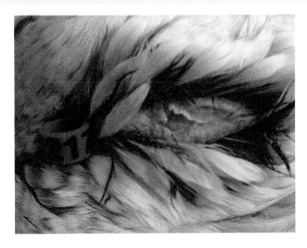

Fig 16.2 Birds which are unable to stand on land are prone to sternal ulceration during hospitalization. Such lesions carry a grave prognosis as the bird cannot be returned to water. (Photo credit IFAW.)

feathers underlaid by thick down cover the whole body apart from the feet and some areas of the face. There is a significant fat (blubber) layer under the skin. Penguins undergo an annual moult during which all feathers are replaced and birds are unable to take to water. During this moult period the bird starves, and up to half its body weight can be lost. With webbed feet, a pelvic limb placed far caudally on a torpedo-shaped body, and a very short tarsometatarsus, penguins have a characteristic upright stance and waddling gait on land. Despite this they are remarkably agile on land or ice and can move over rough terrain and undertake journeys of considerable distance.

Procellariiformes

All except the storm petrels (Hydrobatidae) have long slender wings adapted to soaring flight. They require considerable space to become airborne, and use wind and wave action to aid uplift. Nest sites are often close to cliffs, which are utilized to become airborne. All are oceanic birds that come ashore only to breed and nest, on cliffs or isolated islands. Shearwaters and smaller petrels (Procellariidae) breed in burrows, and often return to the nest site only at night. Legs are placed caudally, and the gait on land is shuffling, utilizing all the caudal aspect of the leg below the hock. The nares are covered dorsally by the operculum, a keratinized flap tubular in structure. The tiny Wilson's storm petrel (*Oceanites oceanicus*) is, surprisingly, one of the world's most numerous birds.

Food consists of fish, invertebrates and plankton. Albatrosses (Diomedeidae) and large petrels will scavenge and often follow ships. Prions (Procellariidae) have hair-like lamellae fringing the bill to aid in straining plankton from the water. Small petrels will flutter close to the surface of the sea, 'walking on the water', whilst feeding.

Fulmars (*Fulmarus glacialis*) are capable of projectile vomiting an oily crop secretion as a defence mechanism. This foul-smelling oil is particularly difficult to remove from plumage, and birds contaminated in the wild frequently die as a result. Captive fulmars often become oiled by their own vomit and require careful washing before release.

Pelecaniformes

Pelecaniformes are fish-eating birds and may be surface divers, such as cormorants and anhingas (Anhingidae), or aerial divers, such as gannets (Sulidae) and brown pelicans (*Pelicanus occidentalis*) (Fig. 16.3). Frigate birds (Fregatidae) are specialized piratical feeders, and harry other birds until they disgorge their stomach contents.

In pelicans (Pelecanidae), the entire floor of the mouth is enormously enlarged for catching fish. The tongue is vestigial in pelicans, cormorants, anhingas and gannets. **Cormorants, gannets, anhingas and frigate birds have no nostrils and breathe through the corners of the mouth, which should not be obstructed during handling or restraint.** The salt gland duct opens directly into the oral cavity. Gannets and cormorants have craniocaudally flattened tarsometatarsi with a teardrop profile, and cormorants have webs on all four digits.

The plumage of cormorants and anhingas is imperfectly waterproof, and after a period in the water they must come ashore to dry out – they are often seen in their typical open-winged posture. Frigate birds also have imperfectly water-repellent plumage. As piratical feeders they do not land on the water, and if forced to do so may become waterlogged and unable to take off again.

Gannets and brown pelicans have air sac diverticula subcutaneously and following the fascial planes between the skeletal muscles over the neck and breast. These are presumed to act as pneumatic shock-absorbers when diving for fish from heights of 35 metres or more. These air sac diverticula can be inflated when stressed, e.g. when handled (Fig. 16.4).

Charadriiformes

The group of birds generally referred to as waders contains 15 families and subfamilies, typical examples being oystercatchers (Haematopididae), plovers (Charadriidae) and sandpipers (Scolopacidae). These are birds of shorelines and estuarine mudflats, and are characterized by long legs and bills suited to feeding on invertebrates in shallow water. There are many adaptations for specialist feeding within this group, e.g. the long downcurved bill of curlews (Tringinae) enabling feeding on invertebrates buried deep in mud, and the long upcurved beak of avocets (Recurvirostridae), which is used in a sweeping movement through the water to sift food from just beneath the surface. They are ground nesters, some taxa favouring

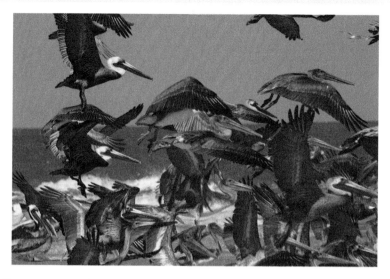

Fig 16.3 Brown pelicans (*Pelicanus occidentalis*).

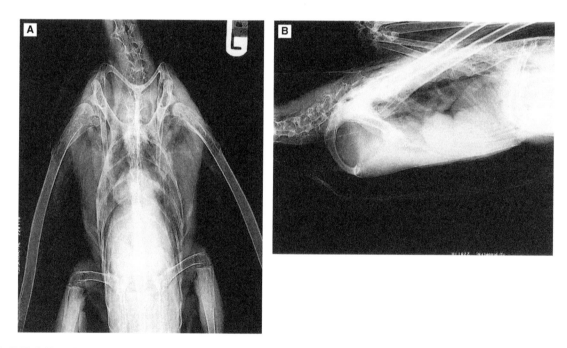

Fig 16.4A, B Normal radiographs of a gannet. This bird has inflated its air sac diverticula, and subcutaneous air can clearly be seen. (Photo credit RSPCA.)

rocky shorelines, others nest on uplands or polar tundra. Many taxa migrate long distances, following traditional flyways between summer nesting sites and winter feeding grounds.

Skuas (Stercorariidae) are aggressive and piratical, but also eat offal and food scraps. Gulls (Laridae) are gregarious and largely coastal. They will often feed on offal, and can be found far inland. Terns (Sterninae) are long-winged and graceful and are totally aquatic in life-style, so they are rarely found far from open water. They

are colony breeders and often migrate long distances. The arctic tern (*Sterna paradisaea*) has the longest migration of any bird, breeding in the Arctic and migrating to the Antarctic.

Auks (Alcidae) are dumpy, wing-propelled diving birds. Their wings are short and narrow, and they can have some difficulty in becoming airborne, paddling the surface of the water with their feet for some distance to build up sufficient speed for take-off. Their legs are placed caudally, and on land they stand upright with their weight resting on the whole of the caudal surface of the leg below the hock. Special rings (bands) have been developed by researchers for cliff ledge nesters such as guillemots (*Uria aalge*) (known as common murres in North America) and razorbills (*Alca torda*). These bands are triangular in section so they present a flat surface to the rock when the bird is standing and thus avoid excessive wear. Puffins (*Fratercula arctica*) are burrow nesters. They have ornate coloured keratinized bill plates, which are shed in sheets at the end of the breeding season. The epithelium of the inside of the mouth of guillemots and razorbills is yellow, and is particularly bright during the breeding season.

Husbandry

Environment

Three separate media – land, water and air – must be considered when providing a captive environment for seabirds. The balance between the three media in an enclosure will vary depending on the anatomical and behavioural specializations of the species under consideration, and the purpose for which the enclosure is intended (display, rehabilitation, captive breeding, etc.). Auks have been successfully maintained in enclosures with water and air only and no access to land, except for artificial breeding ledges during the breeding season (Swennen 1977).

Land

Pool surrounds should be free draining, easy to clean, and have a textured surface to avoid continual pressure on the weight-bearing surfaces of the foot and lower limb.

Concrete surrounds to pools usually become covered with a thin layer of moist guano, which leads to abrasions and pressure necrosis of the feet (and tarsometatarsi and hocks if in contact with the ground), rapidly progressing to pododermatitis (bumblefoot) (Fig. 16.5). To avoid this problem, various substrates have been used, e.g. pea gravel, textured rubber or plastic matting (solid or perforated for drainage), clay, cat litter, natural and artificial turf, and natural and artificial rocks. In general, the floor surface should be free draining and dry quickly, and it should allow the bird to spread its weight over the whole of the weight-bearing surface of the lower limb. If a hard surface is preferred for ease of cleaning, it should be sufficiently textured or uneven to distribute the weight of the bird variably across the weight-bearing surface as it moves, without easily trapping dirt. Perches should be provided for those birds that will use them (cormorants, anhingas and pelicans), and perch surfaces should be chosen for the same characteristics.

Whatever materials are selected for the land surface in a pen or exhibit, it is necessary that adequate cleanliness can be maintained to avoid build-up of excretions, waste food, etc., which may lead to outbreaks of gastrointestinal

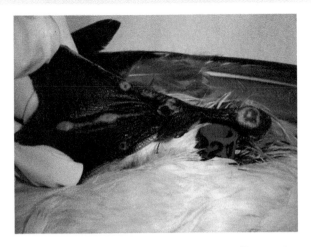

Fig 16.5 Foot and hock lesions caused by poor substrate. (Photo credit IFAW.)

disease and secondary infection of any skin lesions. Care must be taken that disinfectants used are compatible with any pool water biocide. Disinfectants can be toxic if used at excessive concentrations. The new generation of 'oxygen disinfectants' is generally effective and safe.

Water

Seabirds can be kept on fresh water, but if they are to be released onto the sea they may benefit from the addition of salt to the diet (3 g/kg) to maintain the function of the nasal gland.

Water systems can vary from simple pools with a constant through-flow for waste, to highly sophisticated recycling systems. Clean water is essential for the health and welfare of the birds. Clarity of water is often important in display facilities, especially those with underwater viewing. Water treatment systems may work by one or more of the following methods.

Surface skimming

Contamination of the water surface can lead to a reduction in the surface tension or direct contamination of feathers, resulting in a loss of waterproofing. Fish-eating birds are especially prone to contamination with oil from food and faeces. Surface skimming, e.g. draining all or some of the water flow through the pool from the surface, either to waste or into a recirculation system, is an efficient method of controlling this problem.

Pressures andfi ltration

Pressure sand filtration removes inorganic particles and some organic matter. Excess organic matter will rapidly cause compaction and channelling of the filter bed, with water streaming through channels between compacted masses of sand, resulting in reduced efficiency and, eventually, the need to replace the filter bed. If used alone, regular replacement of a proportion of the water is required to prevent build-up of organic matter.

Biological filtration

A biological filter, containing a stable population of autotrophic and heterotrophic microorganisms, will turn nitrogenous waste first into nitrites and then into non-toxic nitrates. In larger units, the filter usually consists of a biotower full of plastic spheres to maximize the active surface area through which some or all of the water will pass on each recirculation.

Biocides

1. *Chlorine.* Free chlorine is an effective biocide at 0.3–3.0 ppm and a pH of not less than 7.6. Free chlorine is usually achieved by the addition of sodium hypochlorite to the water. However, chlorine can combine with organic matter to produce toxic chloramines, especially at lower pH. Chloramines produce skin and eye lesions. Difficulty in monitoring and controlling chloramine levels has led to the abandonment of the use of chlorine in most modern systems.

2. *Ozone.* Bubbled through a tower to allow maximum water contact, ozone is an effective oxidative biocide. In salt water (minimum 2.5% NaCl), ozone can also be used for protein skimming (see later). Ozone is toxic at low levels, so its use is limited to the plant room. Residues in the water returning to the pool must be maintained at below 0.1 mg/L. A suitably calibrated redox meter can be used to control automatically any violations. Unlike chlorine systems, there is no residual biocidal activity in the pool water. This can lead to algal growth on pool surfaces, which may require physical removal or the use of a proprietary algicide.

3. *Ultraviolet light.* Ultraviolet light can be an effective biocide in clear water. Scintillation from particles in the water rapidly reduces the effectiveness of the treatment, so ultraviolet light is generally used after filtration, when water is at its clearest. Ultraviolet light also accelerates the breakdown of ozone, and can be useful in preventing free ozone returning to the pools. Its use is obviously restricted to the plant room.

Algicides

A variety of commercial algicides is available, including those based on copper and bromine.

Protein skimming

First used in saltwater fish farming, protein skimming is now utilized successfully in water systems for marine mammals and birds. Ozone and air are injected into a column of water through a venturi. This ensures good mixing and agitation. Long-chain fat and protein molecules are oxidized and broken down into smaller molecules, which are surfactant and form a stable foam on the surface. This can then be skimmed to waste. If the biological load on the system is very high it is possible that some surfactant may remain on the water surface, resulting in lowered surface tension and wetting of plumage. However, this does not appear to be a problem in well-designed systems.

Air

Larger species that are mobile on land and water may be rendered permanently flightless by pinioning, e.g. cormorants, pelicans.

Surface-diving birds such as auks have difficulty in becoming airborne and need to paddle along the surface of the water with their feet. They are relatively unmanoeuvrable in flight, and are therefore in danger of crashing into enclosure netting. Pinioning is inadvisable, as they use their wings to propel themselves whilst diving. The design of the enclosure must take this into account, although reports of injury are rare despite repeated collisions with enclosure netting (Swennen 1977). Enclosures sited in exposed locations may be subject to high winds, which can blow birds against the netting.

In extremes of ambient temperature, it may be necessary to provide an artificially heated or cooled environment. When conditioned air is recirculated, it should be filtered through a fine particulate filter capable of removing fungal spores.

Breeding

Penguins have been bred successfully in captivity for many years. Amongst other taxa there are relatively few breeding successes, notably of Pelecaniformes – pelicans, gannets and cormorants, and Charadriiformes – various waders, gulls, terns, and auks. Recent trends towards multi-taxa exhibits based on specific habitats has led to the keeping of a wider range of seabird taxa and an increased range of captive breeding.

Although many taxa exhibit breeding plumage, most of the species under consideration are monomorphic and it is difficult to differentiate sexes on appearance alone. A notable exception is the ruff (*Philomachus pugnax*). During the breeding season males develop flamboyant and variable head plumes, which are used to compete for females at ritualized courtships or 'leks'. The subfamily Phalaropidinae exhibit role reversal, the female phalarope being more brightly coloured, and the more subdued male incubating the eggs.

Colony breeders, such as cormorants, may be stimulated to courtship and nesting behaviour by the presence of other birds, and may require a minimum colony size of a dozen or more pairs. Penguins are usually housed in colonies large enough that birds can select their own mates although selective pairing can be achieved if necessary (Beall et al 1994). Sufficient area, materials and, where appropriate, nest boxes (for burrow nesters) or platforms must be available, bearing in mind the territorial behaviour of the species concerned. Nest boxes must be adequately drained and ventilated for disease prevention. Guillemots and razorbills will breed on artificial ledges. The height above the water level of these ledges is not critical (Swennen 1977).

Of the taxa under consideration, only waders are precocial. In the wild, newly hatched wader chicks are heavily reliant on the copious quantities of insects and their larvae present on the breeding grounds for the high energy and protein diet required for their rapid growth, many species more than doubling their weight during the first week of life (Hale 1980). In captivity chicks can be induced to eat artificial diets, but parental care is still an advantage in achieving survival to fledging.

Altricial species are best parent reared whenever possible. Penguins achieve higher growth rates and have fewer health problems when parent reared compared to hand reared, and problems of integration into the colony due to imprinting are avoided. Parents may need two to three times their normal quantity of food during the rearing period (Beall et al 1994).

Handling

Seabirds present no special problems in handling, although some have sharp and pointed beaks and require careful restraint. Cleanliness of operators and equipment is important to ensure that plumage is not contaminated during handling, and care must be taken not to damage or excessively disrupt the feathers. Birds usually require a period of preening following handling to ensure their feathers are correctly aligned for waterproofing.

Soft-rimmed aviary nets are useful for catching birds. Care must be taken to avoid personal injury from sharp pointed beaks, and safety glasses or goggles are recommended. Keeping the bird's head covered with a towel is usually adequate. Light gloves can be used for protection if preferred. Large birds such as penguins and pelicans may be restrained by kneeling astride the bird, using the knees to restrain the wings (flippers) and the hands to control the head. The larger penguin species require two people for restraint. Care must be taken when handling waders to avoid damage to long delicate beaks and legs.

Penguins can be restrained in a light conical plastic tube, open at both ends – traffic cones can be adapted for this purpose.

Sharp beaks may be controlled with tape or a rubber band during more prolonged handling, e.g. washing. In species with no nares the beak must not be taped closed, and a small gag – a matchstick or syringe plunger is adequate – should be taped across the beak to ensure that breathing is not restricted.

Feeding

The majority of seabirds are fed on fresh or frozen fish. Feeding fresh fish may carry an increased risk of transmission of parasitic infestations. Frozen fish are best thawed dry in a refrigerator at 2°C. When available, fish which are blast frozen at sea are preferable. Frozen fish should be stored at −20°C for not more than 6 months. The wet weight required for daily maintenance is variable, as fish can vary greatly in energy density through the season. Most seabirds can be safely fed to appetite, but some (e.g. penguins, gulls and skuas) may become obese. Regular monitoring of body weight and adjustment of the feeding level is preferable. The total daily requirement may be up to 30% of the body weight.

Waders feed on a wide variety of invertebrate prey, including marine worms, crustacea and insects. In summer on breeding grounds berries may be eaten. In captivity live food such as mealworms and brine shrimps, as well as a variety of artificial alternatives such as dog food or trout pellets, can be utilized. Food is best placed in a suitable medium, such as a sand or mud slurry, to stimulate natural feeding behaviour.

Vitamin and mineral supplementation

It is usual to supplement diets for captive seabirds with both mixed B vitamins and oil-soluble vitamins A, D and E. However, alcids have been kept in captivity for years on a diet of frozen fish without any supplementation (Swennen 1977).

There is a danger of thiaminase-induced thiamine deficiency in birds fed stored frozen fish. For adequate maintenance of thiamine levels in the presence of dietary thiaminase, oral supplements (20 mg thiamine/kg body weight) should be given about an hour before feeding. A better alternative is supplementation by parenteral administration. The same dose rate appears to be effective, given once or twice weekly.

Penguins kept on fresh water are frequently given in-feed salt supplementation. However, Mazzaro et al (2004) demonstrated no difference in plasma electrolytes in penguins experimentally maintained with and without salt supplementation, suggesting that penguins do not need to ingest high levels of salt to remain in electrolyte balance, and penguins maintained in freshwater exhibits on a herring, capelin or squid-based diet do not require supplementation.

Nursing

Hospitalization

Hospitalized birds may be kept individually or in groups in cages or pens. In social birds, the behavioural advantage of group housing must be balanced against the necessity for isolation for disease control and clinical monitoring. Usually sick, injured or oiled birds will not be allowed access to water for bathing, to avoid the danger of waterlogging and hypothermia. Damage to the feet and legs, keel and feathers can easily occur. Abrasion and faecal soiling must be kept to a minimum. Birds unable to stand, such as divers and grebes, can be kept on soft nylon netting stretched across a frame inserted into cages or pens to form a false floor (Fig. 16.6). This allows droppings to fall through, reducing soiling, and lessens abrasion on the limbs, keel and feathers. Soft bedding such as rubber mats, deep layers of newspaper, old towels or blankets or even wood shavings can be utilized, but will need frequent changing.

The copious quantities of highly nitrogenous droppings produced by fish-eating birds can rapidly lead to unacceptable atmospheric conditions within the hospital area and the danger of respiratory disease, especially aspergillosis. A ventilation rate of 12 or more air changes per hour is required to prevent the build-up of ammonia in the atmosphere. Such high ventilation rates may necessitate air conditioning to maintain an adequate room temperature.

When birds are kept off water for several days, legs and webbed feet may become dry and brittle. Regular application of petroleum jelly will prevent this, but care must be taken because contaminated plumage will become non-waterproof and require washing before the bird returns to the water.

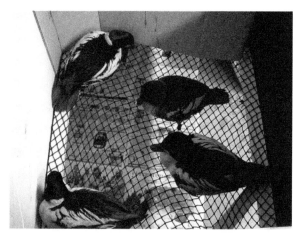

Fig 16.6 Soft net bottomed cages can reduce iatrogenic damage during hospitalization. (Photo credit IFAW.)

Alcidae will climb on rocks placed in a cage or pen, with a beneficial effect on foot condition. Cormorants will perch on anything, even an upturned bucket, which will keep feet and plumage clear of a soiled floor.

Nutrition

Fluid therapy

The detection and treatment of dehydration follow the general principles of avian medicine, although close feathering and thick down can make detection of dehydration more difficult. As a rule of thumb, if dehydration is detectable, the bird is more than 5% dehydrated. More than 15% dehydration is incompatible with life; therefore it is fair to assume a 10% dehydration level. Fluid deficits should be rectified by administration of 10% of body weight (BW) daily in divided doses. This can be considered as 5% BW maintenance + 5% BW (e.g. half the deficit). This dose can be repeated in each 24 h period until there are no signs of dehydration.

Fluids can be administered i.v., s.c., i.o. or p.o. in divided doses. The i.v. route can be used through any accessible vein. If a slow infusion is impossible due to difficulties of restraint or the small size of available veins, an initial bolus of fluid may be given by slow intravenous injection over 1–2 minutes and the rest by an alternative route.

The intraosseous (i.o.) route is possible where i.v. infusion is impracticable (Otto et al 1989). Power- or pressure-driven syringes (e.g. Flowline, Pacific Medical Supplies Pty Ltd, Vic., Australia) are ideal for this method of administration.

Birds should be offered food within 24 hours (Table 16.2), and many will start to eat. If clinical evidence of dehydration persists, administration of fluids should be continued despite self-feeding. Emaciated birds, or birds that fail to self-feed, may be started on a high-energy supplement. Oiled birds may require fluids routinely for 4–8 days despite self-feeding (see also Table 16.3).

Starvation/emaciation

Birds received in rescue centres are frequently emaciated. Clinical investigation is always indicated; however, such birds are rarely suffering from chronic wasting diseases. Emaciated birds may be individual cases or part of a larger incident. There are many reasons why seabirds may suffer from starvation/emaciation, including the following:

- immaturity – immature birds may be naive hunters and fail to meet their nutritional requirements; parasitism and population pressures may be additional stressors
- inclement weather – this may result in reduced feeding opportunities

Table 16.2 Feeding sick birds

Days 1 and 2

Oral rehydration fluid, either as part of rehydration therapy, or as a bland base from which to start any change of diet.

After 24 hours substitute the following mixture given by gavage at 10–20% body weight/day in two to four feeds:

- 50 mL Lectade Plus (SmithKline Beecham) – oral rehydration fluid
- Two tins A/D Diet (Hills Pet Nutrition) – a canine/feline convalescent diet
- 10 mL Ensure Plus (Abbot Laboratories) – a human liquid nutrition product
- ½ Aquavit (International Zoological Veterinary Group) – vitamin supplement high in B_1 and E
- 1× 200 mg ferrous sulphate tablet.

Days 3 and 4

Offer whole fish of a suitable size from Day 3. Birds normally select fish by girth rather than length, and prefer fish smaller than the maximum size they can swallow. Use fish of high calorific value.

Day 5 onwards

If the bird does not start to self-feed, start force feeding fish from Day 5, in addition to gavage, and continue until self-feeding starts. Up to 30% body weight can be given in up to four feeds daily.

However, unless there is weight loss keep force feeding to a minimum to avoid suppressing appetite and delaying the onset of self-feeding. It is rare to force feed more than 20% body weight in two feeds.

Throughout treatment

Weigh bird daily and continue gavage until there is a consistent weight gain over several days, and preferably until the bird has achieved the acceptable minimum weight (AMW) for the species, if known. However, AMW can vary with sex, age, time of year, race or subspecies, etc. and may be difficult to determine.

Table 16.3 Nutritional slurry recipes for oiled birds
3 cups Flamingo breeder pellets
3 ½ cups water
1 multivitamin tablet
100 mg thiamine tablet
Slurry is c. 1 kcal/mL

Source: Oiled Wildlife Care Network/International Bird Rescue Research Centre protocols. These nutritional slurries can also be used as supportive care for sick birds.

- failure of local fish stocks – due to commercial over-fishing, climatic variations or mass mortality events
- long migration
- oiling.

Emaciated birds that have been starving for some time require careful nursing. Overfeeding can result in collapse and death, the physiological demands of a full proventriculus apparently precipitating circulatory failure.

Feeding

Often fish tossed into a tray of shallow water will attract attention and trigger feeding behaviour. The tray should be dark in colour so the silver fish stand out against it. Communal species may be stimulated to eat in the presence of other birds.

Scavengers such as gulls can be treated in a similar way, but offered chopped fish or day-old chicks, or dog or cat food. It may be difficult to persuade invertebrate or plankton eaters to self-feed. However, mealworms, live brine shrimp or artificial diets for plankton-eating fish available through the aquarium trade are worth trying. Some may eat chopped fish or shrimp.

'Die-offs' or 'wrecks'

These are terms used to describe mass mortality events in wild birds. Often the first sign of a large-scale mortality in seabirds will be the discovery of large numbers of sick, dying and dead birds, either at a breeding site or washed up along the shore.

Trauma

Traumatic injuries can be treated according to the basic principles of avian medicine, and present no special problems. Commonly encountered problems in wild seabirds include:

- entanglement in or ingestion of fishing tackle (hooks, monofilament line and nets) or general marine debris such as cargo nets and six-pack plastic rings
- gunshot wounds
- attack by predators, birds, mammals or fish
- laceration by boat propellers, collision with speedboats, jet skis, etc.

Commonly encountered problems in captive birds include:

- pododermatitis and sternal ulceration (Figs 16.2 and 16.5)
- ingestion of foreign bodies, either enclosure substrate, or objects thrown into the enclosure
- heatstroke in polar birds kept in warm climates
- frostbite in tropical birds kept in cold climates.

These can all be prevented by provision of a suitable captive environment.

Care must be taken when treating body wounds not to remove excessive numbers of feathers and not to contaminate the plumage if the bird is to be returned quickly to water. For example, keel ulceration can be treated by debridement and removal of necrotic tissue followed by closure of the wound with absorbable sutures, tissue glue or a combination of the two. A non-detergent skin disinfectant is used for skin preparation and a minimum number of feathers plucked from the wound edges, so that after wound closure the breast feathers, once realigned, will completely cover the wound. The bird can then be rapidly reintroduced to water to prevent recurrence of the condition.

Dressings for webbed feet are best applied with the digits extended, to prevent loss of elasticity of the web and flexibility of the foot. A template of stiff cardboard or light plastic is cut in the shape of the extended foot. The required dressing is sandwiched between the plantar surface of the foot and the template, and with the foot extended, a lightly adhesive tape is applied around the dorsal surface of the foot and the template. A protective dressing can then be applied.

Soaring birds with legs far caudal, such as fulmars, may be unable to take off from flat ground, and if they accidentally land they can become stranded. If in good condition, such birds can simply be moved to a suitable elevated location from which they can re-launch themselves. Recently fledged juvenile birds are frequently found many miles inland after severe onshore storms. They are often undamaged but dehydrated and/or starving, and require first aid and feeding before release at a suitable coastal site. Newly fledged petrels and shearwaters leave their nest burrows at dusk and head towards the open sea, which they recognize by its lighter horizon compared to land. Artificial light can confuse them and cause them to fly inshore. If stranded on shore or close to the coast during daylight, they will easily fall prey to predators such as gulls and skuas. Such birds can be collected, confined in safety over the day, and released at dusk in a suitable location away from artificial lights.

Neoplasia

Neoplasia is reported in the literature only in captive penguins, which is probably due to the longevity of penguins in captivity and the degree of clinical attention given to them.

Reported neoplasias are listed in Table 16.4.

Metabolic diseases

Visceral gout

At post-mortem examination, chalky white urate deposits are found on all visceral surfaces and in renal

Table 16.4

Neoplasia	Species affected	Author
Malignant melanoma	Humboldt penguin	Shindu (1998)
		Rambaud et al (2003)
Cholangiocarcinoma	Adelie penguin	Renner et al (2001)
Proventricular adenocarcinoma	Humboldt penguin	Cho et al (1998)
		Yonemaru et al (2004)

tubules. Visceral gout is usually considered to be secondary to dehydration.

Hypothyroidism

Deaths in captive Humboldt penguin chicks in Germany were associated with a high (76%) prevalence of thyroid lesions. Preventative treatment with levothyroxine at 0.2 mg/kg body weight appeared to be successful in reducing mortality (Burkle et al 2002).

Infectious diseases

Bacterial

Bacteria, especially Enterobacteriaceae, are a major cause of death in captive collections (Kaneene et al 1985). In contrast, wild seabirds rarely die of primary bacterial disease. Carcasses recovered during die-offs or mortality surveys are frequently autolysed, and it can be difficult to determine the significance of isolates.

Sudden death and high mortality has been recorded in gentoo penguins (*Pygoscelis papua*) due to infection with *Clostridium perfringens*. Necropsy revealed enlarged friable livers and enlarged congested spleens with mild lymphoid hyperplasia. Histopathology revealed moderate multifocal hepatocyte necrosis with karyorrhexis and granulocyte hyperplasia. Transmission from scavenging seabirds was suspected as the source of infection. An alpha enterotoxin activity was demonstrated, and removing birds to a different environment prevented further deaths (Fielding 2000). A similar mortality of Humboldt penguins (*Spheniscus humboldti*) due to *C. perfringens* was positive for epsilon toxin but negative for beta toxin, indicating a type D infection. Vaccination against *C. perfringens* types B, C and D prevented further deaths. A transient reaction was noted after the first vaccine dose, which was milder after the second dose (Greenwood 2000).

Some bacterial isolates associated with clinical signs and/or pathology are shown in Table 16.5.

Therapy is best matched to in-vitro sensitivity testing when possible, but in the absence of such specific guidelines, the clinician may choose any of the broad-spectrum antibiotics commonly used in birds, bearing in mind the common potential pathogens in seabirds.

Table 16.5 Some bacterial isolates associated with clinical signs and/or pathology

Bacterial isolate	Clinical signs	Pathology	Taxa affected, comments	Source
Escherichia coli	Diarrhoea, dehydration, soiling of vent. Respiratory distress, sudden death	Enteritis, peritonitis, pericarditis, air sacculitis, granulomatous and necrotic pneumonia	Various, including Alcidae, Laridae, Phalacocoridae	Author
E. coli (with *Edwardisiella tarda* and *Staphylococcus aureus*)	Dehydration, drooping wings, sudden death	Septicaemia, swollen liver, necrotic enteritis	Shag (secondary to oiling)	Wood et al (1993)
Klebsiella pneumoniae (with *Yersinia enterolytica*)	Seabird wreck	Diffuse lymphoid infiltration of lungs	Kittiwakes and guillemots	Louzis et al (1984)
Salmonella spp. (with *Clostridium perfringens*, various *Clostridia* spp. And *Pseudomonas* spp.)	Emaciation, dehydration, severe diarrhoea	Haemorrhagic gastroenteritis, peritonitis	Brown pelicans (associated with sewage contamination)	Ankerberg (1984)
Clostridium perfringens	Not known	Severe haemorrhagic necrotizing enteritis	Alcidae	Petermann et al (1989)
Yersinia enterolytica (with *K. pneumoniae*)	Seabird wreck	Diffuse lymphoid infiltration of lungs	Kittiwakes and guillemots	Louzis et al (1984)
Streptococcus zooepidemicus	Die-off, sudden death	Enlarged buff-coloured liver, congested and oedematous lungs	Grebes	Jensen (1979)
Erysipelothrix rhusiopathiae	Die-off, sudden death	Enlarged friable liver, petechial haemorrhage in pericardial and subcutaneous fat	Mainly grebes, some gulls and ducks	Jensen & Cotter (1976)
Erysipelothrix rhusiopathiae	Dull, recumbency, inappetence, death in 24 hours	Pulmonary congestion, intestinal haemorrhage, necrosis of tips of villi, mononucleosis and short Gram +ve bacilli in microvasculature	Little blue penguin	Boerner et al (2004)
Edwardisiella tarda	Weak, unable to fly, rapid death	Necrotic enteritis but no histological evidence of systemic bacterial invasion	Brown pelicans, common loons and ring-billed gulls	White et al (1973)
Pasteurella multocida	Avian cholera, occurring as epizootic, sudden death of wild birds	Generalized congestion, polyserositis, large numbers of circulating bacteria in ovary, air sacs and pleura	Herring gulls and greater black-backed gulls, guillemots	Osterblom et al (2004)
Pseudomonas spp.	Dehydration, collapse, sudden death	Air sacculitis, septicaemia	Oiled guillemots and razorbills	Author
Pseudomonas spp.	Emaciation, inappetence	Multifocal granulomatous hepatitis	Red-throated diver, *Gavia stellata*	Author
P. putrifaciens, P. fluorescens	Emaciation, dehydration, severe diarrhoea	Haemorrhagic gastroenteritis, peritonitis	Brown pelicans, associated with sewage contamination	Ankerberg (1984)
Nocardia asteroides		Adherent plaques in air sacs, fibrinous exudate with branching filamentous bacteria	Laysan albatross (*Diomedea immutabilis*)	Sileo et al 1990
Mycoplasma sphenisci (sp. nov.)	Recurrent mucocaseous choanal discharge		African penguin	Frasca et al 2005

Viral

Newcastle disease (paramyxovirus type 1)

A neurotropic velogenic, Newcastle disease virus (NDV) has caused excessive mortality in breeding flocks of double-crested cormorants (*Phalacrocorax auritus*) (Banerjee et al 1994). Clinical signs included weakness, lethargy, diarrhoea, respiratory distress, paralysis of wings and legs, torticollis and incoordination. On gross post-mortem examination, the most consistent lesions were oedema of the eyelids and periocular tissues, pulmonary oedema and congestion, splenomegaly, hepatic necrosis and scattered haemorrhages in visceral organs. Histological lesions included severe lymphocytic meningoencephalitis and myelitis, and splenic lymphoid necrosis with haemorrhage.

Paramyxovirus type 1 of unknown clinical significance has also been isolated from guillemots, tufted puffins and European cormorants (Stoskopf & Kennedy-Stoskopf 1986, Petermann et al 1989). A single gannet (*Sula bassana*) died of nephritis apparently associated with Newcastle disease (Wilson 1950).

Tick-borne viruses

A large number of viruses have been isolated from seabird ticks, and in some cases have been shown to infect their host (Holmes 1995). Occasionally such viruses have been implicated in clinical disease. For example, Soldado virus, an arbovirus isolated from the tick *Ornithodoros capensis*, was implicated in the die-off of thousands of sooty terns (*Sterna fusicata nubilosa*) on Bird Island in the Seychelles (Converse et al 1975).

However, many isolations are from ticks only, either from dead birds, or from ticks recovered at nest sites.

Puffinosis

Manx shearwaters (*Puffinus puffinus*) breeding on the islands of Skokholm and Skomer off southwest Wales annually suffer significant mortality amongst fledglings. Large vesicles develop on the webs of the feet, and rapidly rupture. There may be unilateral or bilateral paresis, particularly a spastic paralysis of the legs. Some birds develop a purulent conjunctivitis. There are no pathognomonic lesions on gross post-mortem. Histology of the developing vesicles reveals enlarged nucleoli and vacuolation of the cytoplasm.

Morbidity is highest in late fledging chicks, and may be up to 25%. Mortality may average 4% of total fledglings annually, and does not appear to affect the total population (Brooke 1990).

It is believed that the disease is caused by an uncharacterized virus and spread by the trombiculid mite (*Neotrombicula autumnalis*), which infests breeding burrows. Use of doxycycline has been found to reduce mortality in affected chicks (Brooke 1990).

Other taxa have shown similar foot lesions, including oystercatchers (*Haematopus ostralegus*), various gulls, and shags (*Phalacrocorax aristotelis*). Foot lesions combined with conjunctivitis have been seen in fulmars, but with no associated mortality. Significant mortality has occurred in some penguin species (Stoskopf & Kennedy-Stoskopf 1986).

Avipox

Cutaneous lesions caused by avipox viruses have been described in guillemots (Hill & Bogue 1978), white-tailed tropic birds (*Phaethon lepturus*) (Wingate et al 1980) and royal terns (*Sterna maxima*) (Jacobson et al 1980). Lesions are typically dry, crusty, raised papules, usually occurring on unfeathered skin. Although persistent in the environment, particularly in dried scabs, the virus cannot penetrate intact epithelium. Aggressive pecking during territorial disputes at the nest site can cause small traumatic skin lesions that become infected with virus, which can persist from year to year or be shed in faeces, skin or feather quills from birds with latent infection. Biting insects, particularly mosquitoes, are also a possible mode of transmission.

The diphtheroid form of pox, which produces caseous lesions in the oral cavity, has been recorded in a guillemot (Hill & Bogue 1978). Cutaneous lesions were also present. The large amount of necrotic exudate in the nasal and oral cavities caused inanition and death by asphyxiation.

Adenovirus

Adenovirus-like particles have been identified in kidney tissue from an oiled guillemot. The infection was thought to have been latent and activated by stress, and not a significant cause of disease (Fry & Lowenstine 1985).

Avian influenza

Waterfowl (Anseriformes) are a natural reservoir for influenza A viruses. As waterfowl and seabirds frequently share the same environment there is plenty of opportunity for spread of infection. Highly pathogenic influenza viruses can cause explosive epizootics in both mammals (including humans) and birds. More than 1300 migratory common terns (*Sterna hirundo*) died in an explosive epizootic of avian influenza in South Africa (Becker 1966). Death was peracute, and of 16 carcasses examined histologically lesions were found in only three, all of which showed a meningoencephalitis.

Migrating waterfowl and seabirds have been implicated in the global spread of highly pathogenic avian influenza (HPAI) H5N1, and have been linked to outbreaks in domestic poultry. Biosecurity, including the prevention of contact between domestic poultry and migratory birds, is seen as an important preventative measure against further spread of disease into domestic poultry flocks. Mass mortalities of waterfowl have been reported from Asia, as have deaths of humans and domestic mammals in close proximity with affected poultry. Amongst seabirds, HPAI H5N1 has been reported in cormorants (*Phalacrocorax carbo*), black-headed gulls (*Larus ridibundus*), and herring gulls (*Larus argentatus*). Scavenging on affected carcasses is considered to be the means of spread from waterfowl to gulls and also raptors. Clinical signs are not described for seabirds, as most isolations are from birds found dead, or killed as part of monitoring schemes. However, there is growing evidence of a carrier state amongst both wildfowl and scavengers such as gulls (Sabirovic et al 2006).

Herpesvirus

Small eosinophilic inclusions of Cowdry type A, typical of herpesvirus infection, were found in the liver of oiled birds during the Arabian Gulf oil spill. The damage caused to hepatocytes was assumed to have been present before the ingestion of oil, and may have increased the susceptibility to toxic damage (Greth et al 1995).

Eastern equine encephalitis

Sixty-four per cent of a colony of African penguins in a US aquarium developed clinical signs, including anorexia, lethargy and vomiting, progressing to ataxia, recumbency and grand mal-like seizures. There was a heterophilic leucosis and mild anaemia, and later a monocytosis. All but one juvenile recovered with supportive therapy only. The juvenile was euthanized and on necropsy revealed a bulging left cerebral hemisphere with diminished visibility of blood vessels. On histopathology there was a severe chronic multifocal non-suppurative encephalitis. The pattern of spread of infection was indicative of mosquitoes acting as a vector rather than bird to bird (Tuttle et al 2005).

Other viruses

African and macaroni penguins, with a history of weakness, lethargy and ataxia, which died at a zoo in the UK were found to have both a birnavirus and a reovirus-like agent present as well as *Plasmodium* spp. Although schizonts were found in lung liver and spleen, there was no evidence of parasitaemia, so it is unclear what role the various infectious agents played in the mortality (Gough et al 2002, Jackwood et al 2005).

Antibodies to infectious bursal disease, influenza A and Newcastle disease viruses were found in king penguins in the arctic. Although there were recorded outbreaks of coughing and conjunctivitis in the colony it is not possible to know if the viruses found were linked with clinical signs seen (Gauthier-Clerc et al 2002).

Fungal

Seabirds are a particularly high-risk group for aspergillosis. Housed birds are very prone to infection, especially if ventilation and/or hygiene are suboptimal. **Oiled seabirds frequently develop acute aspergillosis during rehabilitation as a complication of rescue and hospitalization.**

Clinical signs of acute disease include inappetence, respiratory distress and open mouth breathing, and sudden death.

Gross post-mortem signs are varied, depending on the stage and severity of disease. Early cases show small irregular dark foci with a dry appearance in lung tissue. On histology, septate branching fungal hyphae can be seen. These lesions have been noted in rescued guillemots within 8 days of housing. Later, 12–14 days after housing, classic yellow focal lesions develop on air sac surfaces, and fluffy white fungal hyphae may be seen (Fig. 16.7).

Treatment is rarely effective once clinical signs are established, but prophylactic treatment with itraconazole has been effective in preventing further losses among birds at risk. Pre-emptive treatment may be worthwhile, and itraconazole 10 mg/kg p.o. b.i.d. for up to 1 week, followed by 10 mg/kg p.o. s.i.d. for up to 3 weeks, is recommended for divers (Redig 1996). Itraconazole is widely available as capsules containing sustained-release granules. It has been suggested that dividing the number of granules in a capsule to obtain the required dose is unreliable and may lead to toxicity due to the uneven concentration of drug in each granule (Forbes 1992), but the author has experienced no problems.

Aspergillus fumigatus is the most common isolate. More rarely, *A. flavus* may be isolated. *Mucor* spp. have been isolated from puffins, *Geotrichum candidum* from a pelican (Stoskopf & Kennedy-Stoskopf 1986) and blastomycosis from a guillemot (Stoskopf 1993).

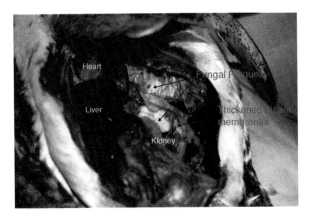

Fig 16.7 Fluffy white fungal hyphae of aspergillosis in a penguin.

Parasites

Ectoparasites

A large number of hard and soft ticks have been associated with seabirds and their nesting sites worldwide. Although associated with transmission of bacteria and viruses, they are rarely themselves a cause of clinical disease. However, king penguins have been shown to have lower incubating success and reduced success in rearing chicks to 1 year in heavily infested areas during high tick (*Ixodes uriae*) infestation years (Mangin et al 2003). Infestation with *Amblyomma loculosum* ticks reduced growth rate and prolonged fledging time in roseate terns (*Sterna dougallii*). Tick infestation appeared to accelerate nestling mortality during periods of food shortage (Ramos et al 2001).

Ixodes uriae is a common ectoparasite of seabirds. It infests a wide range of hosts, although the guillemot is considered the preferred host in the northern hemisphere (Barton et al 1995). It has a far-reaching distribution in the temperate regions of both hemispheres. The life cycle of the tick takes 2–4 years to complete (Steele et al 1990), depending on seasonal constraints and the length of the nesting season and fledging times for available hosts. Duration of attachment and engorgement of each individual tick is up to 6 days (Barton et al 1995). Off the host, the tick may be found in soil around nests and nesting burrows, and in cracks and crevices of the cliff face of breeding ledges, rather than in nests (Steele et al 1990). Spirochaetes of the genus *Borrelia* (*B. burgdorferi* and *B. garinii*), responsible for Lyme disease in humans, have been demonstrated in *Ixodes uriae* ticks (Olsen et al 1993, 1995). It has been suggested that seabirds could play an important role in the spread of borreliosis around the globe. There have been no reports of clinical signs associated with *Borrelia* spp. infection in seabirds.

Death of Laysan albatross chicks (*Diomedea immutabilis*) has been associated with infestation with 'chiggers' (*Womersia midwayensis*). Oedema and focal haemorrhage and necrosis were associated with the ectoparasites. There was secondary bacterial cellulitis and anaemia (Sileo et al 1990).

Both lice and feather mites infest seabirds. Louse species of 16 genera have been described in Procellariiformes alone (Palma 1994). Feather mites tend to favour the distal barb in the trailing vane of the ventral surface of the flight feathers, where they are least likely to be dislodged by airflow or preening activity (Choe & Kim 1991).

High maximum daily temperatures and high numbers of mosquitoes caused breeding failure and adult mortality in Brunnich's guillemots (*Uria lomvia*) in northern Hudson Bay. Both factors needed to be present simultaneously, suggesting that the birds had not had time to adjust their behaviour to climate change and the resultant timing of peak mosquito breeding (Gaston et al 2002).

Ectoparasite infestations rarely require treatment. However, if treating with an acaricide, care must be taken to choose a product that will not affect waterproofing (see earlier). Excessive application of powders or oily sprays can clog feather barbules. Ivermectin injection (Ivomec, MSD Agvet) diluted 1:10 in propylene glycol and a few drops applied topically is usually effective and safe.

Endoparasites

Avian malaria

Avian malaria is a major cause of mortality in captive penguins both in zoological collections and in rehabilitation. Prevalence in the wild is uncertain, but is restricted to temperate climates and habitats with suitable standing fresh water, where the mosquito vectors (mostly *Culex* sp.) can survive. Not all *Plasmodium* species are pathogenic; deaths are most commonly attributed to *Plasmodium relictum*, with a lower prevalence of *P. elongatum* and *P. juxtanucleare* (Grim et al 2003). In captivity, avian malaria can be responsible for outbreaks of disease with up to 60% mortality. Wild birds act as a reservoir of infection and mosquitoes and biting flies as vectors. Clinical signs vary from peracute death to lethargy, dyspnoea and pale mucous membranes. Once clinical signs are present, treatment is often ineffective. Necropsy findings include pulmonary oedema, hydropericardium and hepatomegaly, with organisms demonstrable on smears of spleen and liver. On histopathology, schizonts can be found in lung, spleen, liver and brain, amongst other organs. Both ELISA and PCR tests are available. PCR can also be used to detect the presence of parasites in mosquitoes, which has led to the discovery that the prevalence rates of malaria in mosquitoes can be as high as 50%, and that over the summer there are waves of different *Plasmodium* species present (Cranfield 2003). Survivors carry the parasite subclinically in a tissue phase, which can recrudesce at times of stress such as movement or moulting, but mortality is usually lower (3–4%).

As treatment is of little value once clinical signs are developed, prevention is the preferred option. Several alternatives have been tried:

- Housing birds throughout the risk period. Birds remain susceptible to disease.
- Prophylactic dosing with 1.25 mg/kg primaquine throughout the risk period. Again, birds remain susceptible and treatment must be repeated annually.
- Allowing exposure to infection and monitoring blood films weekly for signs of infection. At the first sign of parasitaemia and before clinical signs are seen, treatment can then be instigated with 10 mg/kg chloroquine b.i.d. on day one, followed by 5 mg/kg and 1 mg/kg primaquine daily for 10 days. In this way birds build up some natural immunity to infection.

Preliminary results of a trial with an anticircumsporozoite DNA vaccine reduced the occurrence of parasitaemia from 50% to approximately 17% despite intense parasite pressure, measured in mosquitoes trapped within the penguin enclosure (Grim et al 2004).

Avian malaria has been recorded in guillemots contaminated with oil (Roertgen 1990), but does not appear to be associated with primary disease.

Babesiasis

Babesia piercei is found commonly in young wild African penguins, and is thought to be spread by *Ixodes* ticks. Clinical signs include lethargy, anorexia, vomiting and anaemia, but most infections are subclinical. Diagnosis is by blood smear, although there is a danger of confusion with malaria. Treatment is with 1 mg/kg primaquine daily for 10 days then weekly for 10 weeks, or 10 mg/kg doxycycline daily for 10 days (van der Merwe 2001).

Gastrointestinal parasites

A wide range of cestodes, trematodes, acanthocephala, nematodes and protozoa has been recorded in seabirds. Some are host-specific, others infect a range of hosts. These parasites are rarely a cause of primary disease. However, young birds, which are most frequently heavily parasitized and in poor body condition, may succumb more easily to the effect of other stressors, such as oiling, disease challenge, severe weather or food shortage. Nematodes of the genus *Contracaecum*, found in the proventriculus, are perhaps the most common parasites. In such birds it is best to treat symptomatically, paying particular attention to correction of dehydration and the instigation of nutritional therapy and ensuring the bird is stable before using anthelmintics.

Other nematodes

Gapeworm (*Syngamus tracheae*) has been the cause of respiratory distress in gulls feeding on agricultural land where they have access to the earthworm intermediate host. Diagnosis is made by the presence of blood-red nematodes in the trachea and large bipolar nematode ova in faeces. Treatment with benzimidazole anthelmintics at standard avian doses is effective.

Nematode worms identified as *Dirofilaria immitis* were isolated from the lumen of the right atrium of the heart and connective tissue of the lung of a captive Humboldt penguin (*Spheniscus humboldti*) (Sano et al 2005).

Coccidiosis

Renal coccidiosis occurs in several taxa, most notably in the colonies of short-tailed shearwaters (*Puffinus tenuirostris*) in Tasmania. Young birds are emaciated, with diarrhoea and soiling of the down. This disease, known as 'Limey disease', was first noticed when the birds were of economic importance as a source of meat and down.

Free-living trematodes

Free-living metacercaria of the trematode *Distomum filiferum*, a parasite of crustacea, have been responsible for the death of white-faced petrels (*Pelagodroma marina*). It was considered that, as the petrels paddled along the surface feeding, large numbers of metacercaria attached to their legs. Long elastic filaments trailing from the metacercaria bound together round both legs, forming 'shackles' of fibrous material that restricted leg movement. Once on land in the breeding colony, the birds were unable to manoeuvre and therefore to take off again, as they rely on launching themselves into the air from a cliff or other suitable vantage point. The birds therefore starved to death. Some 200 000 birds died out of a colony of at least 1 million pairs (Claugher 1976).

Toxins and poisons

Synthetic organic chemicals

Halogenated hydrocarbons (HHCs) are totally artificial compounds, and are not found in nature. They are very persistent in the environment and in living organisms, having an affinity for high-fat tissues including the nervous system. Some of these man-made chemicals can disrupt normal endocrine physiology in animals. Bio-accumulation occurs in the food chain, resulting in the presence of far higher levels of chemicals in top predators such as fish-eating birds than in the environment generally. Fish-eating marine birds and mammals accumulate these toxic dioxin-like compounds in much higher concentration than humans, which seems to be attributable to their lower capacity to metabolize toxic persistent contaminants, and implies that they are at higher risk from exposure. Extremely high concentrations have been found in animals afflicted with diseases and/or the victims of mass mortalities (Tanabe 2002). Although they can be shown to affect the immune system, the exact role of these toxic chemicals in mortality in the wild is often difficult to ascertain, especially as seabirds are exposed to multiple stressors simultaneously, including heavy metals, the effects of fisheries, oil and climate change. The overall health of seabird populations can be used as an important monitor of the health of marine ecosystems (Thompson & Hamer 2000).

Bio-accumulation of HHC residues in birds first became an issue in the 1960s, particularly in relation to the decline in raptor numbers, but the effects were just as dramatic in aquatic environments. HHCs used as agricultural pesticides, such as lindane, DDT, aldrin, dieldrin, etc., caused eggshell thinning, resulting in reduced hatchability and population decline.

HHCs such as dieldrin, DDT and DDE have been implicated in seabird die-offs (Scott et al 1975, Bourne 1976). Healthy herring gulls (*Larus argentatus*) can normally lose up to 30% of their body weight in 17 days without losing vigour (Gilbertson 1988), but such periods of starvation and weight loss can result in signs of acute poisoning due to release of HHCs from body fat depots. Clinical signs of acute pesticide poisoning include nystagmus and clonic convulsions. HHCs can also have an immunosuppressive effect, and deaths may be due to multiple environmental factors.

With the banning of agrochemicals containing lindane, DDT and the 'drin' family, the effects of another equally persistent toxic HHC group, the polychlorinated biphenyls (PCBs), became evident. These chemicals have a wide range of uses, but are not used as agricultural pesticides. They accumulate in the environment mainly through industrial pollution. PCBs have been implicated in embryonic mortality and poor hatching success. Pathological findings associated with high PCB levels include reduced embryonic size, enlarged livers, porphyria, and accumulations of peritoneal and pericardial fluid and subcutaneous mucoserous exudates (Gilbertson & Fox 1977).

Environmental legislation controlling the use and disposal of toxic substances has led to greatly reduced concentrations of HHCs of the 'drin' family and of PCBs. However, a study of the livers of birds killed in mortality incidents in the UK between 1991 and 1996 found similar mean concentrations of PCBs to those recorded in the North Sea in the 1970s and 1980s, although lower than in the Irish Sea in the late 1960s and early 1970s (Malcolm et al 2003).

In the Great Lakes of North America, despite reduced environmental concentrations of total HHCs, increased mortality rates in chicks and embryos of double-crested cormorants have been linked to yet another HHC group, planar halogenated hydrocarbons (PHHs). This group contains the highly toxic dioxins. Selective enrichment of individual HHC congeners (especially those with dioxin-like activity) and interaction between them in the environment may have caused this toxic effect. The ecological significance of such effects is as yet poorly understood (Tillet et al 1992).

Pollution of the environment with persistent synthetic organic chemicals, and their effects on wildlife, will no doubt remain a major environmental issue for the foreseeable future.

Heavy metals

Mercury

High levels of mercury from industrial pollution have been detected in a variety of seabirds, but have not directly been related to disease or mortality. Mercury intoxication has been suspected of contributing to emaciation and death in loons (Brand et al 1988).

Lead

The accidental ingestion of lead from shotgun cartridges or anglers' weights is not generally a problem in fish-eating seabirds. Lead poisoning has been recorded in Laysan albatross chicks due to ingestion of flakes of lead paint from building debris used as nesting material. Symptoms were drooping wings in birds of good nutritional status. On post-mortem there was yellow watery bile and paint chips in the proventriculus (Sileo et al 1990).

Botulism

Botulism is a paralytic disease that affects vertebrates, and is caused by the toxin of the anaerobic bacterium *Clostridium botulinum.*

Avian botulism is an intoxication, not an infectious disease. It is contracted only by the ingestion of toxin pre-formed in suitable media. Type C toxin causes sporadic deaths in birds worldwide, but type E toxin is largely restricted to the Great Lakes of North America. *C. botulinum* cannot survive, nor its toxin persist, in a saline environment equivalent to seawater (Ankerberg 1984). However, deaths of seabirds in fresh or brackish water environments have occurred. High temperatures, shallow, still or slow moving water and decaying organic matter creating a nutrient-rich anaerobic environment predispose to outbreaks of botulism from the germination of *C. botulinum* spores found naturally in soil. Carcasses of botulism casualties and maggots feeding on them are rich sources of toxin, and will cause further deaths if ingested.

Rubbish tips are a common source of toxin for scavenging gulls of many species. Gulls and terns may ingest toxin from shallow stagnant pools used for bathing and loafing (Lloyd et al 1976).

Perhaps most difficult to understand is an outbreak of type E botulism among common loons (*Gavia immer*) in Michigan in 1983 (Brand et al 1988), as loons appear to feed exclusively on live fish. It was considered possible that dead or moribund fish contaminated with toxin were consumed.

Clinical signs of botulism are the acute onset of flaccid paralysis of voluntary muscles. Long-necked seabirds may show classic 'limberneck', as seen in wildfowl, but gulls show uncoordinated gait, become unable to stand, and may show respiratory distress with open mouth breathing before the head carriage becomes affected.

Forbes (1996) links the prognosis to the severity of symptoms in waterfowl, but gulls seem less predictable, often recovering with basic care despite severe clinical signs.

Treatment consists of fluid therapy (oral and parenteral), administration of intestinal adsorbents such as activated charcoal and/or bismuth, and good nursing. Type C antitoxin is produced experimentally in small quantities and has been effective in the treatment of birds, but any such treatment must comply with national legislation regarding the use of such serum-based products.

Confirmation of diagnosis can be made by detection of the toxin in serum or stomach contents. However, the author has found that samples from birds showing classical clinical signs frequently fail to reveal the presence of the toxin.

Algal blooms

Phytoplankton are algae, usually single-celled plants, which survive by photosynthesis and absorption of nutrients directly from the water. They are prey for zooplankton, and both taxa exist in equilibrium. Algal blooms can be part of natural cycles. For example, in the temperate regions of the northern hemisphere, algal blooms can occur naturally in spring as the daylight length increases and surface water warms up, and in autumn when strong winds and tides push nutrient-rich water to the surface (upwelling), while there is still sufficient daylight length for rapid algal growth.

Some species of phytoplankton produce potent toxins, especially neurotoxins. Blooms of phytoplankton can occur in such local abundance that the toxins reach a concentration at which fish and invertebrates are killed. Some toxic phytoplankton are coloured, and in particularly profuse blooms they can reach densities of $20–30 \times 10^6$ cells/L (MacGarvin 1990), causing the sea to be discernibly coloured red, yellow or brown, leading to the term 'red tide'. Toxic phytoplankton include *Chrysochromulina* spp., *Dynophysis* spp., *Gonyaulax* spp. and *Gymnodinium* spp. The latter two are particularly associated with red tides. In Argentina, recurrent blooms of the toxic phytoplankton *Alexandrium tamarense* have coincided with mortality in Magellanic penguins and other marine birds (Gayoso & Fulco 2006).

Shellfish, especially mussels, appear to be immune to the toxin but temporarily concentrate it in their flesh, leading to outbreaks of poisoning – including 'paralytic shellfish poisoning' (PSP) in humans who consume them. Similarly, birds that consume affected shellfish, dead or dying invertebrates, or affected fish during a bloom can be poisoned. The disease is characterized by sudden death, with a high mortality (>80% has been recorded), which is localized and of short duration – the toxins can build up and decline again in as little as 2 weeks. Taxa affected include fulmars, cormorants, eiders (*Somateria mollissima*), gulls, terns and auks (Armstrong et al 1978). Nutrient enrichment of coastal waters with nitrogen and phosphates, particularly from agricultural run-off into rivers, can lead to a significant increase in the quantity and frequency of algal blooms to the point where in some sea areas die-offs of seabirds due to PSP are recurrent and shellfish for human consumption must continually be monitored.

Field diagnosis is by clinical signs and circumstantial evidence. Peracute mortality of diverse taxa (which can include birds, marine mammals and fish) is suspicious, and often adults in good physical condition are worst affected because they consume most prey and therefore most toxin. Confirmation of diagnosis is by detection of lethal levels of toxin in very fresh carcasses or stomach contents, although toxins tend to be labile and degrade rapidly. Some toxins are associated with specific brain lesions that can be detected histologically, but generally histology is useful in elimination of other differential diagnoses. Detection of high numbers of toxic phytoplankton in water samples, or high toxin levels in the food chain, is suspicious. As the disease is characterized by sudden death, treatment is rarely an issue, but if birds are recovered alive they should be treated symptomatically. Specific antitoxins have been used successfully experimentally in marine mammals and humans, but are not commercially available.

Oil

Although any bird can become contaminated with oil, for example pet birds falling into cooking oil, by far the largest problem is created by pollution of the sea with crude or heavy fuel (bunker) oil. The taxa worst affected are surface-swimming and diving birds. Major oil spills are not the only cause of oiling of seabirds. Many minor pollution episodes, such as leakage at off-shore wells, accidental spills and illegal dumping, combine to cause a background pollution level that results in annual seabird casualties in the UK equivalent to those caused by one major tanker disaster.

When a bird swims into an oil slick the oil becomes distributed on the feathers, clogging the feather structure and causing loss of waterproofing. Water penetrates to the skin and the layer of air normally trapped in the down feathers is lost, resulting in loss of insulation and buoyancy. Birds become hypothermic and may drown. Normal behaviour (including feeding) is disrupted, and there is an increase in metabolic requirements to maintain body temperature. Survivors rapidly lose weight.

The net effect of oiling of the plumage is to make water a hostile environment, and survivors of the spill will seek refuge on the shore, where they may be picked up and brought to a rescue centre for treatment.

The behavioural response to feather contamination is vigorous preening, which leads to ingestion of oil and oil toxicosis.

The toxicity of different oils varies greatly, most obviously with the ratio of 'light' aromatic hydrocarbons to

the 'heavy' tar-like fraction. Refined oils, having the tar fraction removed, are the most toxic. Crude oils vary considerably; Arabian oils have a large heavy fraction, North Sea oils have a large light fraction. Once spilt, the oil starts to 'weather' – i.e. the light fraction evaporates and disperses, leaving the less toxic heavy tars, which often end up as tar balls on the beach. Thus the degree of toxic effects of ingestion will depend not only on the volume ingested, but also on the type of oil and how long it has been spilt.

The ingestion of crude oil prevents the uptake of water and electrolytes by the intestinal mucosa, resulting in diarrhoea and dehydration. In a saltwater environment, this in turn prevents the functioning of the nasal gland, rapidly exacerbating dehydration. Birds experimentally dosed with crude oil died rapidly from dehydration in a saltwater environment, but survived on freshwater (Flemming et al 1982).

A primary toxic effect of crude oil ingestion is haemolytic anaemia (Leighton et al 1983). The haemolytic crisis occurs between 3 and 6 days post-exposure, and recovery starts from day 7 (Fry & Lowenstine 1985).

Other sequelae of oil ingestion reported include:

- hepatic haemosiderosis (especially in Kuppfer cells); dissociation of hepatocytes and hepatic necrosis
- renal tubular degeneration and necrosis (Fry & Lowenstine 1985, Khan & Ryan 1991, Greth et al 1995)
- lipid pneumonia (Hartung & Hunt 1966)
- hyperaemia, oedema and venous thrombi in lungs (Greth et al 1995)
- adrenocortical hyperplasia (Holmes et al 1978) and necrosis (Greth et al 1995)
- lymphoid depletion of the spleen (Greth et al 1995)
- immunosuppression (Holmes et al 1978)
- embryonic death and reduced hatchability of eggs (Leighton et al 1995).

A wide range of gastrointestinal lesions has been reported, with and without occult blood. Severe necrotic enteritis is often associated with secondary bacterial infection (Wood et al 1993).

Black fluid in the gastrointestinal tract, a black residue lining the gizzard, and red/black mucus at the isthmus of the gizzard are frequently seen on post-mortem in both oiled and non-oiled birds, but are not oil residues. The origin is unclear, but may be associated with poor body condition (Holmes 1995).

In practice, veterinary treatment and nursing of survivors of oil pollution must first be directed at maintaining hydration and body condition. Although the first 4 days are most critical, auks have become dehydrated up to 8 days after hospitalization despite good appetite and access to fresh water. Birds that appear bright and eat well can rapidly become dull, with drooping wings and hunched appearance. Collapse and death can occur within 2 hours of the onset of clinical signs.

On post-mortem examination, carcasses appear dry, with lack of elasticity of the skin, which is tightly adherent to the underlying musculature (Wood et al 1993). Histological examination of the kidneys commonly reveals urate tophi.

Routine examination and treatment should include:

1. Body temperature. Less than 32.5°C carries a poor prognosis. Hypothermic birds should be warmed gradually until normal body temperature is reached, and blown hot air is the method of choice. Care must be taken to avoid hyperthermia and dehydration by increased evaporation from the respiratory tract. Once normothermic, birds are best maintained in an air temperature of 22–25°C. Higher ambient temperatures may create heat stress, and social birds kept in groups show marked aggression at higher temperatures.
2. State of hydration. Many oiled birds will be severely dehydrated and diarrhoeic. Adsorbents and activated charcoal mixed with oral rehydration fluids can be administered routinely. Fluid therapy may have to be continued, with or without nutritional support, for 4–8 days.
3. Body condition. This should be assessed and the weight compared to a normal for the species, if available. Normal body weight can vary with age, sex and time of year, and if in doubt condition is better assessed by examination than by absolute weight. When assessing the prominence of the keel bone, care must be taken to penetrate the thick down over the breast to the skin beneath.
4. Prophylactic antibiotics. Prophylactic use of antifungals is indicated if birds are considered at risk of aspergillosis, either through species susceptibility or high environmental challenge.
5. PCV and total solids (Tables 16.6, 16.7). Monitoring packed cell volume (PCV or HCT) and total solids (TS), which correlates with total protein (TP), is possible on site with minimal equipment (haematocrit, refractometer) and can be performed using one drop of blood. This is a very useful way of monitoring haemoconcentration due to dehydration, anaemia due to haemolysis and hypoproteinaemia due to negative calorific balance. Even if birds are eating well, additional fluid and nutritional therapy can be administered accordingly.

Only when birds are stable, bright and active, and of adequate body weight and health status, should they be

Table 16.6 Haematology and clinical chemistry. Reference values from clinically healthy birds are available for some seabird species, although often from very limited numbers of individuals

(a) Haematology

Parameter	Units	African penguin (Cranfield 2003)	Humboldt penguin (Cranfield 2003)	Guillemot (common murre) (Newman & Zinkl 1996)	Manx shearwater (Kirkwood et al 1995)	Herring gull (Averbeck 1992)	American white pelican (*Pelicanus erythrorhynchos*) (Bennett et al 1991)	Cormorant (Bennett et al 1991)
Total haemoglobin (Hb)	g/dL	13.7 SD 3.5 (n = 176)	15.2 SD 2.2 (n = 404)	10.2–16.8[b] (n = 10)	14.8 SD 1.8 (n = 10)	13.0 SD 1.9 (n = 109)	10.7–17.3 (n = 12)	8.4–13.1[b] (n = 5)
Red blood cell count (RBC)	10^{12}/L	1.86 SD 0.48 (n = 0.48)	2.15 SD 0.54 (n = 113)	2.43–3.94[b] (n = 10)	2.87 SD 0.38 (n = 9)	2.1 SD 0.4 (n = 143)	1.91–3.0 (n = 12)	1.62–2.30[b] (n = 5)
Packed cell volume (PCV)	L/L	0.46 SD 0.74 (n = 345)	0.49 SD 0.67 (n = 875)	0.33–0.58[b] (n = 10)	0.48 SD 0.05 (n = 9)	0.41 SD 0.01 (n = 109)	0.32–0.47 (n = 12)	0.27–0.41[b] (n = 5)
Mean cell volume (MCV)	FL	249 SD 50 (n = 178)	242 SD 52 (n = 111)	136–179[b] (n = 10)	166 SD 13.7 (n = 9)	200.6 SD 36.0 (n = 109)	139.3–185.4 (n = 12)	164.8–180.4[b] (n = 5)
Mean cell haemoglobin (MCH)	Pg	79.7 SD 16 (n = 129)	81.4 SD 17.8 (n = 69)	36.3–48.3[b] (n = 10)	53.4 SD 5.3 (n = 9)	62.7 SD 10.0 (n = 109)	51.19–61.86 (n = 12)	51.9–57.0[b] (n = 5)
Mean cell haemoglobin concentration (MCHC)	g/dL	31.4 SD 5.1 (n = 172)	30.9 SD 27 (n = 401)	26.0–30.9[b] (n = 10)	32 SD 1.6 (n = 9)	31.5 SD 3.3 (n = + 109)	29.94–39.96 (n = 12)	31.1–33.0[b] (n = 5)
Total white cell count (WBC)	10^9/L	16.1 SD 8.1 (n = 232)	26.5 SD 11.4 (n = 812)	2.0–9.5[b] (n = 10)	5.39 SD 4.26 (n = 10)	15.5 SD 3.1 (n = 103)	2.55–18.7 (n = 12)	6.10–15.5[b] (n = 5)
Heterophil count	10^9/L	8.95 SD 4.93 (n = 229)	14.85 SD 6.82 (n = 812)	1.26–4.86[b] (n = 9)	2.81 SD 2.53 (n = 10)	5.4 SD 2.8 (n = 103)	0–16.28 (n = 12)	5.37–13.2[b] (n = 5)
Lymphocyte count	10^9/L	6.2 SD 4.72 (n = 230)	9.58 SD 6.29 (n = 812)	0.08–1.68[b] (n = 9)	1.19 SD 2.24 (n = 10)	9.4 SD 3.0 (n = 103)	0.38–4.5 (n = 12)	0.4–2.17[b] (n = 5)
Monocyte count	10^9/L	0.73 SD 0.88 (n = 150)	1.37 SD 1.28 (n = 668)	0[b] (n = 10)	0–0.87[a] (n = 10)	0–1.4[a] (n = 103)	0–0.34a (n = 12)	0–0.12[b] (n = 5)
Eosinophil count	10^9/L	0.44 SD 0.37 (n = 103)	0.64 SD 0.80 (n = 430)	0.48–4.46[b] (n = 9)	0–0.23[a] (n = 10)	0–1.6[a] (n = 103)	0–0.41a (n = 12)	0
Basophil count	10^9/L	0.42 SD 0.37 (n = 108)	0.68 SD 0.53 (n = 455)	0–0.24[b] (n = 10)	0–0.76[a] (n = 10)	0.5–1.4[a] (n = 103)	0–0.40a (n = 12)	0–0.49[b] (n = 5)
Thrombocyte count	10^9/L				11.5 SD 4.8 (n = 10)		12.46–34.08 (n = 11)	25–50[b] (n = 5)
Fibrinogen	g/L	2.93 SD 2.56(n = 14)			2.01 SD 0.42 (n = 6)		0–3.5 (n = 11)	2.06–3.86[b] (n = 5)

[a]*Parameters that are not normally distributed and are therefore expressed as ranges rather than standard deviations.*

[b]*Small datasets expressed as standard deviations can result in parameters so widely spread they are of little practical value, and these are also expressed as ranges.*

(continued)

selected for washing, as the process itself is stressful and vigorous preening afterwards is essential. There have been many different ways of removing oil from birds' feathers suggested; one of the few that has been the subject of scientific research is the use of iron filings and magnetism (Orbell et al 2004). However, to date the only practical treatment method presently available is the use of detergent solution.

Several detergents are used worldwide by different rehabilitation groups. In-vitro testing (Brynza et al 1990)

Table 16.6 (continued)

(b) Biochemistry Parameter	Units	African penguin (Cranfield 2003)	Humboldt penguin (Cranfield 2003)	Guillemot (common murre) (Newman & Zinkl 1996)	American white pelican (Bennett et al 1991)
Urea	mmol/L	0.66 SD 0.33 ($n = 123$)	0.66 SD 0.17 ($n = 926$)		0–1.5[b] ($n = 6$)
Creatinine	µmol/L	35.4 SD 17.7 ($n = 73$)	35.4 SD 177 ($n = 865$)	35.4–70.2[b] ($n = 10$)	22–51[b] ($n = 6$)
Bicarbonate	mmol/L	31 SD 25 ($n = 3$)		17–33[b] ($n = 10$)	7–30[b] ($n = 6$)
Chloride	mmol/L	111 SD 4 ($n = 107$)	112 SD 5 ($n = 914$)	103–121[b] ($n = 10$)	110–116[b] ($n = 6$)
Sodium	mmol/L	150 SD 5 ($n = 114$)	152 SD 6 ($n = 1150$)	152–163[b] ($n = 10$)	149–157[b] ($n = 6$)
Potassium	mmol/L	4.5 SD 1.4 ($n = 1110$)	3.9 SD 1.0 ($n = 1026$)	3.3–10[b] ($n = 10$)	1.7–3.1[b] ($n = 6$)
Total protein	g/L	53 SD 9 ($n = 210$)	55 SD 7 ($n = 1059$)	39–48[b] ($n = 10$)	24–42[b] ($n = 6$)
Albumin	g/L	21 SD 6 ($n = 144$)	17 SD 3 ($n = 962$)	11–14[b] ($n = 10$)	10–16[b] ($n = 6$)
Globulin	g/L	34 SD 6 ($n = 146$)	38 SD 7 ($n = 954$)	26–34[b] ($n = 10$)	
Calcium	mmol/L	2.68 SD 0.58 ($n = 187$)	2.78 SD 0.58 ($n = 1142$)	2.08–2.77[b] ($n = 10$)	2.14–2.65[b] ($n = 6$)
Inorganic phosphate	mmol/L	1.26 SD 0.68 ($n = 141$)	1.30 SD 0.65 ($n = 979$)	1.41–2.94[b] ($n = 10$)	0.22–1.66[b] ($n = 6$)
Total bilirubin	µmol/L	5.13 SD 3.42 ($n = 63$)	8.55 SD 10.26 ($n = 785$)	0–5.13[b] ($n = 10$)	2–4[b] ($n = 6$)
Conjugated bilirubin	µmol/L			0–1.71[b] ($n = 10$)	0–1.0[b] ($n = 6$)
Urate	µmol/L	666.2 SD 487.7 ($n = 185$)	469.9 SD 315.2 ($n = 1163$)	267–1118[b] ($n = 10$)	341–601[b] ($n = 5$)
Alkaline phosphatase	IU/L	193 SD 253 ($n = 123$)	168 SD 119 ($n = 980$)	22–149[b] ($n = 10$)	300–1052[b] ($n = 6$)
Alanine transaminase	IU/L	127 SD 111 ($n = 123$)	36 SD 21 ($n = 977$)	53–216[b] ($n = 10$)	23–75[b] ($n = 6$)
Gamma glutamyl transferase	IU/L			0–10.0[b] ($n = 10$)	0–5[b] ($n = 4$)
Aspartate transaminase	IU/L	183 SD 103 ($n = 189$)	191 SD 83 ($n = 1087$)	117–1491[b] ($n = 10$)	56–464[b] ($n = 6$)
Creatine kinase	IU/L	455 SD 593 ($n = 132$)	236 SD 219 ($n = 310$)	537–3801[b] ($n = 10$)	
Iron	µmol/L	8.1 SD 0.13 ($n = 5$)	26.5 SD 10.0 ($n = 68$)		8.2–28.1[b] ($n = 6$)
Cholesterol	mmol/L	7.95 SD 2.51 ($n = 123$)	6.79 SD 2.00 ($n = 956$)	8.22–10.95[b] ($n = 10$)	
Glucose	mmol/L	12.9 SD 2.2 ($n = 192$)	13.6 SD 2.6 ($n = 1081$)	12.26–17.19[b] ($n = 10$)	

[a]Parameters that are not normally distributed and are therefore expressed as ranges rather than standard deviations.

[b]Small datasets expressed as standard deviations can result in parameters so widely spread they are of little practical value, and these are also expressed as ranges.

Table 16.7 Oiled bird treatment guidelines based on PCV and total protein (based on Tseng 1993)

Parameter	Comments
PCV >55%	Require fluid therapy
TS <2.0 g/dL	Require nutritional therapy, even if self-feeding
PCV <15%	Require nutritional therapy, even if self-feeding
TP >2.0 g/dL	Before selecting for washing
PCV >25%	Before selecting for washing

has indicated that the surfactant of choice is 'Dawn' or 'Fairy Liquid' (Proctor and Gamble). A 2% solution is adequate, but in practice small amounts of neat detergent are applied to difficult residues. Well-weathered tar,

fulmar oil or other difficult residues may be pretreated to soften the residue, which is then washed with detergent in the normal way. Vegetable oil, methyl oleate and a variety of biodegradable detergents used in the offshore oil industry have been used successfully.

Technique for washing

Two people are required, one to hold and one to wash. Suitable personal protective equipment, including nitrile gloves which cover both hands and arms, and protective glasses or goggles, must be worn to protect against contact both with toxic oil and with detergent, which can rapidly cause contact dermatitis with constant exposure. The bird is immersed in a solution of detergent at 42°C (range 40–45°C). The holder keeps as much of the bird's body as possible immersed and in contact

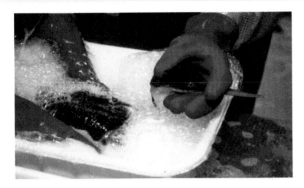

Fig 16.8 Washing oiled birds. The bird, a western grebe (*Aechmophorus occidentalis*), is restrained by the handler while the washer uses both hands to manipulate the feathers. (Photo credit IBRRC.)

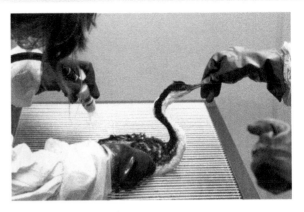

Fig 16.9 Rinsing. The water pressure must be sufficient to lift the feathers and ensure all detergent is removed. Water should bead and run freely off feathers at the end of the rinse. (Photo credit IBRRC.)

with the detergent whilst the washer ensures that the detergent solution reaches all the feathers, including the down, with a gentle agitating movement. Flight and tail feathers are rubbed between fingers and thumb from base to tip until they are all clean. It is essential that no oil residue remains. It is important to follow a standard routine so that no feathers are missed. It is usual to start with the head, using a toothbrush or cotton bud if necessary to remove oil from around the nares and inside the beak (Fig. 16.8). The neck, back and dorsal surface of the tail are then cleaned, followed by each wing and flank. Each time the detergent solution becomes contaminated it should be replaced. To ensure this is done speedily to avoid excess stress, and the danger of hypothermia in a wet bird exposed to the air, it is usual to prepare several tubs of detergent solution at the right temperature, and simply move from one to the next. Heavily contaminated birds may be washed in this manner several times, discarding the soiled detergent solution each time until no more oil comes off the feathers and the water remains visibly clean, as well as there being no visible oil remaining on the bird.

The bird is now clean of oil but thoroughly covered in detergent, which in turn must all be removed. During oil spills when many birds are being washed it is normal at this point to pass the bird to a separate pair of operators for the rinsing process. The operators must ensure that their hands and clothing, and the working surfaces, are free of detergent contamination before commencing to rinse. Using a high-pressure shower jet at 42°C, the washer rinses against the lie of the feathers until all detergent is removed and water is beading on the feathers. Water pressure must be sufficient to lift the feathers and fluff up the underlying down (Fig. 16.9). As detergent is removed the feathers begin to shed water, which beads and runs off leaving feathers dry. Water pressure between 345 and 620 kPa (60 and 90 psi) is ideal. A standard domestic shower attachment can be used,

but if water pressure is a problem, using a commercial spray head with a more restricted flow rate (a smaller jet) may give better results. However, a minimum acceptable flow is required, depending on the size of bird, to avoid prolonged rinsing time. Spray heads designed for 'drive through' car washes come in a variety of suitable sizes and have proved effective. Specialized equipment, including water-holding tanks and booster pumps, is required if a water main of suitable size and pressure is not available.

It is the job of the holder to ensure that contaminated water always flows off the bird away from areas already rinsed. The same methodical routine should be used for rinsing to ensure that no feathers are missed.

On completion, water should be beading freely on all areas of the bird's plumage and the underlying down should look fluffy and dry (Fig. 16.10). Water from the showerhead can be run over the plumage. Any area where water is seen to penetrate the feathers is not 'proofed' and needs further attention. Because of the danger of recontamination by detergent residues, the whole body should be rinsed again, concentrating on areas of water penetration.

Total time taken can vary from 15 to 40 minutes, depending on the size of the bird, the degree of contamination and the skill of the washers. Very large birds such as swans or penguins may take longer.

Once completed, the bird is placed in the drying area and left in a current of warm air until dry. Commercial pet driers used in the dog grooming industry are ideal. The pen or cage can be partially covered with a blanket or sheet to maintain a warm atmosphere of 30–35°C. Care must be taken not to overheat birds in the drying area. Most birds will quickly start to preen to align their feathers correctly. As soon as they are completely dry, which can be from as little as 30 minutes for small birds, or as long as several hours, birds can be put on water.

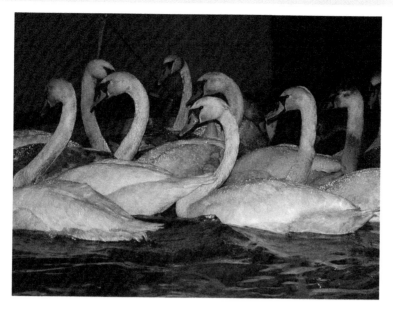

Fig 16.10 Mute swans (*Cygnus olor*) showing water beading and running off the feathers. (Photo credit IFAW.)

Once on water, it is essential that the bird preens. Failure of waterproofing can be due to residual contamination with oil or detergent, failure to preen, or contamination of the surface of the pool. Efficient surface skimming pools (see earlier and Figs 16.11 and 16.12) are important to remove oily faeces, and the bottom of the pool should be kept free of debris and uneaten fish etc. This can easily be achieved without excessive disturbance to the birds using a simple siphon. Large fish-eating birds such as pelicans can be fed in shallow trays away from the water to ensure the water surface is not contaminated with fish oil. The pool sides should be fitted with platforms which slope gently into the water for an easy exit if the birds become wet. There must be sufficient perching space for all birds to come off the water without becoming overcrowded, which leads to birds trampling and defecating on each other, with resultant contamination of feathers and loss of waterproofing. Birds should be observed closely and those which become excessively wet removed and re-dried before reintroducing to the pool.

Birds usually require 4–5 days on water to preen sufficiently to restore the feather structure adequately, although some may take up to 10 days before their plumage shows no water penetration and they are fit for release. Suitable release criteria are that a bird must be bright, alert and reactive, have haematological parameters within normal range, and show no sign of water penetration after being restricted to water without the chance to leave for a suitable period of time (Fig. 16.13). Pelagic birds should be able to swim on a pool with perches and platforms removed for 48 hours without visible signs of water penetration.

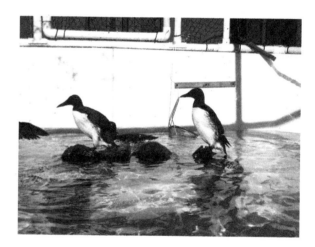

Fig 16.11 After drying overnight the birds are placed on a surface skimming pool, where preening will restore any remaining disrupted feather structure. (Photo credit IFAW.)

An integrated automatic process using a purpose-designed machine and detergent has been developed (Basseres et al 1995). Birds are restrained in a frame, which is lowered into a tank within which are rotating bars carrying spray nozzles. The bird's body is sprayed first with the detergent, then with fresh water, while the head, which is left protruding from the top of the apparatus, is cleaned by hand. In this way a reduction in cleaning time to 7 minutes can be achieved. The use of such a machine during an oil spill enables the rapid

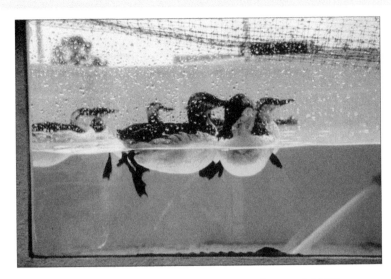

Fig 16.12 Birds should float high on the water and no water should penetrate the plumage. (Photo credit IBRRC.)

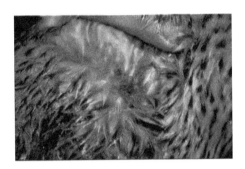

Fig 16.13 Checking the breast plumage to ensure that no water is penetrating prior to release. (Photo credit IFAW.)

deployment of washing facilities to the site of the spill. Also, variability in expertise in washing technique and the need for large numbers of skilled washers can be eliminated. However, the numbers of birds that can be rehabilitated, and the time they must spend in captivity, will be determined not by the speed at which they can be washed but by the facilities for nursing before washing, and pool facilities for holding birds after washing before they become fit for release. These are the most important factors to consider in the siting of any washing facility, manual or automated.

Survival to release

Survival of oil spill victims depends on many factors – the type of oil, species involved, weather conditions, facilities available for collection and treatment of casualties, skill and experience of staff, etc. However, overall survival rates of over 60% are now regularly achieved. For example, when the tanker *Sea Empress* ran aground in Milford Haven, Wales, in February

1996, the Royal Society for the Prevention of Cruelty to Animals (RSPCA) coordinated a rescue effort which resulted in 2266 live oiled casualties of 15 species admitted to RSPCA wildlife hospitals. A total of 1434 birds (63.3%) were released. Of the 18 000 oiled African penguins rescued in a joint effort by the Southern African Foundation for the Conservation of Coastal Birds (SANCCOB) and the International Fund for Animal Welfare (IFAW) when the tanker *Treasure* sank off Robben Island near Cape Town, South Africa, in June 2000, 90% survived to be released to the wild (Nel & Whittington 2003).

Post-release survival

The simplest way of monitoring post-release survival of rehabilitated birds is by the use of numbered leg rings (bands). Use of the same ringing system as for monitoring healthy wild birds provides a natural comparison. However, ring returns from pelagic seabirds are generally low, and therefore a large sample size is required before sufficient returns are obtained for a significant statistical analysis. Of the species of seabirds commonly rehabilitated, only guillemots and African penguins have been ringed in sufficient numbers for such analyses.

Recent statistical analyses of ring returns from rehabilitated oiled guillemots in both North America and Britain have suggested that post-release survival is very low. In a statistical review of 127 ring returns from 3200 released rehabilitated oiled seabirds in North America, Sharp (1996) concluded that guillemots had a post-release life expectancy of only 9.6 days and a negligible number survived more than 12 months. Wernham et al (1997) found that of 309 returns from 2834 released rehabilitated guillemots in Britain, the median survival time was 7 days, equating to an annual survival of 0.6%. This compares to 599 days and 88% respectively for non-rehabilitated adults. Anderson et al (1996) radio-tracked oiled rehabilitated and unaffected brown pelicans. The rehabilitated birds disappeared from the population faster than unaffected birds, and also failed to breed.

Following the *Stuyvesant* spill in 1999 both oiled, rehabilitated and non-oiled common murres were radio-tracked. Rehabilitated birds had a survival rate of 68%, much higher than reported in banding studies, but were still four times less likely to survive than unoiled birds. Eighty per cent of mortality occurred between 15 and 40 days post release. After 40 days survival appeared to be comparable to non-oiled birds until the radios failed. Blood samples taken prior to release indicated that inflammation and secondary infections subsequent to oiling and/or captive care are likely to have contributed to the deaths of some of the murres (Newman 2003).

In contrast, three groups of gulls were radiotracked in southern California: oiled and rehabilitated; non-oiled and rehabilitated for other reasons; and normal controls. There was no difference between the survival of the three groups, only one (control) bird dying before transmitters failed. There was no statistically significant difference in the geographical areas used by the three groups of gulls following release (Golightly et al 2003). Mute swans (*Cygnus olor*) contaminated with light fuel oil and treated conservatively without washing suffered higher mortality than unaffected birds for 5 months and failed to breed that year, after which mortality and breeding returned to normal (Collins et al 1994). At least 87% of oiled and rehabilitated African penguins return to their breeding colonies and post-rehabilitation annual survival rates are no different from those of unaffected birds. At least 60% of rehabilitated birds that were resighted at their colonies have been recorded breeding. A simple deterministic model shows the rehabilitation of oiled

African penguins has resulted in the present population being 19% larger than it would have been in the absence of rehabilitation, and the future cost to the population of ceasing to rehabilitate oiled birds ranges from 17% to 51%.

The remarkable success of rehabilitation reported in penguins and swans in sharp contrast to the almost complete failure reported in auks would suggest that death in non-survivors is not directly due to the effects of contamination with or ingestion of oil. Many suggestions for non-survival have been put forward, including stress during rehabilitation, persistent immunosuppression and the failure to find an adequate food source after release. At present, all suggestions are purely conjecture. Although survival rates during rehabilitation have improved remarkably in recent years, Sharp (1996) and Wernham et al (1997) found no evidence that improved techniques during rehabilitation have had any effect on post-release survival. However, there is a growing body of evidence that suggests that modern rehabilitation programmes have the potential to reduce the impacts to seabird populations from marine spills by returning some affected birds back to wild populations (Golightly et al 2003).

It can be seen from these studies that the rehabilitation of oiled seabirds is a controversial field. The cost of rehabilitation of birds after a major spill can be high, and the cost-effectiveness and conservation value of such efforts have been questioned (Anderson et al 1996, Sharp 1996). However, the rehabilitation of oiled seabirds is perhaps best considered primarily as a welfare issue. The welfare of oil spill victims is only best served by attempted rehabilitation when an acceptable chance of post-release survival can be achieved, and suitable post release monitoring must be considered as an essential part of any oiled bird rehabilitation programme.

References

Anderson D W, Gress F, Fry D M 1996 Survival and dispersal of oiled brown pelicans after rehabilitation and release. Marine Pollution Bulletin 32(10):711–718

Ankerberg C W 1984 Pelican deaths in the vicinity of a sewage lift station: a bacteriological investigation. Microbios Letters 26:33–42

Armstrong I H, Coulson J C, Hawkey P, Hudson M J 1978 Further mass seabird deaths from paralytic shellfish poisoning. British Birds 71:58–68

Averbeck C 1992 Haematology and blood chemistry of healthy and clinically abnormal great black-backed gulls (*Larus marinus*) and herring gulls (*Larus argentatus*). Avian Pathology 21:215–223

Banerjee M, Reed W M, Fitzgerald S D, Panigrahy B 1994 Neurotropic velogenic Newcastle disease in cormorants in Michigan: pathology and virus characterization. Avian Diseases 38:873–878

Barton T R, Harris M P, Wanless S 1995 Natural attachment duration of nymphs of the tick *Ixodes uriae* (*Acari: Ixodidae*) in Kittiwake (*Rissa tridactyla*) nestlings. Experimental and Applied Acarology 19:499–509

Basseres A, Verschuere B, Jacques J-P. et al 1995 A new cleaning product for oiled birds and an integrated automated process. Oil Spill

Conference. Poster Session W3, Evolving technologies. Tri-State Bird Rescue and Research Inc, Delaware, USA

Beall F, Branch S, Cramm A 1994 Penguin husbandry manual. American Zoo and Aquarium Association

Becker W B 1966 The isolation and classification of tern virus: influenza virus A/Tern/South Africa/1961. Journal of Hygiene 64:309–320

Bennett P M, Gascoyne S C, Hart M G et al 1991 The Lynx database. Department of Veterinary Science, Zoological Society of London

Boerner L, Nevis K R, Hinckley L S et al 2004 Erysipelothrix septicaemia in a little blue penguin (*Eudyptula minor*). Journal of Veterinary Diagnostic Investigation 16(2):145–149

Bourne W R P 1976 The mass mortality of common murres in the Irish Sea in 1969. Journal of Wildlife Management 40(4):789–792

Brand C J, Schmitt S M, Duncan R M, Cooley T M 1988 An outbreak of type E. botulism among common loons (*Gavia immer*) in Michigan's upper peninsula. Journal of Wildlife Diseases 24(3):471–476

Brooke M 1990 The Manx shearwater. T & A D Poyser, p 144–167

Brynza H E, Foster J P, McCartney J H et al 1990 Surfactant efficacy in removal of petrochemicals from feathers. The Effects of Oil on Wildlife Oil Symposium. The 13th Annual Conference of the International Wildlife Rehabilitation Council. International Bird Rescue Research Center, Berkeley, CA

Burkle M, Crosta L, Gerlach H 2002 Thyroid lesions in growing parrot and penguin chicks. Tierarztliche Praxis 30(6):467–471

Choe J C, Kim K C 1991 Microhabitat selection and adaption of feather mites (Acari: Analgoidea) on murres and kittiwakes. Canadian Journal of Zoology 69:817–821

Cho K O, Kimura T, Ochiai K, Itakura C 1998 Gizzard adenocarcinoma in an aged Humboldt penguin (Spheniscus humboldti). Avian Pathology 27:100–102

Claugher D 1976 A trematode associated with the death of white-faced storm petrels (Pelagodroma marina) on the Chatham Islands. Journal of Natural History 10:633–641

Collins R, Brazier H, Whelan J 1994 Rehabilitating a herd of oiled mute swans (Cygnus olor). Biology and Environment: Proceedings of the Royal Irish Academy 94B(1):83–99

Converse J D, Hoogstraal H, Moussa M I et al 1975 Soldado virus (Hughes group) from Ornithodoros (alectorobius) capensis (Ixodoidea: Argasidae) infesting sooty tern colonies in the Seychelles, Indian Ocean. American Journal of Tropical Medicine and Hygiene 24:1010–1018

Cranfield M R 2003 Sphenisciformes (Penguins). In: Fowler M E, Miller R E (eds) Zoo and wild animal medicine, 5th edn. Elsevier Science, USA, p 103–110

Croker A D, Cronshaw J, Holmes W N 1974 The effects of a crude oil on intestinal absorption in ducklings (Anas platyrhynchos). Environmental Pollution 7:165–177

Fielding M J 2000 Deaths in captive penguins. Veterinary Record 146(7):199

Flemming W J, Sileo L, Franson J C 1982 Toxicity of Prudhoe Bay crude oil to sandhill cranes. Journal of Wildlife Management 46(2):474–476

Forbes N A 1992 Diagnosis of avian aspergillosis and treatment with itraconazole. Veterinary Record 130:519

Forbes N A 1996 Nervous conditions. In: Benyon P H, Forbes N A, Harcourt-Brown N H (eds) Manual of raptors, pigeons and waterfowl. BSAVA, Cheltenham, p 318

Frasca S Jr, Weber E S, Urquhart H et al 2005 Isolation and characterization of Mycoplasma sphenisci sp. nov. from the choana of an aquarium-reared jackass penguin (Spheniscus demersus). Journal of Clinical Microbiology 43(6):2976–2979

Fry D M, Lowenstine L J 1985 Pathology of common murres and Cassin's auklets exposed to oil. Archives of Environmental Contamination and Toxicology 14:725–737

Gaston A J, Hipfner J M, Campbell D 2002 Heat and mosquitos cause breeding failure and adult mortality in and Arctic nesting seabird. Ibis 144(2):185–191

Gauthier-Clerc M, Eterradossi N, Toquin D et al 2002 Serological survey of the king penguin Aptenodytes patagonicus, in Crozet archipelago for antibodies to infectious bursal disease, influenza A and Newcastle disease virus. Polar Biology 25(4):316

Gayoso A M, Fulco V K 2006 Occurrence patterns of Alexandrium tamarense (Lebour) Balech populations in the Golo Nuevo (Patagonia, Argentina), with observations on ventral pore occurrence in natural and cultured cells. Harmful Algae 5(3):233–241

Gilbertson M 1988 Toxic contaminants and ecosystem health: A Great Lakes focus. John Wiley & Sons, New York

Gilbertson M, Fox G A 1977 Pollutant-associated embryonic mortality of Great Lakes herring gulls. Environmental Pollution 12:211–216

Golightly R T, Newman, S H, Craig, E N et al 2003 Post release survival and behaviour of Western Gulls following exposure to oil and rehabilitation. Proceedings of the 7th international Effects of Oil on Wildlife conference, Hamburg, Germany, 14–16 October 2003. IFAW, 290 Summer St, Yarmouth Port, MA, USA

Gough R E, Drury S E, Welchman D et al 2002 Isolation of birnavirus and reovirus like agents from penguins in the United Kingdom. Veterinary Record 151(14):422–424

Greenwood A G 2000 Identification of Clostridium perfringens enterotoxin in penguins. Veterinary Record 146(6):172

Greth A, Rester C, Gerlach H et al 1995 Pathological effects of oil in seabirds during the Arabian Gulf oil spill. In: Frink L (ed) Wildlife and oil spills, response research and contingency planning. Tri-state Bird Rescue and Research Inc, p 134–141

Grim K C, van der Merwe E, Sullivan M et al 2003 Plasmodium juxtanucleare associated with mortality in black-footed penguins (Spheniscus demersus) admitted to a rehabilitation center. Journal of Zoo and Wildlife Medicine 34(3):250–255

Grim K C, Mccutchan T, Li J, Sullivan M et al 2004 Preliminary results of an anticircumsporozoite DNA vaccine trial for protection against avian malaria in captive African black footed penguins (Sphensicus demersus). Journal of Zoo and Wildlife Medicine 35(2):154–161

Hale W G 1980 Waders. William Collins, Glasgow, p 82–99

Hartung R, Hunt G S 1966 Toxicity of some oils to waterfowl. Journal of Wildlife Management 30:564–569

Hill J R, Bogue G 1978 Natural pox infection in a common murre (Uria aalge). Journal of Wildlife Diseases 14:337

Holmes J P 1995 Health of free-living guillemots (Uria aalga) and razorbills (Alca torda): the value of detailed post-mortem examinations in a sample of beached seabird carcases. MSc thesis, University of London

Holmes W N, Cronshaw J, Gorsline J 1978 Some effects of ingested petroleum on seawater-adapted ducks (Anas platyrhynchos). Environmental Research 17:177–190

Jackwood D J, Gough R E, Sommer S E 2005 Nucleotide and amino acid sequence analysis of a birnavirus isolated from penguins. Veterinary Record 156(17):550–552

Jensen W I 1979 An outbreak of streptococcosis in eared grebes (Podiceps nigricollis). Avian Diseases 23:543

Jensen W I, Cotter S E 1976 An outbreak of erysipelas in eared grebes (Podiceps nigricollis). Journal of Wildlife Diseases 12:583

Jacobson E R, Raphael B L, Nguyen H T et al 1980 Avian pox infection aspergillosis and renal trematodiosis in a royal tern. Journal of Wildlife Diseases 16:627

Kaneene J B, Flint Taylor R, Sikarskie J G et al 1985 Disease patterns in the Detroit Zoo: A study of the avian population from 1973 through 1983. Journal of the American Veterinary Medical Association 187(11):1129–1131

Khan R A, Ryan P 1991 Long-term effects of crude oil on common murres (Uria aalge) following rehabilitation. Bulletin of Environmental Contamination and Toxicology 46:216–222

King A S, McLelland J 1984 Birds, their structure and function. Baillière Tindall, London

Kirkwood J K, Cunningham A A, Hawkey C et al 1995 Haematology of fledgling Manx shearwaters (Puffinus puffinus) with and without 'puffinosis'. Journal of Wildlife Diseases 31(1):96–98

Leighton F A, Peakall D B, Butler R G 1983 Heinz-body haemolytic anaemia from the ingestion of crude oil: A primary toxic effect in marine birds. Science 220:871–873

Leighton F A, Couillard C M, Lusimbo W S 1995 Recent studies on the toxicity of petroleum oils to avian embryos. In: Frink L (ed) Wildlife and oil spills, response research and contingency planning. Tri-state Bird Rescue and Research Inc, p 115–118

Lloyd C S, Thomas G J, Macdonald J W et al 1976 Wild bird mortality caused by botulism in Britain, 1975. Biological Conservation 10:119–129

Louzis C, Guittet M, Richard C et al 1984 Un example desequilibre naturel au sein d'un ecosysteme marin: la mortalité de mouettes triactyles. Bulletin de l'Académie Vétérinaire de France 57:315–323

MacGarvin M 1990 The North Sea. Collins and Brown, London

Mahaffy L 1990 The question of avian water repellency: why are some birds more difficult to rehabilitate? Oil Symposium 1990. The 13th

Annual Conference of the International Wildlife Rehabilitation Council. International Bird Rescue Research Center, Berkeley, CA

Malcolm H M, Osborn D, Wright J et al 2003 Polychlorinated biphenyl (PCB) congener concentrations in seabirds found dead in mortality incidents around the British coast. Archives of Environmental Contamination and Toxicology 45(1):136–147

Mangin S, Gauthier-Clerc M, Frenot Y et al 2003 Ticks *Ixodes uriae* and breeding performance of a colonial seabird, king penguin *Aptenodytes patagonicus*. Journal of Avian Biology 34(1):30–34

Mazzaro L M, Tuttle A, Wyatt J et al 2004 Plasma electrolyte concentrations in captive and free ranging African penguins (*Spheniscus demersus*) maintained with and without dietary salt supplements. Zoo Biology 23(5):397–408

Nel D C, Whittington P A 2003 Rehabilitation of oiled African penguins: A conservation success story. Birdlife South Africa and the Avian Demography Unit, Cape Town, South Africa

Newman S, Zinkl J 1996 Establishment of haematological, serum biochemical and electrophoretogram reference intervals for species of marine birds likely to be impacted by oil spill incidents in the state of California. Baseline Marine Bird Project for the California Dept of Fish and Game, Office of Oil Spill Prevention and Response

Newman S H, 2003 Post release survival of common murres (*Uria aalge*). Proceedings of the 7th international Effects of Oil on Wildlife conference, Hamburg, Germany, 14–16 October 2003. IFAW, 290 Summer St, Yarmouth Port, MA, USA

Olsen B, Jaenson T G T, Noppa L et al 1993 A Lyme borreliosis cycle in seabirds and *Ixodes uriae* ticks. Nature 362:340–342

Olsen B, Duffy D C, Jaenson T G T et al 1995 Transhemispheric exchange of Lyme disease spirochaetes by seabirds. Journal of Clinical Microbiology 33(12):3270–3274

Orbell J D, Ngeh L N, Bigger S W 2004 Whole bird models for the magnetic cleansing of oiled feathers. Marine Pollution Bulletin 48(3/4):336–340

Osterblom H, Jeugd H P, van der Olsson O 2004 Adult survival and avian cholera in common guillemots Uria aalge in the Baltic Sea. Ibis (London) 146(3):531–534

Otto C M, McCall Kaufman G, Crowe D T 1989 Intraosseous infusion of fluids and therapeutics. Compendium of Continuing Education for the Practicing Veterinarian 11(4):421–431

Palma R L 1994 New synonymies in lice (Insecta: Phthiraptera) infesting albatrosses and petrels (*Procellariiformes*). New Zealand Entomologist 17:64–69

Petermann S, Glunder G, Heffels-Redmann U, Hinz K H 1989 Post-mortem findings in guillemots, kittiwakes, herring gulls and black headed gulls found ill or dead in the Heligoland Bight between 1982 and 1985. Deutsche Tierarztliche Wochenschrift 96:271–277

Piersma T, Van Eerden M R 1988 Feather eating in great crested grebes (*Podiceps cristatus*): a unique solution to the problems of debris and gastric parasites in fish-eating birds. Ibis 131:477–486

Rambaud Y F, Flach E J, Freeman K P 2003 Malignant melanoma in a Humboldt penguin (*Spheniscus humboldti*). Veterinary Record 153(7):217–218

Ramos J A, Bowler J, Davis L et al 2001 Activity patterns and effect of ticks on growth and survival of tropical Roseate Tern nestlings. Auk 118(3):709–716

Redig P T 1996 Nursing avian patients. In: Benyon P H, Forbes N A, Harcourt-Brown N H (eds) Manual of raptors, pigeons and waterfowl. BSAVA, Cheltenham, p 42–46

Renner M S, Zaias J, Bossart G D 2001 Cholangiocarcinoma with metastasis in a captive Adelie penguin (*Pygoscelis adeliae*). Journal of Zoo and Wildlife Medicine 32(3):384–386

Rijke A M 1968 The water repellency and feather structure of cormorants (*Phalacrocoracidae*). Journal of Experimental Biology 48:185–189

Roertgen K E 1990 Avian malaria in oil contaminated common murres (*Uria aalge*). Wildlife Journal 13(3):3–8

Sabirovic M, Hall S, Wilesmith J et al 2006 HPAI H5N1 situation in Europe and potential risk factors for the introduction of the virus into the United Kingdom. Online. Available: www.defra.gov.uk/animalh/diseases/monitoring/index.htm

Sano Y, Aoki M, Takahashi H et al 2005 The first record of *Dirofilaria immitis* infection in a humboldt penguin, *Spheniscus humboldti*. Journal of Parasitology 91(5):1235–1237

Scott M J, Wiens J A, Claeys R R 1975 Organochlorine levels associated with a common murre die-off in Oregon. Journal of Wildlife Management 39(2):310–320

Sharp B E 1996 Post-release survival of oiled cleaned seabirds in North America. Ibis 138:222–228

Shindu J 1998 Malignant melanoma in a Humboldt penguin (*Spheniscus humboldti*). Japanese Journal of Zoo and Wildlife Medicine 3(1):65–68

Sileo L, Sievert P R, Samuel D M 1990 Causes of mortality of albatross chicks at Midway Atoll. Journal of Wildlife Diseases 26(3):329–338

Steele G M, Davies C R, Jones L D et al 1990 Life history of the seabird tick, *Ixodes (Ceratixodes) uriae*, at St Abbs Head, Scotland. Acarologia 31(2):125–130

Stoskopf M K 1993 Zoo and wild animal medicine: current therapy 3. W B. Saunders, Philadelphia, PA

Stoskopf M K, Kennedy-Stoskopf S 1986 Zoo and wild animal medicine. W B Saunders, Philadelphia, PA

Swennen C 1977 Laboratory research on seabirds. Netherlands Institute for Sea Research

Tanabe S 2002 Contamination and toxic effects of persistent endocrine disrupters in marine mammals and birds. Marine Pollution Bulletin 45(1/12):69–77

Thompson D R, Hamer K C 2000 Stress in seabirds: causes, consequences and diagnostic value. Journal of Aquatic Ecosystem Stress and Recovery 7(1):91–110

Tillet D E, Ankley G T, Giesey J P et al 1992 Polychlorinated biphenyl residues and egg mortality in double-crested cormorants from the Great Lakes. Environmental Toxicology and Chemistry 11: 1281–1288

Tseng F S 1993 Care of oiled seabirds: a veterinary perspective. In: Proceedings of the 1993 International Oil Spill Conference. American Petroleum Institute, p 421–424

Tuttle A D, Andreadis T G, Frasca S Jr, Dunn J L 2005 Eastern equine encephalitis in a flock of African penguins maintained at an aquarium. Journal of the American Veterinary Medical Association 226(12):2058–2062

van der Merwe E 2001 Standard operating procedures. SANCCOB, Capetown, South Africa

Wernham C V, Peach W J, Browne S 1997 Survival rates of rehabilitation. Unpublished report prepared for Sea Empress Environmental Evaluation Committee. SEEEC

White F H, Simpson C F, Williams L E 1973 Isolation of *Edwardsiella tarda* from aquatic animal species and surface waters in Florida. Journal of Wildlife Diseases 9:204

Wilson J E 1950 Newcastle disease in a gannet (*Sula bassana*). Veterinary Record 62:33

Wingate B, Barker I K, King N W 1980 Poxvirus infection of the white-tailed tropic bird (*Phaethon lepturus*) in Bermuda, North Atlantic Ocean. Journal of Wildlife Diseases 16:619

Wood A M, Munro R, Robinson I 1993 Oiled birds from Shetland, January 1993. Veterinary Record 132:367–368

Yonemaru K, Sakai H, Asaoka Y et al 2004 Proventricular adenocarcinoma in a Humboldt penguin (*Spheniscus humboldti*) and a great horned owl (*Bubo virginiansus*): identification of origin by mucin histochemistry. Avian Pathology 33(1):77–81

17

The management of a multi-species bird collection in a zoological park

Lorenzo Crosta and Linda Timossi

Introduction

The management of multi-species collections, which may include ratites to hummingbirds, is obviously far more complex than that of collections including single taxonomic groups such as Psittaciformes, Falconiformes or Galliformes. Furthermore, for a zoo veterinarian it is uncommon to be a real expert in avian medicine, unless he/she is employed in a zoological garden that is primarily a bird park, or when the avian collection in a zoo is a relevant portion of the animal collection. In most cases a well-known avian veterinarian is consulting from a distance, and called upon depending on specific needs. It is important for the avian veterinarian involved in zoological medicine to keep in mind that his/her patients are wild animals. The individual avian species' biological background must be considered, when planning treatment protocol that would involve capturing, handling, delivering anaesthesia, providing medication, or manipulating management protocol (e.g. nutritional plans, mixing different species, designing an exhibit).

Another important aspect, when taking care of a bird collection in a zoological garden, is to define the main purpose for the birds to be displayed: an avian collection maybe private or open to the public, and this simple fact will make a big difference for the appearance of the birds and the aviaries (Fig. 17.1). Zoos are different from private collections in that they must fulfil special legal requirements, which are far more limiting.

Other concerns, which may not be strictly medical in nature, but surely involve the committed professional, are:

- What is the 'theme' of each display, paddocks, aviaries and exhibits (e.g. African birds only, birds of prey)?
- Is there a biologically oriented animal exhibition (e.g. artificial simulation of the specific environment where a given species lives in the wild)?
- Is the park involved in recovery programmes? (e.g. is the maintenance of the genetic pool a major issue?)
- Is the institution involved in research programmes in biology, behaviour, nutrition and diseases, and publication of the obtained data?

Part 1: General information

Working in a zoo as an avian vet

The involvement of the zoo veterinarian in avian medicine depends on the importance of birds versus other taxonomic groups in a given collection.

Regardless of the avian caseload, a veterinarian's responsibility in a zoo is based on strict routine: clinical and prophylactic actions are combined with record keeping and understanding the general problems of a collection (Fig. 17.2). This routine involves daily, weekly, monthly and yearly work schedules based on the bird species within the collection, exhibit conditions, presence of bird shows, presence of a breeding centre, and local weather conditions.

Most veterinary clinics in zoo settings have a complete complement of required medical equipment allowing for a full range of diagnostic test and surgical procedures. The 'in-house' laboratory normally includes microbiology, haematology, blood chemistry and cytology. Other diagnostic tests (e.g. histopathology, toxicology, virology, specific biochemistry analysis) have to be forwarded to off-site laboratories.

Specific medical equipment

Although there may be some differences, the medical equipment used by the zoo/avian veterinarian does not

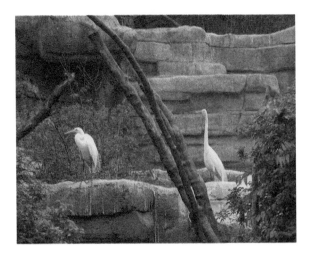

Fig 17.1 A pleasant exhibit may reproduce the birds' natural environment.

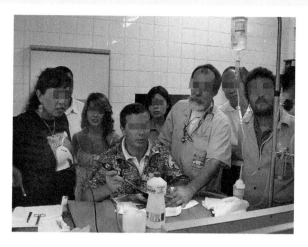

Fig 17.2 Teaching new techniques in the institution where one works, or being invited by other zoos for teaching purposes is one of the duties of zoo veterinarians.

Table 17.1 Equipment for birds in the zoo clinic

Cages, aviaries and hospital cages	The choice of the different enclosures depends on the bird species in the collection
Anaesthesia	A transportable anaesthesia machine is important if there are patients that are difficult to move, or for which moving is risky
	A small animal ventilator is a must when performing long surgeries in birds
Endoscopy	A standard avian rigid endoscopy set is a must. If larger birds are present, a flexible endoscope is also indicated
Surgery	Standard surgical tools for avian patients
X-ray machine	Zoos often need portable X-ray machines
Ultrasound machine	An ultrasound machine equipped with different probes is useful for birds. For smaller patients a 10 MHz probe may be necessary; for most patients a 5–7.5 MHz probe is OK

differ significantly from that found in any avian veterinarian's office (Table 17.1). Different equipment needs may be related to the presence of birds with very specific needs (e.g. Struthioniformes, Sphenisciformes, largest birds of prey). In some cases, if the collection has a limited budget, it is better to have collaborative agreements with well-equipped veterinary clinics in the vicinity, for the use of equipment/staff.

Medical equipment required for the avian veterinarian servicing a large zoo collection should include special cages for specific patients, such as birds of prey, long-legged birds (including water birds), and birds with specific climate needs (e.g. penguins) (Table 17.2).

Planning enclosures

Individuals involved in planning the habitat of zoological avian collections often have different ideas about developing the perfect enclosure for a given avian species. Teamwork is the basis of a well-designed, psychologically stimulating, and educational display or aviary. The different ideas should be discussed and combined in the preplanning phase: once the building work has started it is often impossible or too difficult to make any changes.

The working team must include people that directly interact with the animals, through daily contact, such as keepers, curators and veterinarians, but will also include technical advisers that do not necessarily work with the animals, such as architects, engineers, gardeners, electricians and plumbers.

An important point, when managing a bird collection as a veterinarian, is to ensure optimum care to the animals that live in a captive situation through social and physical welfare. Environmental enrichment can help fulfil the goals of providing the most favourable enclosure.

Environmental enrichment is the improvement of the cages where the animals are kept, to stimulate their natural behaviour. **Further, a natural environment is much more interesting and will promote the life and the natural behaviour of the animals.**

When refurbishing/building a cage, aviary or exhibit, the natural behaviour of the species should be considered, together with other facts regarding animals to be housed in that enclosure (Table 17.3a).

Moreover, particular attention should be focused on the selection of animals occupying neighbouring cages, as there could be incompatibility between species or individuals, including aggressive or challenging behaviour during the breeding season.

Exhibit compatibility is particularly true for most raptor species, which with few exceptions require individual territories. Some parrot species, such as some *Amazona* spp. and macaws (*Ara* spp.), are very protective of their partners during the breeding season.

Conversely, there are birds that need the presence of the group for breeding (e.g. flamingoes). Monk parakeets (*M. monachus*) build very complicated nests in a communal setting. Also cockatoos (*Cacatua* spp.) and African grey parrots (*Psittacus erithacus*) benefit from the visual and vocal contact of co-specific birds.

Housing (cages, aviaries and paddocks)

Most bird species have individual housing requirements. When placed in a zoo environment, there are common parameters regarding avian housing requirements that must be considered. Some of the housing parameters are a matter of common sense while others are based on experience. The committed avian veterinarian must always remember

Table 17.2 Facilities for the hospitalization of birds in a zoo

Critically ill birds	A warmed cage is needed, better if O$_2$ can be delivered in the cage and relative humidity can be controlled.
	Intensive care units (ICUs) are available for the average avian patient. Only the largest birds (i.e. ratites) are too big for commercially available ICUs.
Birds with infectious diseases	Should be isolated in a special room/area. This is not the same as the zoo quarantine.
Anseriformes	Ducks, geese and swans may be very different in size, may have different needs for access to water and can have different diets.
	They all produce a considerable amount of soft stools, which are often diluted with water from their soaked feathers. For this reason it is important that they have: a pool with good quality water a good cleaning system for the floor.
Birds of prey	Raptors, either diurnal or nocturnal, should be maintained in cages with solid walls, as they might damage their feathers.
	If a collection is mostly based on birds of prey, indoor blocks and perches for the different species should be available.
Columbiformes	Doves and pigeons are distributed worldwide. Hence, they are very variable in size, needs and diet.
	For short-term hospitalization, they like cages similar to those for psittacines or birds of prey.
	Some species, e.g. crowned pigeons (*Goura* spp.), are extremely shy and need a very quiet cage.
Galliformes	Originate from very different areas and may vary greatly in size and behaviour.
	Galliformes can be kept in English-type cages, of the appropriate size.
	If several Galliformes are kept in a pen, then a very efficient floor cleaning system is needed.
Long-legged birds (storks, flamingoes, cranes)	Although the exhibition areas for long-legged birds are very different, depending on species, these birds share similar needs when kept in the hospital.
	Primary importance is given to the flooring, which must be soft enough to avoid sores and bumblefoot, hard enough to last long time, and should stand the strongest disinfectants.
Penguins and auks	Sphenisciformes and Alcidae are rather different, but both need to swim in cold, good quality water.
	Furthermore, they all are sensitive to fungal diseases and are fish eaters.
	Ideally a hospital (or quarantine) room for penguins and auks needs to have: a salt water pool a filtration system for water and air a water and air temperature control system.
Psittaciformes	Cages of various sizes are needed for psittacine birds, as they vary a lot in size, diet and behaviour.
Small birds (mostly passerines)	English-type cages (walls are all solid, except the front) are preferred for these shy species, in order to minimize stress.

that birds are kept in a zoo for exhibition and education; therefore the following are important points to consider:

1. The exhibition must be pleasant for the visitors to see.
2. The appearance of the animals must be in a natural setting.
3. The environment should be optimum for birds.
4. Any risk factors must be minimized.

In order to achieve the above results, some factors will be managed accordingly:

Temperature and humidity

When possible, birds should be kept in outdoor exhibits. Indoor facilities have the advantage of being totally controlled, in terms of temperature and humidity, but there are several risks associated with keeping birds indoors (high fungal and bacterial environmental counts are a typical example of what can be observed when indoor facilities are not properly managed). **The high maintenance and increased disease risk factors of indoor facilities require planners to develop outdoor enclosures whenever possible.** Nevertheless, some birds

Table 17.3a Important facts when planning an enclosure

Safety: for the animals, workers and visitors

Routine cleaning: must be easy and effective and prevent bird escapes

Educational requirement of the public

Size and shape of the enclosure

Barriers

Substrate, litter material

Resting area: to rest/hide from public, or from cage mate

Shelters

Temporary elements (perches, ropes, platforms, nests, nesting materials etc.): must be easy to change or renovate)

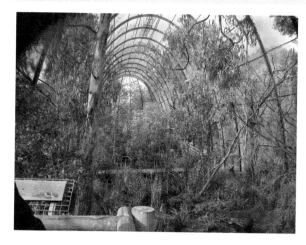

Fig 17.3 Adequate planting is very important in large and walk-through aviaries.

must be housed inside during the coldest (or rarely the warmest) months (e.g. the smallest passerines and psittacines, penguins, snowy owls, gyrfalcons).

Air and water quality

For bird species that require significant quantities of water (e.g. ducks, flamingoes, penguins, auks), and for those kept in an indoor facility, it is of primary importance to routinely monitor the quality of water and air. Air and water must be filtered and changed according to several factors including bird species, biomass load, available room per bird, and outside/inside temperature. Water and air within the enclosure must be checked for the presence of bacteria and fungi, which may indicate either a source of possible pathogens, or a deterioration of the filtering system.

Photoperiod

Most of the bird species originating from temperate areas are dependent on the light cycle for their reproduction activity. Moreover, some physiological cycles (e.g. moulting), are dependent on photoperiod. Species originating from extreme latitudes may have exacerbated light-cycle-dependent issues and this should be taken into consideration when designing exhibits for these animals. When artificially provided light quality is an important husbandry consideration special lamps and bulbs may be necessary for certain avian species and most of those lamps have to be replaced frequently, in order to maintain their healthful properties.

Plants

Most bird species like plants and branches for hiding, nesting, displaying or simply perching. Not all trees are appropriate for planting in an aviary. Most zoos employ botanists, biologists and gardeners who provide veterinarians and curators with advice on selecting the most suitable trees for a given bird species (Fig. 17.3).

Flooring

This is another topic of primary importance. A proper floor is more important for ground-dwelling birds predisposed to infectious pododermatitis lesions (bumblefoot).

The avian veterinarian must always remember the following regarding bird feet:

- When one foot is damaged, 50% of the standing surface is lost.
- In birds weighing more than 150–200 grams, the healthy foot bearing all the bird's weight will soon be compromised.
- Bird feet cannot be used properly if damaged (e.g. walking, swimming, perching, capturing prey, and bearing the weight when the contralateral foot is used to eat).

Roofing

In zoos and bird parks there are birds that do not need a roof to enclose the exhibit because they are flightless (e.g. ratites), or they have been pinioned, or their feathers are routinely trimmed. Nevertheless, most birds do maintain their ability to fly, which is important to some species, as flight is part of more complex behaviours, such as courtship, or raising chicks.

When a roof is needed, several factors are taken into consideration (Table 17.3b).

Nests

The presence of a nest plays a key role in most species' behaviour (Fig. 17.4). For this reason bird curators and veterinarians have to clarify whether they want specific animals to be given the opportunity to reproduce. It should be stressed that birds be placed in an environment

Table 17.3b Suitable roofing according to birds and zoo type

1. Will birds be exhibited to visitors? —————————————→ No

Yes

Roof will simply have to be effective

Roof has to be effective AND must have a nice, natural look. 'Invisible' nets are available and do well for the purpose.

2. Will birds bite and chew the roof? —————————————→ No

Yes —————————————→ Select a material/shape, that cannot be bitten.

3. Will birds climb/hang from the roof? —————————————→ No

Yes —————————————→ Avoid roofs made with wire mesh.
Avoid solid roofing.
Design roof made with wooden lathing strips, 2 cm thick and 10 cm high. Arrange the strips vertically, 5 cm apart: this allows resting birds to see the sky and receive fresh air, rain (and snow). When the birds are flying, this roof will appear as a solid wall and the birds won't fly into it.

that is conducive to reproduction whenever possible. Animals in a reproductively active enclosure gain psychological and physiological benefits.

A nest should be made available for a breeding pair of birds. Nesting considerations for birds include:

- Shape: most bird species have a preferred nest shape. With species that do not have a specific nest shape, two or three different nest selections are provided to improve the chances of selection.
- Size: size is important and should be appropriate for the particular birds' size.

- Material (of which the nest is made): generally speaking most nests are made of wood. Nevertheless, there are birds that prefer different materials, such as mud, stones, rocks, hay and grass. Finally, there are species (e.g. king penguins (*Aptenodytes patagonicus*)) that do not build nests, but incubate their single-egg clutches on their feet, covered by a skin fold.
- Building/filling material: some birds will accept a nest that has been pre-filled with some bedding material (e.g. wood shavings), but other birds prefer to build their own nest, or to fill a nest box

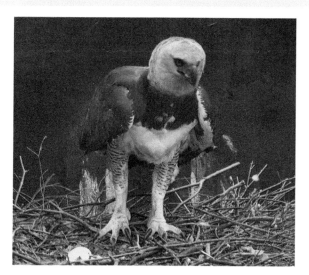

Fig 17.4 A simple nest platform for large birds of prey is adequate provided the aviary environment is relatively quiet. Harpy eagle (*Harpia harpyja*).

with suitable material which may be considered part of normal courtship behaviour. The lack of proper nest-building material for a given species (i.e. stones for some penguins, mud for flamingoes, grass for some psittacine and passerine species) will lead to breeding failure.

- Location: this is especially important when working with very shy species, or with bird flocks, or in multi-species exhibits. Shy species (e.g. crowned pigeons (*Goura* spp.)) prefer a hidden area for nesting with the area often surrounded by plants and bushes. Bird flocks may be willing to share the same area for nesting (e.g. flamingoes), or prefer to interact during the day, but maintain their privacy when in the nest cavity (e.g. lovebirds). When working with a multi-species exhibit, it is important to avoid competition for nest sites and nesting materials. Exhibit competition must be considered when planning the enclosure, mixing only species that are fully compatible. Finally, the nest must be put in a place that is not risky to offspring when taking their first flights. Promoting offspring safety in this manner will help avoid dangerous 'learning crashes'.

- Hygiene: nests are easily soiled with excrement from the offspring, allowing parasites and bacteria to find the perfect environmental conditions for growth: heat, humidity and plenty of organic material for nutrition. Consequently, when present, the bedding material plays an important role when trying to maintain a clean nest environment. In general, bedding material should be clean and free

of pathogens. Inadequate bedding material may increase the birds' exposure to *Aspergillus* spp. organisms. Ectoparasites may be avoided by adding 5% carbaryl powder to the bedding material at the beginning of the breeding season. Bedding material should be routinely tested for bacterial and fungal organisms. Toxic substances within the bedding material may contribute to disease. Wood shavings, widely used as nest bedding, must be checked for paints and wood preservative contamination. The condition of the bedding material must be monitored when the nest is active. Any nest box monitoring should be undertaken in cooperation with the curator or animal keeper in order not to disturb the breeding pair and risk chick mortality. Cleaning and disinfecting the nest after the breeding season should be properly conducted. Wooden nest boxes might require replacement. Natural trunks should be cleaned as carefully as possible with appropriate disinfecting solutions, which will allow the birds to use the nesting site again. In species that use stones for nesting (e.g. gentoo penguin (*Pygoscelis papua*)), the stones should be removed and carefully cleaned after the breeding season. Permanent nesting sites including caves for puffins (*Fratercula arctica*) have to be designed for ease of cleaning and disinfecting. For proper disinfection, the disinfectant has to contact the surface to be cleaned. All organic material must be removed from the surface to be cleaned prior to application of the disinfecting solution. Dirt and/or organic material cannot be disinfected. The design of a nest should always be a compromise between the natural breeding behaviour of the species, its specific hygiene requirements, and the captive situation.

- Access for inspection: ideally a nest for birds in captivity should be easily inspected by the zoo staff. For this reason, not only the location and design are important, but also birds should be trained to allow routine inspection of the nest. If training begins outside of the breeding season, then inspection during egg incubation and chick rearing will be easier and almost without risks.

Quarantine

Quarantine guidelines have been established by several zoo associations (AZA, EAZA); furthermore several articles have been written about quarantine regarding zoological collections. Common sense is very useful when introducing new birds into a well-established collection.

All incoming birds will have to spend at least 6 weeks in quarantine. This also includes birds that have been removed from the collection, then returned (e.g. breeding loan).

Ideally a zoo should have a designated building to be used as a quarantine facility. This building should include various different-sized rooms that will host single birds, small flocks, or even large flocks. It is better to split a large shipment and fill several rooms, than to waste a large room on a single bird. All quarantine rooms should have separate, low-pressure ventilation systems (Fig. 17.5).

Birds must undergo a simple physical examination upon entering a facility, but there is little diagnostic value to the test results generated immediately after the animal's arrival. After a 2 to 4 day conditioning period each bird should be subjected to an intensive medical check-up. Samples for testing should be collected after the conditioning period. Diagnostic tests to be submitted depend on birds' species and origin; the following test protocol is recommended:

- Microbiology (bacteria and fungi from cloaca, choanal and trachea).
- Parasitology (endo- and ectoparasites). Remember to look for protozoan parasites (e.g. coccidia, *Giardia* spp., *Trichomonas* spp.).
- Virology (circovirus, polyomavirus, herpesvirus and possibly adenovirus in the case of psittacine species, avian influenza and Newcastle disease for all birds). Different testing technologies (e.g. PCR, serology, virus isolation) will be used in different situations.
- Checking for *Chlamydophila psittaci* (test for antigens and antibody titres).
- Haematology and blood chemistry, in order to assess the health status of birds, besides the transmission of infection diseases.
- Other tests, depending on the species.

The birds may be integrated into the collection after the quarantine period only if all of the diagnostic tests are negative (i.e. indicate the absence of any detectable disease or infection).

Special attention to behaviour and feeding of new animals should be addressed in the first weeks of quarantine. Before the birds arrive it is very important to get detailed information about their feeding habits, in order to provide food to which they are accustomed, thereby contributing to a smooth transition between facilities.

Ideally, to avoid transmission of diseases from the quarantine facility to the rest of the collection, a separate keeper for the quarantined birds is preferred. Hygienic measures, such as separate clothes, boots, and hand and shoe disinfection baths, should be provided.

Bird nutrition in a zoo setting

Working in a zoo presents the veterinarian with a variety of avian species, often with unusual or specialized diets, and, unfortunately for many bird groups specific

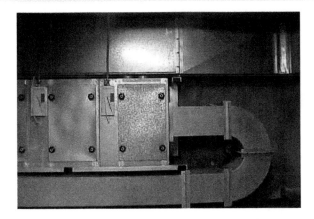

Fig 17.5 Part of the air filtering system in a zoo quarantine facility.

commercial diets are not manufactured. **Hence, the importance of working jointly with other professionals (e.g. zoologist, biologists, nutritionists) in an effort to customize the most appropriate diet for a given avian species.**

To date, specific diets are commercially available for psittacine birds, mynah birds, canaries, small finches, pigeons, thrushes, cranes, emus, flamingoes, game birds, ostriches, waterfowl, sea ducks and toucans.

In some zoos, diets are provided according to 'local traditions,' 'avicultural myths' and keepers' experiences, which may or may not be ideal. Most keepers are open minded and very committed to their animals; therefore, if dietary changes are needed and will benefit the birds, cooperation regarding nutritional improvement is usually forthcoming. The authors have found it beneficial to invite curators and bird keepers to assist with avian necropsies, when the cause of death is suspected to be malnutrition.

Imitation of a species' diet is the best option in a captive environment, but this may not always be possible for several reasons:

- Some or all diet components are not available.
- Nutritional requirements in captivity are different from those in the wild.
- Some food cannot be digested in the absence of other unknown or unavailable items.
- Birds do not recognize the offered diet as food.

A more reasonable approach to avian nutrition is to hire a nutritionist and have available a computer program that helps design a diet for a given species. These programs will not provide the answers to all nutritional questions, but are extremely helpful in avoiding gross mistakes, especially when attempting to balance a diet.

If a diet for birds has to be revised, especially regarding avian species for which there is a paucity of scientific nutritional data available and when birds have

been fed for a long time according to other customs, the best way to evaluate the nutritional value of a diet is to use common sense and professional veterinary skills. Generally speaking, even if a bird flock has been fed a locally developed diet for a long time, it can be assumed that diet and general management were adequate if the birds are in good physical condition; do not show any disease signs; feathers and skin are normal; they moult regularly; sexual behaviour is displayed and reproduction occurs; no pathogenic microorganisms are cultured and blood tests do not show unusual variations; and, finally, in cases of fatalities, no gross lesions related to nutritional problems are observed.

Zoo veterinarians and bird conservation

For many endangered species there exist coordinated breeding programmes and international studbooks (Fig. 17.6). Furthermore, it is generally accepted that diseases may play an important role in the extinction of traditionally small avian populations. Therefore zoo veterinarians are becoming more involved in bird conservation programmes, both in situ and ex situ.

Conservation activities in which avian veterinarians are involved include:

- *Clinical care for individuals belonging to conservation programmes.* **In the case of highly endangered species the individual bird and its genetics are of the highest importance for the survival of viable populations in captivity (Fig. 17.7). Therefore, when sick animals present, the highest standard veterinary procedures are used, as they should be with any patient treated in a veterinary hospital.**
- *Development of nutrition and preventative medicine programmes.* Together with zoo

nutritionists, biologists, curators and animal keepers the development of nutritional standards and preventative medicine programmes plays an important role in conservation. Nutrition of endangered species should have the goal to provide birds with the most adequate food, not only to fulfil their nutritional requirements, but also to provide a diet that would allow the bird to recognize native food sources if released through a reintroduction programme.

Any preventative medicine programme for an endangered species, which will eventually be released into the wild, needs to fulfil special reintroduction requirements (Fig. 17.8). Populations should to be kept free of *known* infectious agents (e.g. viruses, bacteria, parasites). Furthermore, pre-release quarantine programmes must take into consideration those diseases that are still *unknown*. In other words, the professional involved with

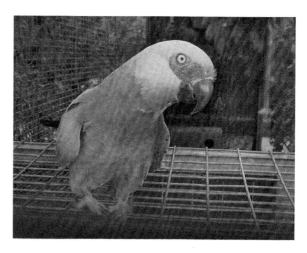

Fig 17.7 The Spix's macaw (*Cyanopsitta spixii*). This species has not been observed in its native habitat since 2000.

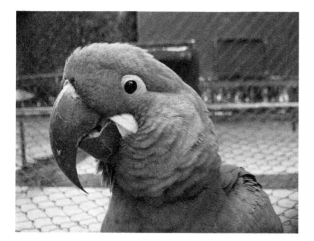

Fig 17.6 The Lear's macaw (*Anodorhynchus leari*), one of the most endangered psittacine birds.

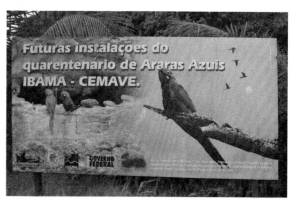

Fig 17.8 Most institutions involved in bird conservation and recovery programmes financially support the building of facilities in situ.

conservation efforts must do all that is possible to avoid introduction of disease in the pre-existing wild populations.

- *Improvement of fertility and reproduction, including new techniques for the evaluation of breeding performance of endangered species.* **For some endangered species captive management and breeding will be the only and last chance to survive.** Especially with small avian populations, the reproduction of every single individual plays an important role for the genetic variability of the population. Therefore all measures should be undertaken to improve fertility and reproduction. There are many reasons for poor reproduction and low fertility rate: poor aviculture management, inadequate nutrition and medical problems.

The task of an avian veterinarian should be to exclude and control the medical reasons for non-reproductive animals and develop, together with the curator, a strategy to improve environmental and management conditions in order to achieve a higher breeding rate (Fig. 17.9). Medical reasons for low reproduction include: obesity, oophoritis, salpingitis, cloacitis, cloacal papillomas, orchitis (often caused by *C. psittaci* infections) and other diseases not related to copulation.

Part 2: Group-specific guidelines

Birds of virtually all orders have been kept in captivity; most of them have also been exhibited in zoos or bird parks (Fig. 17.10). Several avian species have been bred in captivity, and attempts have been made to reproduce many more.

It is clear now that within each taxonomic group there are bird species more adaptable to captivity and therefore more suitable for captive breeding and exhibiting.

Although a few very passionate and committed aviculturists have eventually had breeding success with even the most difficult of avian species, this success with captive reared birds does not apply to every species. The aviculture breeding successes may partially explain why some birds are kept more frequently than others.

Psittaciformes

Parrots are one of the most widely exhibited bird groups. There are roughly 350 species of Psittaciformes ranging from the very small lorikeets and hanging parrots to the huge hyacinth macaw, and each group is very different from the others.

This phenotypic and genotypic variability helps explain why parrots are widely maintained in captivity: not only do they provide companionship, but also there are species suitable for each different house, each garden, and even different budgets.

Parrots are kept in cages or aviaries of different sizes depending on the species and the purpose for which the birds are exhibited. For example, the budgerigar can be easily bred in a home environment, while macaws need long flying aviaries, and cockatoos are known to develop aggressive behaviours when kept in cages that are too small resulting in little psychological stimulation.

Design of the aviary depends on the native geographic location and the species (e.g. keas (*Nestor notabilis*) are known to thrive in a cold climate, even in presence of snow, while birds of the same size, like the palm cockatoo (*Probosciger aterrimus*), are known to have problems when the temperature drops below 10°C (±50°F) (Fig. 17.11). Palm cockatoos require a winter enclosure connected to the outside aviary, while the kea can be hosted in a large light cage or aviary year round.

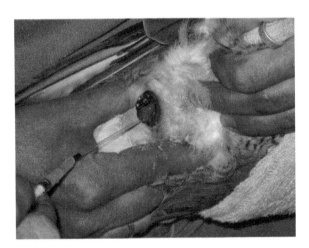

Fig 17.9 Artificial insemination is widely used in reproduction of selected bird families (e.g. Falconiformes, Galliformes, Gruiformes).

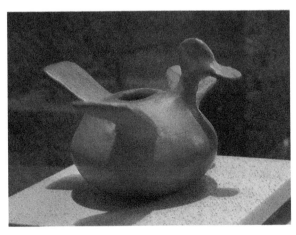

Fig 17.10 Birds have been bred by humans since the ancient times: Aztec duck-shaped pot.

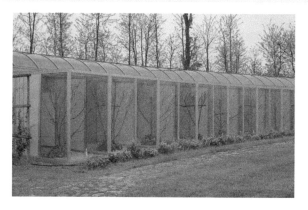

Fig 17.11 Newly built aviaries for a bird park in a temperate climate.

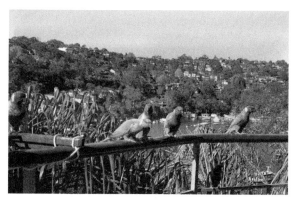

Fig 17.12 Lories are so social that even wild ones can learn to come to private houses. Moluccan lorikeets (*Trichoglossus h. moluccanus*).

Common sense and knowledge of the individual bird species is required to properly care for birds in captivity.

There are sources of information for the minimum requirements for breeding some selected avian species. The minimum requirements for space allowances do not necessarily provide for all of the birds' needs and hence may not result in good management.

Nests are also a key point to psittacine reproduction and aviculture: an aviary that offers the wrong nests will be not successful.

Furthermore, nutrition of the different species may vary significantly. Besides the specific needs of some families, like the lories (Loriidae), even parrot species that are similar in size (e.g. Amazon parrots and cockatoos) should be fed different diets. Conversely, some nutritionists believe that, at least with the more common species, one can improve a commercially formulated diet by adding selected organic seeds, grains, fruit and vegetables.

A nursery has to be organized to care for the baby psittacine birds. The facility would include a room for egg incubation, a room for hatching (or at least special incubators for hatching), and one to three rooms for hand rearing the young.

Lories and lorikeets

Due to their beautiful coloration and gentle nature, which often brings them to the front of aviaries, lories and lorikeets have become popular exhibits in many zoological parks.

This group of psittacine birds, forming the subfamily Loriidae, originates from Southeast Asia, Papua New Guinea, Australia and Polynesia. They are referred to as the brush-tongued parrots, because the tip of the tongue has elongated papillae that give it a brush-like tip. The tongue's papillae have developed because, in nature, Loriidae collect nectar and pollen from flowers as a significant part of their diet. Another important dietary element for lories and lorikeets is fruit. Since Loriidae

eat a diet high in sugar, fruit and water, their stool is often very liquid and difficult to clean.

Almost all of the Loriidae are brightly coloured, and this family includes some of the most beautiful birds in the world (Fig. 17.12). Apart from their coloration, lories and lorikeets are attractive to keep as companion animals because of their positive response to human contact. They are also good breeders and often nest three or four times a year in warm climates, especially if the chicks are removed and hand raised from about 2–3 weeks of age.

Housing

Aviaries suitable for pairs of lories or lorikeets are 1–1.2 m wide, 3 m long and 2 m high. These birds can also be kept very successfully in suspended cages 1 m × 1 m × 3 m long, which of course are not suitable for display purposes. They are very aggressive when mating, so only breeding pairs should be maintained in reproductive flights.

Nest boxes vary in size from 20 × 20 × 30 cm to 25 × 25 × 50 cm, depending on the size of the lorikeet. Entrance holes are placed 10 cm from the top of the box, and observations indicate that birds prefer holes that are just big enough for the body to squeeze through.

Approximately 10–15 cm of coarse wood shavings should be placed in the bottom of the box as nesting material. It should be noted that wood shavings may be a source of bacterial and fungal infections. Since lories and lorikeets feed on a liquid-based diet, it might be necessary to change or add new bedding material when the young are being fed.

For this family of birds, a specially designed nest box has proven to be effective against contamination: Instead of a wooden floor, the nest box floor is constructed of wire mesh, allowing the liquid faeces to drop and ensuring better ventilation.

Feeding

'Easy' lories and lorikeets species (e.g. *Trichoglossus* spp., *Eos* spp., *Pseudeos* sp.) are fed a commercial lory diet, which may be a dry formula, or a nectar to be reconstituted with warm water. There are indications that food intake of lories is dependent on energy intake and not on food volume, so a too diluted nectar does not fully meet their nutritional requirements. This explains why lories may eat (or drink) a large amount of loose nectar, expanding their crop to capacity. Along with nectar, there should be fresh fruits such as apples, pears, grapes, papaya and guavas and edible flowers (e.g. hibiscus). Several of the smallest and 'difficult' species do not do well when fed only commercial diets and fruits, and must receive a small amount of seeds. Also, a few well-known lory breeders have developed special 'home-made' recipes for feeding difficult lory species which seem to provide adequate nutrition for these birds.

Since nectar is an ideal medium for bacterial and fungal growth, especially in hot weather, the feed dishes and trays must be sterilized. A strict routine should be adopted in this respect and a double set of feeding dishes and bowls is recommended, to alternate one set while the other is being cleaned.

Breeding

Loriidae usually lay two eggs, with the incubation period varying from 22 to 26 days. Depending on the species, chicks leave the nest boxes between 55 and 85 days of age. When there are chicks in the nest, the shavings become very wet and soiled. It is recommended to change the nest substrate every 3–4 weeks. A 1–2 cm layer of old shavings should be placed on top of the new shavings to encourage the parents to return to the chicks. Special nests can be used for lories, to limit humidity and mould growth inside the nest box (see above).

Pathology

Almost all pathology noted in lory species appears to involve the liver (Fig. 17.13). It is not known whether the liver is a specific target organ with this avian family, after exposure to infectious organisms through food contamination, poor hygiene, wrong management practices, and contamination from rodents, or if liver failure is the result of a long-term unbalanced diet. Whatever the cause, liver failure and liver tumours are fairly common in the Loriidae.

Other common medical problems encountered with lories are bacterial infections with *Salmonella enterica* serovar *Typhimurium*, *Escherichia coli* and *Klebsiella* spp. Less frequently, *Streptococcus* spp., *Staphylococcus* spp. and *Pseudomonas* spp. have been associated with disease presentations. In the winter, lories have been

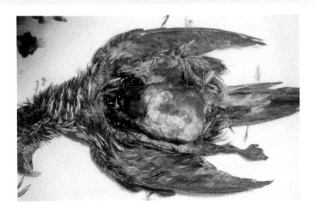

Fig 17.13 Striated lorikeet (*Charmosyna multistriata*), liver abscess.

known to develop intestinal infections from which *Clostridium perfringens* was isolated.

The lorikeet diet predisposes these birds to *Candida albicans* infections. Candidiasis lesions are mainly found on the mouth and tongue, the commissures of the beak, and crop. Clinical signs noted with *C. albicans* infections include regurgitation and frequent licking around the mouth. Lorikeets are also prone to superficial dermatomycoses infections primarily located around the commissures of the beak, cere and forehead, again most likely due to sugary nectar sticking to the feathers in the affected areas. This problem can be prevented by regular prophylaxis treatment with antifungal medication in the nectar (e.g. nystatin, amphotericin-B, miconazole or itraconazole)

Trichomonas gallinae infections also affect lory species. The main clinical sign associated with trichomoniasis infections is vomiting, similar to candidiasis. *Trichomonas* spp. organisms have been recovered from damp swabs of the crop and oesophagus, and the organisms were also found in adult lorikeets showing no clinical signs. There is thickening of the mucosa of the crop and oesophagus and, in some cases, yellow caseous material. Treatment with nitroimidazole drugs usually gives a satisfactory and reasonably rapid response. In some institutions prophylaxis with metronidazole is routinely used, and may be rotated with antifungal medication.

A possibly separate strain of psittacine circovirus, psittacine beak and feather disease virus (PBFDV), has been described in the Loriidae in recent years. Even if this is not a different virus, and lories are simply more resistant to PBFDV, they seem to recover fully from the clinical form of the disease.

Medium and large psittacine species

These include the widely known macaws, cockatoos, African greys, Amazon parrots and less common species including *Pionus* spp., *Eclectus* sp., *Tanygnathus* spp. and *Alisterus* spp. (Fig. 17.14).

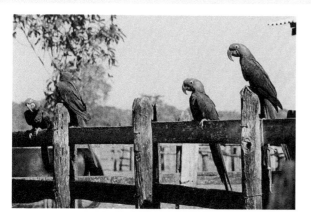

Fig 17.14 A small flock of hyacinth macaws (*Anodorhynchus hyacinthinus*), the largest and one of the most beautiful parrots.

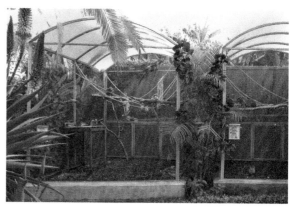

Fig 17.15 Weaning parrots are put together in outside aviaries, in order to socialize and build their flying muscles.

Although the primary purpose of any zoological institution is to exhibit birds in a manner that is attractive to visitors and provides environmental enrichment, birds should always be placed in an enclosure where they have the opportunity to reproduce. Some zoo curators erroneously think the likelihood of birds breeding in exhibition aviaries in front of thousands of visitors is so remote that it is not worth providing nest logs or boxes. Many bird species have successfully reproduced in display exhibits at zoological parks.

In large multi-species collections, management and feeding has to be rationalized wherever possible, as it is not practical to cope with minor variations for individual species. Nevertheless, good zoo keepers are able to know what an individual bird, or pair, will prefer regarding husbandry and nutritional offerings during the different seasons.

Housing

Breeding pairs of macaws and large cockatoos are housed in aviaries 2 m wide, 6–12 m long and 2.5–3 m high. African greys, Amazons, medium and small cockatoos, *Pionus* and *Eclectus* parrots are kept in aviaries 2 m wide, 4 m long and 2–2.5 m high. At one or both ends of the aviary there is a covered area above which the nest log or box and feed tray are placed. The floor of the rest of the aviary is covered by 10–15 cm of coarse river sand so that it drains well. Some institutions provide a seed mixture over this sand to give an attractive green cover. This is not just for the sake of appearance, but also affords a diverse environment and diet to counter boredom, as the birds spend hours on the ground digging out the sprouted seeds.

To counteract the possibility of the birds picking up severe worm infestations (particularly *Capillaria* spp.) during this activity, antiparasitic medication should be administered three or four times a year, with regular faecal examinations being part of the management protocol.

The top 10 cm of soil is renewed once a year to reduce exposure to parasites and/or their intermediate hosts.

Feeding

There are basically two ways to feed a large collection of parrots in a zoo or bird park:

1. A traditional way (seed mixture), improved with fruits, vegetables, nuts, beans and sprouts.
2. Using a formulated diet.

The decision regarding parrot nutrition will depend on bird curator, zoo nutritionist and veterinarian.

Handfeeding

The success or failure of any hand-raising operation will depend largely on the staff involved (Fig. 17.15). There are certain prerequisites for any prospective baby bird 'hand feeder', and these include the following:

- The diligence and dedication required to feed the babies at the correct times.
- Acute observation and the ability to detect signs that a chick may be developing a problem as early as possible.
- Being meticulous over matters such as brooder and food temperatures.
- A good understanding of hygiene requirements.

Hand rearing will take place for basically three reasons:

1. Having tame birds to be used for the show in the park, or to be sold for the pet market. In this case, psittacine chicks are hand raised after being removed from their parents at any time before 2–3 weeks of age.
2. Same as above and increase the number of clutches per year. For this purpose, chicks are

removed younger (at hatching), or better, the eggs are removed and artificially incubated.

3. Rescue one (or more) chicks that are in distress, or whose parents are having problems caring for the young. Those chicks may show clinical disease signs, or may be much smaller than their clutch mate. Their parents may have become sick, or died. Finally parents might be aggressive towards the chicks themselves, or other chicks in the clutch. Whatever the reason problem chicks are to be considered 'suspect' and should not be mixed with healthy chicks, until their health status has been evaluated.

There are reliable, scientifically prepared commercial parrot-rearing foods available in most countries, and these remove much of the guesswork from hand feeding. **Bird breeders must avoid the temptation to add some of their favourite ingredients of past home-made concoctions to 'improve' commercial diets.**

Allowing breeding pairs to raise one clutch a year is a practice that may have merit if the birds have proved in the past to be competent parents. Having a pair of birds raise a clutch is the only way in which an aviculturist may assess whether they are breeding a strain of birds that has the ability and instinct to raise young (Fig. 17.16). Often aviculturists mention that they have had to hand raise babies from a particular pair of birds because the parents never seem to be able to raise them beyond a certain age, or because they only raise about 25% or less of the clutch. This does prompt the question of whether breeders should be perpetuating that line of birds at all, but unfortunately, in the case of valuable birds, economics will usually dictate policy.

There are three ways of administering food to psittacine chicks:

1. Placing a syringe into the back of the mouth.
2. Placing the syringe and tube directly into the crop – this is more suitable for the administration of fluids or medicines than routine feeding, as inexperienced hands will cause crop injuries.
3. By spoon, which has the tip pinched in to form a groove.

In the authors' experience, even in bird parks where more than 1000 baby birds are hand raised each year, the preferred technique is syringe feeding, without the crop tube. Several trials show that there is not much difference in terms of time, chicks learn the right swallowing technique (this does not happen when tube fed) and are much cleaner than when spoon fed.

It is of primary importance to follow a consistent time and procedure schedule in the baby nursery.

First, it is important to keep the chicks (there are few species exceptions) at the right temperature, at a given age (Table 17.4).

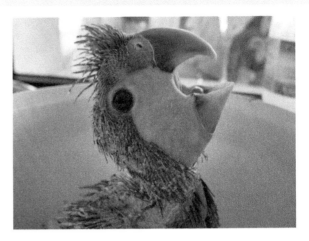

Fig 17.16 Young palm cockatoo (*Probosciger aterrimus*).

Table 17.4 Brooder temperature at different ages

Age in days	Temperature (°C)
1	Hatcher (37)
2	34
10	32
20	30
Feather shafts are opening	28
Feather shafts are open	No heating

Second, a time schedule must be organized, in order to have the right formula ready at the right time. It is not necessary to feed baby parrots at night. Even for the smaller chicks, an interval between midnight and 6 a.m. is adequate (Table 17.5).

Third, each commercial formula has a different dilution (grams of dry formula, in warm water up to 100 grams) that must be used at a different age of the chick. The given dilutions will work for most commercial hand-feeding diets (Table 17.6).

Ratites

There are 10 species of ratites. They all belong to the order Struthioniformes, and are divided in four suborders and five families: Struthionidae (African ostrich, 1 species); Rheidae (rheas, 2 species); Casuariidae (cassowaries, 3 species); Dromaiidae (emus, 1 species) and Apterygidae (kiwis, 3 species).

Ratites are widely exhibited in zoos and bird parks, although several species should not be kept in private parks, either because they are too big and dangerous for visitors, or they are too difficult for non-professionally trained staff to handle.

Table 17.5   Timetable for hand-feeding babies

No. of meals	Timetable									
10	6:00 a.m.	8:00 a.m.	10:00 a.m.	Noon	2:00 p.m.	4:00 p.m.	6:00 p.m.	8:00 p.m.	10:00 p.m.	Midnight
8	6:00 a.m.	8:30 a.m.	11:00 a.m.	1:30 p.m.	4:00 p.m.	6:30 p.m.	9:00 p.m.	11:30 p.m.		
7	6:00 a.m.	9:00 a.m.	Noon	3:00 p.m.	6:00 p.m.	9:00 p.m.	Midnight			
6	6:00 a.m.	9:30 a.m.	1:00 p.m.	4:30 p.m.	8:30 p.m.	11:00 p.m.				
5	7:00 a.m.	11:00 a.m.	3:00 p.m.	7:00 p.m.	11:00 p.m.					
4	6:00 a.m.	Noon	5:30 p.m.	11:00 p.m.						
3	7:00 a.m.	2:00 p.m.	10:30 p.m.							
2	9:00 a.m.	7:00 p.m.								
1	7:00 p.m.									

Table 17.6   Dilution and schedule for hand-feeding formulas

Age in days	Dilution (%)	No. of meals per day	Intervals (hours) between each meal
1–2	10–14	8 or more	2.5
3–5	12–16	7 or more	3
6–10	16–20	7 or more	3
11–20	20–25	6 or more	3.5
21–29	20–25	5	4
30+ feathers opening	20–25	4	5
Feathers opening	20–25	3	6
Starts to eat alone	20–25	2	12
Eats alone	20–25	1	At night

Rheas

Rheas can be maintained in groups, preferably in large areas, since they place great demands on the enclosure's environment and vegetation. An area of at least 200 square metres per bird is recommended to prevent the enclosure from becoming a barren wasteland.

Although the male rheas display some competitiveness for females during the breeding season, they are not aggressive birds, either amongst themselves or with other species within the same enclosure (e.g. cranes, waterfowl) (Fig. 17.17).

If the intention is to allow the birds to incubate their eggs and raise their young, it is acceptable to have a sex ratio of more males than females in the group since the males undertake all parental duties. The males make shallow hollows in the ground in which they encourage the females to lay their eggs. A normal clutch size is 10–12 eggs, but males can cover as many as 15 eggs and are very protective of their nests. In some areas (e.g. South Africa) it has been found that most of the eggs left for parental incubation become rotten. The rhea

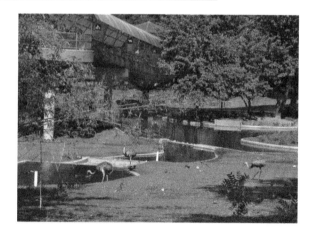

Fig 17.17   Rheas are good birds for mixed species exhibits.

breeding season coincides with the local rainy season in South Africa, which results in the development of rotten eggs. When non-native birds are being maintained as a zoological exhibit, local environmental conditions must be monitored to maintain breeding success and optimum health.

The eggs are incubated at 36.2°C and turned automatically 48 times a day. The humidity control in the incubators is turned off, as the ambient humidity during this period of the year is more than sufficient for incubation. On the thirty-eighth day, eggs are placed in the hatcher at 36.4°C and turning ceases. The incubation period varies from 38 to 40 days for rheas, but the incubation process is monitored during the whole period by noting weight loss and candling of the eggs.

Many rhea chicks seem to need a little assistance when hatching. If the egg has not hatched by the fortieth day, it should be candled and if the chick has pipped internally into the air sac, a hole 1–2 cm in diameter is made through the shell into the air sac. The chick can be assisted to leave the shell over a 12-hour period, taking care not to rupture blood vessels in the egg membranes.

The adult rheas are fed a commercial food for rheas, but they also like a large amount of green food and grains. As with other ratites, care must be taken when raising young rheas that one does not literally 'kill them with kindness' by providing an excessive plane of nutrition, resulting in extremely rapid growth, which can lead to osteodystrophia, fractures and deviations at the growth plates. These musculoskeletal disorders can occur despite feeding a diet with adequate levels of calcium and phosphorus.

Exercise is also of considerable importance in raising rheas as well as other ratites and long-legged walking birds (e.g. cranes, secretary birds). To encourage walking and running as much as possible, they are raised in long narrow pens with a shelter at one end and the food and water at the opposite end of the pen.

Another important requirement in raising baby rheas is gravel chips 0.5–1 cm in diameter, which are an important aid to digestion. These may be scattered on the floor of their pen, where the young birds can pick them up with their beak.

Cassowaries

These solid, heavy, wedge-shaped birds with coarse hair-like plumage are well suited to crashing through the dense forests of northern Australia and New Guinea at great speed. **Cassowaries are reputed to be aggressive and bad-tempered, and have caused many deaths to humans, both in their natural habitat and in zoological gardens.** Their method of causing injury is to leap feet first at their victim, slashing downward with their powerful toes and long sharp nails.

In captivity, cassowaries need large enclosures and, because they are secretive in nature, undergrowth is required in which they can rest and hide. Fencing for cassowaries has to be far more robust than that used for rhea and emu pens. These strong birds can easily damage normal fencing with their kicking. It is very difficult to introduce adult birds even of the opposite sex into one enclosure. For this reason birds often have to be kept singly in adjoining enclosures, and are put together only at breeding time and then separated again when the male commences incubation. The male takes on the entire responsibility of incubating the eggs, which takes 56–58 days, and raising the young.

Cassowaries can be fed commercial diets for emus, and they like chopped or diced fruit of various types (e.g. apples, pears, bananas, melons, grapes) along with grated carrot. The birds have also been observed to eat insects and rodents. The aggressive nature of these birds prohibits them from being used in mixed collections with species such as cranes.

Emus

The natural habitat for this species is the open semi-arid plains of Australia, where they can run at considerable speed over short distances. These birds therefore need spacious enclosures where they can be maintained in groups. Caution must be exercised when introducing a strange adult into an established group unless the area of the enclosure is very large.

In disposition, the emu is less placid than the rhea but not as aggressive or bad-tempered as the cassowary. Emus can therefore be used in mixed exhibits. In captivity, emus can be fed the same diet as cassowaries. Like rheas and cassowaries, the male emu undertakes all parental responsibilities, incubating (for 59–60 days) and brooding the chicks.

Handling and restraint of ratites

Handling and restraint are important considerations when working with adult ratites, as their nervous, fractious nature can result in injuries to both birds and handlers.

Adult rheas may be moved by having two or three curators quietly link hands and closely crowd the birds, or by having one big strong handler straddle the rear of the bird with the arms clasped around the bird's sternum. This technique is not likely to work so well with cassowaries, ostriches and emus due to their more aggressive dispositions, and would probably result in severe kicks to the handlers. For these birds, the use of permanent or portable crush pens erected in one corner of their enclosures is a safer option. These crush pens must have solid sides to the height of the hips to avoid the risk of birds kicking sideways through gaps, which may result in tibiotarsal or tarsometatarsal fractures. Although rheas can be quietly shepherded from one part of the zoological park to another along pathways, this is a risky procedure for cassowaries, emus and ostriches, which invariably panic and race headlong through gardens and fences, injuring themselves in the process. These birds are best moved in crates with sliding doors, which are placed at the end of the crush pen. The birds must not be given too much room in the crates, as they are less likely to injure themselves if slightly cramped. Placing a hood over the head and upper part of the neck will also help to quieten the birds when in the crush pen or crate. Ostriches may be restrained by grasping the neck and pulling it downwards until the head is close to the ground thereby preventing the bird from kicking the handler.

When total restraint is necessary (e.g. surgical procedures), anaesthesia is induced by injecting a combination of ketamine hydrochloride and xylazine into the right jugular vein. Anaesthesia is maintained with isoflurane. Birds should be allowed to recover in a crate or a small room with the floor and lower walls well padded with straw or a sponge material. Subdued light is recommended for recovery to reduce excitement and subsequent injury.

Health problems

Due to the space requirements and generally aggressive dispositions of ratites, zoological institutions do not maintain many animals – generally only a pair of each species and possibly a small group of rheas. For this reason, the veterinary problems encountered amongst ratites in zoological institutions are not necessarily the same as those found on commercial farms where large numbers of young birds are raised together and there is a far greater concentration of adults.

When well managed, adult ratites are remarkably disease-free and healthy. Young chicks may succumb to bacterial infections, mainly caused by *Escherichia coli* and *Clostridium* spp. The great majority of the problems observed in ratites are associated with trauma or foreign body ingestion. Routine treatment of the adult birds for internal parasites twice a year, more often for young birds in groups, results in healthy animals.

Capturem yopathy

Extreme caution must be taken to limit the movement of ratites, whether adult or young, during capture, as stress caused by excitement due to too much chasing by handlers may lead to injury or death associated with capture myopathy. Staff must be aware that if a bird starts to show stress, it is better to abandon the mission temporarily, leave the bird in a cool environment and reassess the whole procedure. Signs noted in birds diagnosed with capture myopathy include panting, increased respiratory and cardiac rates, difficulty in rising and walking, lying on the side and kicking followed by morbidity and death.

The use of selenium and vitamin E injections and aggressive fluid therapy is the suggested treatment option, but if severe signs are already apparent the treatment will yield limited success. When ratites are being transported to other destinations, requiring a several-hour layover in crates, a prophylactic injection of selenium and vitamin E may have some benefit.

Flamingoes

There are five (or possibly six) flamingo species in the world: *Phoenicopterus ruber*, *P. chilensis*, *P. (Phoeniconais) minor*, *P. (Phoenicoparrus) jamesi* and *P. (Phoenicoparrus) andinus*. The taxonomic position of the greater (or pink) flamingo is debated: some authors consider it to be a separate species (*P. roseus*), while others believe it is a subspecies of the Caribbean flamingo (*P. ruber roseus*). Whatever the systematic, the first three (four) species are commonly kept in captivity and until recently, many wild caught lesser flamingoes (*P. minor*) were regularly imported from Africa (Fig. 17.18).

Wild flamingo species are easy to catch and readily available on the market for purchase. Flamingoes have been maintained in colonies in several different zoological settings, both private and public. They are amongst the most popular park birds.

Flamingoes have a specialized feeding method, as they filter from the water the microfauna of their diet (e.g. algae, insect larvae, small crustaceans (brine shrimp), protozoa, fine aquatic plants). **Although there are several specialized companies that produce food for flamingoes, in most collections they are fed a soft, watery blend of different ingredients, such as meat, cereals, poultry and trout pellets, shrimps and canthaxanthin or astaxanthin.** It is also important to add a certain amount of Spirulina to the diet, as this is the primary component of most flamingo species' diets (especially *P. minor*).

For the care of flamingoes in captivity, one should review their biology and use some common sense. The minimum requirements are:

- Presence of water (e.g. pool, lake, pond). There are no data concerning the minimum water surface per bird. The ponds do not need to be very

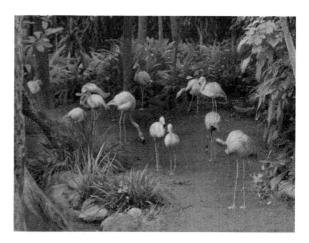

Fig 17.18 Flamingoes may be kept in flocks of different species: Caribbean flamingoes (*Phoenicopterus ruber*) and Chilean flamingoes (*P. chilensis*).

deep – 30–40 cm in the deepest part and sloping up very gently at the edges to minimize injury to feet and legs. As flamingoes spend a great deal of their lives standing in water, the contamination of the water by faeces is considerable. When planning and building flamingo ponds, it is essential that the ponds be designed for cleaning at least twice a week with relative ease. The ideal situation is to have a continual flow of water through the pond.

- Number of birds high enough to make a real flock (at least 20 birds). Flamingoes like to live in a flock and feel protected by the group.
- Even sex ratio. Some flamingo species are more easily bred than others, but in order to breed, they must have the right sex ratio. Flamingoes are easily sexed, either by morphometry, or by endoscopy, and the cock and hen number must be similar.
- Correct food. As stated previously, flamingoes have a specialized bill, and eat a specific food through bill filtration. Thus, if one wants to breed flamingoes, it is necessary to provide them with the most appropriate diet.
- Correct nests and nesting material. Flamingoes will nest readily, provided that:
  – there are good invitational nests, made of mud or concrete
  – there is mud enough to complete the invitational nests
  – there is an appropriate nesting area, with a certain amount of privacy.

Flamingoes are gregarious birds, and like to be together in relatively large numbers. **This gregarious nature can produce problems when sick or injured flamingoes need to be removed from the flock and hospitalized. Isolated birds may become depressed and their health condition will steadily decline, even if there appears to be no medical explanation.** For this reason it is a common policy that if a flamingo has to be isolated in the hospital or recuperation area, one or two other birds are utilized for psychological therapy.

Breeding

In order to breed, flamingos need to be kept in relatively large groups with an approximately equal number of male and female birds. The generally accepted minimum flock size required for breeding is 20 birds. It is necessary to provide a nesting area with a mud bottom close to the concreted pond. The soil is removed from this area to a depth of 25 cm, and 5–10 cm of clay is then placed over the floor so that it will retain water. To save the birds some effort and time, clay is mixed with soft grass and grass roots and mounds are made approximately 30 cm in diameter, 30 cm high and about 1 m apart over the whole nesting area. Coarse salt is then sprinkled over the whole mud pond, which is filled with water to a depth of 10–15 cm. Short pieces of soft grass and roots are scattered in the water and around the edge of the pond. The birds then use their beaks to pack the clay and grass pieces onto the existing mounds to create a crater-shaped nest, which in the case of the Caribbean flamingoes can be 40 cm in diameter and 40 cm high. Water must be added to the mud pool every few days, as well as clay and grass, until nest building is complete.

Just before the breeding season flamingoes become very noisy, and display while quarrelling over nest sites. This display takes the form of 'head flagging', when the birds twist their heads from side to side in jerky movements, and 'flashing', when they quickly extend their wings downwards or above their backs to expose their pink covert feathers and black primaries.

A single egg is laid on top of the mound, and both sexes assist in the incubation. The chick takes 28–30 days to hatch, and thereafter spends 5–7 days in the nest. The chick is fed a secretion, initially red but later straw-coloured, from glands in the upper digestive tract of the parents. The adults can be seen dribbling this secretion into the open upturned mouth of the chick, whose bill is still straight at this stage. The chicks grow quickly, but in captivity they are still seen being fed by their parents at 4 months of age.

Pathology

Although flamingoes often quarrel amongst each other, there is no likelihood of injury to a bird by one of its own kind or to any other species in the same enclosure. For this reason, flamingoes are well suited to mixed exhibits with other species.

Flamingoes live very long lives, both in the wild and in captivity. If they are well managed and fed, it is rare to observe diseases that affect the whole flock. Single-bird problems may occur, but they are generally linked to bad management and lack of critical observation by the keepers. The authors have observed an outbreak of pox (a pox virus was isolated, but not typed) that caused disease and death in young birds, but was self-limiting in adult birds.

With wild-caught flamingoes, there are several reports of bacterial diseases and septicaemia occurring in birds in quarantine. Bacterial isolates from these cases included *Salmonella typhimurium*, *E. coli*, *Klebsiella pneumoniae* and *Pseudomonas* spp. Aspergillosis has also been documented in quarantined flamingoes.

In the authors' experience, visceral gout, has been observed especially when the flamingo diet was too high in protein, and the temperature dropped below 4–5°C. The few problems encountered with flamingoes have been associated with the legs. Bumblefoot periodically occurs and usually necessitates surgical intervention.

The most common fractures have been tibiotarsal fractures and epiphyseal fractures of the femorotibiotarsal joint. Tibiotarsal fractures are frequently compound fractures and have a very poor prognosis due to vascular compromise to the limb distal to the fracture site. Generally fracture repairs in flamingo legs yield poor results, as the legs are thin and delicate. **Even if reasonable apposition of the fracture ends is achieved by either external or internal fixation, postoperative restraint and support presents a problem because flamingoes do not adapt to slinging or isolation.** If flamingoes are hospitalized in a situation where they cannot get their legs in water, it is important to sponge down their legs twice a day to prevent the skin from becoming excessively dry.

Gallinaceous birds

The order Galliformes includes almost 300 bird species, divided into seven families. Galliformes are distributed worldwide and are very variable in size, diet, habits and needs. Some species are far more represented in bird collections and zoos. Most of those are very impressive and beautiful birds, such as peafowl and pheasants. Some semi-tame specimens are often free ranging in large parks and zoos (Fig. 17.19).

Housing

Peafowl, pheasants, partridge and guinea fowl are often kept in well-planted aviaries. The size of the enclosure depends on the species on display. For exhibition purposes, compatible species such as mynahs, pigeons and jays are included with the pheasants in order to provide viewing interest in the top section of the aviary. Care must be exercised in choosing suitable softbills (e.g. non-egg-eaters) to live with the pheasants.

Guinea fowl may be kept in flocks, because there is only mild aggression between competing males during the breeding season. Conversely, pheasants cannot be kept in groups except as juveniles. At the onset of the breeding season, male pheasants will fight to the death over hens and territory.

Most pheasant species, such as the eared pheasants, peacock pheasants, great argus, monals, fireback pheasants, tragopans and Kalij, are best kept in pairs. Some species, such as golden, Lady Amherst's, Reeves's and silver pheasants, may be displayed as trios. The common ringneck may be kept in groups of one cock to four or five hens.

Indian and Javanese green peafowl can coexist in groups until the breeding season, at which time the males will start fighting. Breeding peafowl should be separated in smaller groups of one male to three or four females. Peafowl are very tolerant of other nongallinaceous bird species, making them an excellent bird to be used in mixed exhibits with flamingoes, cranes, waterfowl and rheas.

The floor of aviaries housing gallinaceous birds should be covered with 10–15 cm of coarse river sand into which seeds such as rye grass and oats are regularly planted to provide green food for birds (Fig. 17.20). Being a coarse sand, it dries out rapidly and hopefully desiccates worm eggs quicker than a substrate that retains moisture. This soil should be replaced several times a year.

Feeding

Pelleted diets for exotic and wild Galliformes are commercially available. **If the marketed feeds are unavailable, commercial poultry, pheasant, turkey, or Japanese quail diets may be fed.** Most commercial poultry diets containing anti-coccidic, or other drugs, should be used judiciously, as some drugs may be toxic for exotic species, and especially for non-Galliformes housed together with wild fowl. In addition to the normal base diet,

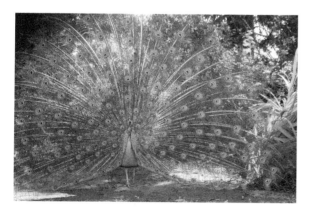

Fig 17.19 Some large gallinaceous birds can be kept as semi-tame animals. Male peacock (*Pavo cristatus*).

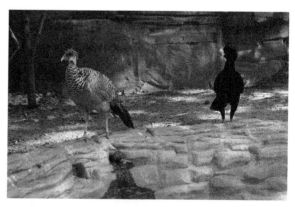

Fig 17.20 Great curassow (*Crax rubra*).

during the breeding season, minerals are supplied in the form of oyster shell grit, ground-up eggshells and cuttle-fish bone. A small amount of green food in the form of lettuce, cabbage, spinach, green alfalfa or just succulent green grass is supplied daily.

When the birds are reproductively inactive, 50% of the pellets are replaced by a mixed poultry grain that includes crushed corn, oats and sorghum.

Apart from the gallinaceous birds that are easy to care for, there are difficult species 'food-wise', like Roul Rouls, peacock pheasants and grouse.

Breeding

When breeding starts, eggs are collected daily and stored on trays in an air-conditioned room at 14–16°C. When the temperature rises over 14–16°C embryos may start to develop abnormally, and below 10°C embryos will die. It has been proven that storing eggs properly, between 2 and 7 days, will increase the hatching rate. After eggs have been stored for 10 days, hatch rates will quickly decrease.

If during the rainy season eggs are brought in dirty, it is advisable not to wash the shells. Washing dirty eggs may enhance bacterial migration through the shell pores, infecting the developing embryo. Rotten eggs usually explode in the incubator at some stage during incubation, thereby spreading the infection throughout the incubator (Fig. 17.21). With a dirty egg, it is preferable to allow the mud to dry and then dry brush, removing as much of the dirt as possible before dipping the egg in a chlorhexidine solution or similar suitable antiseptic. It is appropriate to dip all eggs in such a solution after collection and before being placed in the incubators whether they are soiled or not. **Any egg-dipping solution should be slightly warmer than the egg temperature, again to prevent contamination across the eggshell.**

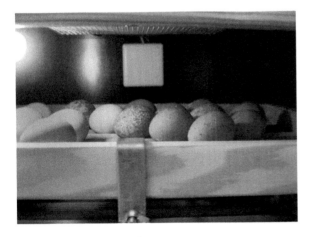

Fig 17.21 Eggs being incubated.

For routine disinfection of incubators between egg settings or after a rotten egg has exploded in the incubator, 45 mL of formalin should be added to 30 g of potassium permanganate for each cubic metre of incubator space and the mixture placed in a container in the incubator. Most gallinaceous birds' eggs are incubated at a temperature of 37.5°C and a humidity of 29.5°C wet bulb, but certain species such as fireback pheasants require a slightly higher humidity (30.5°C wet bulb). The eggs are turned several times a day automatically, and 48 hours before hatching the eggs are placed in a hatcher, at which time turning ceases. During the incubation period, all eggs are regularly weighed and candled so that infertile eggs or eggs showing embryonic death may be removed. **With valuable eggs, the weight loss is plotted on a graph to compare with a normal 14–15% weight loss until 48 hours before hatching.** If the weight loss is excessive the humidity in the incubator will have to be increased, and vice versa. Most pheasant eggs hatch between 22 and 28 days, but some, like the palawan and grey peacock pheasants, hatch after 18 days.

After hatching, the chicks are left in the hatcher for 12–18 hours to dry off and are then placed in brooders on coarse wood shavings. A 250 W infrared bulb suspended about 30 cm above the floor provides heat for the chicks. This should be placed at one end of the brooder to provide sufficient space allowing the chicks to move away from the lamp should they become too hot, as overheating produces several stress-related problems.

If a large number of fully developed chicks do not hatch, or a high mortality of chicks within a few days of hatching occurs, bacterial cultures should be taken from the chicks' internal organs, including the yolk sac. Cultures are also taken from equipment, including the inside of the hatcher and incubator, and a random sample from the external surfaces of eggs being incubated.

Severe mortality may occur in young gallinaceous chicks as a result of:

1. Dietary problems – starter rations that are too low in protein may lead to cannibalism, which takes the form of pecking around the toes, wing tips, vent, cere and the base of the beak.
2. Brooder temperatures – if chicks are huddled in the corners of brooders, this is an indication that the brooder temperature is too low and chicks are feeling cold. On the other hand, overheating also produces stress if the chicks cannot move away from the heat source to a comfortable temperature. Temperature stress can initiate cannibalism.

Overcrowding is probably the prime cause of cannibalism in chicks. If cannibalism is noticed in a batch of chicks, remedial measures must be taken immediately before it becomes a vice throughout the group. Any of the causes of cannibalism mentioned above must be corrected and instigators in the batch isolated. If the instigators are too numerous, the entire group will have to be 'de-beaked' (approximately 20% of the beak is snipped off). Any bleeding is easily controlled with the use of a styptic solution. If cannibalism is taking place, a small bunch of green food (such as lettuce or spinach) should be tied together and hung just out of reach of the chicks so that they have to jump up to peck at it. This food bundle provides a diversion, exercise and nourishment.

Chicks should be fed a 28–30% starter crumble or mash during the first week of life. In nature, their initial diet is almost entirely insectivorous. After 1 week the ration is gradually converted to a 22% protein broiler starter crumble. Some chicks, such as palawan peacock pheasants and Roul Rouls, may need encouragement to develop feeding skills. To teach feeding skills, some termites or mealworms (cut into very small pieces) are scattered on top of the starter mash for a few days. To attract the chick's attention to the food the keeper should scratch around in the bowl with a pencil or stick.

The chicks are moved to outside brooders at about 2 weeks of age, where they have access to a run. Heat must be provided at night for another 1–2 weeks, depending on prevailing weather conditions.

Hornbills

This family, the Bucerotidae, only occurs in Africa and Asia. Hornbills vary in size from 30 cm to over 1 m in length, and in general do not have bright body colours, being a combination of black, white, brown and grey. Usually it is their beaks that are colourful, and many species have large casques on the top beak, often extending above the level of the head. The head and neck regions frequently have interesting patterns and colours. Hornbills are also noted for their long 'eyelash'-like feathers surrounding the eye.

Hornbills feed on a variety of fruits, berries, nuts, insects, rodents, small mammals, eggs, reptiles and birds. Ground hornbills are entirely carnivorous and insectivorous, and may walk up to 10 km daily in their search for food.

Probably the most remarkable feature about hornbills is their breeding habits. All breed in hollow trees, and the female of all species except ground hornbills is walled into the nest chamber after she has laid the eggs. This is done mainly by the female, with some assistance from the male, using faeces, food, clay and saliva, all of which become very hard, leaving a narrow slit through which the female and the babies are fed until the latter are about 3 weeks old. This is obviously a defence mechanism against predators.

When the chick are about 3 weeks old, the female breaks out of the nest and assists the male with the continued feeding, although at this stage she may be quite scruffy and not able to fly well. The chicks in the meantime re-close the hole until they have developed sufficiently to be able to fly. Both the female and the chicks defecate through the slit, but while chicks are very young the female will be seen to drop their faeces and food residues through the slit to the outside.

In captivity hornbills are fed a variety of chopped up fruits such as apples, bananas, pears, guavas, grapes and papaya, and soaked dog-food cubes. The dog-food cubes must not be allowed to get too soft because, in order to feed, hornbills toss the food particle in the air, then open the beak and allow the particle to drop to the back of the throat for swallowing. When they have chicks, a protein supplement is sprinkled on the food and strips of ox heart are also placed on top of it.

Ground hornbills have a basic diet of dead day-old chicks plus rodents and snakes, when available. It has also been observed that they are very fond of any wild birds (e.g. sparrows, doves) which are unfortunate enough to find their way into the enclosures. **Interestingly, attempts to hand raise hornbill chicks with their 'natural diet' (e.g. grasshoppers, mealworms, scorpions) have been far less successful than rearing them with dietary substitutes that are not part of the natural hornbill food (e.g. chopped pinkies, geckos, strips of ox heart).**

Hornbills are both mischievous and aggressive birds. The larger Asian species can only be housed in pairs if a serious breeding programme is being established. Ground hornbills may be kept in family groups if introduced together at a young age. A dominant female is less likely to tolerate other females in the group than a dominant male is to tolerate subservient males.

The smaller hornbill species may be exhibited in large walk-through aviaries or in mixed collections, but are not above killing smaller species if provided with the opportunity.

Hornbills have proved to be tough, long-lived birds with few medical problems. A few cases of aspergillosis have been diagnosed. These fungal infections may have been associated with contaminated fruit.

Most zoological institutions have rodent extermination programmes where the use of warfarin poison is routine. **It is not advisable to use anticoagulant products in the vicinity of hornbill aviaries.** If poisoned rodents can get into the hornbill enclosures this extermination policy should not be used, since these birds have died from eating warfarin laced rats.

Toucans

The family Ramphastidae, which includes 33 species of toucans, toucanettes and aracaris, is native to an area that extends from southern Mexico through Central and South America to northern Argentina. Their natural habitat is rainforests, where they fly from tree to tree

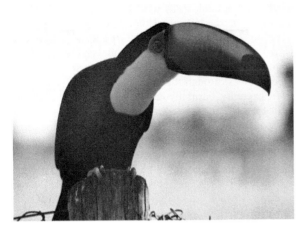

Fig 17.22 Toco toucan (*Ramphastos toco*).

in their quest for food. Generally they are seen in small family groups of two to five individuals (Fig. 17.22).

Toucans are intelligent and interesting birds whose unusual beak shape, beautiful colours and continual activity make them a highly desirable species for zoological institutions. The larger species are basically black in colour, with white, yellow or red breasts, some with transverse colour bands. Red patches under the tail in the vent area are also common to several species, as well as an area of blue surrounding the eyes. The primary physical characteristic that makes the members of this family so distinctive is their incredible beak. Although the beaks are large, they are very light and strong due to their internal support matrix. Usually the beaks are extremely colourful, featuring amazing combinations of streaks, patches or dots, such as are found in keel-billed, channel-billed, Swainson's and spot-billed toucanettes, among others.

Housing

Toucans should be kept in large, well-planted aviaries for exhibition purposes. These birds are most attractive when viewed actively moving in vegetation. They can be housed in aviaries 4 m wide, 7 m deep and 2–3 m high, which afford ample room for exercise, and have a covered area 2 m deep at one end, under which the food and nest log are placed. It is important that toucans have a 'private' part of the aviary where they can rest and hide from visitors. Also, some species, such as the toco toucan (*Ramphastos toco*), are very cold sensitive and may suffer frostbite in winter. When these species are kept in areas with cold winters, they should be housed in a warmed aviary, or a part of the enclosure that is climate controlled.

Feeding

In nature, toucans feed on a wide variety of fruits, berries, eggs and baby birds, reptiles, insects and small rodents.

Commercial toucan diets are available for ramphastids in captivity. Further, fruit such as papaya, pears, guavas, apples, melons, peaches and grapes may be used, diced into 1 cm pieces. Citrus fruits are not recommended as ramphastid food, as they are reputed to increase the absorption of iron. Like hornbills, toucans toss the food in the air before opening their beaks and allowing it to drop into the back of the throat for swallowing, so they are unable to manipulate food particles that are too soft and mushy. Diced vegetables such as beet and carrots may also be included in the toucans' diet.

Along with birds of paradise and mynah birds, toucans are extremely prone to iron storage disease. If no suitable commercial extruded or pelleted toucan diet with low iron content is available, it is vital to select a dog kibble or cube with an iron content of less than 80 ppm (less than 60 ppm if possible).

Breeding

Toucans prefer natural logs for nest locations rather than artificial nest boxes of the type used for psittacine species. For the larger toucans, a log approximately 1.2 m deep with an internal diameter of 25–35 cm is suitable, whereas for toucanettes and aracaris a log 60–80 cm deep and 15–20 cm in internal diameter is adequate. The birds prefer a side entrance to the log, just large enough for that particular species to enter, with a wire ladder down from the entrance to about 25 cm from the bottom. Toucans do not like nest material in the log, but prefer a dish-like hollow in the base of the log in which they lay their eggs.

The Ramphastidae are not easy birds to breed, and breeding requires more effort and expertise than in other species such as psittacines. Naturally, lucky opportunistic breedings occur in zoos and private collections, but regular large-scale reproduction of toucans requires attention to detail for success. One management area that needs close monitoring is the dietary requirements of parents feeding young.

The incubation period for toucans is 16 days, and the chicks fledge at 7–8 weeks.

Ibis

The family Threskiornithidae, in the order Ciconiiformes (storks), includes 32 species of ibises and spoonbills.

Scarlet ibis (Eudocimus ruber)

Originating from northern South America, Scarlet ibises are housed in a very large walk-through aviary with a marsh-type environment. They spend a considerable amount of time digging in the mud with their long, thin beaks and on the water edges looking for food organisms. The food shelter should be within a few metres of the edge of the ponds to allow the birds to take food particles and dip them in the water before swallowing them. They have also been observed catching small fish, frogs and tadpoles in the ponds. **The diet supplied to scarlet ibis consists of soaked dog-food cubes and chopped fish, sardines and ox heart. In order to maintain the brilliant red colour of this species, it is necessary to sprinkle canthaxanthin, or astaxanthin, onto the dog cubes and allow it to soak in, at the rate of 3g per 20 birds per day.**

For nesting, wire platform baskets 10 cm deep and 30 cm in diameter are attached to trees 4–5 m off the ground. Coarse grass and thin sticks are used for nesting material. Ibis breed readily, and prefer to nest in colonies where the nests are grouped together about 1.5–2 m apart. Both sexes share incubation duties, which last for about 24 days. Normally two or three eggs are laid.

Glossy ibis (Plegadis falcinellus)

These birds also like wetland conditions and may be managed in the same manner as scarlet ibis, except they do not require any red pigment in their diets. They also breed in colonies using platform nests with coarse grass and twigs, and have a similar clutch size and incubation period.

Bald ibis (Geronticus eremita)

The natural habitat of these birds is cliff faces, preferably in the vicinity of waterfalls. Most institutions include high rocky cliffs to exhibit bald ibises.

Their diet consists of soaked dog-food cubes and pieces of ox heart or other types of meat on which a vitamin and mineral supplement is sprinkled, particularly when they are breeding. These birds are often found on the ground foraging for insects, worms, snails, frogs and small reptiles.

Bald ibis breed in colonies, creating flimsy platforms of sticks on the cliff ledges. Clutches average two eggs, and the incubation period is 25–28 days, with both sexes sharing the duties of incubation and feeding the chicks. At this institution, bald ibis are usually given the opportunity to raise their own young.

No aggressive tendencies have been noted among the above ibis species, either towards each other or to other avian species maintained in the same mixed collection.

Roseate spoonbill (Platalea ajaja) and European spoonbill (Platalea leucorodia)

They are managed in exactly the same manner as scarlet ibis, with whom they have a very compatible existence.

Gruiformes

There are 15 crane species, distributed worldwide. These elegant, handsome birds form an important exhibit in

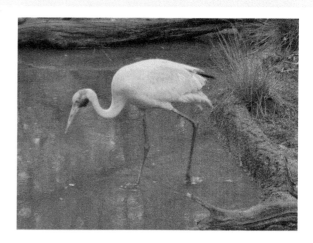

Fig 17.23 Most exhibits for cranes must have a natural look. Brolga crane (*Grus rubiconda*).

any zoological collection, but there are management problems (Fig. 17.23). Most crane management problems relate to their excitable nature, and are often referred to as 'accidents waiting to happen'.

Cranes are best kept in pairs in grass enclosures approximately 10 × 20 m in area. The goal of having a crane pen this size is to optimize breeding results and minimize problems associated with the aggressive nature of some species. The enclosure fencing must be at least 2 m height, to prevent wing-clipped or pinioned birds from climbing over. One must remember that the average crane stands at a very convenient height to peck at children's eyes, and this can happen quickly with very dangerous consequences.

Experienced researchers claim that pinioned or wing-clipped male cranes have a lower fertility than full-winged birds. Perhaps it is not so much the fertility as the act of copulation that is affected, maybe by imbalance of the wings. However, if this is a concern, the enclosure fencing should be higher (up to 4 m) and a nylon shade cloth or large aperture bird netting stretched on top. This allows cranes to dance and display, jumping as high as they like, and also to copulate in a more balanced manner. For aesthetic reasons, most zoological institutions would not build a totally enclosed crane pen and would aim, wherever possible, to incorporate the birds into mixed exhibits with other species.

It is very risky to put larger crane species such as wattled or sarus cranes into mixed collections. During the breeding period large crane species become aggressive, not only to other species but also to curators. These birds may live in a mixed exhibit of birds such as waterfowl and flamingoes for some time with no apparent problems, and then suddenly turn on a bird such as a flamingo and kill it.

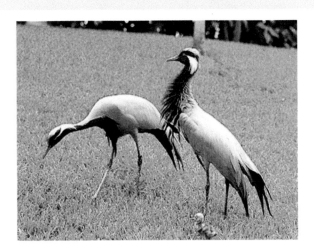

Fig 17.24 Demoiselle cranes (*Anthropoides virgo*) are not too big and not too aggressive. They can be left ranging free in the zoo, and will even reproduce in this setting.

Demoiselle cranes are very gentle and may be kept in a group of two to four pairs (Fig. 17.24). These cranes may be maintained in a mixed collection exhibit with species such as flamingoes and waterfowl if the enclosure is of a reasonable size.

Crowned cranes and blue cranes may also live together in groups of two or three pairs, combined with other avian species such as storks and flamingoes if the enclosure is large enough. These cranes need some privacy at nesting time to ensure breeding success. Occasionally aggressive individuals will be observed, and must be removed from mixed exhibits.

The adult cranes are fed a commercial poultry breeder pellet with a 22% protein concentration and a mixed poultry grain containing mainly corn and sorghum. With the approach of the breeding season, the grain component is eliminated and only the pellets are fed. In mixed exhibits, it is impossible to restrict cranes' feeding. Birds have been observed feeding in the flamingo food dishes, helping themselves to soaked dog-food cubes and even ingesting day-old chicks. They also catch a certain number of insects, small rodents, frogs and tadpoles. The self-generated diet is desirable, as the overall protein analysis should be higher than 22% at breeding time.

The nesting habits of cranes vary considerably: wattled, crowned and sarus cranes build grass mounds up to 20 cm high; demoiselle cranes make virtually no nest but select a bare piece of ground where they gather a few small stones to place around the eggs; blue cranes make a very shallow nest in grassland then gather a small amount of grass around the eggs.

Cranes lay either one or two eggs, and have a wide range of incubation periods from 27–30 days for demoiselles to 35–38 days for wattled cranes. Many crane species will successfully hatch and rear two chicks, but the wattled crane abandons the second egg after the first chick hatches. For artificial incubation eggs are incubated at 37.5°C with a wet bulb reading of 30–30.5°C, in a horizontal position, and are turned automatically every 30 minutes. Forty-eight hours before hatching, the eggs are placed in a hatcher at a high humidity, and turning ceases. Frequently the hatching process will take another 48 hours from the onset of external pipping before the chick is out of the shell.

After hatching, the chick is left in the hatcher for about 12 hours to dry off before being placed in a brooder at a temperature of 32–35°C. A suitable covering for the floor of the brooder is required to prevent leg injuries. Wood shavings or coarse river sand have worked well as a substrate for crane chicks.

Although small crane chicks can be very aggressive and peck each other to death, a single chick can get very lonely and depressed. In these situations, it can be very comforting to the crane chick (and indeed gallinaceous birds) to hang a feather duster near the heat source in the brooder. Chicks will be seen standing between the feathers of the duster.

The chick will not eat for the first 24–36 hours while the yolk sac is being reabsorbed. The starter feed used for crane chicks during the first 7–10 days is a 1:1 mixture of 22% broiler starter crumble with soaked dog-food cubes that have been crushed. Only a small amount of this food is mixed at one time, to prevent the risk of souring. Small mealworms are sprinkled on top of the food, as well as thin strips of ox heart cut to the size of mealworms. The movement of the mealworms attracts the chicks' interest. Food attraction can also be accomplished by scratching around in the food dish with a pencil or piece of wire to draw the chicks' attention to the contents.

When the chick has started to feed readily, a vitamin and mineral supplement is also added to the food mixture. After about 10 days of age, the diet is gradually changed to the straight broiler starter crumbles and then the pelleted form.

Care must be taken to prevent rapid weight gain of the chick. If the growth rate becomes too fast, lateral deviation and rotation of the legs occurs, ultimately causing an inability to walk. As soon as the lateral leg deviations are noticed, the tibiotarsal/metatarsal joints must be bandaged using Elastoplast so that there is still movement of the joint. A strip of thick elastic rubber is incorporated in the bandage in the medial aspect of the joint, allowing tension to pull the leg inward distal to the joint. The bandages are changed and tightened weekly, and it takes a period of about 6 weeks to correct the lateral deviation.

After 3 months of age, the instinct amongst chicks to kill each other diminishes and they may be placed in communal groups. Management skills must be in place when introducing new chicks because disasters can rapidly occur.

Handling

The capture and restraint of birds with long thin legs housed in relatively large enclosures is always a nightmare for curators. One procedure is to erect some 1.8 m high portable wooden frames covered with shade cloth to form a small enclosure in one corner of the pen. Similar dense shade cloth is stretched out from the entrance to the enclosure, forming a funnel similar to that used in game capture. The birds are then quietly walked into the funnel by staff linking hands or holding 1.2 m high shade cloth between them. When erecting the capture enclosure, care must be taken to see the shade cloth is on that side of the wooden frame closest to the birds to prevent wing injuries on the frames.

Birds of prey

Falconiformes

All diurnal birds of prey belong to the order Falconiformes, which includes five families (Fig. 17.25):

- Cathartidae (New World vultures), with 7 species
- Pandionidae (osprey), 1 species
- Accipitridae (hawks, vultures and eagles), 237 species
- Sagittaridae (secretary bird), 1 species
- Falconidae (falcons and caracaras), 61 species.

A few years ago falconry and hawking were exclusive hobbies for a limited number of passionate people; today falcon and hawk breeding has become rather popular. To date there are several thousand owners of birds of prey in the EU.

Furthermore, birds of prey are always impressive animals and they have been exhibited in zoological collections for many years. Today, besides raptors displayed in large flight aviaries, most bird collections have a bird of prey show.

Contrary to what was observed some years ago, when falconers and falcon breeders were actually the same people, today besides those 'mixed' hobbyists, there are fanciers with specific interests: people who fly the birds (e.g. hunting, show, pest control in airports, farms); and there are people who breed and sell birds of prey.

Breeding birds of prey involves a deep knowledge of their biology and taxonomy (Fig. 17.26). Generally speaking one limiting factor is room: large aviaries are needed to host the birds. Furthermore, even larger aviaries are needed for young birds to exercise and open fields must be available in the area for training the birds. This is obviously related to the species, but the majority of breeders are focused on the most commercial raptor species, such as the peregrine falcon (*Falco peregrinus*), the saker falcon (*F. cherrug*), the gyrfalcon (*F. rusticolus*), the Barbary falcon (*F. pelegrinoides*), and the Harris hawk (*Parabuteo unicinctus*). Besides these more common birds, there are people who breed very large birds, like eagles, or rather small raptors, like the Eurasian and the American kestrel (*F. tinnunculus* and *F. sparvirus*).

The average breeding pair requires aviaries approximately measuring 4 × 4 × 3(h) meters, but 'difficult' species, like the goshawk (*Accipiter gentilis*), may need

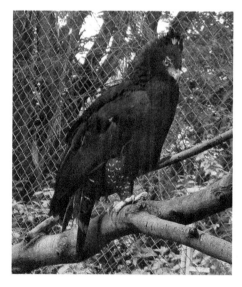

Fig 17.25 Guiana crested eagle (*Morphnus guianensis*); dark morph.

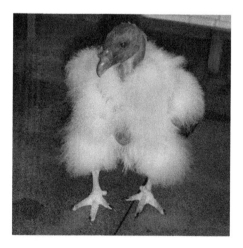

Fig 17.26 Young king vulture (*Sarcoramphus papa*).

separate (or separable) aviaries for the male and female. In most cases the breeding aviary will not be accessible to people in the sense that birds will not be able to see people from inside. This can be achieved by several methods, ranging form hidden eye-holes to one-way windows.

Another issue regarding the welfare of raptors is the hygiene of food. Birds of prey are carnivorous and their food is extremely perishable. There are licensed suppliers of frozen animals (e.g. day-old chicks, quails, mice, rats) who guarantee the quality of their food.

Finally, and this is particularly true in the case of hybrid falcons, where artificial incubation is a must, a dedicated nursery is needed to incubate and hatch the eggs and hand rear the chicks (Fig. 17.27). The nursery should be composed of at least two rooms: one for incubation and hatching and one for rearing. Strict hygiene measures are a must in these rooms, as previously described for Psittaciformes.

Strigiformes

Nocturnal birds of prey are divided into two families:

- Tytonidae (barn-owls and bay-owls), 16 species
- Strigidae (typical owls), 189 species.

Compared to falcons and hawks, breeding nocturnal birds of prey is a hobby for a very limited number of people (Fig. 17.28). In some cases, falcons' fanciers like owls, as well, but there are also people who breed and/ or keep only Strigiformes.

Some of the most emblematic owls, like the Eurasian eagle-owl (*Bubo bubo*), great horned owl (*Bubo virginianus*) and snowy owl (*Bubo (Nyctea) scandiacus*), are often used in bird of prey shows.

The facilities used for breeding owls do not differ much from those described for diurnal raptors, but Strigiformes rarely need to be isolated from human sight as with falcon species. This is probably due to the fact that most of their activity is at night time, when human contact is limited. Nevertheless owls are shy creatures and privacy must be provided and stress factors have to be avoided, or reduced to a minimum (Fig. 17.29). Strigiformes and Falconiformes share the same problems associated with unhygienic conditions within their flights.

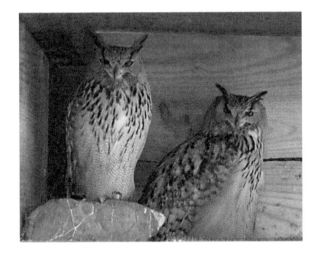

Fig 17.28 Rock eagle-owl (*Bubo bengalensis*) pair.

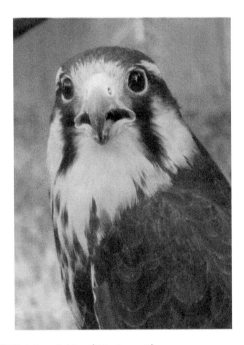

Fig 17.27 Aplomado falcon (*Falco femoralis*).

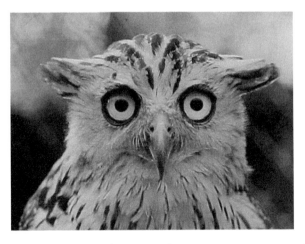

Fig 17.29 Buffy fish-owl (*Ketupa ketupu*).

Penguins

All penguin species belong to the family Spheniscidae, the only one in the order Sphenisciformes. There are 17 living species of penguins, divided into 6 genera:

- *Aptenodyptes* (2 species)
- *Eudyptes* (6 species)
- *Pygoscelis* (3 species)
- *Eudyptela* (1 species)
- *Megadyptes* (1 species)
- *Spheniscus* (4 species).

All the penguin species live in the southern hemisphere; the Galapagos penguin (*Spheniscus mendiculus*) is the species that lives at the most northern latitude (latitude 00° 30′, longitude 90° 30′), close to the equator.

The study of the origin of this family shows that these wingless birds descend from the Procellariiformes, rather than from ratites. In fact the penguins have a keeled breastbone that supports the potent pectoral muscles, but they also have very strong dorsal muscles that play an important role in their efficient underwater flight. Further, as flying birds, penguins have a cerebellum with structures specific to three-dimensional movement. Penguins are pelagic predators spending much of their time in the ocean water. They are agile swimmers and very good divers, they return to land to breed and moult.

Anatomy and physiology

The morphology of the 17 penguin species is very uniform in shape and colours. The body size is the most variable characteristic of the species, ranging from 1 kg weight and 41–45 cm long for the little blue (*Eudyptula minor*) to 23–29 kg up to 38 kg weight (depending on the physiological stage) and 110–130 cm height for the emperor penguin (*Aptenodytes forsteri*).

The wings are modified into flippers with a limited movement in the joints, except the shoulders. Diving penguins reach a speed of 8–12 km/h (there are reports of 27 km/h); in case of need they also can dive deep with an average of 100 m (emperor penguin have been recorded to reach a depth of 560 m).

Feathers cover all the body and overlap extensively to form a waterproof cover. The feathers are slightly curved, short, stiff, lanceolate and uniform in shape. Within the plumage a layer of air is preserved, ensuring buoyancy; the air also helps to insulate the birds in cold water.

Thermal insulation is provided by a subcutaneous fat layer that is thicker in southern species. Circulatory specialization, including the retia mirabilis, allows penguins to maintain normal body temperature in cold water and during winter on land, and to shed heat when hot. Penguin chicks are poikilothermic; the thermoregulation system develops very slowly in these avian species and is complete around the age birds are ready to enter to the water.

The bill is made of horny plate with a shape slightly different according to the preferred prey, those species more specialized for eating fish having a longer and thinner bill than those that eat plankton. The eyes are adapted for underwater vision, but the birds also can see properly out of water.

Penguins are able to drink salt water and filter the excess salt using a specialized nasal salt gland. Interestingly, salt glands are histologically similar to renal tissue. The lack of salt during captive life seems to be responsible for the atrophy of these glands.

Penguins' muscles and blood (i.e. high levels of myoglobin and haemoglobin) seems to be very resistant to changes in physiologic pH that occur during apnoea associated with prolonged dives.

Bones of the penguin are denser than those of flying birds, which is considered an adaptation to their amphibious lifestyle.

Moult

Penguins have a single annual moult, usually after breeding, but Galapagos and king penguins moult before breeding. All feathers are pushed out by the new forming papillae and they simultaneously moult. During moulting penguins must stay on land because they lose their waterproofing capabilities; thus during this period, 2–4 weeks, they have to fast. Moulting is a high energy process for which the penguins prepare themselves with a long foraging period at sea, increasing their body weight by 50–70%. This additional weight is lost during the moulting fast.

Housing

Penguins are becoming increasingly popular in zoos and bird parks. These animals are particularly challenging to maintain. Their special needs are not easily achieved; therefore specific facilities have to be designed because their health is strongly related to the captive environment. Special attention should be given to the air and water quality, land space, substrate, nesting area and lighting (light cycle and intensity).

Water quality

The water may be salt or fresh water, as long as salt is provided in the diet when fresh water is used in the exhibit. It is advisable that the water surface should be three to four times the land space; pool depth should be at least 1 to 3 m with areas that provide easy access to the dry areas of the exhibit. Filtration and frequent turnover of the water is very important to remove excrement and food litter. The use of a surface skimmer is also recommended to remove excess fish oil that could interfere with the natural metabolism of feather development. The surface skimmer also helps in removing excess feathers from the surface of the water during the moulting period. The water temperature should be maintained at around 10–19°C and in outdoor facilities constructed in cold climates particular caution should be observed when the water partially freezes because penguins are known to enter in this water and be unable to spot the entry hole. The water must be monitored for the presence of possible pathogenic organisms (e.g. fungi, bacteria). Microbial monitoring of the water is done through periodical analysis and microbiological cultures using a Dipslide (Oxoid S.p.A. Garbagnate Milanese – Italy). The following parameters are also examined on a routine basis: conductivity, temperature, redox, pH, nitrates and nitrites.

Air quality

With indoor exhibits the filtration system should be accomplished using pre-filters and followed by HEPA filters. **It is imperative that routine monitoring of the air be performed to scan for the presence of potentially pathogenic agents.** The air turnover within the exhibit should be high (15–20 cycles/hour) to help maintain low ammonia levels and reduce the risk of respiratory disease. The air temperature requirement will vary with the species that are exhibited: *Aptenodytes* need a temperature approximately 0°C or below, *Pygoscelis*, *Eudyptes*, *Megadyptes* and *Eudyptela* require a temperature range of 9°C or below, dictating that all of these species are best kept in an indoor climate-controlled facility. Then again, penguins of the *Spheniscus* species are more tolerant of higher temperatures as long as shelter, shade, swimming area and misting system are provided.

Lighting

The light cycle is particularly important for the more southern species and should be as similar as possible to that of their natural habitat, which improves their reproductive rate.

Landspace

The gregarious nature of penguins has led to the recommendation from the SSP (Species Survival Plan) that penguins should not be housed alone or with fewer than three couples. The amount of land provided within a penguin enclosure depends on the number of penguins living together. The Penguins Taxon Advisory Group recommends a minimum space of 550 cm² per bird.

Nesting area

The nesting species of penguins need appropriate material to build their nest (Fig. 17.30). It is useful to know a penguin species' natural behaviour in order to satisfy their reproductive needs. For example, the burrowing species do very well in plastic pet carriers, but when maintained in exhibits with public viewing it is important to provide an appropriate aesthetic appearance of their environment. A naturalistic looking habitat has more educational value for the public and is much more psychologically stimulating for the animals. Moreover the Papua penguin must have an area large enough to build their nest. This species prefers to group nest and they pass the time stealing nest stones from other nests. Therefore stones should be offered in abundance during the breeding season of Papua penguins. To improve the space limitations a whalebone-shaped separation could be offered so the birds within the exhibit can easily build four to five nests in a small space. There are institutions that offer ring-shaped separations, but the concept is the same, improving the space restrictions within an exhibit. Offering adequate nesting material and preparing an adequate nesting area are minor changes to an exhibit that will stimulate a bird's breeding behaviour.

Substrate

Historically, concrete has been used as a substrate; it is easy to clean and readily available (Fig. 17.31). The abrasive nature of concrete can predispose the penguin's feet to pododermatitis (bumblefoot). For this reason concrete, or any substrate, that is to abrasive and remains wet for long periods of time should be avoided. Many zoos have found it advantageous to use matting over concrete in selected areas of the exhibit. Some facilities place a protective coating of lacquer over concrete surfaces to reduce abrasiveness and to fill in the small pores where bacterial colonies can become established; others institutions completely or partially cover the surface with smashed ice 'artificial snow'. In designing or renovating an exhibit, a variety of materials and textures should be provided for the birds. These can be natural rocks, sand,

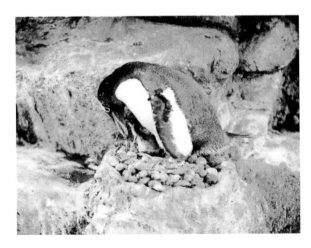

Fig 17.30 Gentoo penguin (*Pygoscelis papua*) on nest.

grass, pebbles and matting. An uneven surface causes a different distribution of the bird's weight on the feet during standing and walking, which is of vital importance in avoiding bumblefoot. **One must remember that some species of penguin, such as *Spheniscus eudyptes*, are good climbers and therefore additional rocky slopes are recommended for exercise.** This behaviour also has an attractive and educational value to the public.

Physical examination of penguins

The physical examination goes through an evaluation of the general body condition, birds are weighed, eyes are checked for lesions, beak, and oral cavity are examined for colour changes, focal lesions or diffuse alteration. Wings are checked for presence of bruising or other lesions. Feet must be carefully examined and if bumblefoot lesions are suspected to be starting, these must be immediately addressed.

Routine checks

Penguins must be examined on a routine basis, so that every bird is carefully evaluated at least once per year. The examination is performed preferably before the breeding season in order to address any problems before reproductive activity begins. It is very important to determine an individual baseline for each bird, so in case of disease, the collected samples can be compared with the 'normal values' for that specific animal. Important penguin baseline data include:

- CBC (WBC/estimated WBC, PCV, differential count of WBC)

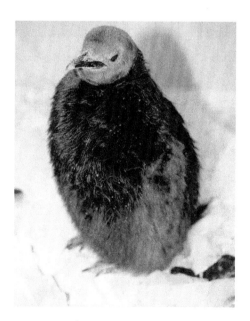

Fig 17.31 King penguin (*Aptenodytes patagonicus*) chick.

- blood chemistry (aspartate aminotransferase, uric acid, lactate dehydrogenase, cholesterol, creatine kinase, bile acid, total protein, protein electrophoresis)
- *Aspergillus* spp. titres
- Choanal and cloacal cultures.

Sex determination

Due to the excessive amount of perivisceral fat, penguins are difficult to sex endoscopically. DNA-related techniques are currently used and are the preferred method of sex determination of penguins.

Breeding

It is very important to have the appropriate nesting areas in order well before the breeding season for each penguin species. In our experience penguins do not have significant problems with egg laying, but low fertility rates are more commonly observed.

Medical control of the chicks

Chicks must be weighed at day one. The umbilicus must be disinfected and sealed if open. Typical problems of penguin chicks are poor growth rate, often resulting from the parents' misbehaviour or inexperience. Also omphalitis and subsequent septicaemia may sometimes be encountered. The chick may be weak and not able to hatch; therefore assisted hatches are one of the typical emergencies performed on young penguins.

Viral diseases

Very little is known about viral diseases specific to this avian order and only a few viral diseases are reported in penguins. Most of these reports involve captive birds. Although paramixovirus-1 infections have been documented in Sphenisciformes, and cutaneous pox lesions have been reported in otherwise asymptomatic penguins, in the Loro Parque exhibits we have never experienced viral outbreaks.

Bacterial pathogens

Penguins are susceptible to the pathogenic bacteria that affect other birds. *E. coli*, *Pasteurella* spp. and *Klebsiella* spp. can affect adult penguins as well as chicks. *Clostridium perfringens* and *Pseudomonas* spp. are also reported to be possible pathogens for Sphenisciformes.

Fungal pathogens

Fungal diseases, especially aspergillosis, are very well-known and serious diseases of penguins. **These birds, as with other avian species from extremely cold climates, are particularly susceptible to *Aspergillus* spp. infections.** Environmental prophylactic measures, as well as early diagnosis, are the keys to successful *Aspergillus* spp. management in the modern penguin exhibit.

Parasitology

Although some parasites have been reported in literature, they are not considered a typical problem of penguins. **The most studied penguin parasite is *Plasmodium spp.*** Malaria, like aspergillosis, is a typical disease of captive penguins and also this disease can be controlled by strict management measures. This explains why a closed environment, similar to those that house the penguins in our institution, can be extremely helpful in controlling this disease.

Non-infectious disease of penguins

Environmental contaminantsa ffecting penguin health

Penguins, like all the fish-eaters, are exposed to intoxication by pesticides accumulated in fish. This includes polychlorinated biphenyls (PBCs) and 2,3,7,8 tetrachlorodibenzo-*p*-dioxin (TCDD). Mortality can be high and strict control measures are necessary. One important consideration is the choice of the fish provider. The fish provider should be able to sell tested and certified fish and be insured for diseases or deaths that result from poor fish quality.

Foreignb ody

Penguins are very curious and playful birds. They easily swallow new objects offered or lost accidentally in the exhibit or pool (Figs 17.32, 17.33). Particular attention should be paid to the quality of new nesting material to prevent introduction of hidden objects that may be ingested.

Show birds

Most bird parks and zoos have a bird show (Fig. 17.34). Most shows are monothematic (they display only one bird group, such as psittacines, or birds of prey), but there are also mixed shows, where birds belonging to different families take part and 'work' (Fig. 17.35). The term 'work' is not inappropriate, since those birds are trained together with their keepers and play a significant role in a show and produce an income for the park. This does not mean that show birds are exploited. On the contrary, in most cases they love being cared for by their trainers and have a very full life, with a lot of interaction with other birds and humans (Fig. 17.36).

The veterinarian employed in a park where bird shows take place (and this applies to any other animal group running a show, like dolphins, sea-lions, seals, etc.), must always remember that there are diseases that are stress

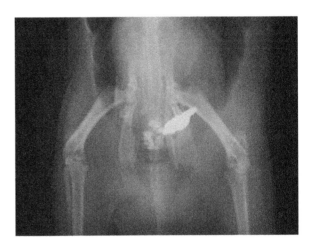

Fig 17.33 X-ray of a metal foreign body in a Humboldt penguin (*Spheniscus humboldti*).

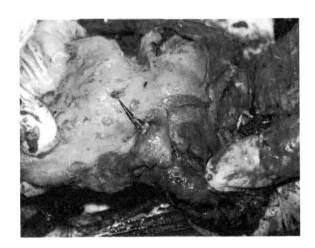

Fig 17.32 Gastric foreign body at necropsy of a gentoo penguin (*P. papua*).

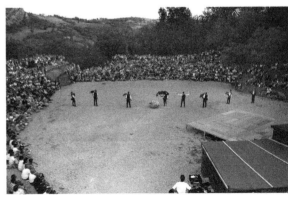

Fig 17.34 Falconers during a bird of prey show.

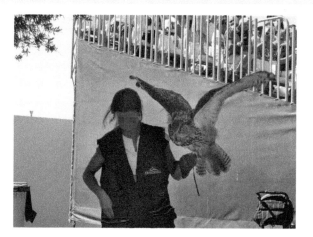

Fig 17.35 Nocturnal raptors are used for shows, as well. Eagle-owl (*Bubo bubo*).

related. The stressful conditions may be derived from over-exploiting working animals, diseases/accidents associated with park visitors (i.e. feeding wrong things to the birds), and finally diseases that birds may pass to humans (i.e. psittacosis).

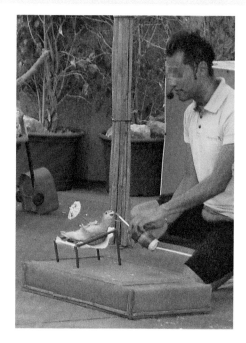

Fig 17.36 The interaction between show birds and their trainer may be very strong.

Suggested reading

Abrey A 2000 The management of a multi-species bird collection in a zoological park. In: Tully T N, Lawton M P C, Dorrestein G M (eds) Avian medicine. Butterworth-Heinemann, Oxford, p 364–385

Aguilar R F 2001 Order Falconiformes (hawks, eagles, falcons, vultures). Raptor medicine and surgery. In: Fowler M E, Cubas Z S (eds) Biology, medicine, and surgery of South American wild animals. Iowa State University Press, Ames, IA, p 118–124

Angel R, Plassé R D 1997 Developing a zoological avian nutrition program. Proceedings of the Annual Conference of the American Association of Zoo Veterinarians, p 39–43

Baer J F 1998 A veterinary perspective of potential risk factors in environmental enrichment. In: Shepherdson D J, Mellen J D, Hutchins M (eds) Second nature, environmental enrichment for captive animals. Smithsonian Institution Press, Washington, DC, p 277–301

Bailey T A et al 2000 The medical dilemmas associated with rehabilitating confiscated wildlife: experience at the environmental research and wildlife development agency, Abu Dhabi, monitoring the recovery of Houbara bustards (*Clamydotis u. macqueenii*) from avian pox and Newcastle disease. Proceedings of the European Association of Zoo and Wildlife Veterinarians:237–241

Bauck L 1998 Psittacine diets and behavioral enrichment. Seminars in Avian and Exotic Pet Medicine 7(3):135–140

Beklova M, Pikula J 2000 Hazards of rodenticidal baits to game birds. Proceedings of the European Association of Zoo and Wildlife Veterinarians:249–252

Bradbury S P 1996 2,3,7,8 Tetrachlorodibenzo-p-dioxin. In: Fairbrother A, Locke L N, Hoff G L (eds) Noninfectious diseases of wildlife, 2nd edn. Iowa State University Press, Ames, IA, p 87–98

Breitweiser Mullins B A 1992 Fluid therapy in penguins. Proceedings of the Annual Conference of the Association of Avian Veterinarians, p 158–160

Clubb S L 1997 Aviculture medicine and flock health management. In: Altman R B, Clubb S L, Dorrestein G M, Quesenberry K (eds) Avian medicine and surgery. W B Saunders, Philadelphia, PA, p 101–121

Coles B H 2000 Galliformes. In: Tully T N, Lawton M P C, Dorrestein G M (eds) Avian medicine. Butterworth-Heinemann, Oxford, p 266–295

Cranfield M R 2003 Spheniciformes (penguins). In: Fowler M, Miller E (eds) Zoo and wild animal medicine, 5th edn. Elsevier Science, St Louis, MO

Cranfield M R, Graczyk T K, McCutchan T F 1995 Molecular technology and avian malaria in the black-footed penguin. Proceedings of Joint Conference American Association of Zoo Veterinarians – Wildlife Disease Association – American Association of Wildlife Veterinarians. East Lansing, MI, p 208–210

Crosta L, Timossi L, Bürkle M, Trägårdh L 2004 Sex determination in two flamingo species by measurement of tarsometatarsus length. AAV Newsletter & Clinical Forum March–May:19–20

Crosta L, Timossi L, Bürkle M 2006 Management of zoo and park birds. In: Harrison G J, Lightfoot T et al (eds) Clinical avian medicine. Spix Publishing, Palm Beach, FL, p 991–1003

Cubas Z S 2001 Order Piciformes (toucans, woodpeckers). Medicine: family Ramphastidae (toucans). In: Fowler M E, Cubas Z S (eds) Biology, medicine, and surgery of South American wild animals. Iowa State University Press, Ames, IA, p 188–199

Curro T G, Langenberg J, Paul-Murphy J 1992 A review of lameness in long-legged birds. Proceedings of the Annual Conference of the Association of Avian Veterinarians, p 265–270

Degernes L A 1994 Introduction to wild bird medicine. Proceedings of the Basic Avian Medicine Symposium, Association of Avian Veterinarians, p 97–41

Degernes L A 1995 Toxicity in waterfowls. Seminars in Avian and Exotic Pet Medicine 4(1):15–22

Doest, O E A 2000 Macaw reintroduction to prevent extinction: fiction or reality? Proceedings of the Annual Conference of the Association of Avian Veterinarians, p 145–148

Dorrestein G M et al 2000 Iron in zoo-animals, frequency and interpretation of the findings. Proceedings of the European Association of Zoo and Wildlife Veterinarians, p 243–248

EAZA (European Association of Zoos and Aquaria) Spheniscus penguin husbandry manual, 1st edn. Edited and compiled by the Penguin TAG

Eulenberger K 1995 Taucher, Pinguine, Röhrennasen, Ruderfüßer. Wat- und Möwenvögel. In: Göltenboth R, Klös H G (eds) Krankheiten der Zoo- und Wildtiere. Blackwell Wissenschaft-Verlag, Berlin, p 488–502

Fowler M E 2001 Order Phenicopteriformes (flamingos). Biology, management in captivity, and medicine. In: Fowler M E, Cubas Z S (eds) Biology, medicine, and surgery of South American wild animals. Iowa State University Press, Ames, IA, p 95–102

Fowler M E 2001 Order Anseriformes (ducks, geese, swans). Captive management and medicine. In: Fowler M E, Cubas Z S (eds) Biology, medicine, and surgery of South American wild animals. Iowa State University Press, Ames, IA, p 105–114

Fowler M E 2001 Order Strigiformes (owls). Biology, medicine, and surgery. In: Fowler M E, Cubas Z S (eds) Biology, medicine, and surgery of South American wild animals. Iowa State University Press, Ames, IA, p 125–132

Fowler G S, Fowler M E 2001 Order Sphenisciformes (penguins). Biology, captive management, and medicine. In: Fowler M E, Cubas Z S (eds) Biology, medicine, and surgery of South American wild animals. Iowa State University Press, Ames, IA, p 53–64

Fox N 1995 Managing a breeding program. In: Understanding the bird of prey. Hancock House Publishers, Surrey, BC, p 58–110

Fox N 1995 Equipment and facilities. In: Understanding the bird of prey. Hancock House Publishers, Surrey, BC, p 112–174

Frey H, Zinc R 2000 Aspects of management within the European bearded vulture (Gypaetus barbatus) reintroduction. In: Lumeij J T, Remple J D, Redig P T et al (eds) Raptor biomedicine III. Zoological Education Network, Lake Worth, FL, p 281–288

Gerlach H 1997 Galliformes. In: Altman R B, Clubb S L, Dorrestein G M, Quesenberry K (eds) Avian medicine and surgery. W B Saunders, Philadelphia, PA, p 944–959

Gerlach H 1997 Anseriformes. In: Altman R B, Clubb S L, Dorrestein G M, Quesenberry K (eds) Avian medicine and surgery. W B Saunders, Philadelphia, PA, p 960–972

Greenwood A G 1995 Veterinary support for in situ avian conservation programs. Proceedings of the Annual Conference of the Association of Avian Veterinarians, p 163–169

Harper J E, Skinner N D 1998 Clinical nutrition of small psittacines and passerines. Seminars in Avian and Exotic Pet Medicine 7(3):116–127

Hatt J M 2000 Nutrition research in zoo animals. In: Nijboer J, Hatt J M, Kaumanns W et al (eds) Zoo animal nutrition. Filander Verlag, Fürth, Germany, p 11–19

Heatley J J, Mikota S K, Olsen G, Tully T N 2000 Antipredator conditioning of Mississippi sandhill cranes (Grus canadensis pulla). Proceedings of the Annual Conference of the Association of Avian Veterinarians, p 143–144

Heidenreich M 1997 Management of raptors in captivity. Birds of prey, medicine and management. Blackwell Science, Oxford, p 5–23

Heitzmann-Fontenelle J 2001 Order Ciconiiformes (herons, storks, ibises). Ciconiiformes Medicine. In: Fowler M E, Cubas Z S (eds) Biology, medicine, and surgery of South American wild animals. Iowa State University Press, Ames, IA, p 84–87

Hooimeijer J, Dorrestein G M 1997 Pigeons and doves. In: Altman R B, Clubb S L, Dorrestein G M, Quesenberry K (eds) Avian medicine and surgery. W B Saunders, Philadelphia, PA, p 886–909

Houston D C 2000 Digestion strategies in meat and fish eating birds. In: Nijboer J, Hatt J M, Kaumanns W et al (eds) Zoo animal nutrition. Filander Verlag, Fürth, Germany, p 57–62

Jenkins J 1996 Ratite medicine and surgery. In: Rosskopf W J Jr., Woerpl R W (eds) Diseases of cage and aviary birds. Williams & Wilkins, Baltimore, MD, p 1002–1006

Jones M P 1998 Developing a veterinary care program for captive birds of prey. Proceedings of the Annual Conference of the Association of Avian Veterinarians, p 183–187

Joseph V 1995 Preventive health programs for falconry birds. Proceedings of the Annual Conference of the Association of Avian Veterinarians, p 171–178

Joseph V 1996 Selected medical topics for birds of prey. Proceedings of the Annual Conference of the Association of Avian Veterinarians, p 261–266

Kirkwood J, Bailey T, Samour J, Keymer I F 2000 Management-related diseases. In: Samour J (ed) Avian medicine. Mosby, London, p 170–218

LaBonde J 1992 The medical and surgical management of domestic waterfowl collections. Proceedings of the Annual Conference of the Association of Avian Veterinarians, p 223–233

LaBonde J 1996 Private collections of waterfowls. Proceedings of the Annual Conference of the Association of Avian Veterinarians, p 215–223

LaBonde J 1996 Medicine and surgery of mynahs. In: Rosskopf W J Jr, Woerpl R W (eds) Diseases of cage and aviary birds. Williams & Wilkins, Baltimore, MD, p 928–932

LaBonde J 1996 Medicine and surgery of gallinaceous birds. In: Rosskopf W J Jr, Woerpl R W (eds) Diseases of cage and aviary birds. Williams & Wilkins, Baltimore, MD, p 951–956

LaBonde J 1996 Medicine and surgery of Anseriformes. In: Rosskopf W J Jr, Woerpl R W (eds) Diseases of cage and aviary birds. Williams & Wilkins, Baltimore, MD, p 956–964

Langenberg J 1995 The role of a veterinarian in an avian conservation program. Proceedings of the Annual Conference of the Association of Avian Veterinarians, p 157–161

Martínez I 1992 Order Sphenisciformes. In: del Hoyo J, Elliott A, Sargatal J (eds) Handbook of the birds of the world, Vol. 1. Lynx Edicions, Barcelona, p 140–161

Meredith A 1997 Prophylactic administration of itraconazole for the control of aspergillosis in Gentoo penguins (Pygoscelis papua). Fourth Conference of the European Committee of the Association of Avian Veterinarians, London, p 227–232

Morgan K N, Line S W, Markowitz H 1998 Zoos, enrichment, and the skeptical observer: the practical value of assessment. In: Shepherdson D J, Mellen J D, Hutchins M (eds) Second nature, environmental enrichment for captive animals. Smithsonian Institution Press, Washington, DC, p 153–171

Norton T M et al 1995 Bali Mynah Captive Medical Management and Reintroduction Program. Proceedings of the Annual Conference of the Association of Avian Veterinarians, p 125–136

O'Hara T M, Rice C D 1996 Polychlorinated biphenyls. In: Fairbrother A, Locke L N, Hoff G L (eds) Noninfectious diseases of wildlife, 2nd edn. Iowa State University Press, Ames, IA, p 71–86

Olsen G H 1993 Common infectious and parasitic diseases of quail and pheasants. Proceedings of the Annual Conference of the Association of Avian Veterinarians, p 146–150

Olsen G H 2000 Cranes. In: Tully T N, Lawton M P C, Dorrestein G M (eds) Avian medicine. Butterworth-Heinemann, Oxford, p 215–227

Olsen G H, Carpenter J W 1995 Andean condor medicine, reproduction and husbandry. Proceedings of the Annual Conference of the Association of Avian Veterinarians, p 147–152

Olsen G H, Langernberg J A, Carpenter J W 1996 Medicine and surgery. In: Ellis D H, Gee G F, Mirande C M (eds) Cranes: their biology, husbandry, and conservation. Hancock House Publishers, Blaine, WA, p 137–174

Olsen G H, Carpenter J W 1997 Cranes. In: Altman R B, Clubb S L, Dorrestein G M, Quesenberry K (eds) Avian medicine and surgery. W B Saunders, Philadelphia, PA, p 973–992

Pokras M A 1996 Clinical management and biomedicine of sea birds. In: Rosskopf W J Jr, Woerpl R W (eds) Diseases of cage and aviary birds. Williams & Wilkins, Baltimore, MD, p 981–1001

Prudente do Amaral P, Sanfilippo L F 2001 Order Ciconiiformes (herons, storks, ibises). Management in captivity. In: Fowler M E, Cubas Z S (eds) Biology, medicine, and surgery of South American wild animals. Iowa State University Press, Ames, IA, p 83–84

Redig P T 1992 Health management of raptors trained for falconry. Proceedings of the Annual Conference of the Association of Avian Veterinarians, p 258–264

Reding P T, Ackermann J 2000 Raptors. In: Tully T N, Lawton M P C, Dorrestein G M (eds) Avian medicine. Butterworth-Heinemann, Oxford, p 180–214

Reidarson T H, McBain J 1995 Serum protein electrophoresis and Aspergillus antibody titers as an aid to diagnosis of aspergillosis in penguins. Proceeding of the Annual Conference of the Association of Avian Veterinarians, p 61–64

Reidarson T H, McBain J, Burch L 1999 A novel approach to the treatment of bumblefoot in penguins. Journal of Avian Medicine and Surgery 3(2):124–127

Robinson I 2000 Seabirds. In: Tully T N, Lawton M P C, Dorrestein G M (eds) Avian medicine. Butterworth-Heinemann, Oxford, p 339–363

Roudybush T E 1999 Psittacine nutrition. Veterinary Clinics of North America (Exotic Animals) 2(1):111–125

Routh A, Sanderson S 2000 Waterfowl. In: Tully T N, Lawton M P C, Dorrestein G M (eds) Avian medicine. Butterworth-Heinemann, Oxford, p 234–265

Seidensticker J, Forthman D L 1998 Evolution, and enrichment: basic considerations for wild animals in zoos. In: Shepherdson D J, Mellen J D, Hutchins M (eds) Second nature, environmental enrichment for captive animals. Smithsonian Institution Press, Washington, DC, p 15–29

Stahl S, Kronfeld D 1998 Veterinary nutrition of large psittacines. Seminars in Avian and Exotic Pet Medicine 7(3):128–134

Stonebreaker R 1997 Ratites. In: Altman R B, Clubb S L, Dorrestein G M, Quesenberry K (eds) Avian medicine and surgery. W B Saunders, Philadelphia, PA, p 929–943

Stoskopf M K, Kennedy-Stoskopf S 1986 Aquatic birds. In: Fowler M E (ed) Zoo and wild animal medicine, 2nd edn. W B Saunders, Philadelphia, PA, p 293–313

Stringfield C E 1998 Medical management of the California Condor (*Gymnogyps californianus*). Proceedings of the Annual Conference of the Association of Avian Veterinarians, p 173–174

Swengel S R, Carpenter J W 1996 General husbandry. In: Ellis D H, Gee G F, Mirande C M (eds) Cranes: their biology, husbandry, and conservation. Hancock House Publishers, Blaine, WA, p 31–43

Timossi L 2002 Enriquecimiento Ambiental. Proceedings 'Simposium Internacional, Mamíferos Salvajes en Cautividad', AVAFES, León, March 2002

Timossi L, Crosta L, Bürkle M 2002 Management and general medical issues of a mixed species penguin collection in closed environment. Proceedings of the European Association of Zoo and Wildlife Veterinarians and European Wildlife Disease Association:283–285

Tully T N 2000 Ratites. In: Tully T N, Lawton M P C, Dorrestein G M (eds) Avian medicine. Butterworth-Heinemann, Oxford, p 228–233

Worrell A B 1996 Medicine and surgery of toucans. In: Rosskopf W J Jr, Woerpl R W (eds) Diseases of cage and aviary birds. Williams & Wilkins, Baltimore, MD, p 933–943

Worrell A B 1997 Toucans and Mynahs. In: Altman R B, Clubb S L, Dorrestein G M, Quesenberry K (eds) Avian medicine and surgery. W B Saunders, Philadelphia, PA, p 910–917

Worrell A B 2000 Ramphastids. In: Tully T N, Lawton M P C, Dorrestein G M (eds) Avian medicine. Butterworth-Heinemann, Oxford, p 296–311

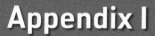

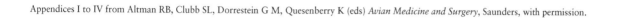

Appendices I to IV from Altman RB, Clubb SL, Dorrestein G M, Quesenberry K (eds) *Avian Medicine and Surgery*, Saunders, with permission.

Appendix IA: Haematological and plasma biochemical reference ranges of common psittacine species

Table 1 Haematological reference ranges of common psittacine species*

Value	African grey parrot	Amazon parrot	Budgerigar	Cockatiel	Cockatoo	Conure	Eclectus parrot	Jardine's parrot	Lovebird	Macaw	Pionus	Quaker parrot	Senegal parrot
Haematocrit (%)	38-48	37-50	38-48	36-49	38-48	36-49	35-47	35-48	38-50	35-48	35-47	35-46	36-48
	42-53†	43-49†	44-54†	43-58†	42-51†	43-56†	43-50†		43-55†	43-54†	43-54†		
Red blood cells (×10⁶/μL)	2.4-3.9	2.4-4.0	2.4-4.0	2.2-3.9	2.2-4.0	2.5-4.0	2.4-3.9	2.4-4.0	2.3-3.9	2.4-4.0	2.4-4.0	2.3-4.0	2.4-4.0
	2.80-3.36†	2.33-2.95†	3.90-4.70†	3.8-4.58†	2.50-2.95†	3.13-3.94†	2.7-3.1†		2.63-3.50†		2.7-3.5†		
Haemoglobin (g/dL)	11.0-16	11.0-17.5	12-16	11-16	11.5-16	12-16	11.5-16	11-16	13-18	11-16	11-16	11-15	11-16
	15.1-16.9†	14.4-16.7†	13.4-15.3†	12.1-14.6†	12.0-14.8†	12.1-14.8†	14.1-16.0†		11.9-15.1†		14.2-15.5†		
Mean corpuscular volume (fL)	90-180	85-200	90-200	90-200	85-200	90-190	95-220	90-190	90-190	90-185	85-210	90-200	90-200
	143-155†	163-170†	115-124†	128-142†	154-170†	135-147†	157-170†		155-166†		154-164†		
Mean corpuscular haemoglobin (g/dL)	28-52	28-55	25-60	28-55	28-60	28-55	27-55	26-56	27-59	27-53	26-54	26-55	27-55
	32.3-45.6†	49.8-58.2†	25.9-30.9†	24.9-36.0†	45.0-55.5†	30.0-40.1†	51.3-54.2†		40-48†		41.4-46.0†		
Mean corpuscular haemoglobin concentration (g/dL)	23-33	23-32	23-30	22-33	21-34	23-31	22-33	21-33	22-32	23-32	24-31	22-32	23-32
	23.16-31.78†	32.8-35.31†	19.80-26.75†	18.91-25.61†	24.12-32.91†	23.5-28.6†	31.2-34.0†		21.9-29.3†		25.8-28.7†		
White blood cells (×10³/μL)	5.0-11.0	6.0-11.0	3.0-8.5	5.0-10.0	5.0-11.0	4.0-11.0	4.0-10.0	4.0-10.0	3.0-8.5	6.0-12.0	4.0-11.5	4.0-10.0	4.0-11.0
	6.0-13.0†	5.0-12.5†	3.0-8.0†	5.0-9.0†	5.0-12.0†	4.0-9.0†			3.0-8.0†	7.0-12.0†			
Heterophils (%)	55-75	55-80	50-75	55-80	55-80	55-75	55-70	55-75	50-75	58-78	50-75	55-80	55-75
	45-72†	32-71†	41-67†	47-72†	45-72†	45-72†			41-71†	48-72†			
Lymphocytes (%)	25-45	20-45	25-45	20-45	20-45	25-45	30-45	25-45	25-50	20-45	25-45	20-45	25-45
	25-50†	20-65†	22-58†	27-58†	20-50†	22-49†			28-52†	18-52†			
Monocytes (%)	0-3	0-3	0-2	0-2	0-1	0-2	0-2	0-2	0-2	0-3	0-2	0-3	0-2
	0-1†	0-1†	0-2†	0-1†	0-1†	0-1†			0-1†	0-1†			
Basophils (%)	0-1	0-1	0-1	0-2	0-1	0-1	0-2	0-1	0-1	0-1	0-1	0-2	0-1
	0-1†	0-2†	0-2†	0-1†	0-1†	0-2†			0-1†	0-1†			
Eosinophils (%)	0-2	0-1	0-2	0-2	0-2	0-2	0-1	0-1	0-1	0-1	0-2	0-1	0-1
	0-1†	0-0.05†	0-0.05†	0-2†	0-2†	0-1†			0-1†	0-1†			

*Except where noted by (†), values from the Avian and Wildlife Laboratory, University of Miami School of Medicine, Miami, FL 33136. Haematological determinations were done by Unopette method (Becton-Dickenson, Rutherford, NJ) from EDTA samples 24 hours after collection. Slides for the differential cell count were made at the time of collection.
†Values from the California Avian Laboratory, Citrus Heights, CA 95621

Table 2 Plasma biochemical reference ranges of common psittacine species*

Value	African grey parrot	Amazon parrot	Budgerigar	Cockatiel	Cockatoo	Conure	Eclectus parrot	Jardine's parrot	Lory	Lovebird	Macaw	Pionus	Quaker parrot	Senegal parrot
Alanine aminotransferase [ALT] (U/L)	5.0–12.0	5.0–11.0	–	5.0–11.0	5.0–11.0	5.0–13.0	5.0–11.0	–	–	–	5.0–12.0	–	–	–
Albumin (g/dL)	1.57–3.23†	1.90–3.52†	–	0.7–1.8† 0.3–0.9‡	1.8–3.1† 0.3–0.9‡	1.9–3.6† 0.3–0.9‡	2.3–2.6†	1.85–2.23†	1.26–1.96†	2.0–2.8† 0.3–0.9‡	1.24–3.11†	2.19–3.19†	1.26–2.52†	1.45–2.28†
Alkaline phosphatase (U/L)	20–160	15–150	10–80	20–250	15–255	80–250	150–350	–	–	10–90	20–230	–	–	–
Amylase (U/L)	210–530	205–510	–	–	–	100–450	150–645	–	–	–	150–550	–	–	–
Aspartate aminotransferase [AST] (U/L)	100–365 112–339†	130–350 155–380‡	145–350 160–372‡	95–345 130–390‡	145–355 145–346‡	125–345 147–360†	120–370	150–275	150–350	110–345 130–343‡	100–300 60–165‡	150–365	150–285	100–350
Bile acids (μmol/L)	13–90 12–85†	18–60 35–144‡	15–70 35–110‡	20–85 45–105‡	25–87 37–98‡	15–55 35–90‡	10–35	25–65	20–65	13–65 34–88‡	6–35 30–80‡	14–60	25–65	20–85
Blood urea nitrogen (BUN) (mg/dL)	3.0–5.4	3.1–5.3	–	2.9–5.0	3.0–5.1	2.8–5.4	3.0–5.5	–	–	–	3.0–5.6	–	–	–
Calcium (mg/dL)	8.5–13.0 8.3–11.7†	8.5–14.0 8.5–13.0‡	6.5–11.0 8.5–11.0‡	8.0–13.0 8.3–10.9‡	8.0–13.0 8.4–11.0‡	7.0–15.0 8.4–11.0‡	7.0–13	7.0–13	6.5–13	8.0–14.0 8.6–11.5‡	8.5–13.0 8.3–11.0‡	7.0–13.5	7.0–12.0	6.5–13.0
Carbon dioxide (CO₂), total (mmol/L)	13–25	13–26	14–25	13–25	14–25	14–25	14–24	–	–	14–25	14–25	–	–	–
Cholesterol (mg/dL)	160–425	180–305 150–220‡	145–275 120–220‡	140–360 90–195‡	145–355 90–200‡	120–400 83–190‡	130–350	–	–	95–335 125–195‡	100–390	130–295	–	–
Creatine kinase (CK) (U/L)	165–412 120–410†	55–345 120–410‡	90–300 120–360‡	30–245 167–420‡	95–305 150–400‡	35–355 150–397‡	220–345	–	–	52–245 160–320‡	100–300 90–360‡	–	–	100–330
Creatinine (mg/dL)	0.1–0.4 0.1–0.5†	0.1–0.4	0.1–0.4	0.1–0.4 0.1–0.5‡	0.1–0.4 0.1–0.8‡	0.1–0.4 0.1–0.8‡	0.1–0.4	–	–	0.1–0.4 0.1–0.8‡	0.1–0.5 0.1–0.7‡	0.1–0.4	–	0.1–0.4
Gamma glutamyltransferase [GGT] (U/L)	1–10	1–12	1–10	1–30	1–45	1–15	1–20	–	–	2.5–18.0	1–30	–	–	1–15

(continued)

Table 2 (continued)

Value	African grey parrot	Amazon parrot	Budgerigar	Cockatiel	Cockatoo	Conure	Eclectus parrot	Jardine's parrot	Lory	Lovebird	Macaw	Pionus	Quaker parrot	Senegal parrot
Globulin (g/dL)	–	–	–	2.5-3.8‡	2.5-3.8‡	2.5-3.8‡	–	–	–	2.5-3.8‡	–	–	–	–
Glucose (mg/dL)	190-350	190-345	190-390	200-445	185-355	200-345	145-245	200-325	200-300	195-405	145-345	125-300	200-350	140-250
	280-354‡	250-370‡	210-450‡	230-440‡	210-410‡	230-400‡	–			210-390‡	210-360‡			
Glutamate dehydrogenase (GLDH) (U/L)	0-9.9	0-9.9	0-9.9	0-9.9	0-9.9	0-9.9	0-9.9	–	–	0-9.9	0-9.9	–	–	–
Lactate dehydrogenase (U/L)	145-465	155-425	145-435	120-455	220-550	120-390	200-425	–	–	105-355	70-350	–	–	–
	154-380‡	160-360‡	162-380‡	125-374‡	200-400‡	210-390‡				230-345‡	70-210‡			
Lipase (U/L)	35-350	35-225	–	30-280	25-275	30-290	35-275	–	–	–	30-250	–	–	–
Phosphorus (mg/dL)	3.2-5.4	3.1-5.5	3.0-5.2	3.2-4.8	2.5-5.5	2.0-10.0	2.9-6.5	–	–	2.8-4.9	2.0-12.0	2.9-6.6	–	–
	3.5-6.9‡		3.7-7.1†	4.0-7.7†	4.2-7.8‡	4.0-7.9‡					4.0-7.8‡			
Potassium (mmol/L)	2.9-4.6	3.0-4.5	2.2-3.9	2.4-4.6	2.5-4.5	3.4-5.0	3.5-4.3	–	–	2.1-4.8	2.0-5.0	3.5-4.6	–	–
Protein, plasma (g/dL)	3.0-4.6	3.0-5.0	2.5-4.5	2.4-4.1	3.0-5.0	3.0-4.2	2.8-3.8	2.8-4.0	2.0-3.5	2.8-4.4	2.1-4.5	2.2-4.0	2.8-3.6	3.5-4.4
	3.2-4.5†§	3.2-4.5†§	3.0-4.4†§	2.9-4.2†§	3.1-4.4†§	3.2-4.4†§				3.2-4.4†§	2.7-4.7†§			
Sodium (mmol/L)	157-165	125-155	139-165	130-153	130-155	135-149	130-145	–	–	132-168	140-165	145-155	–	–
Thyroxine (T4) (μg/dL)	0.3-2.1	0.1-1.1	0.5-2.1	0.7-2.4	0.7-4.1	0.5-2.0	0.5-3.5	–	–	0.2-4.3	0.5-2.3	–	–	–
Triglycerides (mg/dL)	45-145	49-190	105-265	45-200	45-205	50-300	70-410	–	–	45-200	60-135	–	–	–
Uric acid (mg/dL)	4.5-9.5	2.3-10.0	4.5-14.0	3.5-10.5	3.5-10.5	2.5-11.0	2.5-11.0	2.5-12.0	2.8-11.5	3.5-11.0	2.5-11.0	3.5-10.0	3.5-11.5	2.3-10.0
	1.9-9.7†	2.3-9.8‡	4.0-12.2‡	3.5-10.4‡	3.6-10.7‡	2.7-10.2‡				3.2-10.2‡	1.5-11.0‡			

*Except where noted (†), values are from the Avian and Wildlife Laboratory, University of Miami School of Medicine, Miami FL 33136. All biochemical determinations at this laboratory were done by Kodak Ektachem and DuPont Analyst systems.

Analysis was done 24 hours after sample collection into lithium heparin. Samples were centrifuged and separated at time of collection.

†Plasma protein electrophoresis measured by the Beckman Paragon system.

‡Values from the California Avian Laboratory, Citrus Heights, CA 95621.

§Measured by temperature compensated refractometer.

Table 3 Plasma protein electrophoresis reference ranges of common psittacine species*

Value	African grey parrot	Amazon parrot	Cockatiel	Cockatoo	Conure	Eclectus parrot	Jardine's parrot	Lory	Lovebird	Macaw	Pionus	Quaker parrot	Senegal parrot
Prealbumin (g/dL)	0.03-1.35	0.35-1.05	0.8-1.6	0.24-1.18	0.18-0.98	0.4-1.04	0.18-0.32	0.48-0.76	0.6-1.2	0.05-07	0.19-0.93	0.48-1.13	0.19-0.64
Albumin (g/dL)	1.57-3.23	1.90-3.52	0.7-1.8	1.8-3.1	1.9-2.6	2.3-2.6	1.85-2.23	1.26-1.96	2.0-2.8	1.24-3.11	2.19-3.29	1.26-2.52	1.45-2.28
Alpha-1 (g/dL)	0.02-0.27	0.05-0.32	0.05-0.40	0.05-0.18	0.04-0.23	0.09-0.33	0.04-0.15	0.04-0.14	0.08-0.21	0.04-0.25	0.10-0.16	0.04-0.25	0.02-0.20
Alpha-2 (g/dL)	0.12-0.31	0.07-0.32	0.05-0.44	0.04-0.36	0.08-0.26	0.11-0.27	0.08-0.15	0.04-0.23	0.08-0.25	0.04-0.31	0.08-0.15	0.05-0.28	0.08-0.16
Beta (g/dL)	0.15-0.56	0.12-0.72	0.21-0.58	0.22-0.82	0.07-0.47	0.17-0.43	0.18-0.38	0.15-0.58	0.19-0.40	0.14-0.62	0.08-0.45	0.20-0.55	0.26-0.58
Gamma (g/dL)	0.11-0.71	0.17-0.76	0.11-0.43	0.21-0.65	0.12-0.61	0.18-0.55	0.12-0.26	0.13-0.29	0.18-0.45	0.1-0.62	0.18-0.40	0.13-0.48	0.14-0.23
A/G ratio	1.6-4.3	1.9-5.9	1.5-4.3	2.0-4.5	2.2-4.3	2.62-4.05	2.9-3.5	2.3-4.0	2.5-4.6	1.6-4.3	3.4-5.5	2.2-3.2	2.2-3.9

*Values from the Avian and Wildlife Laboratory, University of Miami School of Medicine, Miami, FL 33136. Protein electrophoresis was done with the Beckman Paragon system.

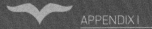
Appendix IB: Haematological biochemical and morphometric reference ranges of selected raptor species

Table 1 Haematological reference ranges of selected healthy adult captive raptors*

Value	Red-tailed hawk (n = 10)	Great-horned owl (n = 10)	Bald eagle (n = 8)	Peregrine falcon (n = 14)	Gyrfalcon (n = 12)
PCA (%)	44.6 (2.6)[†]	43.3 (2.9)	44 (4)	44 (4)	49 (2)
Total protein (g/dL)	4.3 (0.5)	5.1 (0.6)	4.0 (1)	2.65 (1.18)	2.94 (0.38)
White blood cells ($\times 10^3$/μL)	6.0–8.0	6.0–8.0	12.8 (4.8)	8.7 (2.2)	4.6 (1.7)
Heterophils (%)	35 (11.1)	47 (10.7)	75 (13)	65 (12)	51 (5)
Lymphocytes (%)	44 (8.9)	27 (7.0)	18 (10)	35 (13)	47 (5)
Monocytes (%)	6 (3.2)	9 (3.6)	3 (3)	0 (0)	1 (1)
Basophils (%)	2 (1.3)	Rare	Rare	0 (0)	Rare
Eosinophils (%)	13 (3.8)	1 (1.2)	4 (3)	0 (1)	1 (1)

*From Dr. P. Redig, The Raptor Center, University of Minnesota, St Paul, MN 55108.

[†]Standard deviation in parentheses.

Table 2 Haematological and morphometric measurements of wild red–tailed hawk nestlings*

Stage of development	Primary feather length (cm)	Central tail feather length (cm)	PCV (%)	Total protein (g/dL)	RBC ($\times 10^6$/μL)	Haemoglobin (g/dL)
Early (n = 5)	0–10	0–8	28 (1)[†]	3.4 (0.1)	1.74 (0.09)	8.79 (0.40)
Late (n = 5)	11–18	9–16	33 (1)[†]	4.0 (0.1)	2.35 (0.03)	10.98 (0.14)

*From Dr. P. Reding, The Raptor Center, University of Minnesota, St Paul, MN 55108.

[†]Means ± Standard deviations in parentheses.

Table 3 Serum biochemical reference values of selected raptor species*

Value	Bald eagle (n = 8)	Peregrine falcon (n= 14)	Gyrfalcon (n =12)	Red tailed hawk (n = 10)	Great-horned owl (n = 10)
Acetylcholinesterase (delta pH units/h)	0.16 (0.06)	–	–	–	–
Alanine aminotransferase (ALT) (U/L)	25 (13)	62 (56)	–	31 (5)	39 (14)
Albumin (g/dL)	1.09 (0.18)	0.96 (0.13)	0.73 (0.09)	1.34 (0.41)	1.27 (0.35)
Alkaline phosphatase (U/L)	57 (12)	99 (44)	257 (61)	53 (18)	31 (7)
Amylase (U/L)	1158 (376)	–	–	–	–
Aspartate aminotransferase (AST) (U/L)	218 (63)	78 (31)	97 (33)	303 (22)	287 (65)
Bilirubin, total (mg/dL)	0.31 (0.08)	4.57 (2.04)	–	0.16 (0.08)	0.07 (0.06)
Blood urea nitrogen (BUN) (mg/dL)	3.10 (2.47)	3.25 (1.39)	4.67 (0.82)	4.67 (0.47)	5 (2.94)
Calcium (mg/dL)	9.94 (0.45)	8.93 (0.46)	9.61 (0.24)	–	10.19
Chloride (mmol/L)	120 (3)	114.38 (43.36)	125 (2)	125 (3)	122
Creatine kinase (U/L)	383 (300)	783 (503)	402 (163)	1124 (251)	977 (407)
Creatinine (mg/dL)	0.70 (0.26)	0.51 (0.22)	–	–	–
Glucose (mg/dL)	302 (25)	366 (29)	318 (39)	356 (16)	356
Osmolality (mmol/kg)	319 (6)	–	–	–	–

(continued)

Table 3 *(continued)*

Value	Bald eagle (*n* = 8)	Peregrine falcon (*n* = 14)	Gyrfalcon (*n* = 12)	Red tailed hawk (*n* = 10)	Great-horned owl (*n* = 10)
Phosphorus (mg/dL)	3.03 (0.51)	3.35 (0.70)	3.57 (1.13)	3.14 (0.5)	4.34
Potassium (mmol/L)	3.0 (0)	2.04 (0.81)	1.99 (0.56)	2.42 (0.73)	2.8
Protein, total (g/dL) (biuret)	3.51 (0.75)	2.63 (0.48)	2.89 (0.31)	4.17 (0.69)	4.33
Sodium (mmol/L)	156 (4)	143 (54)	160 (3)	157 (1)	156
Uric acid (mg/dL)	5.07 (3.33)	4.50 (4.24)	13.93 (5.64)[†]	10.84 (5.1)[†]	13.7 (10.8)[†]

*From Dr. P. Redig, The Raptor Center, University of Minnesota, St Paul, MN 55108. All samples were collected from healthy adult birds – either display/education or breeders or birds flown in falconry. All samples were collected after the birds had been anaesthetized for a minimum of 10 minutes with isoflurane.
[†]Postprandial samples.

Appendix IC: Haematological and serum biochemical reference ranges of ratites

Table 1 Haematological reference ranges of ratites*

Value	Ostrich adults		Emu adults	
	Mean	Range	Mean	Range
Red blood cells ($\times 10^6/\mu$L)	1.8	–	1.85	–
Haematocrit (%)	45	41–57	47.4	39–57
Haemoglobin (g/dL)	16.92	–	16.04	–
Mean corpuscular volume (fL)	212	–	219	–
Mean corpuscular haemoglobin (pg)	82.19	–	86.51	–
Mean corpuscular haemoglobin concentration (g/L)	37.65	–	39.37	–
Red blood cell distribution width percentage[†] (%)	11.11	–	10.9	–
White blood cells ($\times 10^3/\mu$L)	18.65	10.0–24	14.87	8–21
Heterophils (%)	75.1	58–89	78.8	54–88
Lymphocytes (%)	24.1	12–41	19.8	10–44
Monocytes (%)	0.2	0–2	0.1	0–1
Basophils (%)	1.36	0–3	0.2	0–1
Eosinophils (%)	2.16	0–4	2.58	0–6

*Values from the California Avian Laboratory, Citrus Heights, CA 95621. Values were calculated from samples collected in field conditions and vary somewhat from previously published ranges.
[†]Red cell distribution width (RDW) percentage is a numerical expression of the coefficient of variability of the mean corpuscular volume, calculated by automated erythrocyte analysis (laser flow cytometry). An increase in RDW percentage denotes an increase in anisocytosis; a decrease in RDW percentage denotes a decrease in anisocytosis, as seen in non-regenerative anaemia.

Table 2 Serum biochemical reference ranges of ratites*

Value	Ostrich adults		Emu adults	
	Mean	Range	Mean	Range
Albumin (g/dL)	1.72	1.1–2.3	1.7	1.2–2.4
Aspartate aminotransferase (AST) (U/L)	447.9	226–547	227.2	80–380
Bile acids (μmol/L)	21	2–30	18	2–34
Calcium (mg/dL)	10.7	8.0–13.6	11.1	8.8–12.5

(continued)

Table 2 *(continued)*

Value	Ostrich adults		Emu adults	
	Mean	Range	Mean	Range
Cholesterol (mg/dL)	103	39–172	122	68–170
Creatine kinase (U/L)	3702	800–6600	428.8	70–818
Creatinine (mg/dL)	0.26	0.1–0.7	0.22	0.1–0.4
Globulin	2.21	1.4–3.1	2.23	1.4–3.2
Glucose (mg/dL)	217	164–330	134.1	101–243
Lactate dehydrogenase (U/L)	970	408–1236	778.1	318–1243
Phosphorus (mg/dL)	5.33	2.9–7.7	5.7	3.8–7.2
Plasma protein (g/dL)	3.93	2.4–5.3	3.93	3.4–4.4
Total protein (g/dL)	4.47[†]	2.5–5.2[†]	4.26[†]	2.5–5.6[†]
Uric acid (mg/dL)	8.62	1–14.5	6.3	1–13.7

*Values from the California Avian Laboratory, Citrus Heights, CA 95621. Values were calculated from cases sampled in field conditions and vary somewhat from previously published ranges.
†Measured by temperature-compensated refractometer.

Appendix ID: Haematological and serum biochemical reference ranges of selected non-psittacine avian species*

Table 1 Haematological and serum biochemical reference ranges of selected non-psittacine avian species*

Measurement	Canary	Finch	Greater Indian hill mynah	Toucan	Domestic duck
Haematology:					
PCV (%)	45–60	45–62	44–55	45–60	30–43
	37–49[†]				
Red blood cells (10⁶/μL)	2.5–4.5	2.5–4.6	2.4–4.0	2.5–4.5	2.3–3.5
	2.5–3.8[†]				
White blood cells (10⁶/μL)	4–9	3–8	6–11	4–10	4.5–13.0
	4–9[†]				
Heterophils (%)	20–50	20–65	25–65	35–65	30–70
	50–80[†]				
Lymphocytes (%)	40–75	20–65	20–60	25–50	20–65
	20–45[†]				
Monocytes (%)	0–1	0–1	0–3	0–4	0–3
	0–1[†]				
Eosinophils (%)	0–1	0–1	0–3	0–1	0–4
	0–2[†]				
Basophils (%)	0–5	0–5	0–7	0–5	0–5
	0–1[†]				
Chemistries:					
Alkaline phosphatase (U/L)	146–397	–	–	–	–
	20–135[†]				
Aspartate aminotransferase (AST) (U/L)	45–170	150–350	130–350	130–330	5–100
	145–345[†]				

(continued)

Table 1 *(continued)*

Measurement	Canary	Finch	Greater Indian hill mynah	Toucan	Domestic duck
Calcium (mg/dL)	5.1–13.4	–	9–13	10–15	10–18
	5.5–13.5[†]				
Creatinine (mg/dL)	0.1–1.0	–	0.1–0.6	0.1–0.4	0.1–0.5
	0.1–0.4[†]				
Glucose (mg/dL)	291–391	200–450	190–350	220–350	150–300
	205–435[†]				
Lactate dehydrogenase (U/L)	1300–1816	–	600–1000	200–400	150–800
	120–350[†]				
Phosphorus (mg/dL)	1.6–56	–	–	–	–
	2.9–49[†]				
Potassium (mmol/L)	2.7–4.8	–	0.3–5.1	–	3.0–4.5
	2.2–4.5				
Protein, total (g/dL)	2.0–4.4	3–5	2.3–4.5	3–5	2.5–6.0
	2.8–4.5[†]				
Sodium (mmol/L)	125–154	–	136–152	–	130–155
	135–165[†]				
Thyroxine (T4) (μg/dL)	0.7–32[†]	–	–	–	0.8–3.3
Uric acid (mg/dL)	4.3–14.8	4–12	4–10	4–14	2–12
	4.0–12.0[†]				

*Except where noted, adapted from Carpenter J.W, Mashima T.Y, Rupiper D.J: Exotic Animal Formulary. Manhattan, KS, Greystone Publications, 1996, p 156.

†Values from Avian and Wildlife Laboratory, University of Miami School of Medicine, Miami, FL 33136.

Appendix IE: Plasma biochemical reference ranges for racing pigeons

Table 1 Plasma biochemical reference ranges for racing pigeons

Parameter	$P_{2.5} – P_{97.5}$*
Sodium (mEq/L)	141–149
Potassium (mEq/L)	3.9–4.7
Calcium (mg/dL)	7.6–10.4
Magnesium (mg/dL)	2.7–4.4
Inorganic phosphorus (mg/dL)	1.8–4.1
Chloride (mEq/dL)	101–113
Plasma iron (g/dL)	61–184
Iron binding capacity (μg/dL)	5.4–8.0
Osmolality (mOsm/kg)	297–317
Glucose (mg/dL)	232–369
Creatinine (mg/dL)	0.26–.04
Urea (mg/dL)	2.4–4.2
Uric acid (mg/dL)	2.52–12.86
Urea : Uric acid ratio	1.8 1.8 (mean SD)
CPK (U/L)	110–480

Parameter	$P_{2.5} – P_{97.5}$*
AP (U/L)	160–780
AST (U/L)	45–123
ALT (U/L)	19–48
GLDH (U/L)	0–1
LDH (U/L)	30–205
Bile acids (mol/L)	22–60
GGT (U/L)	0–2.9
Total protein (g/dL)	2.1–3.3
Albumin : Globulin ratio	1.5–3.6
Prealbumin (g/dL)	0.1–0.4
Albumin (g/dL)	1.3–2.2
Alpha globulin (g/dL)	0.2–0.3
Beta globulin (g/dL)	0.3–0.6
Gamma globulin (g/dL)	0.1–0.3

From Lumeij JT: PhD thesis, Utrecht University, 1987.
The inner limits are given for the percentiles P_{25} and $P_{97.5}$ with a probability of 90%.

Appendix IF: Procedures for conducting avian white blood cell counts*

Unopette method for indirect determination of the total white blood cell count (TWC) (phloxine diluent)[†]

1. Count the number of stained cells in each of the four corner squares on both sides of the haemacytometer.
2. Average the counts from the two sides.
3. Multiply the average count $\times$ 80 = the number of granulocytes/μL of blood.
4. Conduct a differential count on a Diff-Quik stained smear.
5. Add the percentages of heterophils, eosinophils and basophils for the total percentage of granulocytes.
6. % heterophils + % eosinophils + % basophils $\times$ total WBC/μL = number of granulocytes.
7. Therefore, total WBC/μL = number of granulocytes ÷ by % granulocytes.

Estimated white blood cell count method[‡] (after L. McEntee)

1. Count all WBCs in five to eight high dry microscopic fields ($40 \times$).[§]
2. Divide the total WBCs counted by the number of fields counted for the average number of WBCs/field.
3. Multiply the average $\times$ 2000 for the total estimated WBCs/μL.

4. To correct for an abnormal PCV, the WBC count is adjusted in the direction of the change in PCV. The formula for this adjustment is:

Divide the observed PCV by the normal PCV and multiply by the total estimated WBC count. This gives you the corrected amount.

Example: Forty WBCs are counted in eight high dry fields and the PCV is 35%.

$$^{40}/_8 = 5 \times 2000 = \text{estimated WBC} = 10\ 000$$
$$^{35}/_{40} \times 10\ 000 = 8500 \text{ (corrected WBC)}$$

Recipes for frequently used haematologic stains

Wright's stain for avian blood

Dry Wright's stain: 3 g
Giemsa stain: 1 g
Add to 4 quarts of **acetone-free** methanol. Begin agitation immediately for several minutes. Continue with intermittent agitation for 10 days. Filter before use.

Wright–Giemsa Buffer

106.08 g KPO_4 anhydrous monobasic
  51.20 g Na_2PO_4 anhydrous dibasic
Dilute to 16 litres in distilled water. Adjust pH to 6.8:
↓pH: add dibasic
↑pH: add monobasic

---

*From Dr. P. Redig, The Raptor Center, University of Minnesota, St Paul, MN 55108.

[†] Unopette, test 5877, Becton-Dickinson, Rutherford, NJ 07070.

[‡] (This determination is predicated on the fact that birds with normal PCVs have approximately 2–4 million RBCs/μL and one leukocyte per 1000 RBCs. There are 1000 RBCs in five to eight high dry fields prepared from avian blood. Therefore, the estimate gives you the average number of leukocytes/μL. This is also based on the assumption that a monolayer blood film area of a properly prepared slide or coverslip is evaluated.)

[§] Typically done on a 'stat' stained slide using Diff-Quik (Harleco, Gibbstown, NJ) or Hema3 (Curtin-Mathisen, Houston, TX).

Table 1 Haematology

Component	Conventional unit	Conversion factor	SI unit symbol	Significant digits[†]
Haemoglobin	g/dL	10	g/L	XXX
Mean corpuscular haemoglobin concentration	g/dL	10	g/L	XX0
	pg	1	pg	XX
Mean corpuscular volume	μm^3	1	fL	XXX
Red blood cell count	$10^6/mm^3$ or $10^6/\mu L$	1	$10^{12}/L$	X.X
Reticulocyte count	/mm^3 or /μL	0.001	$10^9/L$	XX
Thrombocytes	$10^3/mm^3$ or $10^3/\mu L$	1	$10^9/L$	XXX
White blood cell count	/mm^3 or /μL	0.001	$10^9/L$	XX.X

[†] *Significant digits refers to the number of digits used to describe reported results. XX means that results expressed to the nearest whole number are meaningful; XX0 means that results are meaningful when rounded to the nearest 10. Results reported to lower numbers or decimal points are beyond the sensitivity of the test.*

* *Modified from the American Medical Association Manual of Style, 8th edn Baltimore, Williams & Wilkins, 1989.*

Table 2 Clinical chemistry

Component	Conventional unit	Conversion factor	SI unit symbol	Significant digits[†]
Alanine aminotransferase (ALT)	U/L	1	U/L	XX
Albumin	g/dL	10	g/L	XX
Amylase	U/L	1	U/L	XXX
	Somogyi units/dL	1.850	U/L	XX0
Alkaline phosphatase	U/L	1	U/L	XXX
Aspartate aminotransferase (AST)	U/L	1	U/L	XX
Bile acids (total)	mg/L	2.547	µmol/L	X.X
Bilirubin	mg/dL	17.1	µmol/L	XX
Calcium	mg/dL	0.2495	mmol/L	X.XX
Calcium, ionized	mEq/L	0.5	mmol/L	X.XX
Carbon dioxide content (bicarbonate + CO_2)	mEq/L	1	mmol/L	XX
Chloride	mEq/L	1	mmol/L	XXX
Cholesterol	mg/dL	0.02586	mmol/L	X.XX
Cortisol	µg/dL	27.59	nmol/L	XX0
Creatine kinase (CK)	U/L	1	U/L	XXX
Creatinine	mg/dL	88.40	µmol/L	XX0
Electrophoresis, protein	%	0.01	1	X.XX
	g/dL	10	g/L	XX
Fibrinogen	mg/dL	0.01	g/L	X.X
γ-Glutamyltransferase (GGT)	U/L	1	U/L	XX
Glucose	mg/dL	0.05551	mmol/L	XX.X
Globulins	mg/dL	0.001	g/L	XX.XX
Insulin	µU/mL	7.175	pmol/L	XXX
	µg/L	172.2	pmol/L	XXX
Iron	µg/dL	0.0179	µmol/L	XX
Lactate dehydrogenase	U/L	1	U/L	XXX
Lipase	U/L	1	U/L	XX0
Magnesium	mg/dL	0.4114	mmol/L	X.XX
	mEq/L	0.5	mmol/L	X.XX
Phosphate	mg/dL	0.3229	mmol/L	X.XX
Potassium	mEq/L	1	mmol/L	X.X
	mg/dL	0.2558	mmol/L	X.X
Protein (total)	g/dL	10	g/L	XX
Sodium	mEq/L	1	mmol/L	XXX
Thyroxine	µg/dL	12.87	nmol/L	XXX
Triglycerides	mg/dL	0.01129	mmol/L	X.XX
Triiodothyronine	ng/dL	0.01536	nmol/L	X.X
Urate (as uric acid)	mg/dL	59.48	µmol/L	XX0
Urea nitrogen	mg/dL	0.3570	mmol/L	X.X

† Significant digits refers to the number of digits used to describe reported results. XX means that results expressed to the nearest whole number are meaningful; XX0 means that results are meaningful when rounded to the nearest 10. Results reported to lower numbers or decimal points are beyond the sensitivity of the test.

Psittaciformes		
Cockatoos	Citron	283–514 g*
	Goffin's	221–386 g
	Greater sulphur-crested	608–1200 g
	Lesser sulphur-crested	251–412 g
	Major Mitchell's	300–452 g
	Moluccan	640–1025 g
	Palm (Goliath)	990–1057 g
	Rose-breasted	281–390 g
	Umbrella	458–756 g
Macaws	Blue and gold	892–1294 g
	Buffon's	1080–1534 g
	Green-winged	1058–1529 g
	Hyacinth	1185–1529 g
	Military	774–1065 g
	Scarlet	1058–1464 g
	Yellow-collared	223–308 g
Parrots	African grey	300–380 g
	Blue-fronted Amazon	275–510 g
	Blue-headed pionus	238–278 g
	Double yellow-headed Amazon	545 g
	Eclectus	383–524 g
	Hispaniolan Amazon	268 g
	Mealy Amazon	600–685 g
	Orange-winged Amazon	440–470 g
	Senegal	125–150 g
	Yellow-fronted Amazon	260–460 g
Smaller species	Budgerigar	30–60 g
	Blue-crowned conure	84–96 g
	Jandaya conure	118–128 g
	Pennant's parakeet	180–200 g
	Red-crowned parakeet	60–75 g
	Love birds (various species)	50–70 g

Anseriformes	Domestic duck	2–3 kg
	Domestic goose	4–5 kg
	Canada goose	3.5–4.5 kg
Apodiformes	Hummingbirds	2.5–5 g
Columbiformes	Collared dove	150–220 g
	Diamond dove	40 g
	Domestic pigeon	260–350 g
Falconiformes	Harris hawk	574–1000 g
	Kestrel	145–282 g
	Peregrine falcon	560–1500 g
	Red-tailed hawk	698–1350 g
	Sparrow hawk	150–300 g
Galliformes	Domestic fowl	1.75–4 kg
	Domestic turkey	4–15 kg
	Japanese quail	18–42 g
Gruiformes	Crowned crane	3.5–4 kg
Passeriformes	Canary	12–29 g
	English robin	20–30 g
	Glossy starling	74–82 g
	Goldfinch and green finch	15–20 g
	Greater Indian hill mynah	180–240 g
	House sparrow	25–30 g
	Java sparrow	24–30 g
	Zeba finch	10–16 g

(Data from Schubot R M, Clubb K, Clubb SLH: Psittacine Aviculture, pp. 14–19. Loxahatchee, FL, Avicultural Breeding and Research Center, 1992; Arnall L, Keymer IF: Bird Diseases, p 482. Neptune City, NJ, TFH Publications Inc, 1975: Coles BH: Avian Medicine and Surgery, pp 209–213. London, Blackwell Scientific Publications, 1985.)

*Weights are the lowest female weight to the highest male weight.

Amazon

Blue-fronted	*Amazona aestiva*
Cuban	*A. leucocephala*
Green-cheeked	*A. viridigenalis*
Hispaniolan	*A. ventralis*
Lilac-crowned	*A. finschi*
Mealy	*A. farinosa*
Orange-winged	*A. amazonica*
Red-lored	*A. autumnalis autumnalis*
Tucuman	*A. tucumana*
White-fronted	*A. albifrons*
Yellow-crowned	*A. ochrocephala ochrocephala*
Yellow-headed	*A. ochrocephala oratrix*
Yellow-naped	*A. ochrocephala auropalliata*
Yellow-shouldered	*A. barbadensis*

Budgerigar

Melopsittacus undulatus

Caique

Black-headed	*Pionites melanocephala*
White-bellied	*P. leucogaster*

Cockatiel

Nymphicus hollandicus

Cockatoo

Ducorp's	*Cacatua ducorps*
Galah	*Eolophus roseicapillus*
Gang-gang	*Callocephalon fimbriatum*
Goffin's	*Cacatua goffini*
Lesser sulphur-crested	*Cacatua sulphurea*
Major Mitchell's	*Cacatua leadbeateri*
Palm	*Probosciger aterrimus*
Red-tailed	*Calyptorhynchus magnificus*
Red-vented	*Cacatua haematuophygia*
Salmon-crested	*Cacatua moluccensis*
Sulphur-crested	*Cacatua galerita*
White	*Cacatua alba*

Conure

Austral	*Enicognathus ferrigineus*
Aztec	*Aratinga nana astec*
Black-capped	*Pyrrhura rupicola*
Blue-crowned	*Aratinga acuticaudata*
Dusky-headed	*Aratinga weddellii*
Finsch's	*Aratinga finschi*
Golden	*Aratinga guarouba*
Golden-capped	*Aratinga auricapilla*
Green	*Aratinga holochlora*
Green-cheeked	*Pyrrhura molinae*
Jandaya	*Aratinga jandaya*
Maroon-bellied	*Pyrrhura frontalis*
Mitred	*Aratinga mitrata*
Nanday	*Nandayus nenday*
Olive-throated	*Aratinga nana nana*
Painted	*Pyrrhura picta*
Patagonian	*Cyanoliseus patagonus*
Peach-fronted	*Aratinga aurea*
Red-masked	*Aratinga erythrogenys*
Slender-billed	*Enicognathus leptorhynchus*
Sun	*Aratinga solstitialis*
White-eyed	*Aratinga leucophthalmus*

Corella

Little	*Cacatua sanguinea*
Long-billed	*Cacatua tenuirostris*

Kea

Nestor notabilis

Lory

Chattering	*Lorius garrulus*
Black	*Chalcopsitta atra atra*
Black-streaked	*Lorius lory*
Blue-streaked	*Eos reticulata*
Dusky	*Pseudeos fuscata*
Duivenbode's	*Chalcopsitta duivenbodei duivenbodei*
Papuan	*Charmosyna papou papou*

Rainbow	*Trichoglossus haematodus haematodus*
Red	*Eos bornea*
Tahitian	*Vini peruviana*

Lorikeet

Goldie's	*Trichoglossus goldiei*
Iris	*T. iris*
Musschenbroek's	*Neopsittacus musschenbroekii*
Red-flanked	*Charmosyna placentis*

Lovebird

Black-cheeked	*Agapornis nigrigenis*
Fischer's	*A. fischeri*
Grey-headed	*A. cana*
Masked	*A. personata*
Nyasa	*A. lilianae*
Peach-faced	*A. roseicollis*

Macaw

Blue and yellow	*Ara ararauna*
Buffon's	*A. ambigua*
Caninde	*A. caninde*
Chestnut-fronted	*A. severa*
Green-winged	*A. chloroptera*
Hyacinth	*Anodorhynchus hyacinthinus*
Illiger's	*Ara maracana*
Military	*A. militaris*
Red-bellied	*A. manilata*
Red-fronted	*A. rubrogenys*
Red-shouldered	*A. nobilis*
Scarlet	*A. macao*
Yellow-collared	*A. auricollis*

Parakeet

Alexandrine	*Psittacula eupatria*
Blossom-headed	*P. roseata*
Canary-winged	*Brotogeris versicolorus*
Cobalt-winged	*Brotogeris cyanoptera*
Derbyan	*Psittacula derbiana*
Grey-cheeked	*Brotogeris pyrrhopterus*
Monk	*Myiopsitta monachus*
Plum-headed	*Psittacula cyanocephala*
Rose-ringed	*P. krameri*

Slaty-headed	*P. himalayana*
Tui	*Brotogeris sanctithomae*

Parrotlet

Blue-winged	*Forpus xanthopterygius*
Green-rumped	*F. passerinus*
Mexican	*F. cyanopygius cyanopygius*
Pacific	*F. coelestis*

Parrot

African grey	*Psittacus erithacus*
Amboina king	*Alisterus amboinensis amboinensis*
Australian king	*A. scapularis*
Blue-crowned	*Loriculus galgulus*
Blue-naped	*Tanygnathus lucionensis*
Bourke's	*Neophema bourkii*
Bronze-winged	*Pionus chalcopterus*
Brown-headed	*Poicephalus cryptoxanthus*
Cape	*P. robustus*
Desmerest's fig	*Psittaculirostris desmarestii desmarestii*
Double-eyed fig	*Opopsitta diophthalma*
Dusky	*Pionus fuscus*
Edward's fig	*Psittaculirostris edwardsii*
Grand eclectus	*Eclectus roratus roratus*
Great-bill	*Tanygnathus megalorynchos*
Hawk-headed	*Deroptyus accitrinus*
Jardine's	*Poicephalus gulielmi*
Meyer's	*P. meyeri*
Pileated	*Pionopsitta pileata*
Plum-crowned	*Pionus tumultuosus*
Princess	*Polytelis alexandrae*
Red-bellied	*Poicephalus rufiventris*
Red-rumped	*Psephotus haematonotus*
Red-sided eclectus	*Eclectus roratus polychlorus*
Regent	*Polytelis anthopeplus*
Rock	*Neophema petrophila*
Salvadori's fig	*Psittaculirostris salvadorii*
Scarlet-chested	*Neophema splendida*
Scaly-headed	*Pionus maximiliani*
Senegal	*Poicephalus senegalus*
Tanimbar eclectus	*Eclectus roratus riedeli*
Thick-billed	*Rhynchopsitta pachyrhncha pachythncha*
Vasa	*Coracopsis vasa*
White-crowned	*Pionus senilis*

Rosella

Adelaide	*Platycercus adelaidae*	Northern	*P. venustus*
Crimson	*P. elegans*	Pale-headed	*P. adscitus*
Eastern	*P. eximius eximius*	Western	*P. icterotis*

Note: Page numbers in *italics* refer to figures and table.

Printed and bound by CPI Group (UK) Ltd, Croydon, CR0 4YY

08/06/2025

01896875-0012